CW00427748

Clinical Skills in Treating the Foot

This book is dedicated to our parents, Douglas and Betty Tollafield, and Frederick and Patricia Calladine.

We acknowledge their contribution to our education and successful careers—without their love, devotion and sacrifice, our achievements might have been very different.

For Churchill Livingstone:

Editorial director: Mary Law
Project manager: Valerie Burgess
Project development editor: Dinah Thom
Design direction: Judith Wright
Project controller: Pat Miller
Illustrator: Lee Smith
Copy editor: Adam Campbell
Indexer: Liz Granger
Sales promotion executive: Hilary Brown

Clinical Skills in Treating the Foot

Edited by

David R. Tollafield DPodM BSc FPodA
Consultant Podiatrist, Community Health Trust, Manor Hospital, Walsall, West Midlands;
Honorary Lecturer, University of Central England, Birmingham, UK

Linda M. Merriman MPhil DPodM CertEd
Associate Dean, School of Health and Social Sciences, Coventry University, UK

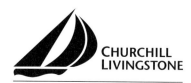

NEW YORK EDINBURGH LONDON MADRID MELBOURNE SAN FRANCISCO TOKYO 1997

CHURCHILL LIVINGSTONE
Medical Division of Pearson Professional Limited

Distributed in the United States of America by Churchill
Livingstone, 650 Avenue of the Americas, New York, N.Y.
10011, and by associated companies, branches and
representatives throughout the world.

© Pearson Professional Limited 1997

All rights reserved. No part of this publication may be
reproduced, stored in a retrieval system, or transmitted in
any form or by any means, electronic, mechanical,
photocopying, recording or otherwise, without either the
prior permission of the publishers (Churchill Livingstone,
Robert Stevenson House, 1-3 Baxter's Place, Leith Walk,
Edinburgh EH1 3AF), or a licence permitting restricted
copying in the United Kingdom issued by the Copyright
Licensing Agency Ltd, 90 Tottenham Court Road, London,
W1P 9HE.

First published 1997

ISBN 0 443 050333 3

British Library Cataloguing in Publication Data
A catalogue record for this book is available from the
British Library.

Library of Congress Cataloging in Publication Data
A catalog record for this book is available from the Library
of Congress.

Note
Medical knowledge is constantly changing. As new
information becomes available, changes in treatment,
procedures, equipment and the used of drugs become
necessary. The editors, contributors and the publishers
have, as far as it is possible, taken care to ensure that the
information given in this text is accurate and up-to-date.
However, readers are strongly advised to confirm that the
information, especially with regard to drug usage, complies
with latest legislation and standards of practice.

The
publisher's
policy is to use
**paper manufactured
from sustainable forests**

Printed in Singapore

Contents

Contributors

Robert L. Ashford BA BEd MA DPodM
Head of School, West Midland School of Podiatry,
University of Central England, Birmingham, UK

Paul Beeson BSc MSc DPodM
Senior Lecturer, Northampton School of Podiatry,
Nene College of Higher Education, Faculty of
Applied Sciences, Northampton, UK

Steven John Avil
Senior Clinical Teacher, Northampton General
Hospital, Northampton, UK

John Richard Carpenter BSc PhD
Senior Medical Editor, Gardiner-Caldwell
Comunications Ltd, Macclesfield; formerly Lecturer
in Pharmacology, University of Manchester,
Manchester, UK

Anne Marie Carr BSc MSc DPodM
Head, School of Podiatry, Central Institute of
Technology, Wellington, New Zealand

John Colin Dagnall LHD FChS SRCh
Member of the Advisory Committee, Center for the
History of Foot Care and Footwear, Pennsylvania
College of Podiatric Medicine, Philadelphia, USA;
Private Practitioner, Bramhall, Cheshire, UK

Joy Dale BSc DPodM MChS SRCh
Lecturer, Department of Podiatry, University of
Salford, Salford, UK

Richard W. Goslin BSc FPodA
Senior Lecturer and Specialist in Podiatric Surgery,
Plymouth School of Podiatry, Plymouth, Devon, UK

Allen Hinde BA MA MCSP DipTP CertED
Senior Lecturer, Nene Centre for Healthcare
Education, Nene College, Northampton, UK

Timothy E. Kilmartin PhD FPodA
Consultant Podiatrist, Doncaster NHS Trust and
Ilkeston Hospital, Derbyshire, UK

Cameron Kippen
Perth, Western Australia

Marylin Lord PhD SMBSc(Eng) Ceng FIMechE
Senior Lecturer, Medical Engineering and Physics,
King's College London, London, UK

Linda Merriman MPhil DPodM CertEd
Associate Dean, School of Health and Social Sciences,
Coventry University, Coventry, UK

Jean Mooney BSc MA DPodM DBiomech CertEd FChS
FSFCP
Senior Teacher, The London Foot Hospital and
School of Podiatric Medicine, London, UK

Robert S. Moore FRCSEd DA FFAEM
Consultant in Accident and Emergency Medicine,
Northampton General Hospital NHS Trust,
Northampton, UK

David Pratt BSc MSc PhD CPhys
Consultant Clinical Scientist, Bioengineering
Research Centre, Derbyshire Royal Infirmary NHS
Trust, Derby, UK

Trevor Dowding Prior BSc FPodA
Specialist in Podiatric Surgery, St Leonards Primary
Care Centre, London, UK

Keith Rome MSc BSc DPodM SRCh
Senior Lecturer in Sports Science, University of
Teesside, Middlesborough, UK

Louise Stuart DPodM MSc
Senior Lecturer, Department of Podiatry, University
of Salford, Manchester, UK

David Tollafield DPodM BSc FPodA
Consultant Podiatrist, Community Health Trust,
Manor Hospital, Walsall, West Midlands; Honorary
Lecturer, University of Central England, UK

Warren Turner DPodM BSc MChS SRCh
Head, Northampton School of Podiatry, Nene
College, Northampton, UK

Preface

Clinical Skills in Treating the Foot has been written as a companion volume to *Assessment of the Lower Limb*. Using the successful style associated with *Assessment of the Lower Limb*, this book focuses on the treatment of foot-related problems.

The terms 'treatment' and 'management' are sometimes used synonymously but many authors see distinct differences between them. Treatment is viewed as a particular process or method to alleviate or cure disease. The term 'management' has a broader connotation in that it is patient- as opposed to disease-focused. This book covers both these aspects: the philosophy and rationale associated with specific treatment strategies, as well as issues related to patient management. An example of the former is Chapter 6, which examines the use of 'operative skills' for the cutaneous treatment of skin lesions. An example of the latter is the concept of the 'elderly person', which is explored in Chapter 15. This looks at some of the specific issues involved in the management of problems associated with the elderly patient.

This book is divided into three sections. The first section is preceded by an introduction which looks at the way in which orthopaedics and podiatry have independently contributed to foot care.

The first section explores issues related to the context in which treatment is delivered, and therefore adopts a patient management approach. It includes chapters on the treatment planning process, the clinical environment, audit, clinical emergencies and foot health promotion and education. All these aspects underpin the management of foot-related problems.

The appropriate selection and implementation of the various strategies used in the treatment of foot problems emanate from *treatment plans*. Treatment plans are devised from information gained from the assessment process. Audit is pivotal in guiding effective and efficient clinical practice. The use of audit tools enables practitioners to undertake objective assessments of their treatment programmes. The safe and effective management of clinical emergencies is an extension of basic first aid. All practitioners should be able to offer immediate care to patients who experience a clinical emergency during treatment.

With the change in perspective from an entirely treatment-focused health care service to one which has started to recognise the inportance of prevention, it is essential that all practitioners play a proactive role in the prevention of foot problems. Chapter 5 explores how the development of health promotion and education can be related to foot health awareness in practice.

The second section focuses on the range of treatment strategies which may be used in the treatment of foot problems. The first chapter documents the operative skills required for the cutaneous treatment of skin lesions and nail surgery. These skills have historically formed the basis of podiatric practice, although, interestingly, they have received scant coverage in other texts. Foot surgery is a rapidly developing aspect of foot health management. The chapter on surgery has been written for practitioners to provide more information when considering referrals. It concentrates on principles of surgery rather than detailing all the likely techniques available. The chapter emphasises preoperative selection of patients, the associated advantages and disadvantages of surgical care, as well as anticipating common problems associated with postoperative care.

Pharmacological preparations have an important role in supporting treatment of the foot. There are very few drugs which can cure foot problems but many which can ameliorate and control symptoms. The judicious use of pharmacological preparations is often combined with other treatment regimens.

Physical therapy plays a key part in managing sports injuries together with mechanical therapy. Mechanical therapy is perhaps a new term to many practitioners. It is a term which was introduced into podiatric practice in 1985, by the editors, while developing the curricula at Northampton School of Podiatry. The need to define this new term arose because there was no collective term which covered the whole field of foot appliances: insoles, orthoses, prostheses, padding and strapping associated with the study of biomechanics. Mechanical therapy has had a considerable influence on the care of the foot. It is, therefore, no strange coincidence that the theme of mechanical therapy frequently arises throughout this book. Three chapters are specifically devoted to it. The chapter on footwear therapy, which also includes modifications which can be made to footwear, complements the material covered in these three chapters. The importance of appropriate and well-fitting footwear in the management of foot problems can never be overstated.

The third and final section considers the management of foot problems related to specific client groups: adults, children, sports injuries and the elderly. This final section also includes a chapter on the management of ulceration and painful feet in groups often considered to be at risk. Where appropriate, case histories and clinical comment have been used to illustrate certain clinical points.

It is hoped that the use of black and white illustrations, figures and tables throughout the text will assist the reader and make the text more meaningful. While this book is undoubtedly biased toward podiatrists, it is hoped that it will appeal to other practitioners interested in the foot. The domain of foot care is not the responsibility of one profession. The contributions made by professionals such as physiotherapists, orthotists, specialist physicians, surgeons and nurses to foot management have been highlighted throughout this book. Together these professionals can form a multidisciplinary team whose joint impact is far greater than that provided by one profession alone.

1996   D.R.T., L.M.M.

Acknowledgements

We are indebted to all those who have contributed to this book. Please accept our thanks for allowing us the distinction of combining your experience in a text which will, hopefully, appeal to those with an interest in the foot.

To Alison Blake, Graham Dickson, Bill Liggins, Sola Oni, Ann Thomas, Jill Tollafield and Adam Campbell (freelance editor)—thanks for providing critical inspiration. Special thanks to Tim Kilmartin who assisted us with Chapter 14 at a late stage in planning.

Many illustrations and photographs in the book belong to the authors of the chapters, but elsewhere we have been grateful for the services of Derbyshire Royal Infirmary, London Foot Hospital, Northampton General and Manor Hospital Medical Illustrations Departments (X-rays and plates); also, to Gary Dockery and colleagues at THC, Fifth Avenue Hospital for inspiring many of the procedures depicted; to Ira Fox for providing advanced technique illustrations; Steve Sandilands with help for his line drawings on Sports Injuries and Julia Flear and Susan Christiansen at Leicester Nuffield Hospital for helping with the illustrations for Chapter 9.

Again, the staff at Churchill Livingstone have not only been helpful, but patient with the many delays brought about by our other duties and unforeseen events.

David Tollafield would also like to acknowledge Yvette Sheward (Walsall Community Health Trust) for providing departmental time and resources, as well as encouragement, during the production of this book.

CHAPTER CONTENTS

Introduction—an historical perspective

D. R. Tollafield
J. C. Dagnall

Whoever seeks information on how people's feet were cared for in past centuries would look in vain in any textbook on history of medicine, or on social history (Seelig 1953).

Exploration of the annals of medical literature reveals little about the treatment of foot disorders before the 18th century. The pursuance of historical material can often address misconceptions of procedural origins. The roots of foot management have been poorly documented and textbooks published during the first two-thirds of the 20th century have often not been followed up or reprinted. This chapter takes a look at the origin of chiropody and orthopaedic surgery predominantly in the UK, although undoubtedly European and American influences cannot be ignored.

PROFESSIONAL DEVELOPMENT

Chiropody—latterly known as podiatry—and orthopaedics comprise the main professional bodies that have had an historical impact on foot health. While other professions undoubtedly claim an interest in some areas of foot management, these two are the most important. (It is, after all, no mistake that *'podos'* and *'pous'*, which form part of the professional titles of both chiro-*pody* and *pod*-iatry, are derived from the Greek meaning 'foot'.)

The term 'chiropody' was changed to 'podiatry' in the USA in the 1950s, in order to alter the perceived image of the profession and to remove the confusion created by the use of two different words to represent much the same thing. The incorporation of the prefix 'pod-' also justified changing 'chiro-', since *'cheir'* relates to the hand whereas *'podos'* relates to the foot. The term 'podiatry' was not adopted in the UK until 25 years later. In the UK a division emerged between those practising chiropody and those wishing to extend chiropody much as had been done in the USA. By the end of the 1980s, however, the use of term

1

'chiropody' in the names of teaching colleges and universities had been replaced by 'podiatry'. It is expected that by the end of the 20th century, the term 'chiropody' will have been completely replaced in the UK. Most English-speaking parts of the world now use 'podiatry', although not all adopt the same scope of practice as the USA.

Emergence of a profession dedicated to feet

From the humble corn-cutters of England and France emerged a chiropodial profession. Nicholas Laurent LaForest published his first book in Paris in 1781, the second edition in 1792, illustrating instruments that resemble many modern instruments of today. The first known depiction of hallux valgus and the mechanical factors involved in the production of corns was described and illustrated in his book entitled *L'Art de Soigner les Pieds* . . .

In the year that LaForest began the rational approach to the disorders of the foot, a Dutch anatomist, Petrus Camper (1722–1789), published a treatise on the best form of shoe in 1781. It contains an account of the structure and function of the foot and laid the basis for its biomechanical study.

The first British contribution to chiropody was by Heyman Lion, in 1802, whose treatise on spinae pedum (his jargon term for corn) added to the work of LaForest. He described a complete dissection technique for removing corns, the space-occupying verruca and the seed corn. Lion gave detailed instructions for the operative treatment of corns and nails.

In 1845, after 30 years' practice in London, Lewis Durlacher (1792–1864), son of a Bath chiropodist, published the classic text which established chiropody as a speciality of medicine. It contained the first description of plantar digital neuritis, the first illustration of onychocryptosis and the first detailed account of the space-occupying plantar wart. Other firsts included conditions such as onychophosis, Durlacher's corn (under the fifth toenail), pre-keratosis inflammation, sectioning operation for onychocryptosis and the description of chronic paronychia. Durlacher gave the best account of corns at that time. He enlarged on Lion's original description of seed corns and differentiated between digital cutaneous and subcutaneous sacs (bursae). The rational use of silver nitrate for corns was described. Amongst all other contributions to the previous scanty literature, Durlacher laid the foundation for what is now called the biomechanics of the foot. He tried to form a dispensary for foot diseases and, possibly, a society of chiropodists. His book is quoted in all the texts on the history of orthopaedics.

Professionalisation of chiropody

The first society of chiropodists was established in New York in 1895, and the Pedic Society produced the first chiropodial journal in 1907, and established the first school in 1911. The first British society appeared in 1912, what is now the London Foot Hospital was opened in 1913 (a school was added in 1919), and its journal first appeared in 1914. With professionalisation, literature expanded on both sides of the Atlantic.

From the last quarter of the 19th century, surgeons specialising in what became known as orthopaedic surgery started to take an interest in the foot, and from then on the chiropodial approach had to consider surgical implications of management (Bick 1948).

The establishment of schools of chiropody in the USA and the UK led to scientific scrutiny of existing chiropodial techniques. Ernest G. V. Runting (1861–1954), the founder, with Dr Arnold Whittaker Oxford (1855–1948), of the first British society and school, brought out his *Practical chiropody* in 1925. He added to the work of Durlacher, rationalising the use of topical preparations such as silver nitrate and monochloroacetic acid specifically for verrucae.

Runting described diseases of the nails and detailed operative techniques. His padding and strapping techniques, to relieve pressure and foot strain, provided the basis for chiropodial practice for many years. He understood the drawbacks of adhesive materials and he used a large range of ingenious replaceable devices from which evolved many of today's orthoses. Runting understood that it was not the appliance that mattered but the principle behind it.

Orthopaedics, in contrast to chiropody, derived its name from the Greek *'orthos'*, suggesting straightness. Paedics is associated with the Greek *'paidion'* (child) and appears to have been coined in Nicolas Andry's (1743) book in which conservative care for childhood deformities using bandaging and bracing was described. The '-paedics' suffix is somewhat misleading, in that it fails to describe the fact that orthopaedics covers a wide range of problems associated with bone, joints and connective tissue, rather than problems with children alone. The well-known illustration in Figure I.1 captures the impression of the role played by a straight pole in straightening a sagging tree. The mechanics involved in influencing changes in tissues forms the basis of orthopaedic biomechanics, although the principle works better in the child than in the adult.

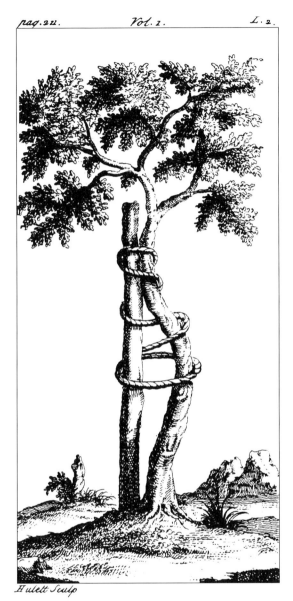

pag. 22. *Vol. 1.* *L. 2.*

Hulett Sculp

Figure I.1 Straightening the crooked trunk of a young tree, depicting the principle of influencing tissue with bracing methods (drawn by Hulett Sculp). (Reproduced from Kirkup 1991a, with permission from Churchill Livingstone.)

Orthopaedic contributions between 1700 and 1900 were dominated by splinting, massage and manipulation. Once surgery had emerged, an understandable dominance arose in this sphere of management over conservative trends, although perhaps not so much in the foot as in other parts of the body. Kirkup (1991a) points out that in regard to surgery, the foot has regrettably become the Cinderella of the orthopaedic

theatre. In contrast, UK podiatry has expanded its own interest in foot surgery and, from the health service viewpoint, some alteration in the balance of foot care provision has taken place between podiatry and orthopaedics since 1975. Changes in such provision are far from well defined, even at this time, but despite the individual views and intolerance of the professions, the use of audit and proven outcomes will ensure that the patient has the best attendant service.

FOOT MANAGEMENT

In the past, management was directed at dealing with injuries and removing foreign objects from the foot. Urgent amputations would have undoubtedly been undertaken, but after 1867, especially with Lister's introduction of the awareness of antisepsis, the number of surgical procedures increased. Ankle tenotomy proved to be the progenitor for elective surgery. It may seem strange that one of the most effective procedures performed for hallux valgus, and one still practised today, was described by J. L. Reverdin as early as 1881. Forms of conservative management seem less well documented than the progress made by surgery. Rather, peculiar remedies emerge to pique our interest, such as the Anglo-Saxon cure for 'angnail' (corn) using 'brass filings, old soap, and oil'.

Orthoses, splints and manipulation

We learn from the limited sources such as Nicholas Andry in the 1700s that conservative views were upheld in managing foot deformity. The thought process concerning flat foot management was then much as it is now; Andry (1743) advises:

If the feet incline too much to one side, you must give the child shoes that are higher on that side, both in the sole and heel which will make him incline to the opposite side.

The use of splints in leather, paste board and metal plates of iron and brass associated with specially constructed footwear were described for day and night use for adducted feet. This information was conveyed by Lorenz Heister (1718) in his paper entitled *A general system of surgery*, which was translated into English in 1743 (Heister 1743).

Kirkup (1991a) suggests that the work of Andry does little to excite modern foot science (sic) and that other sources such as Heister have more practical application.

Of all the variations of foot deformities, club foot has probably had the greatest publicity. Because of the lack of antibacterial technology and general

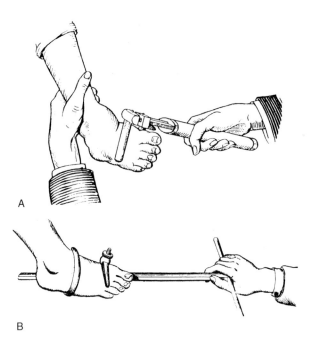

A

B

Figure I.2 A: H. O. Thomas's adjustable manual wrench (1886). B: Bradford's adjustable manual wrench (c.1888). These illustrations represent two of many different designs. (Reproduced from Kirkup 1995, with permission from Churchill Livingstone.)

anaesthesia, manipulation was limited in the presence of bone and soft tissue adhesions. Descriptions of manipulative managements date back to Hippocrates. Further progress was not made until the 19th century when the practice of applying animal fats, strapping and manipulation was recorded for foot treatment. Many 'wrench' type instruments were designed; two such systems were illustrated by H. O. Thomas (1886) and Bradford (1888) (Fig. I.2). The use of manipulative force resulted in complications, as shown later at post-mortem, in the form of haematoma through torn ligaments, fractures and epiphyseal damage. Death could even be associated with periosteal abscess formation. The post-therapeutic discomfort and problems are difficult for us to imagine. One type of compound machine used under general anaesthetic (c. 1890) required two operators exerting a force of 1 ton. While corrective bars for some foot deformities, such as the Ganley bar, are still being used, the popularity of the Denis-Browne bar in the treatment of metatarsus adductus and club foot has diminished in both orthopaedic and podiatric circles. Soft splints for toes are still popular but are applied in a more gentle way than the wrenches above. Manipulation is still used, but often under a short general anaesthetic and with serial casts in children (Ch. 15).

Skin problems, corns and warts

Daniel Turner (1667–1740) published in 1714 what can be regarded as the first textbook on dermatology (Dagnall 1983). Concerning diseases of the skin of the hands and feet, he wrote extensively on 'whitlaws, kibes, warts and corns'. Most of his ideas came from the ancient authorities. He quoted those who warned against the danger of allowing blood from the cutting of corns and warts falling on sound skin, in case new growths should result. His view that corns were caused by disturbance of the humours of the skin, however, missed their mechanical cause. Turner's book confirms the paucity of treatment available from medical sources for foot sufferers. Physicians and surgeons regarded treatment of the corn as an undignified procedure, and so the gap was filled by 'corn-cutters'.

Nicholas Laurent LaForest styled himself as a surgeon-pedicure; in his book of 1781, he gave the cause of corns as 'a thick and sticky humour, hardened in the pores of the skin by a constant pressure which finally forms a hornified mass'. On footwear, he wrote:

It is the short shoe that makes the foot most uneasy. The toes are in arcades, and by this position it makes a thickening of each of them against the toe-cap and particularly at the joint of the phalanx at the tuberosity . . . It is easy to see that the shoes of women with high heels are equivalent to short shoes.

Spirit, in the form of lavender brandy, was recommended for soft corns, together with interdigital padding and rest. LaForest lamented the difficulty in curing corns, 'because the cause always exists' unless the patient can be persuaded to wear shoes suitable to the condition of the feet.

As foot 'orthopaedy' was heavily based upon manipulation of the foot, so chiropody has been heavily associated with corn management. Of all the developments for this multifactorial problem, few have had any long-term effect. The intrinsic pathological process still remains unclear to this day and many theories have been considered. One of the most recent developments, the use of injectable silicone under the skin to replace adipose tissue, was begun 30 years ago by Balkin (1966) of Glendale. However, this method has not yet received official approval and awaits further validation for use with corns.

Surgery[1] and the foot

Amputations

It may seem strange, but therapeutic amputation was

---

[1]Terminology associated with surgery is explained in Chapter 7.

often a forbidden practice in many cultures, whereas judicial dismemberments were permitted (Kirkup 1994a,b). While we are aware of leg amputations, particularly from battles past, early digital amputations around the 17th century may have been carried out using a heavy, possibly curved, chisel for cases of tuberculosis such as dactylitis. Metatarsal amputations using a saw were recommended by Sharp of London in 1739. Presumably, the saw avoided the earlier problem, resulting from the use of chisels, of bone shattering and leaving behind ragged soft tissue. Transtarsal amputations described by Hey of Leeds in 1803 and Lisfranc of Paris in 1815 used a disarticulation method and created a skin flap to cover the cuneiform bones. Arguments between these authors about who was to be accredited went on for some time; today, however, it is Lisfranc's name that is associated with the anatomical structure of the metatarsocuneiform joint.

In 1792, Chopart of Paris provided a description of midtarsal joint amputation, which preserved the hindfoot. With time, variations were described, although in the UK, James Syme of Edinburgh is best known for his supratalar amputation, which leaves the ends of the tibia and fibula (Ch. 7); his keenness for amputation in the presence of *caries*, i.e. bovine tuberculosis, of the calcaneus and talus led to more radical amputations further up the leg around 1831. The wars of 1914–1918 and 1939–1945 ultimately led to many changes and experimentations in amputation technique. Today, however, amputations other than Syme's and those of toes and metatarsals (rays) are rarely practised (Kirkup 1994b).

Functional procedures

Besides amputations associated with the foot, tenotomy provided an early surgical technique for dividing tight Achilles tendons. The popularity of the tenotomy in 1840 did much to encourage the development of orthopaedic surgery. In the UK, William Little successfully underwent a tenotomy operation by Stromeyer in Germany. Influenced by the procedure's success, he published a treatise on club foot and other deformities in 1839. German and French influences were also recorded by William Adams, one of Little's pupils. Adams published material which restored the balance of management after a craze in which tenotomies were undertaken for a wide range of procedures. Adams emphasised the importance of mechanical and physiotherapeutic measures in successful management. In some cases, surgery was unnecessary.

The problems associated with infection, particularly bone infection, probably halted a keen attraction to extensive foot surgery. The aforementioned tenotomy still had an attendant risk of infection, but in successful hands orthopaedic surgery blossomed. Tuberculosis associated with the foot was managed by excision, as recorded in the case of an infected fifth metatarsal: Richard Wiseman wrote in 1676 that he had removed a rotten piece of bone by sawing it when it fragmented with pressure. The use of joint excision allowed sailors to return to their occupation, as illustrated by Henry Park's case history in 1783 where a knee was ankylosed following such surgery for tuberculosis. The use of similar surgical techniques was undoubtedly limited during this period, due again to a lack of available anaesthetic techniques. Nonetheless, as history records, excision of joints became popular in England, leaving stable postsurgical results in many cases.

Arthroplasties have a special part to play in foot surgery. Heuter described excision of the first metatarsal head for hallux valgus in 1871. Davis-Colley of London described excision of the base of the proximal phalanx for hallux flexus in 1887, and this was later modified for a hallux valgus procedure by a US army surgeon, Keller. This latter procedure is still selected in some cases of hallux valgus surgery today. In 1919, Hoffman of St Louis considered a plantar approach for removing all the metatarsal heads in cases of severe (infected) arthritis, so that the digits could still contact the ground afterwards. Modifications to this important salvage procedure have been described by Fowler (1959) of Bridgend and Clayton (1960) of Denver. Replacement arthroplasty was not used until later in the 20th century. Autologous bone as part of a refashioned metatarsal stump was reimplanted by Regnauld of Nantes in 1967. The major success of Swanson's silastic implant has been universal, but this has only been a relatively new development with the evolution of plastic technology (Ch. 7). The stemmed implant has spawned many new designs which take into consideration the attendant biomechanical factors.

As antisepsis and anaesthetic constraints associated with surgery were resolved, instrumentation was developed to cope with the different circumstances that arose. Mallets and chisels (Fig. I.3) were used to fashion cuts through bone.

Osteotomies were described and pioneered by Barton in the US in 1837 to correct knee deformities. Reverdin of Geneva (1881) was the earliest proponent of osteotomy in the foot for hallux valgus, and Gleich of Vienna undertook the first calcaneal osteotomy in 1883.

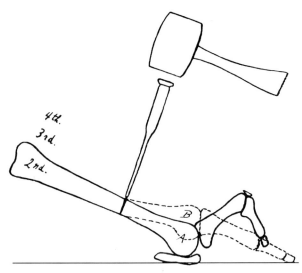

Figure I.3   Many surgical instruments used in orthopaedics bear similarity to carpentry tools. The mallet and osteotome/chisel are still used today, although most foot surgeons favour power saws to incise bone when attempting osteotomies (see text and Ch. 7). (Reproduced from Kirkup 1993a, with permission from Churchill Livingstone.)

SUMMARY

The development of foot care is far from being well documented. Textbooks tend to provide small portions of historical interest, but the whole story of the foot and its management is difficult to relate reliably. Facts which do stand out suggest that many conditions may well have been discovered simultaneously in Europe and the USA. This is best exemplified by Kohler in Germany, who wrote about osteochondritis of the second metatarsal just before Freiberg published his first cases of the same condition in America. Durlacher is now recognised for his original views regarding digital neuroma, but most students attribute the diagnosis and management to Morton in the USA. The French, German and Dutch influence should not go unreported. Language barriers and lack of systematic library referencing probably accounted for many early conditions failing to be recognised until quite late. Through the eyes and painstaking research undertaken by Dagnall (1983) and Kirkup (1991a,b,c, 1993a,b, 1994a,b), we have been able to recreate some sense of the timing of trends of previous centuries. As this century closes, it is interesting to note the huge difference between the dearth of information available before the 1950s and the mass of publications on foot matters today. The avid practitioner is provided now with more literature than can possibly be absorbed by one person alone. Keeping up to date in all aspects of foot health is therefore very difficult.

This chapter has therefore been dedicated to the purpose of bringing together a potpourri of past events that have shaped foot science, if only to remind us how far we need to travel in search of new ideas.

REFERENCES

Andry N 1743 Orthopaedia: or the art of correcting and preventing deformities in children. Millar, London, p 211
Balkin S W 1966 Silicone injection for plantar keratosis, preliminary report. Journal of the American Podiatry Association 56 (1): 1–11
Bick E M 1948 Source book of orthopaedics. Williams & Wilkins, Baltimore
Dagnall J C 1983 A history of chiropody/podiatry and foot care. British Journal of Chiropody 48: 137–180
Heister L 1718 Chirurgie in welcher alles, was zur Wund-Artzney gehoret, nach der neusten und besten Art. J Hoffman, Nurnberg
Heister L 1743 A general system of surgery. Innys II, London, p 289
Kirkup J 1991a The foot, surgery and orthopaedy. The Foot 1 (1): 57–58

Kirkup J 1991b Subcutaneous tenotomy gives birth to orthopaedic surgery. The Foot 1 (2): 107–108
Kirkup J 1991c Bone and joint excisions of the foot. The Foot 1 (3): 165–166
Kirkup J 1993a Osteotomies of the ankle and foot. The Foot 3 (2): 46–48
Kirkup J 1993b Arthoplasties of the ankle and foot. The Foot 3 (2): 93–95
Kirkup J 1994a Foot amputations (1) Fore- and midfoot. The Foot 4 (1): 45–47
Kirkup J 1994b Foot amputations (2) Hindfoot. The Foot 4 (2): 117–119
Kirkup J 1995 Club foot management: manual and instrumental wrenching. The Foot 5 (1): 50–53
Seelig W 1953 Studies in the history of chiropody. Chiropodist 8: 381–397

FURTHER READING

Le Vay D 1990 The history of orthopaedics. Carnforth, Parthenon
Tollafield D R 1986 A podiatric view. The profession of podiatry in the UK. The biomechanics and orthotic management of the foot—1. Proceedings of a conference held at Nene College, Northampton, p 109–114

Essential principles of management

1

Treatment planning

L. Merriman
P. Beeson
C. Kippen
J. Dale

INTRODUCTION

Foot health services make a vital contribution to improving the quality of life. In the very elderly and for the high risk patient, this may mean being able to live longer within the community by circumventing the need for hospitalisation and/or residential care. Maintenance of mobility can reduce the demands on hospital services, social services and welfare support. In children and younger adults, foot health services are directed towards the prevention of acute and chronic foot problems during the developing years.

This chapter explores how the above can be achieved via the treatment planning process. It identifies the components of the treatment plan and the factors, including the role of the multidisciplinary team, which may affect the outcomes of treatment. The chapter concludes by exploring the delivery of foot health services.

THE TREATMENT PLANNING PROCESS

The treatment planning process is informed by, and follows on from, thorough history-taking and examination (primary patient assessment). A thorough assessment is essential in order to:

- identify the aetiology, e.g. trauma, pathogenic microorganisms
- identify any factors which may influence the choice of treatment, e.g. current drug therapy, patient's personal circumstances, vascular status
- assess the extent of pathological changes to inform the prognosis
- establish a baseline in order to identify whether the condition is deteriorating or improving as a result of treatment
- note any previous treatments which have been used, together with an indication of their success or reasons for failure.

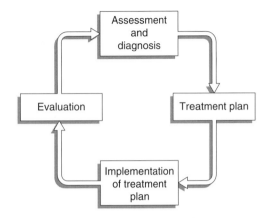

Figure 1.1   The treatment planning process.

Box 1.1   Components of a treatment contract

1. Identification of the problem(s) which require therapeutic intervention
2. The aims and outcomes of the proposed treatment
3. The patient's participation in the treatment, e.g. self-help, change of footwear
4. The practitioner's role in the treatment, e.g. type of treatment to be used, frequency of visits
5. How the outcomes of the treatment will be reviewed

Information gained from the assessment should enable the practitioner to make a diagnosis and identify the underlying cause of the problem. Unfortunately this is not always possible. In these instances, treatment has to focus on the management of the symptoms of the condition, e.g. pain control. Symptomatic relief may be all that can be achieved in certain cases.

All of the above information is used to inform the aims and outcomes of treatment and the selection of appropriate therapeutic modalities. The treatment planning process, however, does not end with the delivery of treatment. It is essential that practitioners evaluate the effects of their treatment in order to ensure that patients receive the most appropriate and effective treatment. It is often necessary, in the light of experience and with the passage of time, to review and update the initial assessment and diagnosis and make changes to the treatment plan. The treatment planning process should, therefore, form an uninterrupted loop, with each stage informing the next stage in the process (Fig. 1.1)

Principles underpinning treatment

The following principles should underpin any treatment plan:

• Practitioners should take into account the patients' psychological, social and personal circumstances, as well as their medical status. A holistic approach should be adopted rather than one which focuses on a specific problem such as a hammer toe.
• Practitioners should be careful not to belittle a patient's concerns, even when they may think these have little substance. The patient should always be listened to. Practitioners can often easily resolve

these concerns by giving appropriate information about the nature of the problem and self-help advice.
• Patients must give their informed consent to any treatment. It is important that patients are fully informed about their treatment in order that they can decide whether they wish to receive it, and, if they do, which treatment they feel is appropriate for them. Practitioners have a duty of beneficence and non-maleficence. A patient's right to refuse treatment should be respected (see Ch. 3). Some practitioners have been accused of paternalism, that is, taking responsibility away from, and not involving, patients with their treatment.
• Treatment plans should be informed by findings from research and audit, i.e. evidence-based health care. It is the responsibility of all practitioners to continually review their practice and ensure that the rationale for their clinical decisions is based on the best evidence available. Practitioners need to know how to evaluate available research evidence and use this evidence to inform their practices.
• A treatment plan involves a contract between the patient and the practitioner. Most treatment contracts are informal, verbal agreements, but in some instances practitioners are using written contracts. The components of a treatment contract are outlined in Box 1.1. It is essential that the patient is fully informed about all aspects of the plan and is willing to actively participate with and undertake their part of the contract.
• Every effort should be made to reduce the likelihood of iatrogenic problems. Iatrogenic problems can occur as a side-effect of many forms of treatment. Practitioners should always inform the patient of the potential risks or side-effects associated with treatment.

Components of a treatment plan

A treatment plan involves the following:

• identification of the problem(s)

- the intended aims of treatment
- the outcome(s) of treatment
- details of the therapeutic interventions
- mechanisms for monitoring and evaluation.

Identification of the problem(s). If a treatment plan is to be effective the patient and practitioner must be in agreement about the need for treatment. It is important that both parties are aware of the purpose of treatment—in other words, why treatment is being provided. If patients present with more than one problem, these should be prioritised in order of need for treatment.

Aims of treatment. The ideal aim of any treatment should be to remove or reduce the effects of the cause of the problem. Unfortunately this may not be possible. As already highlighted, in these instances, the practitioner's primary role is to achieve relief from symptoms. In many cases this involves the relief of pain.

Merriman (1993) identified a range of aims associated with the treatment of foot problems. These are summarised in Table 1.1.

The outcomes of treatment. It is also important that the patient is informed about the likely outcome of treatment. Four outcomes are associated with the treatment of foot-related problems:

1. *Cure*—the complete resolution of the problem. This is usually dependent upon the identification and removal of the underlying cause. For example, a painful, vascular corn on the dorsum of a hammer toe may be cured as a result of an arthrodesis to straighten the toe and reduce the enlarged proximal interphalangeal joint.

2. *Rehabilitation*—a noticeable improvement in the problem but not complete resolution. In this situation it is likely that the symptoms can be satisfactorily addressed but that it is not possible to eradicate the underlying cause completely. For example, a neuropathic ulcer with the aid of operative skills, chemical therapy and appropriate orthotic devices can be resolved. However, it is not possible to resolve the problem completely, due to its underlying systemic nature, although the possibility of reoccurrence may be reduced by education and self-help as well as by routine monitoring and review.

3. *Palliation* prevents a deterioration in the symptoms but does not lead to a noticeable improvement or reduction in symptoms. For example, it may be possible to keep a patient suffering from peripheral vascular disease comfortable with the use of pain-relieving drugs, but due to the underlying disease process, the condition cannot be radically improved

Table 1.1 Aims of treatment

Aim	Commentary
Restore tissue viability	This primarily relates to situations where ulceration has occurred. The main aims of treatment are to promote healing and reduce excessive forces on the foot
Maintain tissue viability in those with 'at risk' feet	A number of systemic and local conditions can adversely affect the tissues of the lower limb. In these cases the main aims of treatment are to prevent loss of tissue and infection and reduce excessive forces on the foot
Improve foot function and maintain tissue viability	Many patients present with painful secondary skin lesions due to abnormal foot function. These lesions, if not effectively treated, may progress to aseptic ulceration and subsequent infection. The aim of treatment in these instances is to improve foot function and thereby prevent loss of tissue viability
Improve foot function	Abnormal foot function may not always result in secondary skin lesions and adversely affect tissue viability. In these instances the aim of treatment is to reduce abnormal foot function
Prevention of abnormal foot function	This relates to preventative work, which is primarily, although not exclusively, carried out with children. For example, abnormal foot function can be avoided with appropriate advice and early intervention in patients involved in sporting activities

unless the patient received surgical intervention such as an arterial bypass.

4. *Prevention* is an important treatment outcome. Often this intervention takes the form of foot health education and promotion. For example, a patient known to be predisposed to chilblains can be given appropriate foot health advice, together with insulating insoles prior to the onset of cold weather.

It is important that the outcomes of treatment are realistic. Research has shown that patients prefer it when they are informed about their health problems and are given an accurate prognosis (Bostrom et al 1994).

> **Box 1.2** Therapeutic modalities used in the treatment of foot problems
>
> - Debridement and enucleation
> - Pharmacology
> - Mechanical
> - Physical
> - Surgical
> - Advice
> - Referral

Therapeutic interventions. An array of treatment modalities can be used to treat foot problems (Box 1.2). Most treatment plans encompass two or more of these modalities. Some modalities primarily lead to symptomatic relief whereas others attempt to reduce or remove the effects of the underlying cause:

1. *Debridement and enucleation*. The use of debridement and enucleation leads to an immediate reduction of symptoms from skin lesions such as corns, calluses and blisters. However, this intervention rarely addresses the underlying aetiology.

2. *Pharmacology*. In many instances pharmacological management is aimed at treating the symptoms of the problem, e.g. anti-inflammatories, analgesics. Antimicrobial drugs are the exception. These drugs aim to eradicate the underlying problem, be it bacterial, fungal or viral.

3. *Mechanical*. Mechanical therapies encompass a broad spectrum of devices. They can be used not only to treat symptoms but also to address the underlying cause. For example, the insertion of a shock-absorbing insole may improve shock absorbency during gait and reduce discomfort in the knees and hips, whereas a splinting device can correct flexible soft tissue deformities.

4. *Physical*. Heat, cold, massage and exercise are primarily used to reduce symptoms. However, in certain instances, physical therapies may remove the underlying cause, e.g. cryotherapy destroys viral wart tissue, and exercise may correct inefficient muscle action.

5. *Surgical*. Surgical intervention can reduce symptoms and also remove or reduce the effects of the underlying cause. For example, the symptoms and broad forefoot appearance associated with hallux abductovalgus deformity can be addressed by surgery.

6. *Advice*. The role of the practitioner as an effective health educator has much to commend it. Advice should be an integral part of any treatment plan. It should include information about the cause of the problem, how to prevent the problem(s) from occurring or reoccurring, and how the patient can self-treat the existing problem.

Clinical consultations are an ideal situation in which to offer advice to the patient. As part of the consultation, interchange of information about not only the well-being of the feet but also specific concerns relating to the general health of the patient may be addressed. Chronic diseases, such as diabetes mellitus or arthritis, may not be preventable at this time, but by identifying their complications early, many of the problems associated with these conditions, such as functional disability, ambulatory dysfunction and pain, can be postponed. The role of health promotion and education in modifying the disease process is essential (see Chs 5 and 18).

7. *Referral*. Sometimes it may be inappropriate for the practitioner to treat the patient, e.g. due to lack of equipment or experience. In these instances, it is important that the patient is referred to another practitioner. Any referral should always be accompanied by a written letter containing relevant details about the patient.

Monitoring and evaluation. Several mechanisms can be used to monitor the effects of and evaluate treatment:

- record improvements/deteriorations from one treatment to the next via the use of a progress chart (Fig. 1.2)
- use of the SOAP format in writing up treatment notes (Weed 1970; Table 1.2). This provides a forum, at each treatment, for the practitioner and patient to assess and review the effects of the

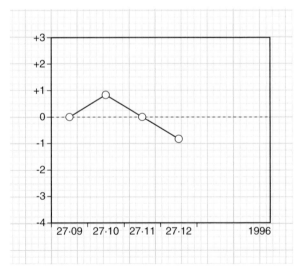

Figure 1.2 Treatment progress can be monitored with the use of a progress chart.

Table 1.2 The SOAP format for monitoring and evaluating treatment

	Term	Description
S	**S**ubjective	The patient's concerns
O	**O**bjective	Signs and features of the condition. This involves undertaking a full or partial examination
A	**A**ssessment	The practitioner's clinical impression in light of the subjective and objective findings
P	**P**lan	The sequential action which should be taken

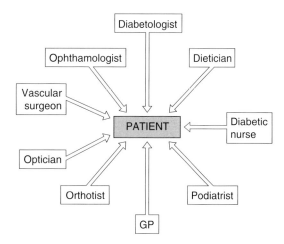

Figure 1.3 Members of the multidisciplinary team involved in the management of the diabetic foot.

previous treatment and update the assessment findings

• set a date to review the outcome of a course of treatment. The practitioner and patient identify a date when they will jointly review the outcomes and effectiveness of the course of treatment. This is helpful for conditions which are known not to show immediate improvement after treatment. For example, it is not appropriate to judge the outcome of a course of ultrasound, for the treatment of enthesopathy, until the end of the course of therapy.

If treatment results in iatrogenic problems, fails to relieve symptoms or to reduce the effects of the underlying cause, the practitioner should always re-evaluate the situation. This involves reviewing and updating the assessment and diagnosis, and evaluating the suitability of the components of the current treatment plan.

The multidisciplinary team approach

Podiatrists, who specialise in the assessment and treatment of foot-related problems, are the main providers of foot health services. However, the management of a number of foot problems benefits from a multidisciplinary approach. For example, it has been shown that the management of the diabetic foot can benefit from an effective multidisciplinary team approach (Thompson et al 1991). The likely membership of a diabetic multidisciplinary team is illustrated in Figure 1.3. There are many other areas where the multidisciplinary approach can be effective, e.g. chronic joint disease, sports injuries and paediatric orthopaedics. Some multidisciplinary teams involve a range of health professionals, whereas others may only comprise two health professions. Mangan et al

(1992) reported on a study looking at the role of the chiropodist and orthopaedic surgeon in the reduction of orthopaedic waiting lists.

Achieving an effective multidisciplinary team requires time, good communication and organisation. It is essential that all members of the team are aware of each other's role and the contribution each member can make. Multidisciplinary teams work best when the members of the team meet on a regular basis to plan and discuss issues. Working in close geographical proximity to each other is very helpful. The team should spend time together away from the patients. This helps the team to develop an understanding and appreciation of each member's role, as well as facilitating the development of sound and effective channels of communication.

Why do treatment plans fail?

This is a question all practitioners find themselves asking from time to time. A multitude of factors may be responsible for failure of a treatment plan. Lack of agreement between the practitioner and the patient about the purpose of the treatment plan is one obvious cause. For example, the practitioner may have failed to communicate to the patient the purpose of treatment and its likely effects. Conversely, the patient may have had unrealistic expectations of what the treatment would achieve.

In some instances the assessment may have failed to reveal contraindications to treatment or, due to lack of relevant information from the patient, may have led to the practitioner making an incorrect diagnosis. The choice of treatment modalities may have been incorrect; other alternative forms of treatment may have been more appropriate.

Many practitioners point to non-compliance as a prime cause for treatment failure. The issue of compliance is mentioned as far back as c. 200 B.C. by Hippocrates in his work 'On decorum': 'Keep a watch also on the faults of the patients which often make them lie about the takings of things prescribed'. In essence, non-compliance is the patient's failure to fulfil the clinical prescription (Haynes et al 1979). Compliance may therefore be defined as one individual agreeing with, or consenting to, another's suggestions, and will usually involve dominant and recessive roles.

A number of studies have been undertaken into patient compliance, and have revealed relatively high non-compliance rates. For example, Ley (1988) found that between 10 and 25% of patients were admitted to hospital on account of non-compliance. Non-compliance or non-adherence is thought to be due to the following factors (Harvey 1988):

- volitional—the individual makes a rational decision not to follow advice; this may be predicated by a number of factors, e.g. cost, perceived benefits
- accidental—the individual forgets or misunderstands the advice
- circumstantial—the individual may be affected by a range of situations which may affect him/her following advice, e.g. painful side-effects, death in the family.

The process by which patients decide whether or not they wish to concur with advice is complex and is influenced by numerous internal and external factors. Patients will be influenced by a number of inherent factors such as personality, affect, social and religious background, age and intelligence. Patients' perceptions of their illness and its prognosis, together with the presence or lack of symptoms, will modify their behaviour. A patient suffering from diabetes whose father died from the same disease may treat her health more seriously than someone of good health with a minor ailment.

Patients' understanding of their illness and of medical advice can indirectly affect their compliance to treatment. Studies have shown that patients do not recall a large proportion of medical information given during consultations (Ley 1983). Ley (1988) also found that the provision of information in the form of leaflets was one of the factors which improved the amount of advice remembered and subsequently led to a good treatment outcome. Advice to patients

may take many forms: details of dressing changes to be carried out, the application of proprietary medicaments, advice on purchasing footwear. The presentation of the information is very important. Short words, short sentences and logical progression are essential for clarity. Medical terminology and jargon are to be avoided or, if used, explained to the patient. The introduction of blank spaces on the leaflet, into which instructions specific to the individual patient are written, is a convenient way of overcoming this deficit.

Practitioners will also influence the patient's decisions. Practitioners develop perceptions about their patients as soon as the patient enters the consulting room. This initial non-verbal assessment may influence or even prejudice how the practitioner approaches the consultation. Accurate assessment requires that the social distance between practitioner and patient is reduced (Plaja et al 1968) and that the barriers created by education, social class, occupational status and ethnicity are identified (Di Matteo & Di Nicola 1982).

Open communication between practitioner and patient is essential to developing a good rapport and mutual respect. Monitoring the patient's response to advice and information is essential. Svarstad (1976) reported that if practitioners neglected to question their patients about compliance, they tended to conclude that the practitioner did not attach much importance to the regimen or did not believe in its efficacy.

Various factors can influence patient compliance. If treatment shows no obvious improvement in symptoms or results, compliance may be impaired, e.g. preventative measures such as diets. The success of treatment versus the resistance to the disease is another important factor. Other factors include:

- costs to the patient
- duration of the course of treatment
- complexity of the treatment process
- side-effects associated with the treatment
- inconvenience to the patient and disruption to the patient's daily living
- prior experiences of treatment which involved pain or were unsuccessful.

If a treatment's obvious effects are to improve symptoms, the patient is likely to respond in a positive manner. This carries a risk, as the patient may stop the treatment too early due to the initial rapid improvement.

Some health educators argue that emphasis should be placed on empowering patients to make decisions and choices about their health and treatment (Totnes

1992). In the past, the emphasis has been on practitioners directing and telling patients what was best for them. Empowerment is achieved when the practitioner works with the patient so that the patient, not the practitioner, identifies what her own needs are. The practitioner's role is to facilitate, not direct, the patient to arrive at a decision. The practitioner has to accept that the patient's informed choice regarding treatment may not be the one the practitioner would have chosen.

Who needs treatment?

Because resources are not unlimited, decisions have to be made regarding the provision of foot health services. How should resources for the management of foot problems be distributed ? Who has the greatest need?

Many authors have attempted to define the term need. Bradshaw (1972) identified four types of need (Table 1.3). Kemp & Winkler (1983) adapted the above classification of need and utilised the following classification in their survey of chiropodial need:

- activated need—a requirement for foot care which is consciously recognised by the sufferer or a third party (demand); action is taken to meet the requirement
- felt need—a requirement for foot care which is consciously recognised by the sufferer or a third party but no action is taken to meet the requirement (potential demand)
- potential need—requirement for foot care which is not acknowledged by an individual. However, a practitioner who undertook a clinical assessment of the individual would consider there was a need.

Two Department of Health (DOH) surveys concerning

Table 1.3 Types of need as identified by Bradshaw (1972)

Type of need	Description
Normative	Need defined by an expert
Felt	A want expressed by the patient or a third party
Expressed	A felt need which is turned into action (demand)
Comparative	Arrived at by studying the characteristics of people in receipt of a service and identifying those with similar characteristics, but not in receipt, as being in need

foot health needs have been undertaken (Clarke 1969, Cartwright & Henderson 1986). Both these surveys adopted similar methodologies and reported a high level of need that was not being met. Other needs-based surveys, although they adopted different methodologies, concur with these findings (Kemp & Winkler 1983, Elton & Sanderson 1987, Wessex Feet 1988).

Research has shown that there are often differences between practitioners and the general public when assessing the level of need. Clarke (1969) commented that practitioners' estimates of unmet needs (or normative needs) exceeded not only people's demands for foot health services but also their perceived needs (felt needs which were not being met). A high percentage of the general public did not consider they were in 'need' of treatment despite practitioners arriving at a clinical decision that treatment was needed. One interesting explanation for this phenomena lies in research undertaken by Dunnell & Cartwright (1972). The authors asked 1400 adults about their general health: 28% said they were in excellent health, 39% good health, 24% fair health, and 9% poor health. When those in 'good' or 'excellent' health were asked if they had experienced any health-related problems in the last few weeks, only 9% said they had not. The common symptoms reported were: 'headaches, skin disorders, accidents and trouble with feet and teeth'. It would appear that the participants accepted that 'trouble with feet' was 'part and parcel of life'.

Epidemiological studies have shown the level of foot health among the general public to be low. Minor foot and foot-related problems of the earlier years are often neglected, but do in many cases go on to become more serious in the middle and later years. An emphasis on the promotion of good foot health and the prevention of disease is as important as the treatment of existing pathologies. Good foot health promotion may reduce the need for foot health services in later life. Unfortunately, the demand for the treatment and care of existing foot pathologies has been so high that little time has been devoted to preventative measures.

The role of the practitioner in foot health promotion/education is examined in Chapter 5. It is essential that practitioners constantly remind themselves of their role as educators. Simple advice on general foot care and hygiene can help prevent a range of foot problems from occurring, e.g. ingrowing toenails, corns, infections.

Need surveys are not always helpful in informing decisions about the allocation of resources. Manning & Ungerson (1990) believe that the incommensurability of different needs makes distribution of resources, according to need, a poor guide to public policy. Factors other than the findings from need surveys should be used in arriving at decisions about the allocation of resources. These factors include:

- demographic trends
- waiting lists
- strategic plans of health commissioning agencies
- public expectations
- political pressure groups
- responsibility for health.

Manning & Ungerson (1990) raised the issue of who should be responsible for the nation's health. For example, who is responsible for the foot problems of the person born with spina bifida or the individual who contracts AIDS—that particular individual, the family or the state?

Foot hygiene, routine nail care and well-fitting footwear should be the responsibility of each individual. The undertaking of these routine tasks can prevent a number of foot problems from arising and, as a result, reduce the need for foot health services. Due to a variety of factors, e.g. poor eyesight and arthritis, some individuals may be unable to undertake these tasks themselves. In these instances, family, friends, and the voluntary, private and statutory services have a role to play.

The annual sales of proprietary products for the self-treatment of some foot pathologies, e.g. corns and verrucae, lead one to assume that a large number of the general public are actively involved in treating their own foot problems. The overall philosophy of a good foot health service should be to promote informed self-care. As long as self-treatment is safe to use and will not lead to unnecessary complications, it can provide a useful adjunct to treatment provided by the health care practitioner.

Many practitioners are faced with long waiting lists and have to make daily decisions as to which patients are in the greatest need and should therefore receive treatment first. Various approaches have been used to prioritise need. In general, priority should be given

Table 1.4 Features of presenting problems which require immediate attention

Feature	Associated signs and symptoms
Pain	Constant weight-bearing and non-weight-bearing Affects patient's normal daily activities
Infection	Raised temperature (pyrexia) Signs of acute inflammation Signs of spreading cellulitis, lymphangitis, lymphadenitis
Ulceration	Loss of skin May or may not be painful May expose underlying tissue
Acute swelling	Unrelieved pain Very noticeable swelling May have associated signs of swelling
Abnormal skin changes	Distinct colour changes Discharge may be malodorous Itching Bleeding

to those patients who present with any of the features outlined in Table 1.4.

SUMMARY

It is the responsibility of all practitioners to inform and regularly update their clinical skills and knowledge. All treatment plans should take into account available evidence from research and audit. When designing and implementing a treatment plan, it is essential that the practitioner bases it on findings from a thorough assessment. Once a treatment plan is implemented, it should be routinely evaluated in order to ensure that patients receive appropriate and effective treatment.

The promotion of good foot health and the prevention of disease is as important as the treatment of foot problems. The overall philosophy of foot health services should be to promote informed self-care so that services can be focused on those patients who require intervention.

REFERENCES

Bostrom J, Crawford-Swent C, Lazar N, Helmer D 1994 Learning needs of hospitalised and recently discharged patients. Patient Education and Counselling 23 (2): 83–9

Bradshaw J 1972 The concept of social need. New Society 19: 640–643

Cartwright A, Henderson 1986 More trouble with feet: a survey of foot problems and chiropody needs of the elderly. DHSS, London

Clark M 1969 Trouble with feet, occasional papers on social administration, No 29. Bell

Di Matteo M R, Di Nicola D D 1982 Achieving patient compliance—the psychology of the medical practitioner's role. Pergammon Press, New York

Dunnell K, Cartwright A 1972 Medicine takers, prescribers and hoarders. Routledge and Kegan Paul, London

Elton P, Sanderson S 1987 A chiropodial survey of elderly persons over sixty five years in the community. The Chiropodist 42 (5): 175–178

Harvey P 1988 Health psychology. Longman, New York

Haynes R B, Taylor D W, Sackett D L 1979 Compliance in health care. John Hopkins University Press, Baltimore

Kemp J, Winkler J 1983 Problems afoot; need and efficiency in footcare. Disabled Living Foundation, London

Ley P 1983 Patient understanding and recall in clinical communication failure. In: Pendleton D, Hasler J (eds) Doctor–patient communication. Academic Press, London, p 89–107

Ley P 1988 Communicating with patients. Croom Helm, London

Mangan J, Ashford L, Murphy J, Beverland D 1992 A multidisciplinary approach to foot surgery waiting lists. The Foot 2: 29–33

Manning N, Ungerson C 1990 Social policy review 1989–1990. Longman, London

Merriman L 1993 What is the purpose of chiropody services? Journal of British Podiatric Medicine 48 (8): 121–124, 128

Plaja A O, Cohen L M, Samora J 1968 Communication between physicians and patients in outpatients clinics, social and cultural factors. Milbank Memorial Fund Quarterly 46: 161–214

Svarstad B 1976 Physician–patient communication and patient conformity with medical advice. In: Mecanie D (ed.) The growth of bureaucratic medicine. Wiley, New York

Thompson F, Veves A, Ashe H, Knowles E, Gem J, Walker M, Hirst P, Boulton A 1991 A team approach to diabetic foot care—the Manchester experience. The Foot 2: 75–82

Totnes K 1992 Empowerment and the promotion of health. Journal of the Institute of Health Education 30: 4

Weed L 1970 Medical records, medical education and patient care. The problem-orientated record as a basic tool. Year Book Medical Publishing Inc., Chicago

Wessex Feet 1985 A regional foot health survey. Wessex Regional Health Authority. The Chiropodist 43 (8): 152–168

2

Audit and outcome measurement

D. R. Tollafield
R. L. Ashford

INTRODUCTION

The Department of Health defines an audit as 'the systematic, critical analysis of the quality of medical care, including the procedures used for diagnosis and treatment, the use of resources, and the resulting outcome and quality of life for the patient' (Ellis & Sensky 1991).

The continuous evaluation of treatment is incumbent upon all who practise in any medical health discipline. While the term 'audit' in general applies to 'accounting', in health circles it has been applied to collecting information about clinical activity in order to measure quality based on predetermined good standards.

The practitioner is required to collect data for a variety of reasons, one of which is for the purposes of an audit. In this chapter, the reasons why it is necessary to audit within the health arena are discussed, and the cyclical nature of audit is described to show its importance within schemes for managing the patient. The term 'outcome' is used a great deal in this chapter, as it is the end result of treatment that is most reported when evaluating the success or failure of a treatment plan. However, while the outcome is obviously of great importance, it should be made clear from the outset that carrying out an audit is more complex than merely looking at the end result. Within the context of an audit, the following questions are uppermost: *why, what, when, who and how to audit?*

Good clinical audit can assist rather than deter good codes of practice. Important goals for designing good codes include ensuring the accurate collection of meaningful data; choosing data that can be measured by recognised methods; and ensuring that the data collected are repeatable and representative of the activity under analysis. How successful one is in accomplishing these goals will determine the real value behind any audit activity.

It is not possible to cover all that there is to know about audit in one chapter. While there are dedicated books that offer much greater detail, few books have been written solely with the practitioner in mind. Since the requirement for greater accountability within our clinical activities will undoubtedly grow, the practitioner should be mindful of the changing trends in the future. Therefore, in this chapter, the emphasis is placed on making the practitioner aware of the potential behind appropriate audit techniques. The measurement of outcome must look towards a number of common scientific methods and these are considered briefly towards the end of the chapter.

The approach to audit preparation has been divided into three parts: lessons learned from an historical perspective, the purpose of clinical audit from the traditional viewpoint, and analysing treatment in order to provide a method with which to carry out the clinical measurement of outcome.

AN HISTORICAL PERSPECTIVE

There has been a distinct lack of audit in past centuries in the area of health and treatment. Few authors in the past have taken account of bad practices. This omission has led to considerable bigotry amongst medical practitioners. Florence Nightingale, known for her opposition to the doctors of her time, reduced mortality to such an extent that her practices were adopted on a greater scale. She used a basic clinical audit that was concerned with daily outcome; this was simply recorded as 'relieved', 'unrelieved' or 'died'. She criticised the case records of that period (c. 1855) as having little value in assisting treatment and bearing a poor correlation with each patient's disorder. By instigating new nursing methods, her mortality figures showed that the death rate was reduced from 40% beforehand to 2% after implementing new techniques. Her figures also showed that the survival rate of patients wounded in battle improved significantly as the distance from hospital increased, because of the delay in encountering the conditions in hospital which actually promoted morbidity. Today these facts are astounding—they seem so obvious that it is difficult to understand how they were not apparent at the time.

One reason for the lack of open practices in the 19th and early 20th centuries may have been that severe criticism or even penalties would have discredited those engaged in seemingly faulty practices.

A further illustration of the problems caused by an intransigent medical community is the case of Ernest Groves at the turn of the 18th century. He criticised the collection of clinical data as being inadequate. He argued that the information collected showed the 'best' results rather than the average results. From his evidence, he believed that records should be collected in a standard way in order to obtain the most authoritative information with no bias. In fact, what Groves was recommending was an Audit Commission of its time. However, not only did the medical profession fail to support any of his ideas, but the British Medical Journal deemed his paper to be unworthy of comment and 'stonewalled' him. This type of activity was not confined to Britain. In the USA, Ernest Codman received similar retribution following publication of his paper on the *End result system*. He was forced to resign from the hospital staff for conduct unbecoming of a physician. Nowadays, he is considered to be the originator of modern health care quality assurance and the concept of medical staff accountability.

Mortality associated with surgery has played a disproportionate role in the history of medical audit. As medicine and the media have matured, events other than death due to disease and medical practice have been notably reported, although not necessarily through audit. Pharmaceutical products undergo far more scrutiny than other treatment practices and have to conform to strict legal codes. The drug industry has only to recall media reporting—as witnessed by the response to the Distiller's drug, Thalidomide—in the 1960s. A drug designed for a different age group was given to pregnant women to help them with morning sickness. The effects on the developing fetus were not appreciated until many children were born with significant limb aberrations.

The changes advocated by Codman and Groves have taken considerable time to be adopted by our health care system worldwide. Indeed, even today, economic and political factors are the real reasons for changes in the current audit perspectives. The political concern about adverse public opinion has led to suppression of sensitive issues in hospitals. The public of today not only expect high standards but are rather intolerant of medical mistakes, no matter how minor.

Audit can offer some prediction of problems and can minimise many issues, by altering standards of care and practices, if implemented soon enough.

The *case conference* offers 'performance review' of medical and surgical management. This type of audit consists of case meetings, known as morbidity and mortality conferences, where doctors consider the effects of treatment in privacy and where notes are limited, if recorded at all. In this manner, doctors can discuss and share information honestly and learn from gaps in their knowledge. *Peer Review Organisations* (PROs) have been developed in order to ensure that cost containment and quality of care are fostered. This particular audit tool is used in the USA. Pro forma criteria are applied when reviewing case records. Any major deviations can be investigated further by senior doctors, and sanctions such as withholding payment can be imposed if the quality of care falls below a certain stated standard.

Cost containment is an issue which has gathered momentum and has accelerated the need for audit. The need for audit systems within the British Health Service has instigated a series of reports and investigations into how to collect data, what data to collect and what to do with it. In 1979, the Merrison Report, supported by a Royal Commission, looked at how data was collected. In the conclusions, collected data was generally felt to be inaccurate, to be produced in the wrong form, and to be gathered too late for any appropriate action to be taken. It is interesting to note that problems of information handling described by Nightingale in the 1850s and Groves in the early 1900s still existed in the 1970s. Korner set out in 1980 to identify and resolve some of the problems arising from poor information systems within the NHS. Seven reports were published between 1982 and 1984, and these started to accelerate the move towards departmental computerisation and the collection of numerous sets of data. However, the issues regarding analysing outcomes of treatment were not addressed by Korner (Pollock & Evans 1993).

The Department of Health and Social Security (DHSS) soon began to work on 'performance indicators'. By 1987, nine consultation papers looked at a wide range of services, including support services, and six areas of health—acute hospital services, support services, community services, services for the mentally ill, services for the elderly, and maternity and children's services. Performance indicators were used to set targets which could be measured and also targets against which comparisons could be made. For instance, in the acute services, numbers of operations for certain groups are now recorded, providing a regional picture of activity. The length of in-hospital stays versus day-case surgery patients is recorded, and the numbers of cancellations and cases per session are noted. The number of avoidable deaths, along with information on age, health and operation code, are also compiled.

Working Paper 6 of the *Working for patients* White Paper (HMSO 1989) recommends that there should be 'an effective programme of audit [which] will help to provide the necessary reassurance to doctors, patients and managers that the best possible quality of care is being achieved within the resources available'. This recommendation makes explicit a programme that promulgates the use of audit as a tool to achieve better levels of care.

This historical narrative gives some idea of how audit has arisen out of changing attitudes and practices. In the past, disease was identified as resulting from poor clinical practices, such as unsatisfactory standards of preparation and care of the patient. By the 1980s, surgeons started to fear contamination from the patient, as blood-borne diseases such as HIV and hepatitis raised concern. These potentially fatal alterations in pathogenesis inflicted by cross-infection thus reversed the belief that patients alone were at risk. Despite modern medicine affording a high quality state of care, we are now increasingly vigilant when dealing with blood and body fluids. The infliction of such cross-infection could prove fatal from an inadvertent stab injury. Regular clinical audit and research of techniques offer a heightened state of awareness.

The quest to cut costs arising from needless waste and inexpeditious treatments has come about as a result of studying health practices in this century. Cost containment has been undertaken by administrative management and by independent bodies rather than by the medical professions.

Cost containment has been politically influenced by the need for accountability and for a form of acceptable practice that lives up to the expectations of an enlightened, better-educated society. 'Waiting times', 'politeness' and 'explanation' are among new standards being enforced upon clinical practice, even though many practitioners may well practise good interpersonal skills anyway.

THE PURPOSE OF CLINICAL AUDIT

This section provides an overview of the audit process, which should help the practitioner to appreciate the preparatory steps that are required when addressing clinical activity. In order to understand the stage that audit has now reached, it is necessary to consider first the traditional views of health care held by managers and hence these will be discussed.

The field of audit has developed a wide lexicon of terms—many of these will be explained in this section.

Terminology

Quality. Donebedian (1966) suggests that there are

three components associated with the quality of health care: good technical care, interpersonal relationships and good amenities. The aims include effectiveness, efficiency, satisfaction and safety. In contrast, Maxwell (1984) identified six dimensions for health care quality, including, in addition to Donebedian's points above, relevance of care (to the whole community), fairness and social acceptability (Pollock & Evans 1993).

When considering quality, Pollock & Evans emphasise the difference between effectiveness and efficiency. *Effectiveness* implies that the correct steps are taken in providing treatment, while *efficiency* relates to the distribution of resources based on need. Of the other two aims, *satisfaction* relates to reaching a desired outcome from treatment and *safety* should include the avoidance of unnecessary problems arising from treatment.

Compassion plays a large role in a patient's perceived quality of care and, to the ill patient, is more important than knowledge of complicated results or impressive diagnostic tests.

Standards of care. Standards are usually set in terms of supplying products or delivering a service; both of these can be applied to health care. Setting standards is one thing, but monitoring and maintaining standards is rather more difficult. This is because specifying standards is demanding, requiring a high level of expertise that can be agreed and understood comprehensively (Ellis & Whittington 1993). Setting standards may be undertaken by a profession, purchaser or institution such as a hospital. Specification is more difficult because each standard has to be defined precisely to account for wide variations of a human, rather than an inorganic, nature. The person setting any standard must have a detailed knowledge of what is achievable. Manufacturers of machine-made items, on the other hand, will have less trouble specifying the tolerance of products. For the purpose of applying quality assurance standards to the clinical setting, these terms will not be separated further, as many of the mechanisms are similar to audit.

Quality assurance. It is important to understand the difference between audit and quality assurance. Quality assurance sets standards and measures compliance. An audit does this too; however, an audit may also be undertaken to identify the standards themselves, against which compliance might be measured, as well looking at the structure, process and outcome which will assist in defining quality assurance.

Since the difference is subtle, consider, for illustrative purposes, the simple example of a product being manufactured to specific standards. In this case, defective items are removed if they fail to meet the required standard of manufacture either because of faulty finish or because of lack of intended function. This whole process could be audited, for example, to see if quality assurance methods were being appropriately applied to minimise customer complaints. The outcome might surmise that no faulty products produced would equate to no customer complaints. In reality, this might be hard to achieve and targets might be set to account for some faults arising. The audit could then be repeated to identify the number of adjusted faulty products expected to reach the shop or customer. Any lowering of the figure would be deemed to be unsatisfactory, and the structure and process of manufacture would have to be reviewed carefully to correct the problem.

Performance indicators (PIs). PIs were set for the purpose of resource efficiency measures. In fact, PIs are linked to quality assurance. As these have been highly confusing in the way that they have been used for internal and external comparisons, they have, not surprisingly, been avoided in the clinical field (Ellis & Whittington 1993).

Performance indicators do not measure outcome. The Department of Health has used PIs in comparing the performance of one hospital with another; a common example uses waiting times for appointments and treatment. The standard initially set may require all hospitals to see new patients within a certain time. Having set this standard, performance is then measured against it. Differences in performance will show up between different hospital services. The reasons for such variations, however, are not explained by simply quoting performance-related figures alone. This lack of discrimination is a point of concern for health care professionals, who, although they may work hard, look less effective on paper. For example, one professional may be in high demand because of his or her success compared with a similar professional in another hospital or centre. The waiting time for the less popular practitioner may look more attractive, creating an unfair bias in any such data collected. This emphasises that the effectiveness (an outcome) is excluded from such a measurement.

Criteria and standards. Criteria and standards are defined by purchasers or managers of the service. It is important to note the difference between the two. Audit criteria are general statements about delivery of patient care. They focus on those aspects that can be used to assess the quality of such care. Criteria-based audit was carried out in the early to mid-1970s in the USA. This work resulted in audits being based on

Table 2.1   Criteria and standards have different implications

Criteria	Standard
The notes of patients on anticoagulant drugs should be clearly marked	The notes of all patients on anticoagulant drugs should be clearly marked i.e. 100%
Patients should not be kept waiting for treatment more than 20 minutes	80% of patients should be expected to be seen in 20 minutes
Patients requiring nail surgery for onychocryptosis should receive an appointment within 3 days	60% of patients should be seen in < 3 days

criteria against which actual practice was compared. From the criteria, standards applicable to the clinic can be developed (Table 2.1).

Why audit?

The broad aims of audit might be considered as:

- improving the quality of patient care
- utilising resources efficiently
- providing an objective assessment of clinical activity
- enabling the practitioner to demonstrate quality of patient care
- reflecting on the effectiveness of care.

The purpose of audit is to gain information so that strengths and weaknesses can be identified. Once data has been collected, improvements in the organisational structure and process can be initiated (Tucker 1995). Changes in patient management need to be identified when clinical practice is at fault. Conversely, this practice should be promoted where it has been shown to be beneficial. In health care, the *product* is the service provided to the patient, and this might be the intended outcome for the NHS. The outcome for the patient, however, is measured in terms of the improvement in their condition. A practitioner will view his or her outcome in a similar manner, i.e. the improvement of the patient's condition. Measurement of this outcome must be considered objectively. This will be considered later in the section on analysing treatment.

All health care individuals may believe that they are doing a good job. How does a practitioner know whether this is indeed the case? Such an assumption raises fundamental questions regarding national standards; the personalities of individuals involved;

the types of training and education that practitioners have received; differences in treatment modalities; different local initiatives; and available financial resources. Performance is based upon the expected standards set down by a profession, which in turn are underpinned by the accepted practice expected by 'society'.

The reasons as to why we want to audit we must accept that quality in health care is dependent upon many facets of our work. These facets require analysing as they have a direct bearing on how a health system can deliver efficient and effective care. Audit comprises the audit of patient care from records, moral and ethical issues of care, economic provision of care, educational responsibilities of care and psychological attitudes of care linked to the whole system of delivery.

Patient records. An audit should show that, in undertaking care, the patient has not been placed at unnecessary risk and that all appropriate investigations have been conducted with safety in mind. The process used in treating a patient should be clearly identified in the case records. A patient with an ankle fracture, for example, would require an X-ray to confirm the diagnosis and identify the best treatment. The use of X-ray reports should be identifiable in the records and it should have been undertaken at the appropriate time during the initial examination routine. Effectiveness can be assumed if no complications arise leading to asymptomatic healing. Effectiveness can be further assumed where the patient with the ankle fracture returns to normal function within a reasonable period. This should include a full unencumbered return to work, ability to walk as before without a limp, good ankle range of motion and freedom from pain. All these recorded results from treatment equate to the desired outcome. Failure to follow the appropriate process, e.g. if the correct diagnostic enquires are omitted, may lead to delays in normal return to daily routines; extending the time off work could have financial repercussions for the patient and for the hospital. Effectiveness can be observed within the case records provided that the method of recording is clear and unambiguous.

Any response to patients' needs and expectations forms the basis of 'patient satisfaction'. Clear ground rules exist as to how patients should be managed; a fair and sensitive approach with sufficient explanation will allow them to contribute to their own care plan. True satisfaction can only be reached when the patient and the practitioner agree that an effective change has occurred.

Moral and ethical. Practitioners are responsible for

recording and reporting information in an honest manner and in an accurate way—in this respect they have a duty. Essential information should be passed on to colleagues where necessary to avoid ineffective management. Standards of expected behaviour can be identified again from case notes, i.e. by the care taken and the conformity to expected practice. Deviation from expected standards of documentation can place a 'legal emphasis' upon practice ethics. Drug reactions or complications from treatment hitherto unknown must be made known. The moral and ethical aspects of clinical activities form part of the overall picture of clinical audit but may not be isolated unless deviation from practice causes serious concern. The use of ethics committees in hospitals provides the correct network for practitioners to set up radical and less accepted types of patient care.

Economic process. Poor structure and efficiency can lead to waste and elevate costs. Areas where waste and inefficiency are experienced are not restricted to the clinic alone but are also found in the administration and support services. Where the practitioner is reliant upon the activities of others and these activities are not carried out properly, the effects upon the service provided can be highly detrimental. The activities of the whole health unit should be monitored, although the specific areas where inefficiency is suspected to lie can be focused upon once they have been identified.

Educational. The practitioner has a professional duty to remain up to date with developments. Altering clinical practice may be implemented by a case conference, publication or research projects. The principal purpose of the audit should be justified on the basis that the result could yield a helpful change in practice or, conversely, could support continuation of a particular practice. Furthermore, if certain standards are expected, the audit will check that such standards are being met.

Psychological. The daily routine can be highly frustrating for the practitioner. Good psychological stability is essential in managing patients, to avoid transposing personal problems to the patient and thereby affecting rapport. A good working environment and administrative support are essential for good service delivery. An audit reviewing daily activities can increase motivation by reporting on achievements as well as problem areas. A change brought about as a result of an audit recommendation can further motivate a practitioner if the change results in positive achievements. It is true, however, that the opposite effect can be created when changes are constantly stipulated. In these situations, one finds

that no sooner has a method been employed than it is changed for a different set of practices. This can lead to disorientation. Achieving the correct balance is essential and important because any deviation in care can affect colleagues and patients.

In conclusion, the reasons for audit are diverse but include general and practical reasons. Practitioners are not encouraged to audit every aspect of their practice at once. Auditing in health care not only accounts for patient management but also includes how the practitioner interfaces with the system of care.

What to audit?

Current convention is to use a framework based upon a model proposed by Donebedian (1966). Donebedian suggested that clinical practice can be classified into three discrete dimensions. They are discrete in terms of their individual characteristics but overlap when considered together in medical care. The three dimensions are as follows:

- *structure*—asks where the service is provided, with what facilities the work is done and who has done it
- *process*—asks what is done and how it is done
- *outcome*—tells what has been done, how well it was done and what the effect has been.

When carrying out an audit it is important that there is an agreed system by which a clinical activity will be examined. The activity should be well defined and the practitioner should be clear about what needs investigating. The *subject* of the proposed audit needs to be defined. Here are several examples which illustrate the point:

- *Why do clinics have so much out-of-date stock?* This refers to the subject of waste and efficiency.
- *Are diabetic patients seen frequently enough to promote the most efficient management of plantar metatarsal ulcers?* The subject is cost and relates to outcome.
- *Consider the diabetic patient ulcer protocol—do all GPs receive a treatment summary following each consultation?* The subject relates to professional ethics communication.
- *Does the complaints system function efficiently?* Again the subject is process-orientated and is related to the effectiveness of clinical protocol.

The structure component relates to what goes on in the clinical setting and tends to be easier to pinpoint. The facility where treatment is delivered should be able to meet the needs being placed on it. For example: are there enough care assistants to manage basic foot care, thus releasing practitioners to attend high risk categories? Are there sufficient examination rooms available to deal with a reasonable number of patients requiring a 3 hour session?

The process of delivery of care should be studied to ensure that the steps taken are in accordance with legal and medical ethics, that case records are up to date and legible, and that treatment plans have been considered and can be shown to be efficient and effective. Then, if the process is followed correctly, it usually follows that the outcome will be satisfactory (Donebedian 1988).

The outcome represents the effects of care on the health status of patients and populations. It is cheaper to audit process and structure than to audit outcome, because outcome depends on following the effects of treatment over a period of time. As a result, outcomes are slower to evaluate. Furthermore, measurement of outcome is complicated, and many of the designs and strategies used are flawed.

Criteria for audit

It has been found that if criteria are defined carefully, it should be possible to obtain an overview of current practice (Table 2.1). The next step would be to agree with colleagues what standards should be applied to a specified practice. It is often the case that standards cannot be agreed until current practice has been analysed and assessed using clear criteria, and the results discussed.

The first attempt at auditing often highlights problems of particular interest. This enables explicit criteria to be clearly defined and standards to be set for the next time around. It is also important when setting criteria and standards not to be too complicated—they should be kept as simple as possible. It is essential that the practitioner collects information that is relevant; the parameters, as with research methods, must be laid down carefully before any data collection commences. A pilot study can provide information valuable to the design of criteria.

In conclusion, the practitioner will be more motivated when analysing the treatment system, the effects of treatment upon patients, the influence of new drugs on specific conditions, the ways to minimise the use of drugs, and the use of new equipment and procedures as a way to reduce treatment costs. The list is endless but one clearly needs to identify areas for analysis that are relevant to treatment delivery.

Standards of care

Standards can be measured. The first Patient's Charter is one example that lends itself to audit. The outcome of the Charter is that patient satisfaction should be reached over a number of stated objectives. Choice, access, information and waiting times are emphasised within statements about the seven basic rights and the nine charter standards. NHS health care delivery now has to embrace the Charter. However, while the outcome of an audit may imply that certain standards are indeed being met, the quality of treatment cannot be assumed to be high, since the Charter is based on quantity, e.g. time, numbers, cost.

When to audit?

If a clinical problem arises for which there is a simple explanation then the use of an audit is inappropriate. Audits attempt to account for problems that are less obvious. Often, it is only once the audit procedure has begun that problems that exist begin to come into focus. In this way a problem might be identified first, and then further study would be required to establish the cause of the problem. For example, a cyclical audit might throw up inefficiency recurring on a monthly or annual basis. Another audit would then be designed to establish where the inefficiency arises and how it might be avoided.

Continuous audit. Certain data needs to be collected continuously, such as the following:

- patient numbers, for example, will fall into treatments performed
- numbers of patients discharged
- numbers of complaints/compliments
- specific treatment comparisons, e.g. number of laser treatments against cryotherapy.

The collection of data is important to make future judgments and predictions about a service. When a service is new and relatively unproven, then the managers of that service will need to ensure that their economic requirements are met to enable their service requirements to be met. An audit in these terms may need to be repeated so that the data can be used to indicate a trend. In this case, structure and process are the subjects of study. Estimates for increasing a clinical provision will depend upon the business plan of that department. Inadequate data will not help to create a strong case for the expansion of a service, and will give rise to poor accountability and highlight poor clinical management. For example, a practitioner may become demotivated when insufficient resources are allocated because a manager, through inadequate audit, has failed to identify the problem.

Sampled audit. An irregular or sampled audit is used to check that a process is being undertaken or that criteria reflecting standards of care are being adhered to. For example, a practitioner may wish to study the effect of a particular treatment if speculative evidence suggests that one type of treatment has risks that have not previously been suspected. In this case the audit does not have to be repeated, and a single sampled audit may be all that is necessary. Conversely, a practitioner may only wish to undertake an audit occasionally to check changing trends.

In a study relating to discomfort from tourniquet pressure around the ankle during surgery, the subject of the study involved placing a cuff around the ankle to obtain haemostasis during surgery (Tollafield et al 1995). The practitioners wanted to know if an anaesthetic infiltrated above the cuff could extend the time of the operation by providing greater comfort. The results showed that a single nerve infiltration above the ankle was insufficient to extend comfort time around the ankle, although most patients were able to undergo surgery quite comfortably for 45–60 minutes using the technique without adverse effects. The *outcome* was measured in terms of effective reduction in discomfort. The evidence supported the use of the technique, providing an objective standard of care for patients undergoing treatment for specific periods of time. These types of clinical audit analysis can be found in most professional journals. The subject does not have to be a patient; for example, a new drug may be compared with an accepted older drug to decide if efficiency or cost might be improved for a specific treatment. While the study has a scientific basis in its design, it will also serve to provide information about the outcome in terms of treatment effectiveness.

Cyclical audit. The use of an occasional or cyclical audit can help the practitioner to monitor trends in practice on a regularly allotted basis, for example every 2, 3, 4 or 5 years. Cyclical audit is therefore useful in deciding when to change a clinical practice, by holding a significant review formally at predetermined points. Any changes that arise from evidence collected can be used to improve the effectiveness and efficiency of the service as well as to monitor many of the selected issues already described.

Duration of audit

Two clear objectives should be aimed for: sufficient data should be collected and a definite outcome should be established. Most audits are determined retrospec-

tively but the concept of prospective design during planning will provide for a more robust analysis.

Collection size. Audit is formed from raw data collected as counts or frequencies in occurrence. When should collection cease? The answer lies perhaps in having sufficient information to predict trends. If a small number of counts are to be made, then the selection should be as random as possible, with the choice of who to select being left to an independent person so as to avoid bias. A group of 50 patients should be small enough to count; on the other hand, 5000 patients may be accurately represented by a proportion, say 10% (500), if they are randomly selected.

Collection period. A period of time is necessary to achieve the required amount of data. If the effects of treatment are to be recorded, sufficient time must be allowed to ensure that the problem does not recur and that side-effects do not arise from management. The period selected for review should ideally be such that some sustained, measurable improvement of the foot condition could reasonably be expected.

In cases following hallux valgus surgery, some sensory loss is normally expected. If the analysis is undertaken over an insufficient period, false negative results might be obtained. Nerve regeneration can take 9 months—an audit completed after 3 months would probably be flawed if nerve regeneration was used as the main criteria for success.

In conclusion, the timing of audit is determined by the aims and objectives of the audit. The results obtained must be complete, the sample size must be large enough, and the period of time selected must consider interfering factors, particularly those associated with outcome, which may extend the study because of the need to wait for full patient recovery.

Who to audit?

In general, practitioners tend to audit *patient groups*. While the practitioner is most likely to want to study the patient, the patient is not in fact the only possible target of study. The 'provider' of the service, or even the 'purchaser', could be the target, depending upon the aims and objectives stated. (These latter terms have been included because they are used in the 1990 NHS reforms associated with Trust management. They refer to the body that delivers the service (provider) and the body that pays for the service (purchaser).) Using the model in Box 2.1, the audit comprised *three* subject groups: GPs (purchasers), patients and patient case records. Equally, the individual or group aspect of an analysis might be an

Box 2.1   Auditing three subject groups. Tollafield & Parmar (1994) undertook an audit on day-care foot surgery. This used the five questions outlined below and each has been amplified as a summary

WHY—the main objectives were to consider the efficiency of foot surgery as assessed by perceptions and attitudes of medical and lay individuals and to record patient outcomes

WHAT—foot surgery was the subject selected. This had a very wide remit, encompassing a range of degrees of complexity of surgery

WHEN—the time interval had been agreed

WHO—this was a closed sample group in terms of patient selection. The patient group had all been referred to, or were already part of, a foot care service

HOW—the methodology was established by collecting data from GPs and patients through open and closed questionnaires. Records of the treatment were then compared to the responses provided by patients

METHOD—forms were filled in by hand by a non-independent researcher and transferred to a mainframe computer for analysis by independent researcher

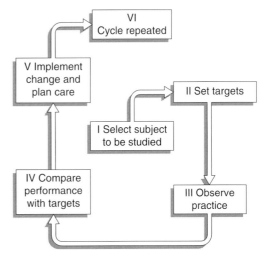

Figure 2.1   Full audit requires at least five stages. Adapted from Lawrence et al (1994).

activity, as might the function of a piece of equipment, or the cost of using a particular pharmaceutical product. The section 'mechanics of audit' in 'how to audit?' considers some of these issues in Donebedian's terms.

In conclusion, the practitioner's needs may be different from those of managers or purchasers, although they are no less important than dealing with service delivery as an overall strategy in terms of who to audit. While managers will want to know that a process is being adhered to and that the outcome is the delivery of that service, the practitioner has the option to qualify or quantify treatment. This is one of the most recent developments in clinical work and the emphasis in the latter part of this chapter will concentrate on treatment outcomes.

ANALYSING THE EFFECTS OF TREATMENT

How to audit?

This is the *procedure* by which audit is undertaken.

Mechanics of audit

Audit questions can be framed in terms of structure, process and outcome. These components can be broken

down so that the practitioner can better understand 'what' as well as 'who' to audit. Unfortunately, 'how' to audit is less clear, because the aforementioned terms tell us nothing about how to measure, how to record data, how to process data and how to present data. The audit procedure will need to encompass planning performance, and the measurement and review of clinical activities as suggested in the list below.

The audit process may involve a number of stages (Fig. 2.1):

- Initial stage
  —plan the study (audit)
  —collect the data
  —analyse the data
  —measure performance (outcome)
- Repeat stage
  —set new criteria
  —measure performance again
  —improve practice
  —monitor changes and effectiveness
  —repeat cycle.

Research and audit. The most robust form of audit follows similar principles as those applied to research methodology. The overlap with research is evident, as the quality of the final analysis depends on there being an adequate number of samples. The design of an audit must be carefully thought out in advance to take account of the type of data needed at the end.

The results of audit and research may well be used differently, though each is designed to bring about a change. Both share a common goal in this respect

Table 2.2   Comparison between audit and research (Bradshaw 1995)

Feature	Research	Audit
Purpose of study	Collects evidence to test a theory	Collects information to measure best practice
Data collection	Prospective	Retrospective
Scientific principles	Rigorous principles are repeatable	Uses audit principles which may not be repeatable
Experiments	May involve humans	Never includes experiments on humans
Results	Factual and will accept or refute hypothesis	Decides whether standard of care has been met and indicates changes needed
Publication	Published	Internal use, but may be circulated widely

and both may refute past attitudes about management of the patient in terms of effectiveness and efficiency. Research should be performed under strict controls; audit has more flexibility but must be equally rigorous if the results are to be taken seriously.

Results should be considered carefully to reflect true change; for example, when introducing a new method into practice, critical analysis is important. For example, a 50% response from a patient survey is inconclusive. The implication suggests that while half may have been helped by the new method, half were not helped. Surveys use questionnaires, and a lack of response must always be assumed to be a response in the negative. Careful interpretation of results must be considered in audit as well as in research.

Table 2.2 attempts to differentiate research from audit, but in practice, when applied to clinical outcome, the difference is small. The comparison in the table (Bradshaw 1995) has been adapted but generally attempts to show that there is a clear division between research and audit. There is an intrinsic flaw here, because there is no reason why research itself cannot be audited. The process of research is often more time-consuming and resource-intensive.

Data collection

The practitioner may elect to use an independent person to conduct an audit. This certainly offers less bias. Data can be collected from responses to a questionnaire or from direct measurement of a clinical activity. Some examples have already been provided under 'when to audit?'. The main terminology concerned with collecting data can be found in all basic statistics texts; however, it is essential that the part played by the data in measuring the outcome is understood. Such data is known as nominal, ordinal and interval.

Nominal data involves a simple 'yes' or 'no' response

which offers one of two choices. Patients can cope with this but often wish to expand their answer over and above what is is effectively a closed response. Did an injection for pain help you—yes or no? The patient may believe that the pain was reduced initially and that as time passed this was less so, with an overall impression that some improvement had been experienced. In this case, the 'yes' response would be correct but unqualified.

Ordinal data is collected in the form of a scale derived from predetermined points of view: 'like' to 'dislike' may have varying strengths of expression with a 'no view', or 'cannot make mind up' type of conclusion as a middle of the road response. The Likert scale, as this is called, is used frequently for questionnaire or interview responses, as shown below. The response is marked, obviating the need for a full written statement, and forms another example of a closed response (Box 2.2).

Ordinal data collection along these lines is easy to carry out and can be computerised and the results analysed relatively easily. Where a facility exists for direct input onto computer at the time of the patient interview, then collection allows rapid analysis. Two problems can arise. Initially the type of data has no mathematical power. There is no way to say that a '1' response for one patient is the same as a '1' response for another. Indeed, a '1' and '2' could mean the same for two different patients; how much worse (or better) a patient feels cannot be ascertained from

---

Box 2.2   Likert scale-type questionnaire

Has the original complaint been made:
1. Much worse
2. Worse
3. The same
4. Better
5. Much better   1   2   3   4   5

the analysis. Secondly, collection from a computer, while desirable, means that the patient does not have time to consider their response in privacy. The issue of whether to use anonymous data collection is considered later.

Interval data and ratio scales. This form of data is considered the most ideal. Measurements that do not have a true zero, such as temperature, are interval scales. Those measurements with true zero points, such as weight, are ratio scales. Mathematically, these scales form more powerful data. Unlike ordinal data, interval and ratio scales have an infinite number of values. Metres can be subdivided into centimetres and then into millimetres. Smaller values can be measured in microns or angstroms. The difference between measurements collected can be compared and will offer more meaning. A reduction in pressure over a metatarsal head from 980 to 150 kPa by the use of an orthosis is a quantitative measurement with greater objectivity than if the patient were to express a nominal or ordinal response. A reduction of 830 kPa represents an 85% improvement. This expression has powerful implications in terms of statistical testing.

Data falls broadly into two categories: *parametric* and *non-parametric*. The former is considered to allow the most powerful statistical analysis. For the purpose of simple discussion, parametric data arises from samples that have a normal distribution, that is to say they fit the ideal shape of a frequency curve with a bell profile (Fig. 2.2). This form of data is predictable and has greatest frequency under the central part of the curve. Height in cm is a good example of parametric data, where the majority of people fall under the curve depending upon sex, nationality and age over a typical range. The ends of the curve never touch the *x*-axis and there is a very small percentage that falls outside the expected 'height'.

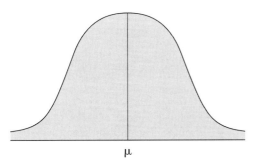

μ

Figure 2.2 An example of parametric data reflected by a frequency curve with an ideal bell-shaped distribution. The centre point μ of a normal curve depends upon the value of the mean and the value of the standard deviation.

The use of parametric data allows statements to be made about how likely data is to fall within bands known as standard deviations. The larger the value of standard deviation (SD), the more distributed or spread out will be the data.

Data that falls outside normal distributions is therefore known as *non-parametric*. Unfortunately much of the clinical data collected falls into this latter category, making it more difficult to analyse statistically.

Questionnaires. Questionnaires are a popular method of collecting clinical information from patients and practitioners. While they may seem simple, their implementation can create problems and these will be discussed below. Reports from questionnaires should ideally show repeatability and offer the recipient a comprehensive summary of activity and outcome.

Fitzpatrick (1991) made a useful comparison between the collection of data via a self-completed questionnaire (Qu.) and collection via an interview. Table 2.3 emphasises that no one method can preclude all the likely problems. An interview will ensure a 100% response from attendees, but may not always achieve the honest or accurate response that a questionnaire filled out in the privacy of home might.

Questionnaires, especially when sent out by post, frequently fail to achieve high return rates. Hicks & Baker (1991) received responses to 76% (*n* = 226) of questionnaires when asking GPs to evaluate patient services. In another case, 48% (*n* = 478) of GPs returned questionnaires that contained six simple questions (Tagoe 1995). Tollafield & Parmar (1994) only received a 38% (*n* = 371) response from GPs to their questionnaire. The difference between these studies (which were unrelated) emphasises the advantages of a simple over a more complex questionnaire. Hicks & Baker (1991) used a basic frame of 11 questions. The design was simple and relatively unambiguous, as shown below, using ratings alone rather than open or closed responses (Box 2.3).

Table 2.3 Comparison between interview and self-questionnaires.

Interview	Self-completed Qu.
Sensitivity to the patient's concerns	Standardisation of items
Flexibility in covering topics	No interviewer bias
Rapport	Anonymity
Clarification of ambiguities	Low cost of gathering data
Response adherence	No training needed
Ability to follow up Qu.	

Box 2.3 An example of a simple questionnaire design (Hicks & Baker 1991). While such questionnaires give little elaboration for each question posed, the likely returns are higher than for questionnaires with multiple domains. Clinical audit must strike a balance between having sufficient information and not having enough

Quantity
1. Over-provided
2. Ample
3. Adequate
4. Inadequate
5. Grossly inadequate
6. Insufficient experience to offer an opinion

Quality
1. Excellent
2. Good
3. Adequate
4. Poor
5. Very poor

Tollafield & Parmar (1994), on the other hand, used 11 open and closed questions with a more complex design. In each of the three cases cited above, a postal survey was used.

The use of questionnaires often affects the quality of the information returned, and a compromise usually needs to be reached. For example, less elaborate questionnaires may provide a higher return rate. The value of marketing questionnaires is important; it is vital that the consumer does not consider the form to be yet another piece of paper!

In conclusion, questionnaire audits should be simple, they should be delivered and collected personally by an independent authority, and they should have a layout that allows easy completion. These factors may motivate consumers to complete and return their questionnaires. Long and complex questionnaires have drawbacks unless conducted by personal interview.

Methods of measuring health and well-being

The best way to collect and evaluate data is to use conventional research methods. The practitioner should always be on the lookout for errors and other factors that have the effect of creating bias, poor repeatability and poor validity.

Generic measurements. These measurements apply to a wide group of practices based upon measuring health in terms of fitness. Fitness itself has a number of domains, which range from physical to psychological well-being. Because the whole body may be involved with a disease process, isolating the foot can cause great difficulty when attempting to measure outcomes objectively, both before and after treatment.

In order to explain the concept of the generic measurement 'instrument', some examples are provided below with an accompanying discussion. Again we find that studies have mainly been carried out in the area of surgery, although the impact of disease on mobility has been studied extensively in physiotherapy and occupational therapy.

Health measures. Anaesthetists use a system of grading patients suitable for induction anaesthesia on an ordinal basis, except that each patient is given a score. This is indivisible and runs from 1 to 5. The American Society of Anesthesiologists' (ASA) score of 1 infers that no organic, physiological, biochemical or psychiatric process exists. ASA 5 infers that the patient is moribund and not expected to survive.

QUALYS. The quality of life index has been measured by workers such as Spitzer, Williams, Kind and Rosser to quantify disability and distress. When applied to cost in terms of how long a patient will live, and how much maintenance will cost for the period of treatment or benefit, the quality of life can be termed 'quality adjusted life years' or 'Qualys'. Radford (in Pysent et al 1993) compares the cost of kidney therapy as cost per Qualy. A kidney transplant costs £1413 per Qualy, as against haemodialysis which costs £9075 per Qualy. The years gained per patient are calculated from an index. The cost of the treatment for the period expected is worked out: 6.1 years for haemodialysis and 7.4 years for kidney transplant. Dividing the total cost by the number of years produces the cost per Qualy.

Foot care has been studied by Bryan et al (1991). As they point out, Qualys have been considered largely in the area of high-tech treatment (as above). When compared to repetitive maintenance care as seen in the elderly domiciliary chiropody patient, the picture changes. Their figures were as follows: for haemodialysis in hospital, £19 129; for kidney transplant, £4099; for domiciliary chiropody, £229; and for in-clinic chiropody, £694. Chiropody is a low cost service (prices based on 1989/90) and the gain from this type of care arises from preventing deterioration rather than from raising the health status of the patient.

As a measurement instrument, the Qualy can be easily misinterpreted. The application of this 'tool' has been in small populations. Differences arise between patients and workers as to how to interpret their health status, which means that any comparison is likely to have a poor correlation. The Qualy assessment assumes that every patient studied has an equal value for each year of life extended and does not account for the differences of age. An older person may be regarded by society as having less worth than a younger person in terms of extension of quality of life. Of course, the converse may be true, but the point is that difficulties arise when false judgements are made. The fact that workers have very different attitudes to what constitutes health is well covered in Bryan et al's (1991) study. Wide variations existed in the responses of chiropody practitioners, who had more difficulty than nurses in assigning distress and disability ratings. This was put down to a lack of experience on the part of the chiropodists in using this type of assessment.

Health profiles. A number of methods of measuring health have been developed for specific disabilities. In this case, the health status is considered rather than the quality of life. Practitioners should adopt a guarded approach to using such measurements.

Firstly, the profile, which is constructed from a large number of patient responses based on simple life activities, must be applicable to the particular treatment being evaluated. Foot health, for example, may be determined by other systemic, physiological and psychological factors. The omission of one of these groups from the profile could invalidate the overall results and create false assumptions.

Consider the headings shown in Box 2.4, which are taken from the *Nottingham health profile* (NHP). Thirty-eight questions are grouped under six domains, although each domain is weighted differently. The practitioner needs to be clear on what aspect of health needs highlighting in such a study and in this respect the health profiles may be biased.

Several other health profiles of this nature exist. The *arthritis impact measurement scale* (AIMS) includes dexterity but also expands physical activities into nine domains. These include household, daily and social activities as measurements of incapacity against which improvement can be gauged. The *sickness impact profile* (SIP) has 12 rather than six or nine domains, and in

---

Table 2.4 Examples of reliability for three types of health profile (Pysent et al 1993)

Nottingham health profile	0.87
Arthritis impact measurement scale	0.75–0.88
Sickness impact profile	0.97

---

contrast with the previous measures has 130 questions as opposed to 45 for AIMS and 38 for NHP.

Secondly, when studying a new instrument, the repeatability factor should be investigated. Retest reliability coefficients can be measured for these profiles by repeating measurements between workers and comparing the results. A coefficient of 0.80 is promising, while less than 0.70 shows a weaker trend for repeatability. The values for the aforementioned health instruments are given in Table 2.4 (Pysent et al 1993).

Health profiles commonly use questionnaires. The results of repeatability testing show variations between each of the three examples given in the table. The use of an interviewer can make a difference: the SIP was measured at 0.97 with an interviewer but at 0.87 without. Health profiling can offer some elements of quality assurance, but the aim of the measurement should be decided before any recording commences. The real value of health profiling lies in what it can tell you about the effect of management.

Measurement of pain

Problems of measurement. Pain is a subjective response to physical stimuli and is complicated by emotional responses that are less easy to predict. Pain is a useful outcome measure within the context of a clinical audit; it is also useful as an indicator of the effectiveness of treatment—i.e. has pain been diminished as a result? The reduction of pain can be measured in many different ways, depending on the type of treatment: duration of resolution, side-effects (particularly from drugs), mobility improvement, emotional effects, changes in sleep patterns, and the ability to use shoes that were previously abandoned.

Pain scales. A nominal (binary) scale of 'yes/no' can be used. This system offers a method of retrieving data quickly but will collect less satisfactory detail about the effect of pain relief. The question posed may be asked in more than one way. In this case the likely accuracy will be greater and repeatability will be better, as ambiguity can be reduced.

Categorical scales can be used, where a score is attributed to a descriptor such as 'severe pain' or 'moderate pain'. It is interesting to note that the British

---

Box 2.4 The Nottingham profile is an example of a health profile. Six domains are shown, attracting 38 questions. Not all domains have an equal number of questions

- Energy level
- Pain
- Emotional reaction
- Sleep
- Social isolation
- Physical activities

National Formulary uses such descriptors for classifying analgesic strengths. Pain intensity or pain relief is measured using a number, e.g. 0 for 'no pain' and 3 for 'severe pain'. Good correlation has been shown between pain scores and pain intensity offering a simple method for comparing intensity or relief of pain.

Visual analogue scales are favoured in many circles. The patient is asked to put a mark on a line (continuum), having first been told the extreme ranges. This barometer of pain intensity or relief can then be measured in millimetres using a ruler along the predetermined length of line selected (often 10 cm).

Pain charts such as the Oxford pain chart, the Burford chart and the Evans chart use category rating scales. The use of Likert scales can indicate the effectiveness of treatment within categories such as poor, fair, good, very good and excellent. In one sense the chart acts as a focused diary of pain intensity.

Pain questionnaires. Questionnaires have been designed along the lines of the *McGill pain questionnaire* (MPQ). This design is similar to the methods seen previously in the Nottingham health profile. The MPQ uses 102 pain descriptors, although a shortened version uses 78 questions. Patients with limited vocabularies and those classified as 'sick' respond less well than others. The time needed to prepare this type of measurement is lengthy compared to rating and analogue scales.

Physiological methods. Physiological methods can be used to evaluate blood pressure, hormonal activity, respiratory levels and skin temperature. While useful for research, as a general form of audit these methods are less attractive. *Behavioural methods* require careful monitoring of a patient's physical changes. The method requires the practitioner to be available around the clock to assess food intake, alertness, and facial responses such as distortion. However, different patients behave very differently, and the behavioural method system is therefore poor and insensitive as a measure.

In conclusion, the weakness of using pain response alone affects the quality of measurement. The use of a broad range of factors, coupled with other aspects of the disease process or treatment such as healing and reduced doses of analgesics, is more helpful and offers greater sensitivity.

Measuring clinical outcome

Clinical activity measurement is today taken more seriously in health circles than it has been in the past, when many decisions were taken on the basis of empiricism. Pysent et al (1993) have criticised the lack

of available methods for evaluating [orthopaedic] treatment. In point of fact it is not the shortage of methods alone but the specificity and reliability of such methods which lead to an unsuitable system of measurement. The majority of examples used in the latter part of this chapter have been taken from material in recent years.

When measurement forms part of the quantitative analysis, the assessment of outcomes becomes more robust. Once a reliable system has been found for analysing a particular pathology, providing that it is repeatable, valid and reproducible, then that system can be used as a measure of change. Several examples are given below which are specifically related to analysing the effect of treatment on the foot:

- assessment of deformity
- joint motion
- gait analysis.

Deformity. In the foot, lesser toes, hallux, midfoot and hindfoot are the main focuses of problems. Kitoaka et al (1994) looked at a clinical rating system that used partial measurement with subjective features as described in health profiles, but that focused on mobility. No useful repeatability study has been used to formalise the method, although the authors believe it to be a practical system which allows comparability before and after treatment via a method of scoring. Moran & Claridge (1994) have used Kitoaka et al's method to show the changes in 12 patients following a particular surgery. The domains used in the study are shown in Table 2.5. An initial score indicates the extent of the problem, and the second, higher, score shows the average improvement made. The domains used are recognised criteria for identifying patient satisfaction; for example, patients regard an early return to wearing shoes after surgery as a recognisable improvement.

Joint motion. Measuring joint motion suffers from the same problems as measuring deformity. In the case of joints, the excursion of motion is affected by

Table 2.5 Overall improvement can be expressed as a percentage average improvement. Measured before and after operation (Moran & Claridge 1994)

	Symptoms	
	Before	After
Pain	7.2	27.2
Activity tolerance	10.6	14.1
Shoes	5.0	7.8
Cosmesis	2.2	4.4
Overall	4.1	8.8

Table 2.6 When using methods for evaluating change the process should be repeatable. The table shows inter- and intra-class correlation coefficients. The same observer is usually more reliable at repeating the measurement than different observers

Joint	Movement	Inter-observer	Intra-observer
Ankle	Dorsiflexion	0.50	0.90
	Plantarflexion	0.72	0.86
Subtalar	Inversion	0.32	0.74
	Eversion	0.17	0.75

temperature and synovial joint fluid viscosity. Variations in measurement may occur as a result of a practitioner's poor knowledge of anatomy, physiology and joint biomechanics. Relatively large joints of the foot, such as the subtalar and ankle joint, are complicated because their motion has no single dimension of movement. Inter- and intra-class correlation coefficients have been measured by Elveru (Pysent et al 1993) and are given in Table 2.6.

Sufficient care must be taken when interpreting quantitative data. If the technique can withstand scientific rigour, then as an audit tool it has great value. Measurement by goniometer provides a baseline value; if it is accurate then the quantification of disability and improvement after treatment or otherwise may be recorded within the case records.

Gait analysis. In recent years the measuring instruments for foot contact pressures and forces have become more elaborate and more portable. Divided into ink mats, force and pressure platforms, as well as individual sensors used over specific points, these systems have been used to make comments about disability and altered contact phases during gait. Efficiency of oxygen has been measured to assess energy consumption, although it has not been used for routine measurement. Most of these methods are too laborious for the everyday clinical situation and are more appropriate for academic research. Many workers have attempted to use gait analysis methods to measure the effect of orthoses and therefore the effects of treatment.

The common factor in each of the above cases is that the instrument of measurement is physical and needs calibrating to ensure repeatability. Errors arise from both instruments and patients as well as from human handling (examiner). Any valuable conclusion must first include a statement of reliability, repeatability and validity; this is so important that it is worth repeating again and again. Unfortunately some techniques still lack reliability or repeatability in measuring joint position, movement and ground–foot interface pressures, but improvements are encouraging.

Effects of measurement on treatment policy for the future

The advent of research in health has affected the shape of outcomes dramatically, with many more practitioners now questioning the methods of assessment, the interpretation of results and the comparative effects of the different methods. The use of medication, orthoses and surgery is for the first time being questioned, where previously such treatment was accepted empirically. One of the major impacts of this work is directly related to cost of provision of treatment and the likely resources required.

Modern technology is constantly influencing the development of more rapid audit mechanisms. The use of pen-activated linked computers with interfacing microphones will allow medical records to be audited with ease and speed, and will allow the generation of letters, as well as providing reasonable patient data security. Database analysis will provide rapid breakdown on treatment, drugs and complications. The link with clinical economics will drive the development of dedicated systems which are currently being tested particularly in the North American Health Care system.

Presenting data

Case files are probably the commonest source of data in following treatment progress. Retrospective analysis is more frequently employed than prospective analysis. Loss of data is a significant problem leading to potentially incorrect conclusions. The use of computerised information or well-designed data books (similar to accounting books) can overcome this problem as long as they are kept up to date. Stamp pads designed to record simple data such as foot lesions and vascular tree pressure indices are helpful and easily identified within case records.

Practitioners should develop a system of summarising information and recording improvement and deterioration in a systematic way at the end of each entry to allow for occasional audit. Clear writing and minimum use of abbreviations will greatly speed up the process of reviewing case records. A certain amount of standardisation is recommended for such reviews to make comparison more informative.

Setting out the evidence. Tabulated results are valuable when presented with explanatory text. Each

Table 2.7 Auditing the same question – would patients be prepared to have surgery repeated in the same way again? The cycle of audit should be repeated and changes to responses should be monitored for wide variations. Standards need to be maintained. The values below relate to different centres: Tollafield (podiatry) and Tibrewal (orthopaedics).

1991	Tibrewal & Floss	80%
1987–91	Tollafield & Parmar*	93%
1993	Tollafield & Sheward	97%
1993–4	Tollafield & Kilmartin*	97%

section of this text should be clearly marked and numbered, and should have subsections. Consider Table 2.7 which shows how patients responded when questioned about returning to a service. The data were used in an internal report to show the percentage of patients prepared to return for day surgery at three centres having been sent a questionnaire 6 months or longer after the event.

Other forms of reporting may use data, such as a research paper which can be published and cited. Sample sizes should be large enough and ideally include a control or comparison. Graphs, flow charts, histograms and pie charts are valuable tools for reporting trends for large data sets. Complicated statistics are undesirable as in many cases they are used inappropriately.

In conclusion, setting out internal and scientific audit reports requires clarity with a sound structure that has a progressive and logical flow. The *objectives* should be stated, the *method* included and *results* brought together in tables or plots to highlight trends.

The *conclusion* should be based upon the evidence presented without excessive elaboration. A *summary* is valuable, allowing the reader to scan the information quickly for relevance. Where audit requires a large amount of data collection, the report should have more than one section, allowing for unrelated information to be separated. The conclusion can then be used to bring all the sections together, if indeed there is a valid reason for doing this. Scientific audit may be more specific and require greater controls and analysis. Omitting the usual scientific principles and failing to use the style required will usually result in your paper being rejected.

SUMMARY

Audit is a very large subject and in a brief chapter many areas that would ideally be described in greater detail must be left to texts which are devoted solely to this subject. Emphasis has been placed here on audit within health care, with a bias towards measuring clinical outcomes.

The need to implement audit in the clinic is based upon many different requirements. Practitioners must take account of educational, legal, political, moral, ethical and research aspects in conducting their activities. Standards set for practice should ideally be underpinned by proving the effectiveness of treatment. Politics and economics drive medical audit today, leaving health care professionals to justify their selection of treatment.

Audit has come a long way since the days of Florence Nightingale and Ernest Codman at a time when medical dogma refused to recognise that old practices were outdated and ineffective.

REFERENCES

Bradshaw T W 1995 Clinical audit in theory and practice. British Journal of Podiatric Medicine 50: 3–5, 9

Bryan S, Parkin D, Donaldson C 1991 Chiropody and the Qualy; a case study in assigning categories of disability and distress to patients. Health Policy 18: 169–185

Donebedian A 1966 Evaluating the quality of medical care. Millbank Memorial Fund Quarterly, Part 3: 166–206

Donebedian A 1988 The quality of care. How can it be assessed? Journal of the American Medical Association 260: 1743–1748

Ellis B W, Sensky T 1991 A clinician's guide to setting up audit. British Journal of Medicine 302: 704–707

Ellis R, Whittington D 1993 Quality assurance in health care. A handbook. Edward Arnold, London, p 2–3

Fitzpatrick R 1991 Surveys of satisfaction: I—Important general considerations. British Medical Journal 303: 887–889

Hicks N R, Baker I A 1991 A General Practitioner's opinions of health services available to their patients. British Medical Journal 302: 991–993

HMSO 1989 NHS Working for patients. CMNO 555. HMSO, London

Kitoaka H B, Alexander I J, Adelaar R S, Nunley J A, Myerson M S, Sanders M 1994 Clinical rating systems for ankle-hindfoot, midfoot, hallux and lesser toes. Foot and Ankle International 15 (7): 349–353

Lawrence M, Griew K, Derry J, Anderson J, Humphreys J 1994 Auditing audits: use and development of the Oxfordshire Medical Audit Advisory Group rating system. British Medical Journal 309: 513–516

Maxwell R J 1984 Quality assessment in health. British Medical Journal 228: 1470–1477

Moran M M, Claridge R J 1994 Chevron osteotomy for bunionette. Foot and Ankle International 15 (12): 684–688

O'Doherty D 1993 In: Pysent P, Fairbank J, Carr A (eds) Outcome measures in orthopaedics. Butterworth-Heinemann, Oxford p 245–264

Pollock A, Evans M 1993 Surgical audit, 2nd edn. Butterworth-Heinmann, Oxford, p 25–27, 58–63

Pysent P, Fairbank J, Carr A 1993 Outcome measures in orthopaedics. Butterworth-Heinemann, Oxford

Shaw C 1990 Medical audit. King's Fund, London

Tagoe M 1995 Patient satisfaction audit following podiatric surgery. In: Report of Podiatry Association on podiatry & hospital foot services (Appendix B) Podiatry Association, January, p 18–22

Tollafield D R 1993 Podiatric surgical audit. Impact on foothealth—results of a five year study. British Journal of Podiatric Medicine 48 (6): 89–92

Tollafield D R, Kilmartin T E, Holdcroft D J, Quinn G 1995 Measurement of ankle cuff discomfort in unsedated patients undergoing day case foot surgery. Ambulatory Surgery 3 (2): 91–96

Tollafield D R, Parmar D G 1994 Setting standards for day care foot surgery. A quinquennial review. British Journal of Podiatric Medicine & Surgery 6 (1): 7–20

Tucker P 1995 Clinical audit lectures. 20 Watling Street Rd, Preston, Lancs (Personal correspondence)

Turbutt I F 1994 Auditorium. Podiatric surgery audit. Foot surgery survey of 46 centres in the United Kingdom. British Journal of Podiatric Medicine & Surgery 6 (2): 30–31

FURTHER READING

ACCO 1990 Quality assurance. Instep, 5–8

Ariori A R, Graham R B, Antony R J 1989 Results of a six month practice in Podiatric Day Surgery in the NHS. Journal of the Podiatric Association, April, 16

Ashcroft D J, Lavis G J, Russell L H 1979 Retrospective analysis of partial nail avulsions. The Chiropodist 34: 100–108

Beaton D 1990 Ingrowing toenails: a patient evaluation of phenolisation versus wedge excision. British Journal of Podiatric Medicine 45: 62

Bunbridge C A 1993 Survey of patient satisfaction with the quality of service provided by the West Berkshire Chiropody Department. British Journal of Podiatric Medicine 48: 46–48

Crombie I K 1992 Towards good Audit. British Journal of Hospital Medicine 48 (3): 182–185

Difford F 1990 Audit in person. British Medical Journal 300: 92–94

Duncan A 1980 Quality assurance: What now and where next? British Medical Journal 300–302

Gaskell B 1989 Nail surgery—the patient's reaction. Enfield Health Authority Department of Chiropody. The Chiropodist 44: 174–176

Griffiths C 1995 Clinical measurement. In: Merriman L M, Tollafield D R (eds) Assessment of the lower limb. Churchill Livingstone, Edinburgh

Helfand A E 1990 Guidelines for podiatric services in long-term care facilities. Journal of the American Podiatric Medical Association 80 (8): 448–450

Helm P A 1981 Ingrowing toe nails. An evaluation of two treatments. British Medical Journal 283: 1125–1126

Green Park Unit 1992 A guide to medical audit. Medical Audit Department, Musgrave Park Hospital, Northern Ireland

Jones O R, Christenson C J 1992 Podiatric utilization referral patterns at an army medical centre. Military Medicine 157 (1): 7–10

Keefe M 1989 An audit of wart treatment in a Scottish dermatology department. British Journal of Podiatric Medicine 44: 271–274

Kilmartin T E, Barrington R L, Wallace W A 1992 The X-ray measurement of hallux valgus. An inter and intra-observer error study. The Foot 2: 7–11

Kind P, Rosser R, Williams A 1982 Valuation of quality of life: some pyschometric evidence. In: Jones-Lee M W (ed) The value of life and safety. North-Holland, Amsterdam

Kuwada G T 1991 Long-term evaluation of partial and total surgical and phenol matrixectomies. Journal of the American Podiatric Medical Association 81 (1): 33–36

McKee C M, Lauglo M, Lessof L 1989 Medical audit: a review. Journal of the Royal Society of Medicine 82: 474–478

Mangan J L, Ashford R L, Murphy J S G, Beverland D E 1992 Waiting list initiatives: application to foot surgery. Medical Audit News 2 (2): 44–45

Mangan J L, Ashford R L, Murphy J S G, Beverland D E 1992 A multidisciplinary approach to foot surgery waiting lists. The Foot 2: 29–33

Merriman L 1990 Manpower planning in chiropody: what is chiropody? British Journal of Podiatric Medicine 45: 179–182

Merriman L 1991 Manpower planning in chiropody treatment for life. British Journal of Podiatric Medicine 46: 36–40

Palmer B V, Jones 1979 Ingrowing toenails. The results of treatment. British Journal of Surgeons 66: 575–576

Society of Chiropodists 1991 Guidelines on standards of chiropody/podiatry practice. Society of Chiropodists,

Spitzer W O 1987 State of science 1986: quality of life and functional status as target variables for research. Journal of Chronic Diseases 40: 465–471

Tollafield D R, Price M 1985 Hallux metatarsophalangeal joint survey related to postoperative surgery analysis. The Chiropodist 40 (5): 283–288

University of Dundee 1992 Moving to audit. What every doctor needs to know about medical audit.

3

Clinical protocols

J. Dale
L. Merriman

INTRODUCTION

The first part of this chapter looks at the factors which influence how practitioners act and behave in clinical practice. This is followed by examination of four clinical protocols in which practitioners who are involved in the treatment of the foot need to be cognisant (Box 3.1). A protocol states the course of action to be adopted by people working within a particular organisation, profession or service.

Clinical protocols are basically rules of how to proceed in certain situations. They provide health care practitioners with parameters in which to operate. The term 'code of practice' may be used synonymously with clinical protocols. A code comprises a set of laws or rules. Codes of practice may be formulated by statutory organisations, professional bodies, employers or voluntary organisations. They may cover a diverse range of issues or focus on a specific process or issue. For example, codes of practice related to the practitioner–patient relationship cover a broad range of issues, whereas a code of practice for the sterilisation of instruments focuses on one specific issue. All codes of practice should be regularly reviewed and updated in the light of current research in order to ensure the best delivery of clinical services.

Box 3.1   Clinical protocols

- Health and safety
- Infection control
- Liability insurance
- Practitioner–patient relationship

WHAT INFLUENCES HOW A PRACTITIONER PRACTICES?

All health care practitioners are accountable:

- for their own individual actions

- for the care of other people
- to professional organisations
- to the general public.

When treating patients, practitioners must be aware of these obligations and responsibilities. In order to offer the best service to their patients and society in general, it is incumbent on practitioners to ensure that their practice is safe, does not put the patient at harm (i.e. is not maleficent) and is of benefit to the patient (i.e. is beneficent). Each practitioner is accountable and responsible for their own actions, but in deciding how to act they will be influenced by the following:

- current legislation
- the codes of practice/conduct of professional organisations
- the codes of practice/conduct of employing organisations
- their own attitudes and beliefs.

All of the above influence the practitioner, but in some circumstances one may override the others, e.g. current legislation. Each of the above influences will be considered in turn.

Current legislation

Acts of Parliament and judicial decisions, arising from what are commonly known as 'test cases', collectively impose legal responsibilities on practitioners. All practitioners should keep themselves informed about relevant Acts of Parliament which may affect their practice. Box 3.2 lists some of the Acts of Parliament which are relevant to health care practitioners involved in treating the foot. These Acts may be amended or replaced from time to time.

Codes of practice/conduct of professional organisations

The practice of health care professions is influenced by statutory and professional bodies. There are specific statutory bodies responsible for most of the health care professions. For example, the statutory body for doctors is the General Medical Council, that for chiropodists/podiatrists is the Chiropodist Board, and that for nursing is the United Kingdom Central Council. The role of these statutory bodies varies but usually involves responsibility for initial education and issues related to practice and conduct. For example, the Professions Supplementary to Medicine (PSM) Act (1960) requires the Chiropodist Board to prepare a statement as to the kind of conduct and

---

Box 3.2   Examples of relevant Acts of Parliament*
- Occupier's Liability Act 1957 - Health and Safety at Work Act 1974 - Data Protection Act 1974 - Reporting of Injuries, Diseases and Dangerous Occurrence Regulations 1985 - Consumer Protection Act 1987 - Ionising Radiation (protection of persons undergoing medical examination or treatment) Regulations 1988 - Control of Substances Hazardous to Health (COSHH) 1988 - Pressure Systems and Transportable Gas Containers Regulations 1989 - Children's Act 1989 - Access to Health Records Act 1990 - Provision and Use of Work Equipment Regulations 1992 - Manual Handling Operations Regulations 1992 - Management of Health and Safety at Work Regulations 1992 - Personal Protective Equipment at Work Regulations 1992 - Electromagnetic Compatibility Regulations 1992
*Copies of these Acts/Regulations can be obtained from Her Majesty's Stationery Office (HMSO).

---

practice expected of chiropodists/podiatrists. The purpose of this 'statement of conduct' is to enable the Board to fulfil its statutory function of promoting high standards of professional conduct.

The practice of health practitioners, as well as being influenced by statutory bodies, is also affected by professional organisations. Most health professionals are members of one or more professional organisations, for example, the British Medical Association (BMA) and the Royal College of Nurses (RCN). These organisations have no statutory function; their role is to protect and promote the interests of their members. As part of this function, they produce their own codes of practice. The prime purposes of these codes are to:

- reassure the public that they can expect high standards of practice
- provide guidelines on best practice for members.

Codes of practice/conduct of employing organisations

The NHS is by far the largest employer of health care practitioners in the United Kingdom. It produces a range of codes of practice which influence the practice of its health care practitioners. For example, the NHS has a code of practice related to immunisation of first line practitioners for hepatitis B (HSG(93)40).

Box 3.3 Patient Charter standards (Department of Health 1995)

- To receive health care on the basis of clinical need, regardless of ability to pay
- To be registered with a General Practitioner (GP)
- To receive emergency medical care at any time, through your GP or the emergency ambulance service and the hospital accident and emergency department
- To be referred to a consultant acceptable to you when your GP thinks it necessary, and to be referred for a second opinion if you and your GP agree this is desirable
- To be given clear explanation of any treatment proposed, including any risk and any alternatives, before you decide whether you will agree to the treatment
- To have access to your health records, and to know that those working for the NHS are under a legal duty to keep their contents confidential
- To choose whether or not you wish to take part in medical research or medical student training
- To be given detailed information on local health services, including quality standards and maximum waiting times
- To be guaranteed admission for treatment by a specific date no later than two years from the day when your consultant places you on a waiting list
- To have any complaint about NHS services—whoever provides them—investigated and to receive a full and prompt written reply from the chief executive or general manager

---

The Patient's Charter (Department of Health 1991) is another example of a NHS code of practice. Initially, the Charter laid down standards for seven aspects of patient care; in April 1992 a further three were added (Box 3.3). Following the setting of these national standards, individual NHS Trusts have published their own additional local standards.

A standard identifies the required level of practice. Clinical codes of practice are commonly expressed in terms of minimum standards. A minimum standard is the lowest acceptable level of practice necessary for the proper care of patients. Standards are arrived at from a number of sources, e.g. experts in the field, professional organisations, employers and special interest groups.

Individual attitudes and beliefs

We all have our own individual notions about what we consider to be right and wrong, about how we should treat other people, and about what is fair and appropriate. These personal views are influenced by a range of circumstances—upbringing, schooling, religious beliefs and past experiences to name but a few. Sometimes there may be differences between our personal attitudes and beliefs and the law of the land or the codes of practice of the professional organisations of which we are members. In such instances, each individual practitioner must decide what he or she considers to be the most appropriate course of action. However, at all times the interests and needs of the patient should be paramount.

CLINICAL PROTOCOLS

Health and safety

Practitioners' responsibilities for health and safety are governed by the Health and Safety at Work Act (HSW) 1974 and associated Acts and Regulations. In January 1993, the Health and Safety Executive produced a code of practice for workplace health, safety and welfare (Health and Safety Executive 1993a). This code was in response to section 16 (1) of the Health and Safety at Work Act 1974. Under this Act, responsibility for health and safety rests with the highest level of management but all individuals have a degree of responsibility for carrying out health and safety policies. Particular areas of responsibility may be designated to named individuals; for example, the maintenance of clinical equipment may be the responsibility of a chief technician. However, the practitioner is ultimately responsible for the treatment a patient receives, and in the case of equipment the practitioner must be satisfied that it is safe to use at the point of contact.

For the practitioner involved with treating disorders of the foot the following specific aspects of health and safety should be borne in mind. Some of these relate to specific Acts of Parliament, while others relate to a general consensus of what constitutes good practice:

- design of clinical areas
- safe use of equipment
- use of hazardous substances
- responsibilities of employers and employees.

Design of clinical areas

The practitioner's involvement in the design of the treatment area is essential. The general layout of equipment should be decided upon during the initial planning stage. Early decisions prevent incorrect siting of integral fittings such as sinks and power points. Due consideration should be given to lighting, both natural and artificial. The position of light sources in relation to working surfaces is of particular importance.

The conversion of existing premises to provide suitable clinical accommodation can be problematic. Ornate ceilings, picture rails and skirting boards may be in keeping with the property but are not conducive to the creation of an ideal clinical treatment area. Advice from experts, such as architects and builders, can alleviate some of the difficulties. Discussion with colleagues who have experience of similar situations can prove invaluable.

Ease of access to clinical premises is of the utmost importance as patients may be disabled. Ground floor accommodation is preferable unless a lift is available. Consideration should be given to the distance which patients need to walk or be transported from the entrance to the waiting area and then to the surgery.

Careful attention to planning of reception facilities and waiting areas pays dividends. Not only is it important to create a safe environment for patients, but attention should also be paid to ensuring that the reception area is welcoming. First impressions are important; hence the significance of welcoming reception facilities. Natural light and high ceilings provide a 'relaxing atmosphere' (Combs 1992). Adequate seating, particularly for the less agile, a children's play area and the availability of drinks are features appreciated by patients and, at the same time, ensure a safe and healthy environment. Clear signposting to treatment areas and facilities reduces patients' anxiety. It is often useful to involve representatives of users and potential users of the service in the planning of reception and waiting facilities.

A variety of patients' chairs are now on the market (Fig. 3.1). When selecting a chair, it is essential that the back rest is adjustable; chairs with fully reclining back rests are essential for patient examination and the management of clinical emergencies. The height of the chair should also be adjustable; this facilitates easier access for the patient and provides a convenient working position for the practitioner, thus preventing known occupational hazards such as chronic back pain. The manufacturer's manual should be carefully studied to ensure safe usage.

The operating chair must be comfortable for the practitioner. The height of the chair and the position of the back rest should be adjustable. A five star base fitted with casters allows manoeuverability and prevents tipping. The suitability of an operating chair should be assessed in combination with the patient's chair with which it is to be used.

Examination lamps should be installed as additional lighting. These may be wall- or ceiling-mounted

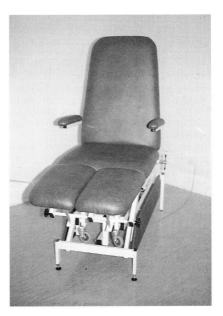

Figure 3.1 Flat-bed couch with adjustable back rest.

or fitted onto work units or mobile bases. The aim is to have a non-distorting, colour-corrected light source which can be focused on a particular site. To achieve this, lamps are extended by means of articulating arms. The length and range of movement of the arm should be assessed with regard to the position in which the lamp is to be mounted. Fluorescent tubes or incandescent lamps are most commonly used in routine clinical practice. The amount of heat generated by the lamp when in use is an important consideration. It is possible to purchase examination lamps which incorporate a magnifying glass; these lamps can be particularly helpful for observing skin changes and for operating.

Adequate storage space for supplies and portable equipment is of prime importance. A separate, lockable store room, adjacent to the treatment room, is desirable but not always possible. Storage racks and cupboards should be used efficiently. Labelling of cupboards with details of their contents is helpful, especially if other practitioners use the area. All drugs, needles and syringes must be stored in a locked cabinet. To promote compliance with this regulation, other items should not be stored in this space.

Safe use of equipment

All surgery equipment should be maintained as per the manufacturer's instructions. Servicing contracts with the manufacturer or specialist contractors ensure that maintenance procedures are not overlooked. Equipment which is to be repaired or serviced must be decontaminated first. For example, nail drill handpieces should be autoclaved and dust bags removed from drills. If adequate decontamination has not been carried out, the service engineers must be notified by appropriate labelling of the equipment.

The individual manufacturer's instructions for the use of specific equipment, such as cryosurgery and ultrasound equipment, must be followed and safety precautions must be strictly adhered to. For example, an exhaust hose to vent noxious waste gas from cryotherapy systems should always be used (see Chapter 9).

The Health and Safety Executive Memorandum of Guidance on the Electricity at Work Regulations (1989) state the legal requirements for the maintenance of portable electrical equipment (including autoclaves). The user is charged with the responsibility for checking that equipment appears to be in a sound condition before use. The establishment of a system for the inspection and testing of equipment is also a requirement of these regulations.

There continues to be significant improvements in the mechanical efficiency of nail drills. An effective dust extraction mechanism is a priority. Drills need to be robust to withstand heavy usage. This is particularly so in clinics used by several practitioners. The size and shape of the handpiece should be appropriate to the operator's hand. Adequate holders are needed to protect handpieces from damage when they are not in use. Autoclavable handpieces are essential. Drills may be fixed to work units by means of a bracket, positioned adjacent to an existing surface or used on a mobile base.

Certain equipment that may be used in diagnosing and treating foot problems, e.g. X-ray and laser equipment, is controlled by separate regulations. Advice on the safety aspects of these procedures may be obtained from authorities such as the National Radiological Protection Board.

Use of hazardous substances

The Control of Substances Hazardous to Health (COSHH) Regulations 1988 provide a framework for the protection of people against health risks from hazardous substances. Under the COSHH regulations, a risk assessment of all the substances encountered in practice must be made and any necessary action taken to reduce identified risks. Examples of hazardous substances used in the treatment of foot problems are strong acids and alkalis, solvents and adhesives.

In 1993, the Health and Safety Executive produced a useful step-by-step guide to COSHH regulations (Health and Safety Executive 1993b).

Responsibilities of employers and employees

If five or more people are employed, the employer must have a written health and safety policy. In situations where complex procedures are undertaken, this policy should refer the reader to other, more specific health and safety documents. Codes of practice dealing with infection control and the use of orthotic laboratories are examples where specific documentation would be required. The law only requires safety policy statements to cover the health and safety of employees (Health and Safety Executive 1990a). However, it is recommended that a strategy for protecting other people (patients, visitors, cleaners, maintenance staff and contractors) who could be put at risk by activities undertaken during the course of practice is established.

Employers must ensure that employees are provided with adequate health and safety training, including refresher training. Changes made to existing policies must be made known to all employees. The implementation of safety policies should be closely monitored. Revision of policies is necessary from time to time in the light of experience or because of the introduction of new or altered practices.

Health and safety regulations also apply to the self-employed. Practitioners who are self-employed have a duty to conduct their practices in such a manner so as to ensure, as far as is reasonably practical, that they and other persons who may be affected are not exposed to risks to their health and safety.

Infection control

Infection control is an integral part of good practice. The prime purpose of any infection control policy is to reduce the likelihood of cross-infection either between the practitioner and the patient or between patients. Practitioners involved in treating foot problems are, at times, likely to come into contact with the body fluids of their patients. Conversely the patient may, under certain circumstances, come into contact with the body fluids of the practitioner, e.g. if a practitioner cuts herself with a scalpel. Of particular concern are the systemic infections transmitted by body fluids, human immunodeficiency virus (HIV) and hepatitis B (HBV). The other main risks of cross-infection are from localised infections of the feet involving bacteria, fungi or viruses.

In practice, there are many differences in the cross-infection procedures adopted by particular establishments or organisations; these differences do not usually present a problem. However, it is most important that each establishment/organisation documents its infection control policy and that copies of this policy are available to all practitioners. An infection control policy should, as a minimum standard, encompass the following areas.

Routine clinical cleansing

Cleaning of the clinical environment is essential to reduce the risk of cross-infection between patients and the personnel involved in the delivery of treatment. The cleaning of equipment and furnishings should be organised in terms of procedure, frequency of use and who is responsible. Cleaning procedures adopted must be justifiable. There is no evidence that the use of disinfectant solutions is of benefit in the cleaning of walls or floors (Maurer 1985, Ward 1990). Detergent solutions are adequate for most general cleaning. The effectiveness of cleaning depends to a large extent on the frictional scrubbing action which is applied to any surface. Walls need to be washed, at a minimum, every 3 months (unless splashing occurs). Floors require washing at least every day.

Infection control procedures are easier to undertake if units are of a simple design. The pristine condition of storage compartments is soon lost with continual usage. The whole unit must be easily cleaned. A durable and easily cleaned top surface of, for example, glass or stainless steel, is necessary to isolate sterilised instruments. The unit should be mobile to allow easy access and to facilitate floor cleaning.

Durable floor covering is essential. Non-slip vinyl, extended to skirting level and with sealed seams, is a relatively safe option and can be easily cleaned. The choice of window blinds should also be influenced by ease of cleaning. Curtaining around changing cubicles should be washable and, in line with Department of Health (DoH) regulations, fire-retardant. Worn furnishings, such as floor coverings, must be replaced before they become dangerous.

The safe removal of debris following each treatment has consistently been debated. Sweeping brushes disperse bacteria into the air (Babb 1963). Vacuum cleaners have been shown to have the same effect (Bate 1961). Wet-vacuum systems are acceptable but wet floors are hazardous. The solution lies in the collection of all debris at source (Fig. 3.2). If reusable debris trays are used, they should be protected by a moisture-proof cover, which is changed after every treatment.

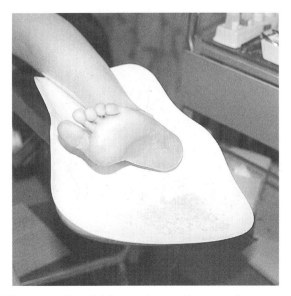

Figure 3.2 Foot debris tray shown without a moisture-proof cover (now recommended).

Handwashing

Evidence strongly supports a causal relationship between handwashing and infection control (Larson 1988). The primary objective of clinical handwashing is to eliminate transient contaminants that have been acquired from patients or the environment and to reduce the resident flora of the skin to as low a level as possible. Transient contaminants are easily removed by thorough washing with soap and water. A vigorous scrub with a non-medicated soap for at least 10–15 seconds will reliably remove gross contamination (Knittle et al 1975). Antiseptic handwashing agents assist the removal of resident organisms. It is important that handwashing agents used for pre-operative scrubbing have rapid and potent antimicrobial activity, that they be well tolerated, and ideally that they exert a residual antibacterial effect for a prolonged period following the scrub (Maki 1989).

Many comparative studies of handwashing agents have been undertaken. Bendig (1991) concluded that a 4% chlorhexidine detergent solution was significantly more effective than 2% triclosan detergent solution. Cremieux et al (1989) found that the immediate efficacy of povidone-iodine and chlorhexidine were equivalent, but that the cumulative efficacy and remnant effects of chlorhexidine were higher than those of povidone-iodine. The properties of a handwashing agent should be evaluated in terms of expected usage.

Use of gloves

Protective gloves are now worn for all procedures which may involve exposure to blood, body fluids or other sources of infection. Non-sterile gloves are adequate for non-invasive work but sterile gloves must always be worn for any invasive procedure.

Practitioners often complain of the poor fit of non-sterile disposable gloves and resort to the use of sterile surgical gloves which are much more expensive. The necessity to discard non-sterile gloves after each treatment is debatable (Baumann 1992). Provided that these gloves are not punctured, washing and disinfection may be adequate. To decontaminate gloves, washing with a hand-cleansing agent for 30 seconds is generally necessary (Douglas 1989). In practice, loose-fitting non-sterile gloves can be difficult to wash satisfactorily. Surgical gloves are damaged by frequent washing and become sticky through loss of talcum and/or starch on the surface (Mitchell et al 1983).

If gloves are to protect the practitioner and the patient against cross-infection, they must be used in the proper manner (Fig. 3.3). Handwashing is necessary before donning gloves and after their removal. When treatment is completed, immediate removal, in the case of an invasive procedure, or washing of gloves, in the case of a non-invasive procedure, is essential. To contain contaminants, gloves must be removed by turning them inside out.

The incidence of hand dermatitis is reputedly on the increase because of the wider and more frequent use of latex gloves in health care practice (Sharma 1991). Gloves can affect skin in different ways, e.g. hands may become dry and cracked or sweaty and swollen. The use of hypoallergenic gloves frequently alleviates these skin pathologies.

Instrument sterilisation

Sterilisation of instruments is an integral part of routine practice. Thorough cleaning of instruments prior to sterilisation is essential. Blood and other adherent material will coagulate and become fixed on instruments as they pass through the heat sterilisation cycle. Instruments should be cleaned in a dedicated sink using warm water and detergent. Robust, protective rubber gloves should be worn during this procedure. A more convenient and efficient method is to use an ultrasonic cleaner (Fig. 3.4A). When washing instruments, excessive amounts of detergent or inadequate rinsing results in residues which can subsequently damage the autoclave mechanisms.

Steam pressure autoclaves provide the most convenient and reliable method of achieving instrument sterilisation (Fig. 3.4B). The cleaned instruments should be spaced out on the autoclave trays and closed instruments should be opened so that all surfaces will be exposed to steam during the sterilisation process (Fig. 3.4C). Prospective purchasers are strongly recommended to consider only models which comply with British Standard 3970 Part 4 *Specification for transportable steam sterilizers for unwrapped instruments and utensils* (see also Health and Safety Executive 1990). The purchaser's choice of autoclave must be influenced first and foremost by compliance with safety requirements. Autoclaves require commissioning before use, and operating instructions must be strictly adhered to. Steam sterilisers are pressure vessels and must comply with the *Pressure systems and transportable gas container Regulations* (1989), whereby the user is required to have a suitable scheme for the periodic examination of the steriliser. The insurers of premises on which autoclaves are being used must be notified.

Small steam sterilisers are generally considered as being only suitable for the sterilisation of unwrapped loads for immediate use (Department of Health 1990). In practice, there may be a short delay before instruments are used. Contamination may then be minimised by placing the trays into an ultraviolet cabinet or by completely covering with sterile paper (British Medical Association 1989; Fig 3.4D).

High vacuum autoclaves are used to sterilise porous items, such as wrapped instruments, dressings and linen. In this type of autoclave, a vacuum is first created to enable the steam to penetrate the load more efficiently. At the end of the sterilisation time, drying of the load occurs by means of the vacuum system. High vacuum autoclaves are installed in central sterile supply departments (CSSDs) and hospital sterilising units (HSDUs). Access to the services of a sterile supplies department is essential for all practitioners.

Sterile packs

Costly sterilisation processes will be negated if packs are wrongly stored or used. Packaging must not be damaged in any way if the contents are to remain sterile. Sterile products are marked with a 'use by' date after which their sterility cannot be guaranteed. Consequently, strict rotation of stock is necessary to avoid wastage. Contamination of the contents can occur if packs are incorrectly opened or misused. Paper autoclave bags should be opened by means of the side folds. Similarly, peelable wrapping must not be indiscriminately cut or torn open.

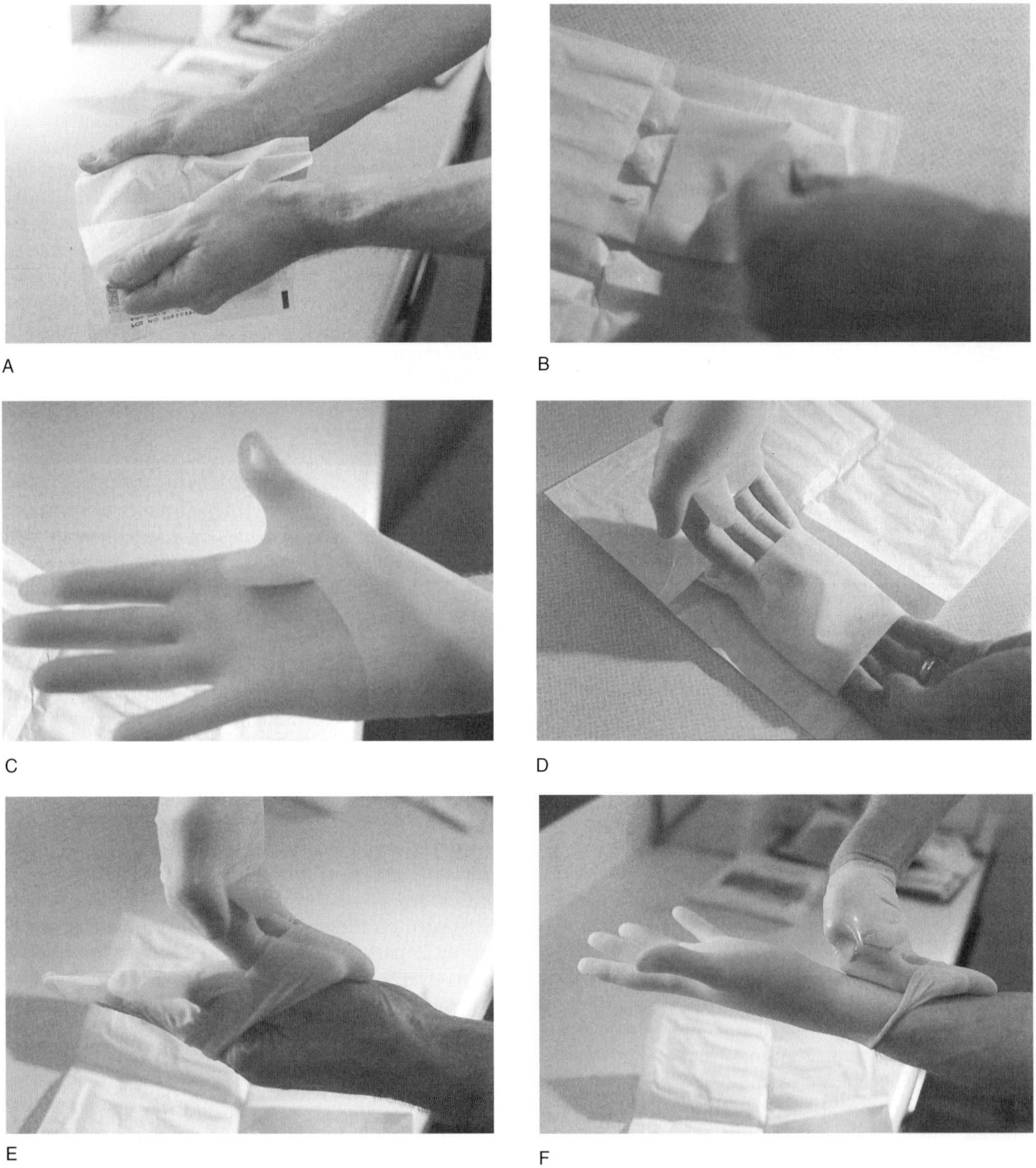

Figure 3.3 A–F: Procedure for putting on sterile surgical gloves.

Single-use items

Instruments and equipment intended for single use, e.g. blades, needles and pipettes, must not be reused. Re-sterilisation of these products is forbidden and failure to comply with this instruction invalidates the manufacturer's product liability. The practitioner then becomes liable if damage is caused to the patient as a result of using the recycled item. To prevent transmission of infection, the unused contents of

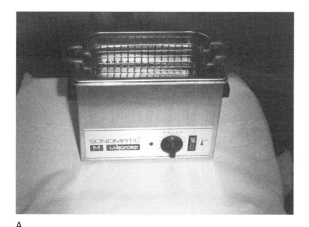

A

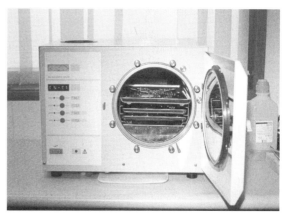

B

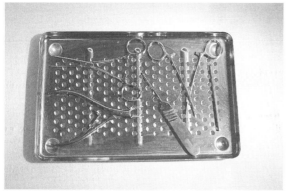

C

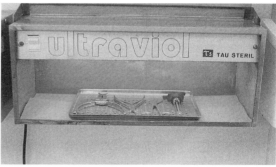

D

Figure 3.4 Procedure for the sterilisation of instruments. A: Ultrasonic cleaner to ensure instruments are clean prior to autoclaving. B: Autoclave. C: Instruments should be spaced out and closed instruments should be opened prior to autoclaving. D: Storage of autoclaved instruments in the ultraviolet cabinet.

single-dose containers and single-use packs should be discarded.

Disposal of clinical waste

Clinical waste generated in practice is segregated into two categories, i.e. sharps and non-sharps.

Immediate disposal of scalpel blades (sharps) is necessary on completion of treatment or if there is contamination with blood, pus or serum during treatment. Safe disposal of scalpel blades begins with careful removal of the blade from the handle. A specially designed instrument or other device gives some protection against injury (Fig. 3.5). Accidental injury caused by recapping hyperdermic needles has been shown to be a common occupational hazard for

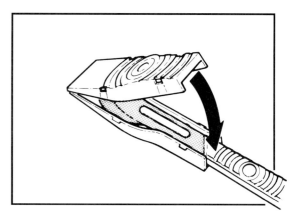

Figure 3.5 Example of a device for the safe removal of scalpel blades.

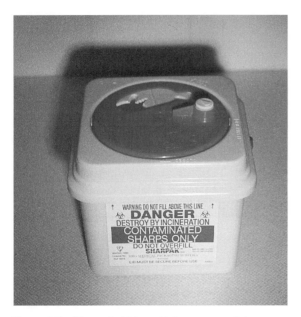

Figure 3.6 Disposal of 'sharps' into an appropriate container.

hospital staff (Neuberger et al 1984). The practice of re-sheathing needles is generally prohibited. Dental needles are an exception, and the use of a finger guard or other safety device is necessary when re-sheathing. Approved sharps containers are manufactured to DoH specification TSS/S/30.015. Blades, needles, syringes, glass and all other sharps are safely disposed of in these containers (Fig. 3.6).

Other clinical waste generated during patient treatment includes human tissue, soiled dressings, swabs and other contaminated material. Appropriately labelled, heavy duty yellow plastic bags are mandatory for the storage and disposal of this type of waste. Double bagging is necessary if waste is known to be infected.

Waste awaiting collection must be stored safely in a lockable container. Responsibility for the safe disposal of clinical waste (including that generated during domiciliary treatments) ultimately rests with the practitioner (Department of the Environment 1991).

Spillages

Spillages should be dealt with immediately and in an appropriate way. Blood or other body fluid spillages should be disinfected with chlorine-releasing agents, i.e. 1% hypochlorite solution (10–000 ppm available chlorine) or chlorine-releasing granules, before the area is cleared. Hypochlorites have antiviral proper-

ties and are active against HIV and HBV. Hypochlorites can damage fabrics and cause corrosion if used on metal surfaces. In these situations, 2% glutaraldehyde is a suitable alternative. Since medical history and examination cannot reliably identify all patients infected with HIV or other blood-borne pathogens, blood and body fluid precautions should be consistently used for all patients.

Health of the practitioner

As part of any infection control policy, it is incumbent on all practitioners to ensure that they do not act as sources of infection. It is usual practice for all health practitioners to undergo occupational health screening and to show that they are up to date in their immunisations.

The NHS Management Executive (HSG(93)40) (1993) requires that all practitioners who are at risk of acquiring hepatitis B are immunised, this includes those practitioners who are at risk of coming into contact with blood or body fluids. Practitioners who do not respond to the vaccine must have routine blood checks to see if they are HBeAg-positive carriers. Any practitioner who is an HBeAg-positive carrier should not perform exposure-prone procedures. Practitioners who are found to be HIV-positive are advised to refrain from undertaking exposure-prone procedures, e.g. invasive surgery.

Liability insurance

Most health care practitioners take out professional insurance in order to provide third party cover in cases of negligence. Technically there is a difference between those practitioners who are employed and those who are self-employed and in private practice. Employers are liable for the actions of their employees who are acting in the course of their employment. This is known as vicarious liability. The employer may also be liable, for example, by failing to set up proper working procedures or provide proper facilities for staff to do their jobs (employer negligence). In cases of vicarious liability and negligence, it is usually the employer who pays compensation to the injured party. However, if the employee is not doing what he is employed to do, he is not protected vicariously. In this instance, the employer is likely to take counter action and make a claim against the employee. It is because of this latter situation that many practitioners in employment elect to take up professional indemnity.

If a practitioner is injured whilst treating patients

in residential care or in their own homes, and she is an employee, then she would be able to claim industrial injury benefit. Injuries due to the state of the premises visited are governed by the Occupiers Liability Act (1957). Unfortunately, problems may occur when attempting to gain compensation under this act. For example, the owner of a private house may not have insurance cover. If a motor vehicle is used in the course of professional practice, as in the case of domiciliary visiting or travelling between clinics, the motor insurance policy must be extended to include business usage.

In the case of a practitioner who operates a private practice, the Occupiers Liability Act (1957) imposes a duty on the practitioner to ensure that premises are safe for visitors (this includes patients). The Occupiers Liability Act (1984) extended this liability to trespassers, i.e. those who unlawfully enter premises. Public liability insurance cover may be obtained as part of a comprehensive policy, extension of a domestic policy (if the practice is part of domestic premises) or by a professional body's third party policy for members.

Practitioner–patient relationship

There are many aspects of the practitioner–patient relationship, most of which are beyond the remit of this chapter. For the purposes of this chapter the issues highlighted in Box 3.4 will be discussed.

Confidentiality

The relationship between the practitioner and the patient is a special one. Special relationships are those in which particular duties and obligations are owed and in which certain duties and obligations go beyond the scope of ordinary social conversation (Fromer 1981). The practitioner may be privy to personal, social and medical information about the patient, and is therefore in a privileged position.

Most patients expect that the information they give will remain confidential and that they will certainly not read about it in the tabloid press the next day. Practitioners should note that, if they disclose con-

fidential information, then the burden of proof is upon the practitioner to prove it was morally justifiable (Beauchamp & Childress 1994).

It is quite legitimate for information about a patient to be shared between practitioners if it is deemed to be in the interests of the patient. In these circumstances, it is important to inform the patient of this prior to the information being passed on. The other instance where confidential information may be divulged is when a court of law requests the information or the patient has a notifiable disease.

Consent

When one discusses consent, a distinction needs to be made between 'informed' and 'educated' consent (Rumbold 1993). Informed consent refers to the information which a person receives, while educated consent relates to the ability of the patient to arrive at a reasoned decision based on that information. It is now generally accepted in health care practice that treatment should not be given without the patient's educated consent. This has not always been the case, and there are still those who consider that the practitioner has a right to undertake treatment which he thinks would be for the benefit of the patient. This is known as 'therapeutic privilege' and is still used when the patient is unable to give educated consent. An example of such a situation is when a patient is unconscious due to a road traffic accident.

Before a patient gives educated consent, full details of the treatment, its indications, risks and contraindications, as well as details of alternative treatments, must be communicated to the patient. The patient has to be able to understand the nature of the information in order to make an educated decision. If a patient is considered unable to give educated consent, it is good practice to discuss the issue with the next of kin. In cases where patients consider they have been treated without their consent, they can claim assault and take out a criminal or civil case against the practitioner. It is then up to a court of law to decide whether there is a case.

With regard to children, it is customary practice that parents or guardians are informed of the procedure and their consent obtained. However, there is no law which states this must be so. Defining who is a child is not easy. In general, anyone who meets the criteria outlined below, whatever their age, can be deemed to be able to give consent to treatment:

- possesses a set of values and goals
- is able to communicate and understand information

Box 3.4 Practitioner–patient relationship

- Confidentiality
- Consent
- Complaints
- Negligence

- has the ability to reason and deliberate about one's choice (The President's Commission 1982).

Consent is not binding; patients may withdraw their consent when they want. Patients' autonomy should be respected—all patients have the right to refuse treatment. Further information on medico-legal aspects of practice is covered in Chapter 4.

Complaints

From time to time, patient complaints may be made against an individual practitioner. Such complaints are usually about the manner in which the patient was treated or the actual treatment received.

At all times it is important that the practitioner acts in a manner to safeguard and promote the interests of the patient. If a patient wishes to make a formal complaint it should be put in writing. The Patient's Charter (Department of Health 1995) specifies that every citizen has the right to 'have any complaint about NHS services (whoever provides them) investigated and to get a quick, full written reply from the relevant chief executive or general manager'. All NHS Trusts should have formal, documented policies and procedures related to the handling of complaints. Staff training should be given on the implementation and operation of these policies and procedures. Similarly, sufficient information about making complaints should be publicised to patients, relatives, carers and the public. Complaints should be regarded in a positive light as they act as valuable feedback on the quality of services provided.

Patients who wish to make formal complaints about a practitioner in the private sector should be referred to the appropriate statutory and/or professional body.

Negligence

Negligence is considered to have occured when the acceptable standards of care towards others are not met. These acceptable standards of care emanate from the customs, policies and practices of that profession. The dividing line between acceptable and unacceptable standards of care is often difficult to draw. Hence, cases of negligence are usually decided by courts of law and involve an array of 'expert' witnesses. Usually practitioners are judged to have been negligent when they knowingly did not observe acceptable standards or when they did not take into consideration known (usually cited in the literature) side-effects or other problems associated with a treatment.

SUMMARY

Health care practitioners are in a privileged position and should not abuse that privilege. At all times the interests of the patient should be of paramount importance. All practitioners should practice within current legislation and observe codes of practice of appropriate bodies. Ovretveit (1992) believes that quality methods and philosophies, adapted to the special circumstances of the health services, will emerge as the most important response to health provision in the future. If practitioners adopt appropriate and effective protocols into their clinical practice, they should be in a position to offer their patients safe treatment and achieve high standards of care.

REFERENCES

Babb J R 1963 Cleaning of hospital floors with oiled mops. Journal of Hygiene, Cambridge 61: 393

Bate J G 1961 Bacteriological investigations of exhaust air from hospital vacuum cleaners. Lancet 1: 159

Baumann M A 1992 Protective gloves. International Dental Journal 42(3): 170–180

Beauchamp T, Childress J 1994 Principles of biomedical ethics, 4th edn. Oxford University Press, New York, p 70

Bendig J W A 1991 Surgical hand disinfection: comparison of 4% chlorhexidine detergent solution and 2% triclosan detergent solution. Journal of Hospital Infection 15: 143–148

British Medical Association 1989 A code of practice for sterilisation of instruments and control of cross infection. British Medical Association, London.

Combs R 1992 Clinic designed for two practices. Dental Economics 82(9): 51–54

Cremieux A, Reverdy M, Pons J, Savage C, Chevalier J, Fleurette J, Mosse M 1989 Standardised method for evaluation of hand disinfection by surgical scrub formulations. Applied and environmental microbiology 55(11): 2944–2948

Department of the Environment 1991 Waste management. The duty of care: A code of practice. HMSO, London

Department of Health 1990 A further evaluation of transportable steam sterilisers for unwrapped instruments and utensils. HEI No. 196. NHS Procurement Directorate, London

Department of Health 1991 The Patient's Charter. HMSO, London

Department of Health 1995 The Patient's Charter. HMSO, London

Douglas C W I 1989 The use of various handwashing agents to decontaminate gloved hands. British Dental Journal 167: 62–65

Fromer M J 1981 Ethical issues in health care. C V Mosby, St Louis

Health and Safety at Work Act 1974 HMSO, London

Health and Safety Executive 1988 Committee for Substances Hazardous to Health. HMSO, London

Health and Safety Executive 1989 Memorandum of guidance on the Electricity at Work Regulations. HMSO, London

Health and Safety Executive 1990a Writing a safety policy statement: advice to employers HSC 6. HMSO, London

Health and Safety Executive 1990b Guidance Note PM73, Safety of autoclaves. HMSO: London

Health and Safety Executive 1993a Code of practice for workplace health, safety and welfare. HMSO, London

Health and Safety Executive 1993b COSHH. A step by step guide. HMSO, London

Knittle M A, Eitzman D, Herman Baer M 1975 Role of hand contamination of personnel in the epidemiology of Gram-negative nosocomial infections. Journal of Paediatrics 86: 433

Larson E 1988 A causal link between handwashing and risk of infection? Examination of the evidence. Infection Control Hospital Epidemiology 9: 28–36

Maki D G 1989 The use of antiseptics for handwashing by medical personnel. Journal of Chemotherapy 1: 5–11

Maurer I M 1985 Hospital hygiene, 3rd edn. Edward Arnold, London

Mitchell R, Cumming C, MacLennan W, Ross P, Peuther J,

Baxter A 1983 The use of operating gloves in dental practice. British Dental Journal 154: 372–374

Neuberger J S, Harris J, Kundin W, Bischane A, Chin T 1984 Incidence of needlestick injuries in hospital personnel: implications for prevention. American Journal of Infection Control 12(3): 171–176

NHS Management Executive 1993 Health service guidelines HSG(93)40. Department of Health, London

Occupiers Liability Act 1957 HMSO, London

Occupiers Liability Act 1984 HMSO, London

Ovretveit J 1992 Health service quality. An introduction to quality methods for health services. Blackwell Scientific, London

Pressure Systems and Transportable Gas Container Regulations 1989 HMSO, London

Professions Supplementary to Medicine Act 1960 HMSO, London

Rumbold G 1993 Ethics in nursing practice. Balliere Tindall, London, p 94–99

Sharma S K 1991 Hand dermatitis from gloves. Occupation Environmental Medicine Reports 5(5): 45–48

The President's Commission for the study of ethical problems in medicine and biomedical and behavioral research 1982 Making health care decisions. US Government Printing Office, Washington DC

Ward K 1990 Dirt in hospitals. All that glitters. Nursing Times 86(24): 32–34

FURTHER READING

The Society of Chiropodists and Podiatrists 1992 Guidelines on Health and Safety at Work. The Society of Chiropodists and Podiatrists, London

4

Clinical emergencies

R. S. Moore

INTRODUCTION

All clinicians have a duty of care to their patients, and when attending a clinic for any kind of treatment, the patient has expectations of safety during treatment. This applies to those visiting a GP, to individuals seeking dental treatment and to others undergoing major surgery. It should therefore equally apply to people seeking the services of a podiatrist. In any branch of medicine, complications can arise as a result of treatment given. On occasion these complications can be life-threatening. Other crises can arise as a result of natural disease processes. It behoves the practitioner to be able to provide initial treatment for the patient until such time as further medical care becomes available. The main difficulty for those who are not routinely exposed to medical crises is one of recognition. Too often, individuals overreact to circumstances which are misconstrued as being life-threatening but which often require simple, yet effective, measures to remedy.

The aim of this chapter is to highlight the nature of medical emergencies, to describe the pathological processes involved, to describe the common modes of presentation and to provide a framework on which to base early treatment. It will also provide the reader with information which should make provisional diagnosis more reliable.

THE NATURE OF MEDICAL EMERGENCIES

The definition of acute medical emergency is not as straightforward as it might at first seem. Doctors tend to regard this status as being one where, without immediate treatment, there will be some irreversible pathological change. This may not necessarily imply loss of life. The difference comes in the time needed to take remedial action. Actions to save sight after a retinal detachment take on an urgency wherein treatment is likely to be necessary in a matter of some few hours, yet if a person suffers a cardiac arrest following myocardial infarction, treatment must be immediate.

The patient will also have his own idea of what constitutes an emergency. Pain is a common reason for attendance at accident and emergency departments, and urgent relief is sought and provided. In these situations, though, it is frequently the case that there is no clinical 'emergency', i.e. there is no immediate danger to life or limb. This difference in perception of the urgency of a situation often leads to difficulties in the busy accident and emergency department. Patients attend with a variety of painful conditions, and because of their pain, all are seeking rapid relief and treatment. However, some kind of sorting has to take place to identify the cases which require rapid intervention.

Triage is a concept that has been known since the period of the Napoleonic Wars. The majority of modern accident units now operate a system of early rapid assessment of all patients soon after arrival at the department (see Fig. 4.1). This is usually carried out by an experienced and adequately trained nurse. This nurse can identify patients who need rapid treatment and/or pain relief. The patient is then categorised into one of four groups, as described in Box 4.1.

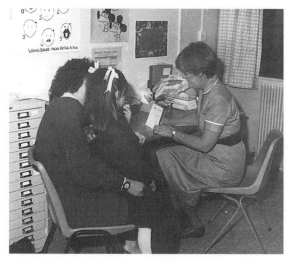

Figure 4.1 Early, rapid assessment is required to determine the urgency of treatment priority on arrival at the Accident and Emergency Department.

Box 4.1 Categorisation of patients upon arrival at accident and emergency department

- *A, immediate*—death likely without rapid intervention, e.g. cardiac arrest
- *B, urgent*—severe illness or injury requiring treatment as soon as possible, e.g. major fractures, suspected appendicitis
- *C, semi-urgent*—not a clinical emergency but requires hospital treatment; can wait, e.g. lacerations
- *D, minor*—trivial complaints or wholly inappropriate for hospital care; may have to wait some hours for attention

---

The outcome of treatment within the hospital environment for emergencies that arise within the community is frequently determined by the quality of pre-hospital care that is provided, and this is especially true in the case of resuscitation after witnessed cardiac arrest. Studies in the USA (Eisenberg et al 1979) have clearly indicated better outcomes for the management of cardiac arrest in areas where community programmes for the training of citizens in 'basic cardiac life support' have been implemented. Similar schemes in the UK have only been partially successful (Vincent et al 1984). The moral obligation on podiatrists and other health workers is clear. All should to be capable of procedures that can hold a critical situation until such time as a higher level of expertise becomes available. However, this higher level of expertise is no longer confined to medical personnel. Ambulance crews who respond to initial calls are now commonly trained in advanced skills such as endotracheal intubation, defibrillation and intravenous cannulation. These 'paramedics' have undergone systematic training in the theoretical and practical aspects of emergency management at the scene of an incident.

In summary, the management of any medical emergency requires a team of health care workers, as described in Box 4.2 (see also Fig. 4.2).

Box 4.2 Team of health care workers for the management of a medical emergency

- First responder—passer-by, friend, podiatrist, nurse, GP, etc.
- Primary care—paramedic, GP, hospital flying squad
- Secondary care—district general hospital/accident and emergency department
- Tertiary care—regional centre, e.g. burns unit

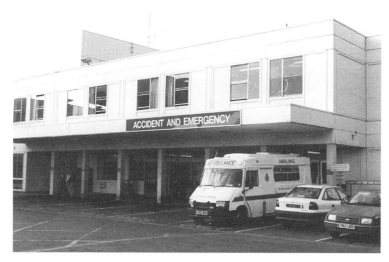

Figure 4.2 A modern accident and emergency department serving a district general hospital.

Medicolegal aspects of practice

In everyday practice, the most important factor to be considered after decisions have been taken regarding treatment is the question of consent. Without the consent of the patient, any act of surgical intervention can be construed as an assault upon the person, whether or not it might be in that person's best interests.

Consent can be implicit or explicit (McClay 1990, Knight 1992). Implicit consent is normally inferred from the cooperation of the patient by his attendance at the clinic or by his compliance during treatment. Explicit consent is necessary for more intimate examinations and surgical procedures. Explicit consent can be obtained verbally but requires a third party to act as a witness. Written consent provides a more secure form of record. In 1985, the concept of 'informed' consent was introduced, which established the need for practitioners to balance the major risks against the potential benefits entailed in a procedure, while still allowing them some discretion with regard to individual cases.

The Family Law Reform Act (1985) laid down that individuals of sound mind were able to give consent from the age of 16, although the advice from the courts concerning the rights of older children has been a little unclear since then. The Gillick case highlighted the need for parental involvement wherever possible in the management of young people. Parental consent can be overruled in special circumstances, where it is thought to be in the child's best interests. This may involve the child being effectively removed to a 'fit person' to allow usually life-saving treatment.

The ability to give consent implies a level of rationality. Unconsciousness prevents this, and in these circumstances close relatives can be approached or, if the situation is life-threatening, treatment may be implemented on the assumption that the practitioner is acting in the best interests of the patient. Low intelligence does not affect the ability to give consent provided that the person can appreciate the nature of the treatment and its indication. Patients detained under the Mental Health Act (1983) forfeit their right of consent to the Medical Officer providing their overall care, but relatives should still be involved. Voluntary patients in a mental institution can give consent provided they have the capacity to comprehend the state of their own health.

CARDIOVASCULAR EMERGENCIES

All tissues of the body rely on an adequate cardiac output to maintain tissue oxygenation and to remove the products of local metabolism. If tissue perfusion is interrupted then injury will follow. The period required for cell death is variable but is most acute in the brain where hypoxic damage begins after only 4 minutes. Other sensitive areas include the kidney and the heart itself. The normal cardiac output in a resting adult is approximately 5 L/min. The ability of the heart to achieve this depends on three physiological variables:

• Preload—this describes the state of filling of the venous circulation and the filling pressure of the right ventricle. This can be assessed by taking measurements of the jugular venous pressure (JVP).

• Afterload—this refers to the resistance against which the heart has to pump. This reflects the tone of the arteriolar and capillary circulation, which in turn responds to changes in the sympathetic nervous system. Systemic blood pressure is an indirect measure of this.

• Contractility of the myocardium—this affects the force and efficiency of myocardial contraction and can be measured as the stroke volume.

Conditions such as myocardial infarction can lead to rapid alterations of these parameters and lead to reduction or loss of cardiac output with serious consequences.

Cardiac arrest

Cardiac arrest will, if not recognised and treated immediately, lead rapidly to death. It is characterised by cardiac standstill detectable by the absence of the central pulses, rapid loss of consciousness and, within a few minutes, respiratory arrest. It is frequently associated with loss of sphincter control, manifest by gastric regurgitation and incontinence. It may arise

as a result of a primary cardiac disturbance, such as acute myocardial infarction, or secondary to some other event such as asphyxia or massive haemorrhage. There are three recognised modes of cardiac arrest:

• *Ventricular fibrillation*. The fibres of the myocardium contract chaotically so that the pumping action of the heart is lost but there remains electrical activity detectable on an electrocardiograph (ECG). This electrical disturbance is potentially reversible, but only if treatment is delivered within a few minutes of onset.

• *Asystole*. There is no activity in the heart at all and no electrical activity is detected. This is rarely reversible and often follows on from prolonged ventricular fibrillation.

• *Electromechanical dissociation*. There is no activity within the heart but there is still electrical activity seen on an ECG. This condition is usually terminal, although, as it can follow certain physical derangements such as cardiac tamponade, it is important for the clinician to look for an underlying cause.

The only effective treatment for cardiac arrest is defibrillation (Fig. 4.3). This technique is at present restricted to medical personnel, trained paramedics and some members of the nursing profession working in coronary care and intensive care units (ICUs). Guidelines for advanced cardiac life support were

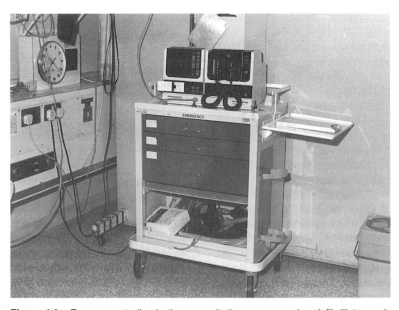

Figure 4.3 Emergency trolley in the resuscitation room carrying defibrillator and emergency drugs.

recently issued by the European Resuscitation Council Advanced Life Support Working Party (1992). The importance of early treatment cannot be overemphasised. If defibrillation is unavoidably delayed, the priority is to maintain some kind of rudimentary circulation to protect the brain. This is achieved by the basic life support measures of maintaining a clear airway, ventilating the lungs and carrying out external cardiac compression. All first aid courses teach these skills. Tuition for the full sequence of management is now being brought together in advanced life support (ALS) courses around the UK.

Acute myocardial infarction

Ischaemic heart disease causes the deaths of approximately 160 000 people each year in England and Wales, and the most common cause of sudden death is myocardial infarction. There is a 40–50% mortality within the first 2 hours of symptoms (Fulton et al 1969). The primary disturbance is of an interruption to the normal perfusion of the myocardium, leading to muscle necrosis and dysfunction. This change in perfusion can arise from a sudden vascular occlusion due to thrombus formation in a coronary vessel or it can sometimes be due to spasm in the wall of an arteriole. The acute event may lead to ventricular fibrillation and other cardiac rhythm abnormalities. In other circumstances, the pump action of the heart may be impaired, leading to heart failure. The area around the dead infarcted tissue is liable to be ischaemic and will lead to chest pain. This pain is characteristically described as being retrosternal, tight and constricting, and frequently radiates into the left arm and up into the neck. It can sometimes be difficult for clinicians to distinguish this pain from that of oesophageal reflux or heartburn. Treatment now depends upon early recognition and diagnosis. This allows the administration of drugs which can re-establish vascular patency by breaking down thrombus (thrombolysis). The first line management comprises calling an ambulance to the scene, administering oxygen, sitting the patient up and giving a single tablet of aspirin if it is known that there is no contraindication. Aspirin in small doses effectively reduces platelet adhesiveness and aids thrombolytic therapy. Adequate pain relief is usually only obtained by the use of morphine or one of its derivatives, although glyceryl trinitrate (GTN) may be of help.

Massive pulmonary embolism

Acute massive pulmonary embolism is a condition characterised by an acute obstruction of the pulmonary circulation caused by a large blood clot impacting in the pulmonary artery. This clot usually develops in the peripheral venous circulation, most commonly in the pelvic bed or the lower limb. The clot then fragments and travels to the heart via the inferior vena cava. The primary event of deep venous thrombosis is associated with prolonged periods of bed rest or immobility such as that encountered after major surgery. It is also linked to cigarette smoking and the use of oral contraceptives.

The mode of presentation is often identical to that of primary cardiac arrest, with severe central chest pain, sudden collapse, lack of pulse and loss of consciousness. However, there may be an antecedent history of chest pains due to earlier minor emboli reaching the lungs. The patient may have a history of recent surgery. Electromechanical dissociation is more commonly encountered on ECG monitoring as the heart vainly attempts to beat against the obstruction. Treatment follows the guidelines for any cardiac arrest, but the results of treatment are poor. Success is more likely in centres equipped with access to thoracotomy and emergency cardiopulmonary bypass.

Massive haemorrhage

Haemorrhage refers to the extravasation of whole blood from the circulation. It can be described as internal (occult) or external (overt). External or overt haemorrhage refers to bleeding that is apparent, such as that due to a laceration or nosebleed. Internal or occult bleeding can arise from injury to abdominal viscera or duodenal ulceration. When haemorrhage is severe, the recognition of the fact is crucial to the early and effective treatment of hypovolaemic shock.

Shock has been defined as 'inadequate perfusion of the tissues', but in all events leads to local hypoxia and cell death. Hypovolaemia is one cause for this state and its treatment is designed to minimise and reduce the duration of tissue hypoxia. The longer the duration of the shock state the more likely the chance that life-threatening complications will ensue. These complications range from early death to adult respiratory distress syndrome and acute renal failure.

The response of the body to haemorrhage is governed by activity within the sympathetic autonomic nervous system. These responses are at their most efficient in youth and become steadily attenuated with increasing age—hence the greater tolerance to haemorrhage in youth. The early response to haemorrhage comprises decreased activity in the baroceptors of the carotid sinus and aortic arch, which then causes a reflex increase in peripheral sympathetic tone. This clinically manifests as vasoconstriction in the skin and kidney with reduced urine output. This increase in peripheral vascular resistance helps to maintain blood pressure and perfusion to important areas. A further increase in sympathetic activity will raise the heart rate. These compensatory changes will usually be adequate for losses of up to 1 litre. When the loss exceeds this amount, or it has been incurred too quickly for the system to cope, then blood pressure will fall. If the fall is profound or prolonged, the problems mentioned earlier will appear. In particular, if haemorrhage is ongoing, then cerebral perfusion fails, leading to drowsiness, coma and death. This is likely with losses of 3 litres if not treated.

It is necessary to recognise life-threatening haemorrhage quickly and to replace fluid losses promptly. This will require early venous cannulation and transfusion. It is perhaps more important, in the first place, to attempt to arrest the bleeding. When the bleeding is due to an open wound, haemostasis can usually be obtained by simple direct pressure over the wound via a simple dressing. This is aided by elevation of the injured part. This is particularly applicable to patients suffering heavy bleeding from rupture of a varicose vein at the ankle. In general, tourniquets are rarely necessary but, if applied, should be released every 20 minutes to prevent tissue ischaemia. When available, oxygen should be given to all patients sustaining a major haemorrhage. The management of hypovolaemia related to haemorrhage has been recognised in recent years as being a leading cause of preventable death after trauma. The implementation of training in advanced trauma life support for clinicians has gone some way to remedying this. Members of the professions allied to medicine are also undergoing training.

RESPIRATORY EMERGENCIES

While the cardiovascular system provides a means of transport of metabolites around the body, the respiratory system is the means for exchange of oxygen and carbon dioxide with the atmosphere. There are a number of anatomical and physiological features which optimise this function. As with the cardiovascular system, if any of these features are suddenly impaired, pathological changes rapidly follow.

Physiology

The most obvious sign of life is breathing. This semiautomatic activity is necessary for ventilation of the lungs and renewal of the quality of alveolar air. It depends on a clear airway from the nasopharynx to the alveolus. It further depends upon an intact neuromuscular system connecting the respiratory centres of the brain stem to the intercostal muscles and diaphragm via the spinal cord. Finally, there is the need for structural integrity of the ribcage and pleural membranes, thereby allowing the mechanical effects of muscular contraction to be transferred to the lungs, enabling inflation and deflation.

Ventilation brings oxygen-rich air to the alveolus, but at this point the determining feature becomes the permeability of the capillary membranes to oxygen and carbon dioxide. This may be impaired by increased secretions, oedema or pathological processes causing scarring and thickening of the alveolar walls.

Pneumothorax

Lying between the lungs and the ribcage is the pleural space enclosed by the pleural membranes. This is usually only a potential space, and the two layers of membrane are separated by a thin film of fluid. The pressure within this space is normally slightly negative with respect to atmospheric pressure, so that when the rib cage expands it indirectly exerts a bellows effect on the underlying lung, causing it to be inflated. If air should leak into this space by reason of breakdown of a congenital bulla on the surface of the lung or by means of a puncture caused by direct trauma from a fractured rib, for example, then the underlying lung will fall back from the ribcage and will not ventilate adequately. This will lead to poor oxygenation of the blood and systemic hypoxia. This condition is known as pneumothorax (Fig. 4.4). If it should happen that a one-way valve effect arises, whereby air can enter the pleural cavity but is trapped, then the intrapleural pressure will rise and quickly impair ventilation of the opposite lung and will later affect the venous return to the heart. This is a life-threatening emergency known as tension pneumothorax and has the capacity to cause death within minutes. It requires the rapid intervention of a clinician to allow escape of air to the exterior and reduce the intrathoracic pressure. This is achieved by placing a sterile plastic tube or chest drain through an intercostal space into the pleural cavity. This is then attached to a one-way valve system to prevent the return of air into the chest.

Spontaneous pneumothorax commonly affects young healthy males but can arise in the elderly population as a complication of chronic obstructive airways disease. Traumatic pneumothorax can complicate almost

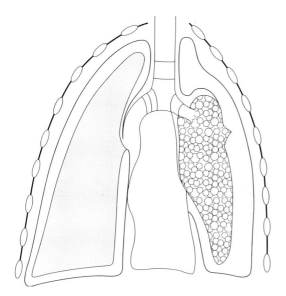

Figure 4.4 Simple pneumothorax with air in the left pleural space.

any insult to the thorax, be it blunt or penetrating in origin. The common symptoms include unilateral chest pain which is worse on inspiration, shortness of breath and a history of a similar event. The patient, particularly if young, may be in little distress. In contrast, the patient with a tension pneumothorax will be extremely distressed by severe breathlessness, cyanosed with hypoxia and will rapidly lose consciousness without treatment.

Asthma

Asthma is common, with a prevalence of between 1 and 40%, depending on geography. It is a condition characterised by a variable and intermittent degree of lower airway obstruction caused by narrowing of bronchioles. This narrowing can arise from smooth muscle hyperreactivity or from oedema of the mucosa. An acute attack is commonly due to a combination of the two. The characteristic symptom is breathlessness associated with an expiratory wheeze. Attacks may be spontaneous but frequently appear to be associated with upper respiratory tract viral infections. Other common associations are with exposure to allergens, such as grass pollen or animal hair, and to exercise. Asthma can vary in severity from a slight wheeze with nocturnal cough to a life-threatening situation where death may rapidly result without the highest standards of intensive care. A significant number of people still die each year from this ailment (1.5–3.0/10 000 per annum in the Western world; Burney 1992) and guidelines have recently been revised for the medical management of this disease.

The control of asthma is tailored according to the severity of symptoms in the individual. At one extreme,

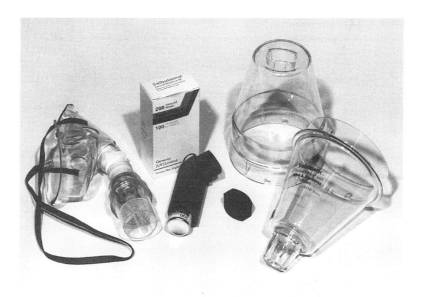

Figure 4.5 Therapeutic tools for asthma (left to right): mask with nebuliser, aerosol inhaler, and spacer to improve the efficiency of the inhaler.

the patient may carry an aerosol inhaler containing a bronchodilator such as salbutamol or terbutaline (see Fig. 4.5). This would be used only when symptomatic. If symptoms were more frequent, sodium chromoglycate might be added as a prophylactic agent. In the presence of recurrent wheeze, an inhaled steroid might also be indicated. When a severe attack intervenes, these drugs may be given in the nebulised state, providing a higher dose and a more reliable means of delivery. If this mode of treatment is implemented in the community and fails to lead to a rapid improvement, then the patient must be referred to hospital without delay. Asthma is unpredictable and dangerous, and whenever there is doubt about the severity of symptoms, medical advice must be sought.

The obstructed airway

The airway is the area extending from the lips or nostrils to the alveoli. Obstruction of the airway will rapidly lead to hypoxia. In contrast to asthma, the wheeze that develops is generally inspiratory and is referred to as stridor. When stridor is acute, the patient will be distressed and there will be signs of rib recession and activity in the accessory muscles of respiration in the neck. Any object, if inhaled, can cause this. Commoner items include nuts, boiled sweets and, in children, marbles and similar trinkets. These may affect the normal healthy individual with normal reflexes, but in the individual whose consciousness is clouded by virtue of disease or drugs, the risk is higher because of attenuation of the normal protective cough reflexes. A common cause of respiratory obstruction in these circumstances is occlusion

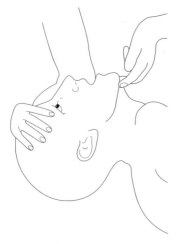

Figure 4.6 Maintaining the airway.

of the pharynx by the tongue dropping backwards through loss of muscular tone. Substances or items which may also be troublesome in these circumstances include broken or false teeth, food and vomit. In all circumstances, the need for early recognition and relief must be emphasised. Simple remedies include safe positioning of the obtunded patient (Fig. 4.6), lifting the jaw to clear the tongue from the back of the pharynx and ensuring that there are no objects obstructing the back of the mouth. Surgical manoeuvres such as cricothyroidotomy are sometimes indicated in extreme circumstances, in order to maintain an airway in life-threatening situations.

NEUROLOGICAL EMERGENCIES

Epilepsy

Epilepsy is a term used to describe a wide spectrum of convulsive disorders that are either idiopathic, or secondary to brain abnormalities like tumour or scarring following injury. Two common forms are Grand Mal and Petit Mal fits. The former is the classic tonic-clonic convulsion, in which the individual suddenly loses consciousness, sometimes after experiencing an 'aura', and collapses. There then follows a period of shaking of all the limbs before the patient relaxes into a period of stupor or unconsciousness (the post-ictal period) for a variable period. This kind of fit is a feature of local anaesthetic toxicity. If the period of convulsing is brief, then all that is required is to put the person into the recovery position (Fig. 4.7) and to remove sources of danger. If the fit has not stopped within 3–4 minutes, urgent treatment is required, and an ambulance must be called.

The other common kind of fit is called Petit Mal and is more common in the young. It takes the form of brief 'absences' where the child suddenly appears to be daydreaming and then, just as suddenly, snaps out of it. It is rarely dangerous, and by virtue of its brief nature, often goes undiagnosed for some time.

Epilepsy can be well controlled by drugs such as Phenytoin and Carbamazepine, but prolonged fits require the parenteral administration of Diazepam. The most rapid route of administration is intravenously, but it can also be given rectally to good effect in children. 5–10 mg iv is usually adequate for adults.

Subarachnoid haemorrhage

The meninges are a membranous covering of the brain and spinal cord which provide support and

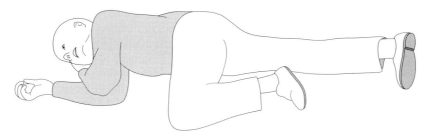

Figure 4.7 The recovery position.

protection in addition to that afforded by the skull and spinal column. They are divided into three layers: the dura mater, which is a thick membrane lying immediately within the skull; the arachnoid mater, a thin membrane lining the dura; and the pia mater, which is very thin and fragile and adheres to the brain surface and spinal cord. Blood vessels supplying the underlying brain traverse the subarachnoid space on their way to the cortex. Occasionally, one of these vessels can rupture, causing a subarachnoid haemorrhage. This may be totally spontaneous, but frequently the site of rupture is a small area of dilatation of an arterial vessel known as a berry aneurysm. This is a developmental abnormality which may be asymptomatic until rupture. Another cause is the presence of an arteriovenous malformation.

The common mode of presentation is a sudden onset of severe headache associated with disturbed consciousness or confusion, nausea and vomiting, and visual disturbance. There is frequently a history of minor headaches in the weeks preceding a major incident, indicating earlier small bleeds. Unfortunately, these earlier episodes often go unheeded. Subarachnoid haemorrhage has a significant mortality and is no respector of age. Its sometimes devastating effects on the brain frequently lead to rapid brain death in an otherwise healthy individual. Families of the victims are frequently approached with regard to organ donation. Conversely, if the disorder is recognised early, before severe brain injury has resulted, then neurosurgical intervention to clip off the offending vessel can be life-saving.

Cerebrovascular accident

The term cerebrovascular accident (CVA) is a collective expression to describe injuries to the brain arising from an interruption to the normal blood supply of the brain substance. The term therefore includes subarachnoid haemorrhage, but it is normally used to describe incidents affecting the older generations. The popular term in the UK is 'stroke'. In older age groups, the development of cerebral ischaemia is a gradual process mediated by disease and degenerative changes such as atherosclerosis and atheroma. The damaged vessels are then more prone to occlusion by thrombus or to rupture. The incidence of cerebrovascular disease is 2/1000 per annum (Wade 1988) and is related to hypertension and cigarette smoking. Typically, in the elderly, stroke presents as an acute onset of weakness affecting one side of the body, with clouding of the conscious level and a variable degree of speech disturbance. The extent of brain injury determines the outcome and long-term morbidity. Early treatment consists of the administration of oxygen and care of the ABCs of resuscitation. In the longer term, the departments of physiotherapy, occupational therapy and speech therapy assume a high profile in rehabilitation.

On occasion, the classical symptoms of CVA may develop, only to pass off again within a few hours. This syndrome is known as a transient ischaemic attack (TIA). These attacks may be frequent and may be the precursor to a complete CVA. At other times, TIA is an infrequent event which does not progress any further. Initial treatment comprises simple observation. Later, intervention may be considered with antiplatelet agents, such as aspirin or dipyridamole, to lessen the risk of thrombotic episodes.

METABOLIC CRISES

Hypoglycaemia

Hypoglycaemia refers to the condition wherein the level of glucose in the bloodstream falls below normal levels. The normal blood glucose level is 2–8 mol/L. The commonest cause for this abnormality is uncontrolled diabetes mellitus. The patient receiving regular insulin supplements may have injected too much insulin or may have missed a meal after a normal insulin dose. In either case, there is a relative excess of insulin, causing a fall in blood glucose. Other causes include the delayed hypoglycaemia associated with excessive alcohol consumption (this is particularly common in the young) and the rare hormone-secreting tumour, insulinoma.

The early effects of hypoglycaemia are due to dysfunction of the brain. Glucose is the only energy supplying substrate for brain tissue and any lack rapidly leads to dysfunction. Signs and symptoms are similar to those of acute anxiety with apprehension and agitation, tremor and clamminess. The patient will appear pale and become confused, and sometimes aggressive, before slipping into coma, if treatment is not quickly given. Treating the early signs is reliant upon the administration of a carbohydrate load or simple glucose. If consciousness is lost, recovery usually follows the intravenous administration of 50% dextrose solution. Another remedy sometimes carried by ambulance paramedics is Glucagon. This is a naturally occurring hormone which, following intramuscular injection, leads to rapid mobilisation of glucose from the liver by stimulating breakdown of glycogen stores.

The need for rapid reversal of hypoglycaemia cannot be stressed too highly, as prolongation will lead to permanent brain injury.

Acute anaphylaxis

This is a life-threatening emergency with a speed of onset of dramatic proportions. It follows the exposure of a susceptible individual to a substance or allergen which triggers a dramatic release of histamine from mast cells throughout the body. There is usually a history of previous exposure and similar, though often less severe, reactions. Common allergens include drugs such as penicillin, some foodstuffs, e.g. nuts and strawberries, some vaccines, e.g. tetanus toxoid, and bee stings. Even a small exposure to allergen can lead to a severe reaction. The widespread release of histamine within the body leads to a catastrophic increase in capillary permeability and vascular dilatation. This is manifest as a dramatic fall in systemic blood pressure. Other more local effects of histamine release include widespread urticaria (hives), flushing of the skin and bronchospasm, causing breathlessness and wheeze.

Without prompt treatment the patient may quickly die. The first line treatment consists of the intramuscular injection of adrenaline (0.5 mg). It may also be given intravenously, but lower doses and more caution are required because of the high risk of cardiac arrythmias. Adrenaline should be followed by appropriate intravenous fluid replacement and the administration of antihistamines (chlorpheniramine) and steroids (hydrocortisone and/or prednisolone). Patients with life-threatening reactions frequently require management on an intensive care unit.

A better method of management, however, is prevention. This can usually be secured by taking a full history before the administration of any new agents, particularly antibiotics. Appropriate alternatives can then be used in treatment. Some patients with a known susceptibility carry supplies of adrenaline about their person for self-administration in the event of an emergency.

SOME SUBACUTE EMERGENCIES
Congestive heart failure

This is a common condition in the elderly and is usually secondary to ischaemic heart disease. It is characterised by a chronic failure of the right side of the heart, leading to fluid retention in the venous side of the circulation and in the pulmonary vasculature. This is manifest as breathlessness on exertion— or at rest in more serious cases—and oedema of the dependent areas such as the ankles and sacrum. It may also be associated with angina. This complaint is usually treated with a combination of diuretics, such as frusemide or amiloride, and digoxin (particularly if the heart rhythm is abnormal with atrial fibrillation). New drugs are becoming available to further improve the efficiency of the heart.

Unstable angina

Patients with angina frequently enter into a steady state whereby their angina is either infrequent or well controlled by medication. In these circumstances, episodes of chest pain follow patterns that depend upon factors such as exertion or stress, or may simply be characterised by a certain frequency of attacks each week. This pattern implies that the quality of perfusion of the myocardium is also steady. If the pattern of pain changes so that episodes of pain are becoming more frequent or severe, the implication is that the coronary circulation is deteriorating. This situation may be the precursor to myocardial infarction. It is for this reason that a history of suddenly worsening angina is taken so seriously by medical staff and often leads to hospital admission for rest, assessment and a review of medication.

WHAT TO DO IF A PATIENT IN YOUR SURGERY SUDDENLY LOSES CONSCIOUSNESS (Fig. 4.8)

1. Ensure a safe environment for you both
2. Lie the patient supine
3. Check and, if necessary, clear the airway. Remember dentures!
4. Check for breathing
5. Feel for a pulse in the neck
6. If your patient is breathing freely and has a good pulse then there is no immediate danger; get help now
7. If either is absent then start 'basic life support' and seek help or call an ambulance urgently
8. In the midst of all this, keep a clear head and try to recall the events leading up to the collapse. This information will be invaluable to paramedics and clinicians who may later be involved in the treatment of your patient.

SUMMARY

From time to time, all health workers will be exposed to a medical emergency of some kind. Not all incidents that may be perceived as emergencies by non-medical staff will be seen as such by clinicians. In a podiatrist's clinic, where equipment and experience may not be suited to these events, the sense of urgency is evident nonetheless.

The key to sensible and safe management of all emergencies is to have a framework on which to base action. To preserve life, that framework is simply A, B, C—maintain **A**irway, **B**reathing and **C**irculation. The rest can wait.

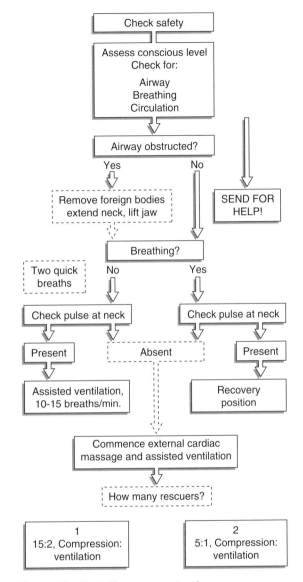

Figure 4.8 Basic life support protocols.

REFERENCES

Burney P G J 1992 Epidemiology. In: Clark T J H, Godfrey S, Lee T H (eds) Asthma, 3rd edn. Chapman and Hall, London

Eisenberg M S, Bergner L, Hallstrom A 1979 Cardiac resuscitation in the community. Journal of the American Medical Association 241: 1905–1907

Fulton M, Julian D G, Oliver M F 1969 Sudden death and myocardial infarction. Circulation 39(iv): 182–191

Gillick (1984) QB 581, (1984) 1 AV ER 365; on appeal (1986) AC 112, (1985) 1 AV ER 533, CA: revised (1986) AC 112, (1985) 3 AV ER 402, 1–12

Knight B (ed) 1992 Legal aspects of medical practice. Churchill Livingstone, Edinburgh, p 39–47

McClay W D S (ed) 1990 Clinical forensic medicine. Pinter, London, p 2–5

Vincent R, Martin B, Williams G, Quinn E, Robertson G, Chamberlain D A 1984 A community training scheme in cardiopulmonary resuscitation. British Medical Journal 288: 617–620

Wade D 1988 Stroke: practical guides for general practice 4. Oxford University Press, Oxford

FURTHER READING

Edwards C R W, Bouchier I A D (eds) 1991 Davidson's principles and practice of medicine, 16th edn. Churchill Livingstone, Edinburgh

Evans T R (ed) 1990 ABC of resuscitation, 2nd edn. British Medical Journal, London

Yates D W, Redmond A D 1985 Lecture notes on accident and emergency medicine. Blackwell Scientific Publications, Oxford

5

Foot health education and promotion

L. Stuart

A wise man ought to realise that health is his most important asset, and learn to treat his illnesses by his own judgement (Hippocrates).

INTRODUCTION

The emergence of the concepts of health education and promotion have brought about radical changes within health care provision. *The health of the nation* (Department of Health 1992) heralds a welcome commitment by the British government to the prevention of disease and the promotion of health. An important feature of this initiative is the achievement of good foot health. This requires the active support from all practitioners involved in the delivery of foot health services. However, there exists a need for more foot care provision and an increased input into foot health education. It is true to say that we ultimately receive up to three pairs of teeth, but only one pair of feet (Fig. 5.1)!

This chapter comprises four sections:

- the concepts and boundaries of health education and promotion
- issues related to foot health education and promotion
- approaches and skills required by foot health educators and promoters
- planning and implementation of foot health educational activities.

WHAT IS HEALTH?

The word 'health' represents not a fact, but a concept. Any definition of health is largely based upon opinion; health means different things to different people. Attempts to define health are numerous and diverse, and are met with extreme controversy and debate. The World Health Organization (WHO) defines it as 'a state of complete physical, mental and social well

You can have 3 pairs of teeth

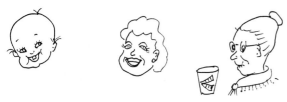

...... but only 1 pair of feet!

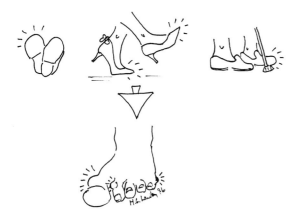

Figure 5.1 You can have three pairs of teeth but only one pair of feet (reproduced with permission from Michael G. Lawley).

being and not merely the absence of disease or infirmity' (WHO 1946). This much quoted definition has been widely criticised, not least for attempting to define health in objective and unrealistic terms. An alternative definition states that 'health is the foundation for achievement' (Seedhouse 1986).

Practitioners must explore and define their own and their patients' perceptions of health. Various studies have shown that the effectiveness of communication between patients and practitioners is limited when both parties have different perceptions of the meaning of health (Helman 1983). Conflict often arises where the patient does not recognise the need for the information given by the practitioner (Coles 1991). This is particularly the case when the individual is symptom-free. For example, a diabetic patient who is suffering from a painless sensory neuropathy may, from a lay perspective, consider the lack of pain to be a beneficial feature of the condition. Such a belief may be held despite the practitioner's attempts to inform the patient of the potential dangers associated with the condition (Binyet et al 1994).

Ultimately, it is an individual's experiences, knowledge, values and expectations which shape their ideas of health and illness. For example, the mother of a toddler may be influenced more by economic factors, peer group pressure, the media or cultural values than the need to purchase well-fitting shoes. Health practitioners should work towards removing the obstacles which prevent the achievement of health. In pursuing such an approach, the individual, as well as the societal influences which are inextricably linked to an individual's health, should be considered. An individual's ability to make choices about personal health is far more complex than it may initially appear. Those attempting to influence health behaviour should be aware that factors surrounding health-related decisions lie outside an individual's control.

A more extensive debate of the concept of health, while important in the context of health promotion, is beyond the scope of this chapter. It should be noted that good health rarely occurs as a result of chance or luck. It is vital that health care practitioners work towards improved standards of foot health. They should be familiar with the complex range of factors which influence an individual's health. The then Secretary of State for Health, in her introduction to *The health of the nation*, stated that '...there is a commitment in this White Paper to the pursuit of health in its widest sense, both in this Government and beyond' (Department of Health 1992). Uncertainty regarding the meaning of the term health complicates this task.

HEALTH EDUCATION OR HEALTH PROMOTION?

The terms 'health education' and 'health promotion' have been extensively debated. Some see no distinction between them, whilst others suggest that both terms are inextricably linked but that they represent different philosophies. The World Health Organization adopts the latter perspective; it considers that health promotion programmes promote health, and that health education is an integral part of that activity (WHO 1986a). Ewles & Simnett (1995) use the term 'health promotion' as an umbrella term which includes health education (Fig. 5.2).

Traditionally health education has been associated with any change in behaviour, conducive to health, which takes place as a result of learning. The majority of definitions of health education share the following characteristics:

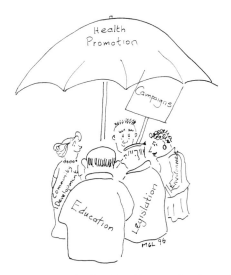

Figure 5.2 The umbrella of health promotion (reproduced with permission from Michael G. Lawley).

1. health education focuses primarily on the individual and lifestyle
2. health education programmes are concerned with the transmission of health-related information
3. any change in behaviour occurring as a result of health education is voluntary.

Since the mid-1980s there has been much debate surrounding the boundaries of health education (Seymour 1984, Tannahill 1985). Traditional health education, which aims to influence individual lifestyle behaviour, has been criticised for 'blaming the victim', or holding the individual solely responsible for their own health. This approach does not take into account factors outside of an individual's control, which may prevent the making of healthy choices. For example, some individuals are relatively powerless, owing to a range of factors, to achieve improved standards of foot health. Furthermore, health education strategies focused purely on the individual often fail to consider the wider issues which influence health. For example, adding VAT to children's footwear may place parents who are already under financial strain in a position where they are unable to afford 'well-fitting' footwear for their children.

Whereas health education is seen as an activity targeted at individuals, health promotion focuses on the population as a whole. It is, therefore, not restricted to individuals or specified groups, and rather than 'conserving health' it is aimed at 'enhancing' it (Nutbeam 1986). This broader approach includes

efforts to change legal, socio-economic and environmental factors which affect health.

The key principles of health promotion have been outlined by the World Health Organization (1986a) as follows:

1. health promotion involves the population as a whole
2. health promotion is directed towards action on the determinants or causes of health
3. health promotion combines diverse but complementary methods or approaches
4. health promotion aims particularly at effective and public participation
5. health professionals have an important role in nurturing and enabling health promotion.

The principles of health promotion recognise the need for a change in approach to the prevention of disease and the promotion of health. Implicit within these principles is the message that health is not an area exclusively managed by health care practitioners. To achieve 'health', more value should be placed on the development of public participation and multidisciplinary collaboration, both within and outside the health care sector. Improvements in the provision of foot health services requires the combined influence of service providers, service purchasers, and national and local policy makers. For practitioners working within foot health services, this involves efficient and effective collaboration with individuals and organisations both within and outside the health care setting. Foot health promotion embodies a strategy whereby practitioners should 'cease to see themselves working on the public or doing things to them, but instead see themselves acting with the public' (Dines & Cribb 1993).

BOUNDARIES OF HEALTH PROMOTION

The first international conference on health promotion produced the *Ottawa charter for health promotion* (WHO 1986b). The overall aim of this charter is the achievement of 'health for all' by the year 2000 and beyond. The charter is concerned with enabling individuals and groups to increase control over and improve their health. A 'charter for action' was issued in an attempt to provide sound theoretical guidance to those involved in health promotion. This charter encompasses major areas within which strategies for health promotion are based. These include:

- building healthy public policy
- creating supportive environments

- strengthening community action
- developing personal skills
- reorientating health services.

The five aspects of health promotion activities outlined in the *Ottawa charter* offer a broad framework in which activities relating to foot health may be examined. Unfortunately, there is no widely held consensus regarding which of these activities relate specifically to foot health promotion. Each of the above activities, and their potential implication for foot health, are considered below.

Building health public policy

The *Ottawa charter* states that health promotion policy should combine the diversity of a number of different approaches, which include legislation, fiscal measures, taxation and organisational change. *The health of the nation* demonstrates a commitment by the British government to the prevention of disease and the promotion of health (Department of Health 1992). Specific health targets are identified in *The health of the nation*, two of which, coronary heart disease and stroke, have implications for foot health services.

Increased physical activity is required to reduce the risks of both coronary heart disease and stroke. It is unlikely that anyone who is suffering from foot problems will be willing either to take part in or to increase their level of physical activity. Good foot health is therefore an essential prerequisite in reducing the risks associated with stroke and coronary heart disease. Foot health services have a valuable contribution to make in the overall strategy for improving the nation's health.

Another example of the importance of national and local policies in the overall promotion of good foot health is the provision of transport services. Smith & Jacobson (1990) found that approximately 25% of persons over 75 years of age were unable to use public transport in the UK. Members of this section of the population are known to suffer from more foot problems than younger generations (Cartwright & Henderson 1986). Elderly people are the largest client group who attend for podiatric services (Salvage et al 1988). Clearly there are opportunities here for policy change, at both local and national levels, to maximise the potential mobility of the elderly population, e.g. by the provision of door-to-door bus services, improved concessionary fares and easy access to health centres and clinics.

The exemption of children's footwear from VAT is an example of a fiscal measure which contributes to foot health by keeping the cost of these items to a minimum. It is the role of the policy makers, at national and local level, in health sectors as well as non-health sectors, to remove obstacles which prevent individuals from making health choices. The role of practitioners involved in the provision of foot health services is to inform policy makers of factors which would aid in achieving this aim.

Creating supportive environments

The Department of Health (1992) in its strategy document *The health of the nation* stated that the success or failure of the strategy was dependent, to a large extent, on the commitment and skills of the health practitioners within the National Health Service (NHS). Health practitioners have a responsibility, as health promoters, to appreciate the many factors which have an impact on health. Practitioners involved in the provision of foot health services should not limit their role purely to the foot. They should be aware of the effects of environmental factors and recognise and make use of the various environmental health agencies involved in the promotion of healthy environments. Two examples of major environmental issues which have implications for all health care professionals are:

- smoking and passive smoking
- health and safety issues.

Smoking and passive smoking. It is undeniable that smoking affects the environment in which non-smokers live, work and travel. The Independent Scientific Committee on Smoking and Health (1988) concluded that passive smoking presents a hazard to non-smokers. The report made recommendations for the separation of smokers and non-smokers in the workplace and in other public settings. The NHS has been declared as a 'healthy workplace', and the whole of the health service is working towards a smoke-free environment for staff, patients and visitors.

Health and safety issues. The environment in which people work has potential serious effects on their health. The Health and Safety at Work Act (1974) places responsibility on the employer for ensuring, as far as is reasonably possible, the health, safety and welfare at work of all her employees. Health practitioners are affected by various health and safety regulations, e.g. the *Control of substances hazardous to health* (COSHH). It is the responsibility of practitioners working in the health care services to prevent or, where reasonably practicable, to adequately control, the exposure to patients of substances hazardous to their health.

Strict infection control guidelines should be evident in all related health care settings to minimise the risk of cross-infection. This is particularly the case where patients and practitioners may be exposed to a variety of potentially pathological agents. Infection control policies should include the safe disposal of contaminated waste, sterilisation of clinical instruments and personal hygiene.

Health and safety issues specific to good foot health extend outside the health care setting. Many foot health policies are evident in the workplace. For example, in industrial settings where the foot is at risk of trauma, employees are required to wear protective footwear at all times during working hours. A commitment towards improved standards of occupational health care is widely encouraged in the workplace, in order to provide healthier working environments. As part of this policy, workers are actively taking an interest in their own well-being, which includes the maintenance of good foot health.

Strengthening community action

The major causes of morbidity and mortality in society are associated with chronic diseases such as coronary heart disease, stroke, arthritis and diabetes. The vast majority of chronic illnesses and disabilities are looked after within the community. Health promotion in the community aims to allow people to achieve their maximum health potential by enabling them to take control of some of the many factors which determine their health. Programmes to strengthen community action aim to encourage and empower groups of people regarding issues surrounding their own health. Patients, families and carers are actively encouraged to be involved in their own health care. A vital component of community action is networking, which means establishing good communication links between the various voluntary and statutory agencies that have an impact on health.

The majority of people suffering from chronic debilitating illnesses are over 65 years of age. The concern of those caring for the elderly in the community is to prevent unnecessary loss of functional capacity. This requires a broad response, involving the support of social and welfare policy, and contributions from various statutory and voluntary agencies. Networking between the various agencies, e.g. health, social and voluntary services, maximises the potential of the elderly to function independently in the community.

Foot health services provide a valuable aspect of care for the elderly in the community, by preventing foot problems, wherever possible, and by palliatively managing existing foot problems to promote maximum mobility. This is usually achieved by providing for the regular management of patients in community clinics or in their own homes. This primarily includes podiatric services but may also involve other members of the primary health care team. The voluntary services often play a vital role in maximising the mobility of the elderly, by providing or organising transport for patients attending community clinics for podiatry appointments. Such provision prevents the need for otherwise costly domiciliary visits. Figure 5.3 highlights the various agencies which play a role in promoting good foot health.

Various self-help groups in the community provide general health care support for patients, families and carers, as well as specific foot health information. The local diabetes services advisory groups (LDSAGs) of the British Diabetic Association include specialist representatives, e.g. primary health care practitioners, people with diabetes and their carers. The group work together to advise on how best to implement the *St Vincent declaration* (WHO/IDF 1990). One of the major targets of this declaration is to reduce the incidence of amputation by 50% within a 5 year period. Those working within foot health services have an undeniable role in striving to achieve this target. Educating patients at a community level about foot care demands a multidisciplinary approach, and the information given can range from simple foot care through to exercise programmes and advice on how to stop smoking.

Developing personal skills

Health promotion provides both information and education about health, which aim to increase an individual's options and potential to contribute to their own health. Within the health promotion framework, the aim of any health education intervention is to develop the competence of individuals to be able to make this contribution. Education about health involves an active learning process by which individuals and groups learn to promote, maintain or restore health. Those working within all areas of health care have a vast potential to provide information and promote skills which enable improved standards of foot health and which can prevent the onset of many diseases affecting the foot.

Communication between the various agencies and practitioners involved in promoting foot health needs to be facilitated. All parties need to be aware of the range of services that are available. Practitioners should pass on routine or specific foot health infor-

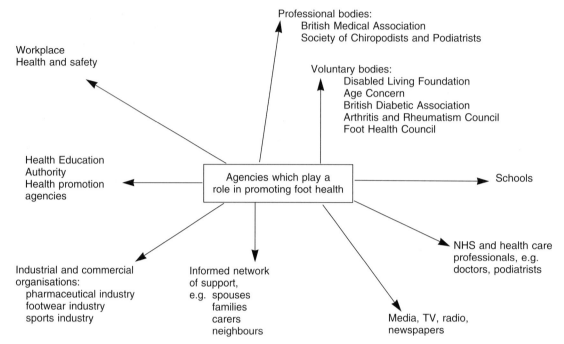

Figure 5.3   The various agencies which play a role in promoting foot health.

mation to others. The importance of prevention within the foot health services is seen particularly within the field of diabetes, where a multidisciplinary team of specialists work together to prevent, where possible, the onset of diabetes-related foot pathology.

Reorientating health services

The *Ottawa charter* (WHO 1986b) states that 'the role of the health sector must move increasingly in a health promotional direction, beyond its responsibility for providing clinical and curative services'. The government's health strategy *The health of the nation* (Department of Health 1992) reflects to some extent the views expressed in the WHO *Ottawa charter*. It recognises that a strategy for disease prevention and health promotion is fundamental to achieving health for all. Although this strategy is specific to England, other UK health promotion strategies exist in Wales, Scotland and Ireland. Other documents and policies that have been influential in the move towards primary health care and health promotion include:

- *Promoting better health* (Department of Health and Social Security 1987)
- *Caring for people* (Department of Health 1989)
- *The Patients' Charter* (Department of Health 1991).

Responsibility for the majority of illness in society lies with the health services. However, the NHS is a health service and not merely a service provided for illness. Everyone in the NHS has a responsibility to promote health, and this means taking greater responsibility in leading and coordinating other agencies that have an impact on health (Department of Health 1992).

Target 36 of the *Health for all targets* (WHO 1993b) states that 'by the year 2000, education and training of health and other personnel in all member states should actively contribute to the achievement of health for all'. If this target is to be met, greater emphasis must be placed on the theory and practice of health promotion, both at undergraduate and postgraduate levels. This need is supported in podiatry, where, at undergraduate level, there appears to be no nationally recognised curriculum for health promotion training. Health education and promotion seems to be regarded as a low priority in the syllabus (Kippen 1988, Axford 1990, Coles 1990).

THE ROLE OF FOOT HEALTH EDUCATION AND PROMOTION

Foot health education/promotion covers a diverse range of activities. Draper et al (1980) identified three types of health education:

• *Type 1.* Education about the lower limb and the body and how to look after it. A great deal of everyday foot health promotion falls within this category, promoting safe self-foot care where appropriate.

• *Type 2.* The provision of information regarding access to, and most appropriate use of, foot health services. *The Patients' Charter* aims to provide comprehensive information for individuals regarding their rights of care in the NHS (Department of Health 1991). The Foot Health Council also contributes to this aspect of health. The role of the podiatrist and other practitioners in promoting good foot health is publicised during national 'foot health week'.

• *Type 3.* The provision of national, regional and local policies, structures and processes aimed at improving foot health. For example, government legislation was responsible for employers having to ensure that their employees wear safety footwear in designated industrial settings. Foot health educational initiatives also have a fundamental role to play in promoting the scope of practice of the various members of the foot health team, both to the public and among health practitioners. Professional bodies play a role in the national promotion of the scope of practice of their respective professions.

Since Draper et al (1980) published their work, a great deal of change has taken place in health education. However, the three types of health education which they identified are essentially still accepted today.

Ewles & Simnett (1995) described three levels of prevention, which can be applied to foot health:

1. *Primary prevention.* This is prevention which is directed towards healthy individuals. The aim is to prevent the onset of disease or ill-health. Foot health education aimed at children falls within this category. Alternatively, communication with other members of the health care team to promote the scope of practice and give general foot care information must also be considered as a form of primary prevention. For example, information targeted at GPs concerning the range of available foot health services aims to promote effective and efficient use of the podiatry services.

2. *Secondary prevention.* This level of prevention is targeted at individuals who already have the early stages of foot pathology. Secondary prevention is indicated when there is a need to prevent the problem from moving into a chronic or irreversible stage. The aim is to restore the individual to an optimum state of health. Giving advice to patients regarding the avoidance of potentially harmful self-treatment would constitute secondary prevention. For example, where

an individual has developed a septic lesion due to the inappropriate use of a corn plaster, appropriate information could be given regarding the future management of this lesion.

3. *Tertiary prevention.* This term is used to describe preventative efforts directed towards patients, professionals or carers of individuals who have foot problems which cannot be prevented or completely cured. Such individuals may have a permanent deformity or may have developed manifestations within the lower limb as a result of a systemic disease. Tertiary stage prevention would be tailored to prevent further deterioration of a pathology, and to rehabilitate and make the patient as comfortable as possible. It often involves a multidisciplinary approach to patient management. For example, a person suffering from the acute symptoms of rheumatoid arthritis, with recurrent vasculitic ulceration of the foot, will require close collaboration among numerous members of the health care team. The team would aim to prevent further deterioration of the patient's condition, to promote healing and to minimise the risks of future vasculitic episodes.

Table 5.1 gives examples of the three levels of prevention applied to diabetic care.

Primary, secondary and tertiary prevention of foot pathology is vital to patient's overall wellbeing. The terms represent a useful framework within which to apply health education principles. However, a person's state of health is open to interpretation and therefore there will always be some degree of overlap between the three levels of prevention.

Implications of foot health education and promotion

Foot health education can take place in a variety of settings and should not be limited to the health care services:

• the workplace
• schools
• the community
• hospitals
• the media, e.g. radio, TV, magazines.

Foot health information is provided by a number of agencies and agents, including the podiatrist, other health practitioners, the footwear industry, the pharmaceutical industry, and voluntary bodies such as Age Concern, the Disabled Living Foundation, the British Diabetic Association and the Arthritis and Rheumatism Council.

Table 5.1 Examples of primary, secondary and tertiary prevention related to the management of the foot in diabetes

Type of prevention	Examples related to the foot in diabetes
Primary	Foot health educational programmes providing information for those without diabetic-related foot complications
	Effective multidisciplinary collaboration between key members of the diabetic team, both within and between hospital and community settings
Secondary	The provision of regular foot screening to allow for the early identification of those factors which place an individual at greater risk of foot pathology
	Provision of intensive diabetes management by the diabetic team for those identified as being at greater risk of potential foot pathology. Management should involve modification or removal of risk factors, where possible, as well as early intervention and effective education
Tertiary	Regular liaison and observation by members of the diabetic team to monitor the patient's foot problems, to promote healing and to prevent further deterioration of the patient's overall condition
	Multidisciplinary rehabilitation of the patient post-amputation/surgery

Foot health education programmes may be targeted at the population as a whole or to certain sections of society. It may be related to generic foot health issues or to specific types of foot problem, as follows:

- the prevention of sports injuries
- general foot health advice
- prevention of foot pathology related to podopaediatrics
- those who are especially at risk of foot pathology
- other individuals and agencies with a contribution to make to the promotion of foot health, e.g. health professionals, self-help groups and the footwear industry
- promotion of good health by the pharmaceutical industry who provide foot health literature to support the use of foot-related products.

Financial stringency in the NHS today is such that all health professionals must constantly consider the economic aspects of the services they provide. It is unlikely that significant reorientation of health services to facilitate greater emphasis on health promotion will be achieved unless there is redeployment of already depleting resources. The economic and social implications of the pain, deformity, dysfunction and immobility which occur in relation to foot pathology are widely documented (Brodie 1989). Cartwright & Henderson (1986) found that 86% of a randomly selected group of elderly people reported some form of foot problem. Further to this, they concluded that the level of podiatric services provided for the elderly alone needed to be doubled. There is little, if any, evidence to suggest that podiatric services have since doubled. Demographic changes over the next 10 years will bring about a significant increase in those over the age of 75 (Thompson 1987). A large number of elderly people require some form of foot care. To meet this need, current foot health services will require extensive review.

Providing ameliorative podiatry care for the elderly is a highly effective intervention for what others may consider a small problem (Bryan et al 1991). There are other groups of patients who require a more specialist approach to managing their foot health. The foot provides a mirror for many systemic diseases, e.g. diabetes mellitus and the complex range of connective tissue disorders and circulatory disturbances which undeniably have an effect on the foot. Patients with systemic disease are at greater risk of developing associated foot pathology, such as ulceration, gangrene or extreme cases requiring surgical intervention. Those considered at risk are a priority group within the foot health services and present potentially serious economic and social implications in health care provision. In particular, patients with diabetes carry an increased risk of amputation (Pecoraro et al 1990). One study suggested that more than 50% of non-traumatic amputations were associated with diabetes and that people with diabetes had a 15-fold greater risk of amputation than those without the disease (Sussman et al 1992). Research undertaken suggests that diabetic patients with circulatory problems represent the largest population of hospital daily admissions (Williams 1985). The need for health education specifically about diabetes is widely noted in the literature (Diabetes Control and Complications Trial Research Group 1993, Fletcher & Jeffcoate 1994).

The socio-economic impact of diabetes may be considered under the headings of direct and indirect costs (Sanger 1992). Direct costs include those associated with medical attention, and include hospitalisation, outpatient or in-patient care, antibiotics and other drugs used to manage the patient's condition and prevent further deterioration, surgical intervention, and pathology and other laboratory facilities required. Further costs include the provision of specialist footwear by the orthotist, the expense of dressings, the manufacture and provision of pressure-relieving devices, and the specialised staff and equipment required. Indirect socio-economic costs include early death and loss of working days, leading to a loss of production and earnings, the impact of which has implications both for the economy overall and for the individuals concerned. Further indirect costs include social security costs in respect of unemployment, supplementary benefits and attendance allowance. Indirect costs have never been reliably estimated, but one study suggested that the average health care cost for diabetic patients undergoing lower limb amputation was $24 700 in 1985 (Reiber 1992).

Child foot health is arguably another key priority area within the foot health services not only in terms of managing existing foot problems but also in terms of screening to identify those at risk of future foot pathologies. However, it is suggested that the role of prevention within the foot health services is restricted, as the vast majority of patients seeking attention, in particular from the podiatrist, are of pensionable age. Therefore, it is argued that the overwhelming bulk of NHS podiatric services are dealing with ameliorative care rather than actively focusing on the promotion of good foot health and the prevention of foot pathology for the rest of the population (Powrie 1992).

The role of screening in foot health promotion

Screening allows the practitioner to identify those patients at greatest risk of foot pathology. Clinics which regularly screen their patients are on the increase, particularly with the increased emphasis which is being placed on clinical audit (Connor 1994). Information obtained from screening is valuable in highlighting areas of particular need. Ward (1988) suggested the use of community registers to identify those individuals with diabetes who require priority care. Cartwright & Henderson (1986) concluded that screening clinics for the elderly were necessary to identify those needing but not receiving podiatric care, as over half of such individuals did not recognise their own needs.

The need for screening is recognised where patients' general health, and neurological and vascular status require regular monitoring and observation. Screening allows for the early detection of potentially pathological foot problems in diabetes and is supported by the *St Vincent declaration* (WHO 1990).

The aim of a diabetic foot screening clinic is to facilitate the early identification of foot complications related to diabetes. This allows for the subsequent prioritisation of the diabetic foot care services, so that those patients considered at greatest risk of developing foot ulceration might receive immediate attention. There is considerable national and international commitment to the provision of foot screening clinics, as stated by, for example, the WHO study group on the prevention of diabetes mellitus (WHO 1994), the *St Vincent declaration* (WHO 1990) and many other recognised specialists involved in the management of the diabetic foot (McKinnes 1994).

Screening clinics must not be set up in isolation; they should be supported by a service to provide treatment for the screened population. This requires the commitment of resources to accommodate the increased costs of those services. For example, screening clinics for child foot health require supportive services to treat diagnosed foot problems. This may involve the manufacture of orthoses to correct detected biomechanical problems. Financial support may not be available to support this initiative, as existing services may already be overstretched.

Screening has the potential to provide valuable information for practitioners to determine the foot health needs of the population, and highlights the need for increased service provisions and a reorientation of existing services. The ongoing evaluation of screening programmes can only strengthen the case for increased commitment to the further development of preventative strategies in the foot health services.

APPROACHES TO FOOT HEALTH EDUCATION

Patient education is a vital component of the broader concept of health promotion. The prevention of foot pathology and the promotion of good foot health are largely dependent on the informed and willing contribution of individuals to their own foot care. This can only be facilitated if practitioners within the foot health services spend more time effectively educating their patients.

A number of different approaches exist within the field of patient education. These can be broadly categorised as compliance-based and patient-centred. The compliance-based approach aims to provide information for people in the hope that they will change their behaviour in the light of knowledge about potential foot problems. In adopting this approach, the most common assumption is that individuals can be treated as empty buckets into which the appropriate information regarding foot health can be poured (Coles 1989). The extent to which patients follow advice given to them poses a major problem for health professionals. The failure of traditional compliance-based educational programmes is widely recognised; indeed a number of journals devote much of their space to this problem, e.g. *Diabetes Education* and *Patient Education and Counselling*.

Frequently, patients with a risk of potential foot problems do not see the relevance of what they are told, particularly when they are symptom-free at the time. In a study regarding the effectiveness of a learning contract in improving levels of foot care knowledge, Stuart & Wiles (1993) found that, despite improved levels of foot care knowledge at the end of the programme, patients did not perceive themselves as being vulnerable to future foot problems as a result of having been diagnosed as diabetic. Compliance-based education is also of limited value where individuals find they are unable to remember much of what has been said (Kippen 1988). Lack of understanding of information imparted by practitioners is also recognised as a reason for poor levels of compliance. A complex relationship between many other factors plays a role in determining whether or not a patient will comply with foot health information. Clearly, a purely didactic approach to patient education only has a limited potential to influence patient behaviour.

Current educational philosophy in health promotion addresses the importance of self-esteem, personal skills and social support in developing health attitudes and behaviours towards improved foot health. Educational programmes are now required to empower individuals, and in doing so to help them to develop their skills and strengthen their decision-making abilities. Health education programmes should aim to increase the individual's health options and so provide them with greater control over their own foot health.

Health education which aims to empower an individual is very different from education which is designed so that patients become compliant and merely obey instructions given to them. The approach to patient education which embodies the concept of self-empowerment is often termed the 'patient-centred approach' (McWhinney 1989). The patient-centred approach aims to help patients to understand their own illness, whatever that may be. This approach aims to enable individuals to identify the benefits and develop the skills of contributing to effective self-care wherever possible. Stuart & Wiles (1993) found that

those individuals who entered into a learning contract developed knowledge levels significantly higher than the control group who received foot health information in the conventional way.

Principles of a patient-centred approach to education include:

1. promoting an individual's sense of ownership over the behavioural changes needed; this may be achieved via a greater understanding of the condition or illness, motivating the individual to want to know more about it
2. helping patients to define their own objectives, to acknowledge their strengths and weaknesses, to decide upon a course of action and to evaluate the consequences of such a decision
3. facilitating the learning process by actively encouraging the patient to contribute to it
4. building upon the patient's existing knowledge; any new information should only be introduced once the learner has identified a reason for needing it.

Whilst the patient-centred approach might seem overly complex, it has widespread implications for foot health education where existing compliance-based approaches have demonstrated limited effectiveness. The patient-centred approach is widely adopted in the management of many chronic illnesses, e.g. diabetes, rheumatoid arthritis and asthma. This approach is becoming increasingly popular with regard to the management of patients with diabetes, where the patients' contribution to their own care, including foot care, is vital to their overall well-being (Funnell et al 1991).

Whatever the approach, it is necessary continually to evaluate and critically analyse its effectiveness. Inevitably, this calls for education of the educators themselves. One way of doing this is through educational workshops. Such workshops are now well established in the field of chronic illness, where practitioners involved in the care of various illnesses are introduced to the principles and skills required to encourage individuals to play a more extensive role in their own health care (Day et al 1985, Coping with Crisis Research Group 1987).

Communication skills and foot health education

Practitioners working in the foot health services generally possess credibility because of their training and expert knowledge. However, the possession of expertise alone does not make a good educator—good communication skills are also essential. Helping individuals to reorganise their own health needs, raising their competence and empowering them to contribute towards improved levels of foot health, is dependent on good communication skills. With the ever-increasing need for foot care provision in the elderly and priority populations, coupled with too few trained health care professionals, effective communication becomes all the more necessary (Kippen 1988). Only through good communication skills can the need for foot health be promoted. Effective communication skills are fundamental to health promotion. It is not sufficient merely to read about them. A number of post-basic courses are available for health care practitioners wanting to develop their agreed health promotional role. The Health Education Authority provides a health education certificate course, and postgraduate diplomas and Masters degrees in health education and promotion are increasingly available. However, it must be recognised that resource constraints can be responsible for hindering many practitioners from achieving their potential in health promotion. For example, staff shortages and the overloading burden of work reduce the time available for health promotion work.

Communicating health information

Much has been written on the principles of communicating health messages effectively. Health messages need to be short, clear and powerful. Language used must be appropriate for the intended audience and should avoid ambiguity. Further, the receiver of the health message must have an interest in the information conveyed if it is to be effective.

Methods of communicating health information used by health professionals include the following:

- one-to-one
- written
- group education
- the media.

One-to-one. This is the most common means of educating patients. There are a number of points to consider when educating an individual on a one-to-one basis. These include the following:

1. It is important to ensure that there is a personal introduction between the patient and the health care provider. This provides a foundation on which the individual's trust in the practitioner can be established. The acknowledgement of the importance of named health care professionals is now a recognised feature of *The Patients' Charter* (Department of Health 1991). In multidisciplinary settings, e.g. the diabetic foot clinic, a patient may assume, incorrectly, that the person wearing the white coat is always the doctor; therefore, introduction of patient and practitioner is especially necessary.

2. It is suggested that patients forget 50% of what is said during a medical consultation (Kippen 1988). Clearly, then, health messages should be brief and simplified. Ley (1992) demonstrated that simplification of health information significantly improves understanding and memory.

3. In providing new information and skills on a one-to-one basis, one should aim to build on what is already known. Therefore the practitioner should find out as much as possible about what the patient already knows, so that additional information can be pitched at an appropriate level—as, for example, when professionals are required to provide appropriate information to athletes regarding the prevention and management of sports injuries. The athlete's level of knowledge and experience of injuries may be comparable to that of the physiotherapist or podiatrist providing the information. Alternatively, the athlete may require basic advice regarding training, warm-up exercises, footwear or general foot health education.

4. Information should be given when the patients are at their most receptive. Kippen (1988) explored one-to-one health education programmes in chiropody clinics. Findings from this study suggest that patients are at their most receptive during the middle phase of a foot care consultation, and are at their least receptive at the beginning and end.

5. Patients should be actively encouraged to contribute throughout the educational session. It is this active communication that empowers them to take increased responsibility for health. It has been suggested, however, that patients are reluctant to ask for health-related information from health professionals (Roter 1983).

6. At the end of any one-to-one educational session, patients should be provided with sufficient information to know when, how and who to contact for the management of any further foot problems.

Written information. This provides a useful means of supplementing, reiterating or clarifying verbal information. Alternatively, written advice may be used as the primary source of education aimed at improving a patient's knowledge. Foot health information is available in a variety of written formats, including information sheets, leaflets, booklets and posters. Many agents and agencies produce written information on foot health in a variety of settings:

- Voluntary and professional organisations
  —British Diabetic Association
  —Age Concern
  —Disabled and Rheumatism Council
  —Foot Health Council
  —Health Education Authority
  —Society of Chiropodists and Podiatrists
- NHS community and hospital trusts
- The pharmaceutical industry
- The footwear industry.

Each of the following points will help to make written communication more effective:

1. Attract attention, particularly when the information is to be used as the primary method of communication; failure to gain the attention of the reader may lead to a loss of the opportunity to provide education
2. Make the information easily readable by using shorter words and sentences and by avoiding unnecessary jargon
3. Use illustrations to explain or enhance the text. Alternatively, if illustrations are the main means of communicating the message, the accompanying text must clearly explain the picture to avoid confusing the reader as to its message
4. Use an attractive format. The colour, design, print and size of typeface all provide valuable contributions to the overall effectiveness of written communications. For example, a mass photocopied, wordy information sheet will hardly inspire an individual to read it. Equally, leaflets which lack colour and provide overwhelming amounts of written details will not attract the reader's attention either.

Some advantages and disadvantages of providing information in a written format are outlined in Table 5.2.

Group education. Promotion of foot health may involve groups of individuals, formally or informally. Formal foot health programmes may be targeted towards specific health professionals, e.g. podiatrists providing information regarding diabetic foot health for district nurses. Alternatively, a great deal of informal foot health education may take place in a group setting, e.g. antenatal classes, school foot health education programmes and foot health educational programmes targeted at athletes. Many of the principles previously considered in the sections on one-to-one and written communication also apply to group education.

Table 5.2 Advantages and disadvantages of written health information

Advantages	Disadvantages
Provides a recognised means of increasing knowledge	May be too difficult for patients to understand
Target group can read at their own pace	Can end up unread if the reader is not motivated to read it
Relatively easy and inexpensive to produce	Can be expensive if commercially made
Can be passed on to others	May be lost or put in the bin
Can reach a large number of individuals at relatively low cost	Not suitable for everybody to read
Provides a valuable method of reiterating and clarifying a health message	Provides no feedback

The media. A wide range of mass media are available to communicate foot health information, including television, radio, newspapers, journals and videos. Those involved in foot health education are likely to become involved with mass media when undertaking promotional campaigns for the public, e.g. the annual foot health week organised by the Foot Health Council. A more extensive review of mass media in foot health promotion is not possible within the scope of this chapter, but other useful information can be found in a number of health promotion texts.

PLANNING AND IMPLEMENTING FOOT HEALTH EDUCATION AND PROMOTION ACTIVITIES

The success of any foot health educational activity is largely dependent on careful strategic planning. Before embarking on any activity which aims to promote foot heath or prevent the onset of foot disease, the practitioner must identify the needs and priorities of those at whom the activity is targeted. It is important to identify whether or not health education will provide an effective means of addressing the particular problem or issue. It is widely recognised that inaccurate or inappropriate assessment of health needs is responsible for the failure of many health education or promotional activities. This is particularly the case when the practitioner provides information which patients do not feel is relevant to their own condition (McWhinney 1989).

Once the need for an educational intervention has been established, planning of the programme may

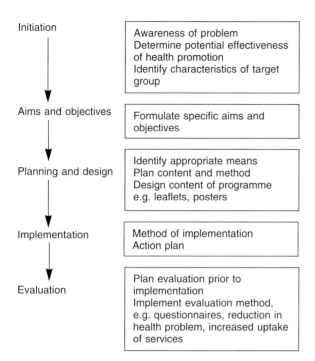

Initiation

| Awareness of problem
| Determine potential effectiveness
| of health promotion
| Identify characteristics of target
| group

Aims and objectives

| Formulate specific aims and
| objectives

Planning and design

| Identify appropriate means
| Plan content and method
| Design content of programme
| e.g. leaflets, posters

Implementation

| Method of implementation
| Action plan

Evaluation

| Plan evaluation prior to
| implementation
| Implement evaluation method,
| e.g. questionnaires, reduction in
| health problem, increased uptake
| of services

Figure 5.4 A flowchart for planning health promotion activities.

usefully be considered under the following headings (Fig. 5.4):

- initiation
- aims and objectives
- planning and design
- implementation
- evaluation.

Initiation

Initiation of a programme involves identifying the extent of the problem which requires educational intervention. The initiation of a health education activity may result from:

- the practitioner's own experience of areas requiring greater educational intervention
- epidemiological data highlighting the increased incidence or prevalence of a particular problem; alternatively, this data may provide evidence as to the levels of morbidity (illness) and mortality (death) occurring as a result of the problem
- NHS data providing information regarding waiting lists, service planning, etc.
- public demand for particular aspects of podiatric services, as expressed by individuals

themselves, voluntary bodies or community groups
- public and professionals understanding of the scope of practice of the podiatrist; this is vital if effective use of podiatry services is to take place
- Government policy, e.g. *The health of the nation* (Department of Health 1992)
- findings from research and audit into foot health practices and services.

Once the extent of the problem has been assessed and documented, the practitioner must then assess the characteristics of the client group for whom the educational intervention is intended. As well as considering the age, culture and attitudes of the client group, this should include determining whether or not the target group perceive a need for the intervention. Where the target group do not see the need for educational intervention, effectiveness in influencing attitudes or behaviour will be limited.

Aims and objectives

It is important to establish clear aims and objectives for the activity, not least because the outcomes can be assessed against these. Aims and objectives should be realistic and achievable. For example, the aim of a diabetic screening clinic would be to develop and implement a diabetic foot screening clinic to allow for the early identification of foot complications which place an individual at risk of foot ulceration. The objectives would include:

- provision of a comprehensive foot screening programme for diabetic patients attending the GP practice on an annual basis
- prioritisation of those patients at greater risk of potential foot ulceration
- referral of patients identified as 'at risk' to the appropriate foot health services.

Planning and design

The planning and design of a foot health activity involves:

- identifying the most appropriate means of targeting client groups
- designing the structure and content of the activity.

When choosing and designing an appropriate educational programme, the practitioner, as the health educator, must place himself within the context in which the preventative strategy is to take place. The design of specific material, e.g. leaflets and posters, may require specialist input. Numerous methods may be employed to promote preventative strategies, e.g. displays, informal or formal lectures, or campaigns. All preventative strategies require careful design to achieve maximum effectiveness.

Whatever the design selected, the practitioner must consider whether or not it is appropriate for the target group it is intended to reach. For example, a leaflet given to patients identified as being at risk of potential foot ulceration is unlikely to be effective if those patients are not motivated to read it. Once the most appropriate means of delivering health education information has been selected, the health educator should ensure that the information is tailored to reflect the age, culture and perceived needs of the target group.

If a foot screening clinic was to be established, it would be necessary to prepare written information, to be given to patients and practitioners, regarding the purpose of the clinic. A mechanism would also have to be agreed which allowed for the early referral, to the appropriate practitioner, of patients identified as being at specific risk of foot pathology.

Implementation

Key aspects of the process of implementation should include monitoring the preventative strategy to ensure that it is being implemented as planned. This is particularly important in the screening of the diabetic foot, where inconsistencies in screening can miss vital complications or invalidate the results obtained from the screening programme. Prior to implementation, a detailed action plan should be drawn up. This should include a detailed report of how, when and with what resources the programme will take place. The action plan should also provide a schedule from which the practitioner implementing the preventative strategy can work. This is useful as it should provide deadlines that the health campaign should meet. The plan also helps to clearly identify the various roles of individuals contributing to the programme.

Evaluation

Evaluation is a key aspect of health promotional practice (Tones & Tilford 1994). It provides a tool by which the health promoter can assess the level of success or failure of the programme. Evaluation methods to be used, of which there are many to choose from, should be determined before implementing a promotional strategy. These methods may range from the use of a questionnaire to determine improvements in knowledge, to direct observation to monitor changes in behaviour. Alternative methods include polls, written comments following the programme, overall attendance at a particular programme or, alternatively, future demand for health promotion initiatives.

Whatever the form of evaluation adopted, the results should provide tangible evidence of what has been accomplished. Evaluation also highlights areas which may require future modification. It is often only when viewed retrospectively that useful feedback can be obtained to suggest that the promotional initiative used was worthwhile in terms of what it cost. The success of a foot screening clinic would be apparent from a number of aspects, and these would provide a means of evaluation. In the short term, for example, success might be indicated by an increased demand for priority service provision and an increased need for structured educational programmes. In the long term, success might be indicated by a reduction in foot ulceration or interventional surgery required for patients with diabetes who fall under the care of a community clinic.

Essentially, evaluation is an integral aspect of health promotion activities. It is necessary to ascertain the effects of the programme, to assess the methods used, and to examine the use of resources.

SUMMARY

All members of the foot health services have an active role to play in promoting knowledge of, and the adoption of, good foot care strategies, particularly for those at risk. Foot problems are not divorced from other medical and social problems. The elderly who are economically disadvantaged may be unable to afford footwear which accommodates their foot problems. Furthermore, they may have specific medical problems or lifestyles which have an effect on the foot, e.g. medical conditions such as diabetes and rheumatoid arthritis, and lifestyle factors such as smoking or lack of exercise.

The introduction of a wider health promotional perspective within foot health services can only be achieved by practitioners who have a sound knowledge and understanding of health education and health promotion theory and practice. All practitioners working within the health care setting play a valuable role and, given adequate training and resources, they can make a valuable contribution to reducing the demand on services and to promoting the concept of good health for all.

REFERENCES

Axford G 1990 Chiropody and health education. The Chiropodist 4: 72–76

Binyet S, Aufseeser M, Lacroix A, Assal J P 1994 The diabetic foot: various interpretations by patients of some terms used by physicians in podiatric consultations. Diabetes Metabolism 20: 275–281

Brodie B S 1989 Community health and foot health. Canadian Journal of Public Health 80: 331–333

Bryan S, Parkin D, Donaldson C 1991 Chiropody and the QALY: a case study in assigning disability and distress to patients. Health Policy 18: 169–185

Cartwright A, Henderson G 1986 More trouble with feet. A survey of foot problems and chiropody needs of the elderly. HMSO, London

Coles C R 1989 Diabetes education: theories of practice. Practical Diabetes 6: 199–202

Coles C 1990 Diabetes education: letting the patient into the picture. Practical Diabetes 7: 110–112

Coles C 1991 How people learn: applying our understanding of human learning to the clinical process and the education of diabetes educators. The Diabetes Education Study Group of The European Association for the Study of Diabetes 2

Connor H 1994 Prevention of diabetic foot problems: identification and the team approach. In: Boulton A J M, Connor H, Cavanagh P R (eds) The foot in diabetes. Wiley, London, p 57–65

Coping with Crisis Research Group 1987 The open university running workshops. Croom Helm, Beckenham

Day J L, Hicks B, Johnson P, Spathis M 1985 Diabetes patient education workshops. Diabetes Medicine 2: 479–483

Department of Health 1989 Caring for people. HMSO, London, CMn849.

Department of Health 1991 The Patients' Charter. Department of Health, London

Department of Health 1992 The health of the nation: a strategy for health in England. HMSO, London

Department of Health and Social Security 1987 Promoting better health. HMSO, London, Cmnd 249

Diabetes Control and Complications Trial Research Group 1993 The effect of intensive diabetes treatment on the development and progression of long term complications in insulin-dependent diabetes mellitus. New England Medicine 329: 977–986

Dines A, Cribb A 1993 Health promotion: concepts and practice. Blackwell, London, ch 2

Draper P, Griffiths J, Popay J 1980 Three types of health education. British Medical Journal 16: 493–495

Ewles L, Simnett I 1995 Promoting health: a practical guide, 3rd edn. Scutari, London

Fletcher E H, Jeffcoate W J 1994 Footcare education and the specialist nurse. In: Boulton A J M, Connor H, Cavanagh P R (eds) The foot in diabetes. Wiley, London, p 69–75

Funnell M M , Arnold M, Donnelly M, Taylor-Moon D 1991 Empowerment: an idea whose time has come in diabetes education. Diabetes Education 1: 37–41

Great Britain Health and Safety at Work Act. Ch. 37. Elizabeth II, London, HMSO

Health and Safety At Work Act 1974. HMSO, London

Helman C G 1983 Communication in primary care: the role of patient and practitioner exploratory models. Social Science Medicine 20(9): 923–931

Independent Scientific Committee on Smoking and Health 1988 Fourth report. HMSO, London

Kippen C 1988 Foot health education – an observational analysis. The Chiropodist 43(4): 57–60

Ley P 1992 Communicating with patients. Chapman and Hall, London, p 79–80

McKinnes A D 1994 The role of the chiropodist. In: Boulton A J M, Connor H, Cavanagh P R (eds) The foot in diabetes. Wiley, London, p 77–79

McWhinney I 1989 The need for a transformed clinical method. In: Stewart M, Roter D (eds) Communicating with patients. Sage, London

Nutbeam D 1986 Health promotion glossary. Health Promotion 1(1): 113–126

Pecoraro R E, Reiber G E, Burgess E M 1990 Pathways to diabetic amputation: basis for prevention. Diabetes Spectrum 5: 329–334

Powrie P 1992 Health education training for chiropodists: need, demand and future development. Journal of British Podiatric Medicine 11: 229–235

Reiber G E 1992 Financial implications and practice guidelines. Diabetes Care 15: 29–31

Roter D 1983 Physician–patient communication. Maryland State Medical Journal 32: 260–265

Salvage A V, Vetter N J, Jones D A 1988 Attitudes of the over 75s to NHS chiropody services. The Chiropodist 43: 103–105

Sanger T 1992 The economics of diabetes core. In: Albert K G M M et al (eds) International textbook of diabetes mellitus. John Wiley, London, p 1643–1654

Seedhouse D 1986 Health: the foundations for achievement. John Wiley & Sons, Chichester

Seymour H 1984 Health education versus health promotion – a practitioner's view. Health Education Journal 43: 37–38

Smith A, Jacobson B 1990. The nation's health. King's Fund, London, p 220–221

Stuart L, Wiles P G 1993 The influence of a learning contract on levels of footcare knowledge. Diabetic Medicine 10(suppl 2): 53

Sussman K E, Reiber G, Albert S F 1992 The diabetic foot problem – a failed system of healthcare? Diabetes Research in Clinical Practice 17: 1–8

Tannahill A 1985 What is health promotion? Health Education Journal 44(4): 167–168

Thompson J 1987 Ageing of the population. Population Trends 50: 18–22

Tones K, Tilford S 1994 Health education: effectiveness efficiency and equity, 2nd edn. Chapman and Hall, London

Ward J D 1988 Essential requirements of diabetic footcare. In: Boulton A J M, Connor H, Cavanagh P (eds) The Foot in Diabetes. Wiley, London, p 151–158

WHO 1946 Constitution. World Health Organization, New York

WHO 1986a A discussion document on the concept and principles of health promotion. Health Promotion 1(1): 73–76

WHO 1986b Ottowa charter for health promotion. An

international conference on health promotion, November 17–21. WHO Regional Office for Europe, Copenhagen

WHO/IDF 1990 Diabetes care and research in Europe: the St Vincent declaration. Diabetic Medicine 7: 360

WHO 1993b (Target 36) Health for all targets: the health policy for Europe, updated edn. WHO, Regional Office for Europe, Copenhagen

WHO 1994 Prevention of diabetes mellitus. World Health Organization, Geneva, p 64–65

Williams D R R 1985 Hospital admissions of diabetic patients: information from hospital activity analysis. Diabetic Medicine 2: 27–32

FURTHER READING

Ewles L, Simnett I 1995 Promoting health: a practical Guide. 3rd Edn, Chapter 15. Scutari, London

Gallup Poll on behalf of the Society of Chiropodists 1992. Research amongst the general public and GPs. Gallup Research

Naidoo J, Wills J 1994 Health Promotion Foundations for Practice. Chapter 13, part 4. Baillière Tindall, London

Methods of managing foot conditions

6

Operative techniques

D. R. Tollafield
L. M. Merriman

INTRODUCTION

This chapter concentrates on the operative techniques used to reduce or remove lesions affecting the skin and nails.

The term 'operative' suggests a requirement for surgical skills. Traditionally, routine skin care and surgery have been differentiated as requiring different skills. In reality, the skills used in both are derived from the same source. The way in which the scalpels are used may be different, but most of the techniques, invasive and otherwise, require the same considerations. The techniques often require adjunct therapies, details of which can be found in the relevant chapters, in order for the condition to be fully resolved. For example, enucleation of a corn may lead to an immediate reduction in the level of discomfort experienced by the patient, but if this reduction is to be maintained and the problem fully resolved, chemical and mechanical therapies, and in some cases physical therapies, may also be required. As with any therapy, the practitioner should always be mindful of the benefits and limitations. Box 6.1 summarises the wide range of operative techniques associated with skin and nail lesions. There may be more than one approach to deal with any given problem.

OPERATIVE TREATMENT

Aims

The aims of carrying out operative techniques are:

- to provide an immediate reduction in the discomfort/pain
- to complement the use of other therapies as part of the management plan
- to prevent complications from arising as a result of non-treatment.

Box 6.1 Direct and indirect operating skills associated with cutaneous forms of treatment.

SKIN
Debridement (cutaneous skin)
• verruca
• fissure
• callus (tyloma)
• ulcer
• onychophosis

Enucleation
• corn (clavus) (Latin: heloma, H.)
  —hard (H. durum)
  —soft (H. molle)
  —vascular (H. vasculare)
  —intractable plantar keratoma (IPK)
  —seed corn (H. milliare)
  —subungual corn (H. subungualis)

Currettage (cutaneous)
• verrucae
• granuloma

Cautery (cutaneous and subcutaneous)
• thermal
  —heat
  —electrical
  —laser
  —cryotherapy (extreme cold below freezing)—
  gases under pressure
• chemical
  —eschar-forming agents, e.g. silver nitrate—self-
    limiting
  —phenol—protein denatured
  —liquid nitrogen—cell destruction

Incisional (subcutaneous)
• stab—osteotripsy
• along a length linear or curved
• excisional skin biopsy (also punch)
• closing defects (multi-lobed/flaps)

NAILS
Nail reduction (length and thickness)
• manual skills
  —long nails
  —onychomycosis
• power drill
  —onychauxis
  —onychogryphosis
  —onychomycosis

Nail ablation (whole or part of structure)
• onychocryptosis
• onychauxis
• onychogryphosis
• onychomycosis
• involuted (incurvated)

Operative techniques should be undertaken following patient assessment; this should include a full medical history. Once the likely cause of the problem has been established, a management plan should be implemented (Ch. 1).

Objectives

When carrying out operative treatment, a number of factors should be borne in mind. Techniques should be performed in a safe manner. The patient should not leave the clinic with more problems than when they entered. For example, if the patient's skin has been accidentally incised or abraded, appropriate measures should be taken to prevent infection developing. Particular attention should be paid to asepsis in high risk groups. The objectives of operative treatment are the same for any patient situation where there is a risk involved. Techniques should be performed:

• in a safe manner
• with the minimum of discomfort to patients
• using appropriate motor processes
• within an acceptable period of time
• such that the outcome results in sufficient removal of the problem.

General considerations

Prior to discussing each technique in detail, the following areas will be considered:

• clinical procedure
• analgesia
• selection of instruments
• ergonomics
• time management.

Clinical procedure. When employing operative techniques, the patient is put at risk if a portal of entry results, whether inadvertently or as an intended outcome of the technique. It is essential, in this case, that a 'minimum touch' approach is used and attention is paid to the sterilisation of instruments, the use of gloves and the postoperative care of any resulting portal of entry, i.e. with antisepsis and dressings (Ch. 3).

Analgesia. In general, most cutaneous techniques should not give rise to discomfort. Optimal skin tension will reduce unnecessary symptoms during debridement. Some patients may experience varying levels of pain, either as a result of a previous bad experience or because of low pain threshold; when this is identified, anaesthetic should be used, e.g. when enucleating a vascular corn with deep fibrosis. Some of the techniques discussed in this chapter should not be performed without the use of local anaesthesia.

The term 'analgesia' refers to an inability to feel pain, and occurs without loss of consciousness (note that the terms 'anaesthesia' and 'analgesia' are often confused). Sensory loss associated with local anaesthetic (analgesic) has the advantage of allowing procedures involving incision to be undertaken painlessly. Most cutaneous procedures do not require local anaesthesia when the scalpel is used in the correct manner. Ethyl alcohol has the effect of cooling the skin and reducing sensation. This can be used in the form of a fine spray prior to infiltrating the skin with a hypodermic needle. Emla (Astra) is another useful agent, in cream form, which contains 2.5% lignocaine with 2.5% prilocaine. This is spread thickly onto the skin at least 2 hours before using a hypodermic infiltration. These agents add time to any procedure but are worth considering in children or very sensitive patients who become anxious.

Infiltration techniques are used to deposit the analgesic agent near a nerve. Regional anaesthesia is reserved for specific operative procedures as described in Chapter 7, although infiltration may selectively prevent sensory information, allowing complete pain relief (analgesia). Long-acting anaesthetics such as bupivacaine (e.g. Marcain) provide a better analgesic effect. The addition of adrenaline to all anaesthetics is highly beneficial and can extend the period of analgesia to as long as that obtained with Marcain, while maintaining a lower toxic dose in the tissues. In the case of adrenaline, caution must be exercised around the toes as it has a vasoconstrictive effect.

Regional blocks, e.g. a common peroneal block, commonly affect both sensory and motor pathways, although direct infiltration into muscle will have a similar effect at the level of application. The patient should experience only a dull touch on the affected part when it is cut with a sharp instrument. Initially, temperature changes may be perceptible. A posterior tibial block will affect most of the plantar surface (Ch. 7). Direct infiltration can be beneficial when there is a disadvantage in producing more extensive anaesthesia.

Selection of instruments. There is a range of instruments at the practitioner's disposal (Fig. 6.1). It is essential that practitioners use the instrument which is most suitable for the technique they wish to undertake; no one blade should be used for all scalpel-based techniques. Some blades are more suited to enucleation, while others are more suited to debridement.

Use of instruments. The techniques deployed to physically manipulate instruments will vary between practitioners. Tensing of muscles or the use of inappropriate muscles when holding instruments may result in premature fatigue. When reducing tissue by debridement, it is quite difficult to explain in words how much should be removed. The end result, however, should be that the patient's situation is improved compared with that prior to any form of management. The expert practitioner will be able to find a balance between over- and under-reduction. This kind of clinical judgement comes through practice and experience.

Ergonomics. When using the techniques outlined in this chapter, it is important for practitioners to consider their own working environment. For example, occupation-related problems such as back pain, eye strain and repetitive strain injury can result from inappropriate or incorrect seating positions.

Time management. Time is another significant factor in a busy routine clinic. A practitioner may have a very good technique and may achieve the aims outlined earlier, yet may take an inordinate amount of time to do this. Good time management is essential for efficient practice.

SUPERFICIAL TECHNIQUES USED ON SKIN

DEBRIDEMENT AND ENUCLEATION

Indications

Debridement is a French term used to denote the removal of unhealthy tissue (lesions). Lesions lending themselves to local debridement are listed in Box 6.1. The term 'enucleation' is used for this technique when referring specifically to corns.

The objective of debridement and enucleation is to reduce excessive keratinous tissue which acts as an external pressure on the numerous nerve endings. In many cases, the effects of these techniques are short-lived. The decision as to whether a lesion should or should not be debrided must be related to the sequence of the treatment plan. The long-term objective must aim to provide minimal debridement, since the technique may in fact damage the tissues further.

Not all calluses need to be debrided. Calluses occur as a result of a combination of excessive friction, shear and pressure on the skin. They are a normal reaction to excessive stresses on the skin, e.g. the hand of a manual worker usually exhibits thickened skin. In these instances removal of the hard skin is not indicated. Corns need to be enucleated because they tend to be painful lesions and constitute the prime reason for the patient's appointment.

There are few contraindications to debridement and enucleation; those that do exist relate to disorders

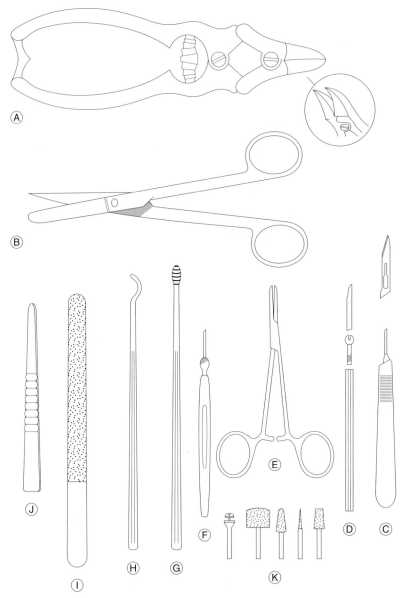

Figure 6.1 Instruments may be selected as preference dictates. A basic set of instruments for superficial cutaneous management is shown. A, nail nippers (cantilever style); B, dressing scissors; C, Baird-Parker handle 3; D, Beaver handle and blade 67; E, grasping forceps, e.g. Spencer-Wells or Halsteads; F, Baird-Parker handle 7; G, Blacks file; H, probe; I, rasp; J, forceps; K, burrs (various) and Moore's disc mandrill.

which affect tissue repair or are related to collagen defects. Patients with vascular impairment, insensate skin or connective tissue disorders, or patients undergoing chemotherapy, are particularly at risk from the complications which may arise from debridement and enucleation. The skin in these cases is easily traumatised and does not heal well. Another category of patient includes those suffering from bleeding diatheses. Patients with conditions such as absent clotting factors, vitamin deficiencies (vitamin C in particular) and fragility of blood vessels should be managed carefully.

Equipment

The scalpel is the most popular and common tool for debridement and enucleation. A nail drill fitted with an abrasive disc can also be used to debride thickened skin. There is a wide variety of differently sized and shaped scalpels and scalpel blades on the market. The 'Beaver' scalpel (Fig. 6.1D) is the one that most closely resembles the traditional solid scalpel, which was used prior to the advent of replaceable blades (Fig. 6.2). The advantage of the Beaver scalpel arises from the ability to fit different styles of 'mini-blade' onto one handle. In Figure 6.1D, only the 67 blade is shown; others do exist, such as blades 61–66, 68 and 69 which have chisel-shaped, pointed or hooked ends. Microblades are also available but they have less application in cutaneous debridement. Blades from the mini-blade system are screwed to a handle of the appropriate design; this offers a greater degree of stiffness over other scalpel handles which are more flexible. Interlocking blades fitted to Baird-Parker (BP) handles (Figs 6.1C and 6.2), for example, have been known to snap when used on dense callosity. In these instances, the sterile disposable blade is dispensed onto the BP scalpel with the appropriate instrument, and removed with safety devices to prevent unnecessary laceration of the practitioner's fingers (Ch. 3).

Interestingly, American podiatrists use chisels, while in the UK, 11 and 15 blades are favoured. The 11 is a straight blade with a sharp point. Both the point and the straight edge are valuable in different situations. The 11 is primarily used for debridement.

In general, a large blade should be used on very thick plantar callus, and a smaller blade should be used on small lesions and lesions on the dorsum or apex of the toes.

For enucleation, a blade with a rounded end should be chosen, as it is this part of the instrument which is used (Figs 6.1D, 6.2[15]). After use on a patient, blades should be either discarded or sterilised. Inevitably the life span of any autoclaved scalpel blade is limited, and only stainless steel blades can be adequately recycled.

Debridement techniques

Using a scalpel

Debridement is not a gross movement; the arm should remain as near to the side as possible. The area surrounding the tissue to be removed is held firmly between finger and thumb as shown in Figure 6.3. Skin tension is important in preventing early blunting of the blade and in maintaining efficient cutting. Movement of the scalpel is achieved through a combination of thumb, forefinger and wrist action. The most common position in which to hold the scalpel is with the distal end between the thumb and forefinger, and the proximal end in the cleft of the fourth and fifth fingers (Fig. 6.4). The practitioner should attempt to make controlled sliced cuts. This is achieved by angling the blade so that it is nearly parallel with the surface. The direction of movement will be dependent upon the site of the callus; usually a distal to proximal action is used.

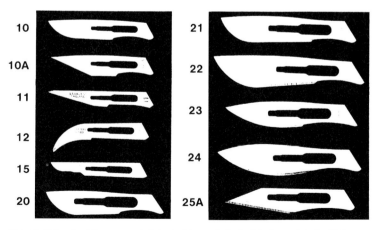

Figure 6.2 A wide range of detachable and sterile blades exists to fit the Baird-Parker (BP handle) systems. A number of variations can be found, such as the Martin and Nova patterns. All blades should be removed with blade removers. (Reproduced with permission from Bailey Instruments.)

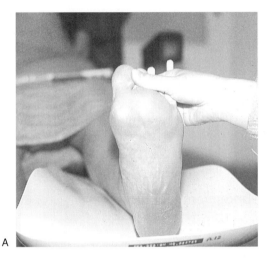

A

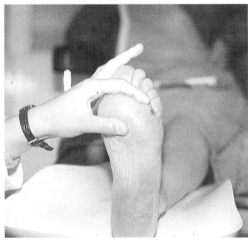

B

Figure 6.3 A, B: In each figure, a different method is shown to achieve skin tension, which contributes to effective use of the scalpel blade and prevents premature dulling of the edge.

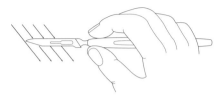

Figure 6.4 Position of the hand when using a scalpel to debride callosity. While the stroke is shown as diagonal to the skin surface, a combined downward stroke improves the cutting efficiency. An 11 blade is illustrated.

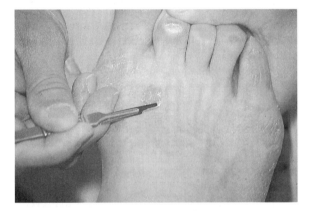

Figure 6.5 Sensitive areas require the practitioner to adopt a different position when holding the scalpel, e.g. debriding on the dorsum of the foot where the blade can inadvertently slip and slice the skin. The backward or reverse position shown offers good control with safety. A 15 blade is illustrated.

The amount of pressure applied to the blade and the angle between the blade and the skin will affect the size of skin particles removed; small particles of the stratum corneum layer should be removed initially, in order to judge the depth of reduction (Fig. 6.5). Deeper and more uneven thickened keratin can prove more difficult. In these cases, especially with uneven callus, an 'ecope' or 'scooping' action can be used. The ecope technique is effective for large areas of callosity complicated by deep furrows. The whole length of the 11 blade is used so that the wrist rotates the scalpel between two ridges.

A callosity comprises skin which has an excessive keratinous build-up and a yellow colour, as opposed to the pinkish colour of skin of normal thickness. Sometimes the skin may be macerated, which makes it look white. Alternative scalpel positions are adopted as necessary, particularly when working in sensitive areas.

Using a nail drill

The sanding disc attachment is fitted to the nail drill by way of a mandrill (Fig. 6.1K). The disc is held parallel to the skin and is moved over the area of thickened skin to be reduced. The practitioner's thumb should be held against the skin to prevent any accidental slippage. A sanding disc is particularly useful where the skin is very dry or fissured, or where the state of the patient's skin is poor; in this case, a scalpel is not as useful because it can pull on delicate skin and, if there are fissures, may exacerbate the situation. The sanding disc can be applied gently to the area and does not result in further trauma.

The area being sanded may become very warm as a result of the friction between the skin and the disc. Sanding discs should be discarded after use on each patient.

Enucleation techniques

For this technique, the scalpel is best held between the finger and thumb, as if one is holding a pencil. Enucleating a corn requires the correct technique and much practice. It is very easy to leave much of the central core behind, causing pain soon after the patient

has had treatment (see Fig. 6.6). It is essential that the overlying callus is debrided prior to enucleation. Failure to do this is one of the most common causes of poor enucleation, resulting in the practitioner enucleating overlying callus.

The term *enucleation* is perhaps a misnomer, as it implies complete removal. Because of this, 'excision' will be used to mean complete removal and 'minute section' will be used for partial removal. With the excision approach, the whole of the corn is removed as one piece without puncturing the dermis which would cause haemorrhage. The blade is held at an

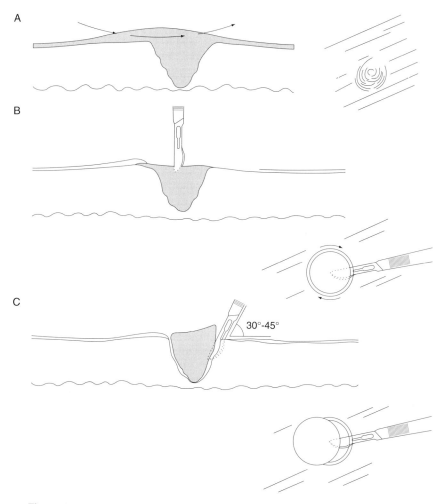

Figure 6.6 A: Debrided overlying callosity should be removed as shown to allow easier access to enucleate the corn. No attempt should be made to incise the lesion until the area has been well demarcated. B: Initially the corn should be incised vertically all the way around its perimeter. C: The blade (D15) should be angled at 45° and moved around the lesion. A grasping forceps may be useful to complete the manoeuvre.

angle of 45° or more to the skin and is worked all the way around the juncture between the corn and normal skin. If the corn is large or if the site of the corn makes enucleation difficult, minute sections can be removed where the patient finds the procedure uncomfortable.

Ultimately, experienced practitioners use the technique they find most acceptable. Variations in the way the scalpel is held will depend upon the site of the lesion. Interdigital lesions are difficult to access, often leading to interdigital cleft injury. The most painful type of corn to enucleate is undoubtedly the intractable plantar keratoma (IPK).

Complications

The following problems may result from both debridement and enucleation:

- haemorrhage
- creation of a portal of entry
- over-reduction/over-enucleation
- under-reduction/partial enucleation
- problems resulting from inappropriate technique.

Creation of a portal of entry. This can be both avoidable and unavoidable. The pathological changes which result in callus and corn formation involve the proliferation of dermal papillae together with small capillary loops. Following debridement, these papillae can be easily damaged, resulting in bleeding. Once this has occurred, further debridement is masked by haemorrhage. Deep and direct pressure with gauze and using gloved hands may stem the flow. Chemical agents of choice can be selected, e.g. styptics or haemostatic dressings; current examples include ferric chloride (15%) aqueous, silver nitrate 20–40% (styptics) or Caltostat, to name but one of many dressings. These types of portal of entry are unavoidable.

Avoidable portals of entry can result from cutting the affected or adjacent unaffected skin either because of poor technique or because the patient suddenly moves. Appropriate aseptic measures should be adopted to dress the wound.

Over-reduction/over-enucleation. If too much of the keratinous build-up is removed, the skin may feel very tender, especially on activity. A thin anti-friction pad, such as fleecy web or moleskin, can be applied to reduce any discomfort. If the over-reduction has been excessive, papillary haemorrhaging may occur, and in this case a dressing will be necessary.

Under-reduction/partial enucleation. Where insufficient keratinous material has been removed, the patient may continue to experience the same discomfort that was being experienced prior to treatment. An aseptic

breakdown due to the presence of bulky keratinous material may occur if this is unattended, especially in patients with poor skin quality or with areas experiencing higher pressures of load.

Problems resulting from inappropriate technique. The use of an unsuitable technique can result in an uneven finish, feathery appearance of the skin and practitioner fatigue. Attention should be paid to the following:

- maintenance of skin tension
- position of the practitioner
- use of muscles and resultant action
- position of the scalpel in relation to the skin
- sharpness of the blade.

Lack of skin tension results in the skin being pulled every time the scalpel blade is laid over the skin; this may lead to a feathery finish. Too much skin tension can give rise to patient discomfort, mask papillary bleeding and lead to practitioner fatigue. The position and action used by the practitioner can also lead to problems. Practitioners must ensure that they are not having to strain or use muscles that should not be used. A blunt blade will result in a feathery appearance to the skin, as the scalpel action will not cut all the way through it. A scalpel which is not held parallel to the skin will result in an uneven appearance when debriding. Failure to use the scalpel correctly when enucleating will produce an unsatisfactory result.

Special considerations

Site. Lesions which require debriding and enucleating may occur on parts of the foot which are difficult to access, e.g. the heel and interdigital clefts. Practitioners should make use of aids, such as foot raisers, to access the heel, especially the posterior surface. It may be necessary to ask the patient to kneel on the chair with his back to you. With subungual corns and calluses, it is necessary to cut back the nail in order to expose the lesion prior to enucleation or debridement.

Excessive callus. Some patients may suffer with extensive callosity. Such occurrences are rare but include conditions such as ichthyosis tylosis where the callosity is present from heel to toes on the plantar surface. These patients may take up to an hour to debride effectively.

Complete excision of corns. Corns can be extremely difficult to manage, even when a range of therapeutic techniques are available. The case history in Box 6.2 illustrates this point, cautioning against the desire for complete removal of corns.

Neuropathic ulcers. These require debridement of

Box 6.2 Case history: removal of callus

A 43-year-old white female nurse presented with a callus under her right foot which failed to resolve with debridement and insoles over a period of years. The patient requested excision, which was performed under regional ankle block. Reoccurrence took 8 weeks. X-rays (with markers) revealed that the site of the corn did not lie beneath any bony prominence. Further surgery was performed using a skin flap to provide a fatty pad covering. The patient gained relief on the second occasion for 6 months, but the lesion returned even though functional orthoses with appropriate redistributive adaptations had been prescribed. Histopathology following both procedures excluded a foreign body or implantation cyst.

Conclusion. The replacement fat was reabsorbed and high shear forces stimulated further hyperkeratotic change. Further surgery has been ruled out because of poor prognosis.

---

the keratinous edges in order to promote healing. Some authorities recommend extensive removal of the keratin in order to stimulate the formation of granulation tissue.

Verrucae. Pathological changes which occur with verrucae bear similarities to changes in callosity, although verrucae have the distinction that they produce papillary haemorrhages. Debridement of overlying callosity is usually indicated before chemical treatment.

Young patients. Most patients will cooperate, but children can be wary, often due to fear of the scalpel. The scalpel is best left out of sight until needed.

Fidgety patients or patients with tremors. Patients with tremors such as Parkinsonism require the scalpel blade and operator almost to move with the tremor to achieve any reasonable result. Attempts can be made to occupy the attention of the fidgety patient by giving them a book to look at.

LANCING AND DRAINAGE

Indications

There are a number of lesions which can benefit from lancing and drainage. This technique is usually employed in acute situations before the condition has become chronic.

Equipment

The pointed end of an 11 blade is most commonly used. In the case of a subungual haematoma, a nail drill and a thin pointed burr are used.

Technique

A blister is usually lanced and drained; the use of two drainage points ensures better reduction of internal pressure than if one drain hole were used, with easier release of pressurised fluid. The epidermal tissue overlying the blister is usually left intact and a compressive dressing applied. Leaving the epidermal surface over the site of the blister gives some protection to the underlying skin and is an attempt to avoid the risks of infection. A septic toe associated with a corn or blister is usually lanced by piercing the skin with the point of the 11 blade. The tip of the blade is placed at an acute angle to penetrate the epidermal surface. If appropriate, the area may then be debrided in order to encourage drainage and remove slough which may impair healing. Particular attention should be paid to antisepsis when undertaking this technique.

Haematoma. A subungual haematoma can give rise to excruciating pain on account of the build-up of pressure under the nail. Within 12 hours of the problem occurring, the fluid can be released by piercing the nail plate. A nail drill with a thin pointed burr is used. The point of the drill is held directly over the lesion and the nail is reduced until the underlying skin is reached, thus allowing the blood to escape.

TECHNIQUES USED ON NAILS

NAIL CARE

Indications

Most people cut their own toenails; however, there are instances when it is either not possible or not appropriate for an individual to undertake this task. The following are examples of patients who may experience difficulty:

- cannot see clearly, e.g. due to glaucoma
- cannot reach their feet, e.g. due to arthritis
- cannot use instruments such as nail nippers
- have abnormal nails which are difficult to cut.

If toenails are not cut on a regular basis, a range of problems may result. Long toenails may pierce the skin of adjacent toes, causing a portal of entry which may result in infection and ulceration. Subungual ulceration may result from pressure caused by footwear pressing onto long nails. These complications are more prevalent in 'at risk' patients.

In general, if patients have normal assessment findings, can see and reach their feet, and can use a pair of nippers, then they should be able to undertake their own routine nail care. Diabetic patients, so long as they have a normal blood supply, normal sensation, no kidney disease, no eye problems and a stable blood glucose level, should also be encouraged to undertake their own routine nail care. Some of the general public, however, are not clear as to how this should be done. People often pick or poke down the sides of the nail, and as a result infections are easy to come by.

This section looks at how routine nail care should be undertaken for those who unable to perform the task themselves and also indicates how the general public should perform this task.

Equipment

A pair of nail nippers and a file are the standard pieces of equipment. Nail nippers offer mechanical advantages over clippers. There are many types available on the market; cantilever styles are probably the most powerful, but can, in the wrong hands, cut through toes. Attention should be paid to the size of the nippers in relation to the size of the hand. Problems with tenosynovitis may result from the combination of a small hand and a large pair of nippers.

A practitioner may also wish to use a Blacks file, probe or scalpel where appropriate. All instruments should be sterilised between patients. In the case of self-care, instruments should be kept clean and washed after use in warm soapy water and dried thoroughly before use on another person.

Technique

An understanding of the anatomy of the nail apparatus, its relationship with the (distal) interphalangeal joint and the contribution made to nail growth by the nail bed, eponychium, hyponychium and sulcal edges is important. Nails should appear smooth—shaped with a slight longitudinal and lateral curvature—dull, and have clean demarcations of the sulci. The nail plate is translucent but will appear pink due to the underlying nail bed. Contrary to common belief, nails should not be cut straight, but marginally curved, depending upon the shape of the distal end of the toe. The nail should not be cut below the free edge. A nail should not be cut in one piece. It is easier, and preferable, to cut a nail in sections. After cutting, the nail should be filed over gently with a nail file, using a one-way action working from proximal to distal. There should be no rough or jagged edges to

catch on hosiery, and the free edge of the nail should be visible. When you have completed the task, check between the digits to ensure that no pieces of nail are present. If left, these will pierce the skin, and lead to an open wound. Unless the patient complains of discomfort, leave the sulci alone.

Complications

Problems may arise if one or more of the following has occurred:

- the skin surrounding the nail has been cut
- the skin of adjacent toes has been cut
- the nail has been cut below the free edge
- a piece of nail has damaged the practitioner's eye.

In the first two cases, appropriate dressing and, if necessary, antisepsis should be used. In the case of cutting below the free edge, long-term problems may result as the skin moulds around the short nail plate and the growing nail presses into surrounding skin. When cut, brittle or thickened nails can act as flying hazards. Eyes are often in danger, due to the position of the practitioner in relation to the patient's foot. Eye goggles can be used to reduce the likelihood of eye damage.

Special considerations

Thickened nails. Some nails may be thickened; the lesser fifth toes are the most likely, due to entrapment against the lateral side of shoes. Thickened nails can be reduced by debridement with a scalpel or by using a nail drill.

Nail tufts. Cutting nails may be a hazard when thick keratin and blood vessels become enmeshed as one, tethering down the nail plate, as in nail tufts or angiokeratoma (Fig. 6.7). Simple nail tufts have a blackened thrombosed appearance and usually arise as a result of previous trauma. Routine care and the use of silver nitrate to chemically cauterise the blood vessels can be helpful. However, this only has a superficial action due to lack of penetration. Serious problems may need to be excised.

Subungual exostoses. Subungual exostoses are not uncommon. The nail plate may be lifted at one end of the nail, so producing a thickened appearance. A lateral X-ray and medial oblique view offer a standard approach to providing a differential diagnosis. Callosity and redness provide all the appearances of an expanding osteochondroma. Surgical excision is the treatment of choice (Fig. 6.8).

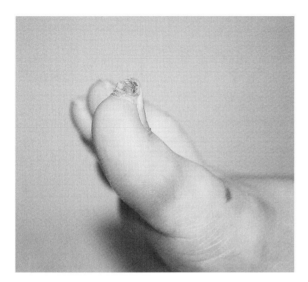

Figure 6.7 An angiokeratoma has caused a problem in trimming the nail. Careful nail management requires the nail to be thinned around the area. Cautery with hyfrecation may be offered, or silver nitrate to attempt to reduce the main vascular involvement. If management fails, surgical excision may be necessary.

Removal of part of the nail may be expedient but may only relieve the patient's discomfort for short periods. An exostectomy should be considered with a view to saving the nail.

Onychomycosis. Nails with this condition vary in appearance and quality, ranging in cross-section from thin to thick and showing varying degrees of discoloration and separation from the nail bed. Some infections produce a brittle, honeycomb appearance in their late stages. Such nails can be removed or reduced so that they are thin enough to allow penetration of creams, ointments and lotions offering an antimycotic action. The nail can be reduced by using a scalpel or, preferably, a nail drill. Borotannic compounds tend to be inadequate in these cases, although they appear to slow fungal growth. The practitioner might also use clotrimazole, miconazole and tioconazole (Trosyl), all of which are painted onto the nail plate. These should be stopped if skin irritation occurs. Medications such as griseofulvin, terbinafine and ketoconazole can be taken systemically, but patients are better off having a nail ablated permanently with phenol if a long period of ingestion is necessary.

Splits and furrows. These are not very common. Median nail dystrophy has the appearance of a 'Christmas tree' rising in the centre of the nail plate. Reducing the asperitous surface so that it is level and smoother can be further assisted by covering with an occlusive cream. Creams might include Calmurid (urea-based) or a flexible collodion such as Opsite (Smith & Nephew).

Painful sulci. Pain may arise from impacted skin debris in the sulci, onychophosis or involuted nails. In the case of debris (shed skin squames), a Blacks file or probe can be used to clear the groove. Prior to using these instruments, the debris can be softened. Shed skin squames will absorb water and swell, so any aqueous solution should assist in softening the debris. Hydrogen peroxide 10–20 vols applied to the sulci is particularly effective. A Blacks file or probe may be used to aid penetration of the hydrogen peroxide and to clear the sulci of debris. Both instruments should be used gently and carefully—if not, the patient may experience severe discomfort and the sulcus can be traumatised, resulting in a break in the skin. Post-

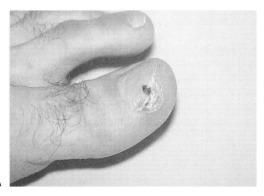

A

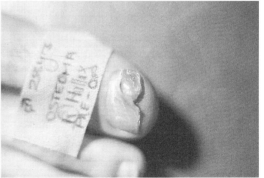

B

Figure 6.8 Two types of exostosis are shown. A: Nail ablation (see later in this chapter) may be offered in the case of mild nail elevation. B: In this case of major nail deformity, the patient should have the bone excised with a view to allowing normal nail regrowth.

operative emollient care is essential to ensure there is not a repeat build-up of debris.

The epidermis can thicken along one or both sides of the nail sulcus, resulting in onychophosis. It is essential that the cause is established and an appropriate management plan implemented. Often the problem is due to lateral pressure from shoes or abnormal foot biomechanics. It may be necessary to cut back the nail in order to expose the lesion; in these instances the minimum amount of nail should be removed. This technique can be quite painful for the patient; local analgesia may have to be used. If a nail has to be cut back, it is essential that the sides are filed with a Blacks file in order to ensure that there are no roughened edges which could lead to further irritation of the sulcus. The callus should be debrided and the corns enucleated. Postoperatively, the sulci can be packed with cotton wool, foam or gauze. A pledget of cotton wool packed with tincture of benzoin (Friar's balsam), although dated, is a cheap and effective method. Other medications such as ichthammol and even clove oil have proven effective as conservative measures. Plastic sulcus gutters are more 'high-tech' but are probably no more effective. Repetitive sulcus pain should be treated by partial nail ablation.

Involuted nails lead to discomfort as a result of the nail irritating the sulcus. In these instances, clearing of the sulci, cutting back the nail and packing of the sulcus are all conservative methods which may be used. However, the deployment of these techniques may result in a vicious circle comprising repetitive conservative treatment, nail regrowth and pain. A partial or, if the nail is very deformed, total nail ablation may be the only way to resolve this problem.

NAIL DRILL

Indications

The nail drill can be used to reduce thickened and deformed nails and hyperkeratosis. Toenails are predisposed to thickening because of the prevalence of traumatic injuries to the foot and the trauma between the foot and shoe. Toenails may also thicken as a result of pathological conditions, e.g. psoriasis. Onychauxis (even thickening) or onychogryphosis (uneven thickening with deformity) may result. If left unattended, subungual ulceration or the piercing of adjacent skin may result.

Equipment

Nail drills can be powered by mains electricity or battery. Battery-powered drills are not as effective as the larger mains-powered drills. The drill can usually operate at variable speeds: 12 000 rpm is perhaps the most efficient. Care should be taken when selecting the speed as the nail plate can become uncomfortably hot if too high a speed is used or if the drill is used for a long period of time. Newer nail drills include a fine water spray. All drills should be fitted with dust extraction in order to prevent occupation-related lung problems and reduce the problem of air-borne contamination arising from nail dust. The dust extraction bags should be changed regularly. Face masks are used by some practitioners in an attempt to reduce inhalation of nail dust, but the efficacy of these is not proven. Nail drills should be regularly maintained.

Burrs which fit into the drill handle come in many shapes and sizes, ranging from fine-pointed burrs to release subungual haematomata, to broad-barrel burrs to reduce nail thickness. The burrs are made from a range of materials, such as steel and diamond. The practitioner should equip the surgery with a selection of burrs (Fig. 6.1). They should be sterilised between treatments. Ultrasonic cleansers can be used to dislodge debris from the burr prior to sterilisation. Care must always be taken to use the correct size. A burr which is too small for the task will result in the drill having to be used for a longer period of time, causing warming of the nail. A burr which is too big may result in periungual damage.

Sanding discs can also be fitted, via an attachment, to nail drills. These discs comprise an abrasive piece of material which is used to sand down hyperkeratosis as previously discussed under debridement.

Burr technique

A one-way action should be used, working from the proximal to the distal end of the nail. The amount of pressure exerted onto the burr will affect the amount of nail reduced. Care should be taken not to apply too much pressure. The pressure should be kept constant, otherwise an uneven nail plate will result. In order to avoid the skin being caught by the burr, the adjacent skin may be masked by covering it with adhesive plaster cut to the shape of the surrounding skin. If the patient experiences discomfort, usually as a result of the nail becoming warm, stop the drill and spray the nail with an alcohol-based spray, returning once the nail has cooled down. It may be helpful to cut the length down and strip off the top layer of keratin with nippers prior to using the drill. In this way the plate is thinned, allowing for easier drilling.

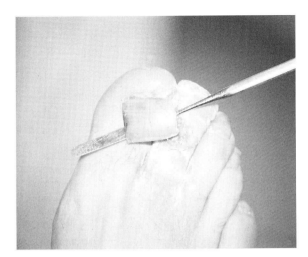

Figure 6.9 This patient presented with total lysis of the nail plate. This should be removed using local anaesthetic if attachment to the nail bed is still evident. All nails should be cut back as far as the nail is separated.

Complications

The main complication from using the drill is the creation of a portal of entry due to removing too much skin or nail, or catching adjacent skin. Appropriate antiseptic and dressing measures should be undertaken to prevent infection. Avoid using cotton wool around spinning burrs, as these can become entangled.

Special considerations

Subungual ulceration. The practitioner must reduce any lytic (detached) parts of nail plate. If the plate is loose, remove it; nails that are lytic should be cut back as much as is allowed (Fig. 6.9). The ulcer heals with little assistance. Pain or infection should settle within a day or two in uncompromised patients. An antiseptic with sterile dressing should be applied.

NAIL SURGERY

NAIL ABLATION

Nail ablation techniques are indicated for a range of nail conditions:

- involution
- ingrowing toenail (onychocryptosis)
- abnormal structure and shape
- hypertrophy
- atrophy
- direct trauma
- minor exostosis
- soft tissue granulation
- onychomycosis
- subungual wart
- discoloration and lysis
- ungual fibromata
- subungual exostosis.

Involuted nails or ingrowing toenails, sometimes abbreviated to IGTN or o/c, are by far the most common reasons for performing nail surgery. Ablation means removal by surgery of a part, while avulsion suggests plucking out or tearing away. A range of ablation techniques may be performed on the nail. For the purposes of this chapter, these techniques will be divided into invasive and non-invasive. Non-invasive techniques relate to those procedures which do not cut into the skin and expose subdermal tissues. Using this approach, nail ablation techniques can be classified as follows:

- Non-invasive
  —partial nail ablation
  —total nail ablation
- Invasive
  —Winograd
  —Frost
  —Zadik
  —Syme's amputation.

The most common *non-invasive technique* is ablation with phenol. This is used in most of the cases which would benefit from removal of part or all of the nail.

Invasive techniques for removing part of the nail are indicated when a large piece of periungual tissue needs to be removed in concert with the nail. Invasive techniques may not have the highest success rates, but the toe does heal faster than is the case with non-invasive techniques. They are therefore useful for those patients who need to recover quickly and for those who, if they failed to heal, might be compromised. This latter group includes steroid users, diabetics and those likely to be over-sensitive to chemical cautery.

Where possible, only part of the nail is removed in order to maintain the cosmetic appearance of the remaining part. Conditions such as involution and ingrowing toenails can be treated by this partial removal. In general, if more than 50% of the nail needs to be removed, a total nail ablation should be considered. The cosmetic appearance of the nail will be worse if only a small amount of nail is left. Some conditions, such as onychomycosis, discoloration and lysis, require the whole nail to be removed if treatment is to be successful.

Healthy vascular perfusion must be the most important criterion for any surgical technique. Presence of dorsalis pedis does not automatically suggest good perfusion to a toe; the posterior tibial artery is more important as it is the larger supplier of blood to the toes.

Non-invasive techniques can be performed in the presence of infection as long as it is restricted to the periungual tissues. When cellulitis is present, affecting more than the nail apparatus, a 1 week course of oral antibiotics is usually recommended prior to surgery. Non-invasive techniques can be undertaken in the second week, provided that the toe has responded to antibiosis. Healing will be more rapid once the source of infection is removed, particularly if drainage of the toe can be established.

Invasive techniques may also be performed in the presence of infection, but again with antibiotic cover. Incisional surgery will release pus that has been walled off. Deeper bone tissue must be protected. Local anaesthetics should not be infiltrated into infected tissue as this may result in the infection spreading. It is best to use proximal blocks wherever possible.

Malignancy

The nail plate should be examined for suspected subungual melanoma; these may take on the appearance of dark streaks. A specialist should be consulted prior to operating if a suspicious lesion around the nail plate is observed; biopsy is essential to confirm diagnosis. The prognosis and survival rates vary depending on speed of diagnosis, thickness of the lesion and the type of melanoma. Radical excision is considered important around the boundary of the melanoma. Usually it is better for toes to be amputated, as grafting skin later can create difficulties with seeding.

Contraindications to nail surgery

The main reasons why invasive and non-invasive techniques may be contraindicated are:

- unsuitability for the administration of local analgesia
- poor healing post surgery
- bleeding disorders
- psychosocial problems resulting in poor aftercare or compliance
- severe uncontrolled organic disease.

Collagen disorders produce thin atrophic skin. In particular, scleroderma is contraindicated in order to avoid circulatory embarrassment. Active skin lesions

---

Box 6.3 Case history

A 47-year-old white female was treated by her general practitioner for 6 months for an infected toe. Exuberant granulation was noted which was subsequently excised. Closure could only be achieved once part of the distal phalanx had also been excised. At 6 months, excellent restoration of the toe was recorded despite loss of fat and bone (Fig. 6.10A).

Conclusion. Histopathology revealed multiple sinuses within a large granular nodule due to abscess formation. Antibiotics had failed to reach the site and the patient would have been placed at risk from osteomyelitis if the lesion remained unattended.

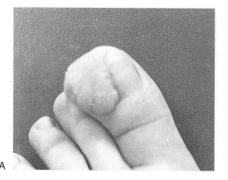
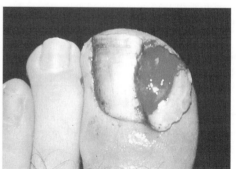

A   B

Figure 6.10 A: Unsuccessful treatment of an ingrowing nail which has formed abscesses.
B: Common presentation of ingrowing nail or onychocryptosis with exuberant hypergranulation.

such as psoriasis or eczema should also be avoided due to increased reactivity of the skin.

Peripheral vascular disease may be a reflection of other disease, of which diabetes is the most common. Failure to heal may give rise to secondary complications such as infection and gangrene. Patients undergoing chemotherapy or radiotherapy, or receiving high doses of steroids are at risk. Failure to heal or produce a normal immunological response to infection may be very serious for at-risk patients.

Patients who are malnourished or who cannot attend to their own hygiene will be unsuitable. Patients who have suffered strokes, who have a mental disability, should be judged on their individual merits. Patients with known violent tendencies tend to be unsuitable for local anaesthetics. Patients should not return home unaccompanied if attending for day surgery. Good support at home is needed for the immediate 24 hour period of postoperative recovery.

Patients with sickle cell anaemia (not the sickle cell trait) should not have tourniquets applied. Current medical convention is that patients with implants, Dacron bypass vessels and faulty heart valves must have prophylactic antibiotics.

Technique

Local anaesthetics. Nail ablation procedures affecting toes should be performed with good anaesthetic techniques (Fig. 6.11). The use of adrenaline is considered to be contraindicated. The effects of vasoconstrictors in digital analgesia may not be as much of a problem as has previously been suggested, and this type of analgesia is commonly used by American podiatrists without detrimental ischaemia; nonetheless, excessive use of any injectable substance around the base of a digit (as in a ring block) may compress vessels. Common sense dictates the utmost caution with vasoconstrictors, although when used as a hemiblock, haemorrhage from granulation tissue is controlled with little risk to the patient, thus dispelling some of the previous concerns about vasoconstrictors. Vascular risks probably increase with age, as digital vessels become less competent with degeneration of

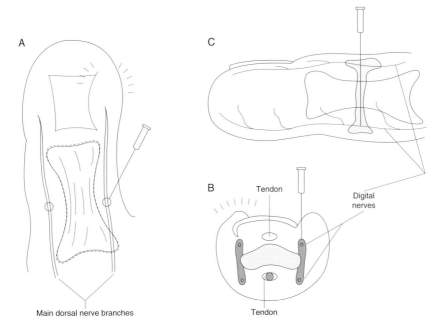

Figure 6.11 Digital blocks. Full ring blocks should be avoided if at all possible. The toes are infiltrated at the base of the proximal phalanx as shown. For a total block, the lateral side should be infiltrated first, as the skin is looser. Dorsal to plantar injections are common for single sides. A full ring block would encompass the whole toe; the volume should be strictly monitored in respect to the toe size and can cause a tourniquet effect. A: Dorsoplantar view. B: Lateral view. C: Cross-section showing position of nerves and tendons. The shaded area shows the deposit of anaesthetic.

the vessel lumen; such findings have been observed when performing amputations without tourniquet.

Local anaesthesia with prilocaine (plain) 1–4% is adequate for most tasks, although many prefer lignocaine or mepivacaine. Most digits require no more than 2 ml, taking some 10–20 minutes to produce numbness for surgical ablation. Bupivacaine is more toxic, and some consider that it should not be used routinely for this type of procedure, although there is no evidence to support this view. Failure to achieve sufficient analgesia may require changing the anaesthetic agent. A useful test is to place a blunt seeker down the painful nail sulcus to establish the depth of analgesia. Pricking the skin with syringe needles for this purpose is not advised and will cause reactive wheals following histamine release; a clean blunt paper clip suffices.

Sterile field. Once anaesthesia has been achieved, the skin is prepared and a local sterile field established. The practitioner should be wearing sterile gloves. Non-invasive procedures can be performed in a clean clinical area with just a local sterile field. In the case of invasive techniques, particularly those affecting bone, a dedicated operating room is required with observation of the correct surgical protocol.

Equipment. Instruments should be freshly autoclaved, or pre-packed by a sterile supply department. A basic set of instruments for nail surgery is illustrated in Figure 6.12.

Tourniquet. It is essential that exsanguination is achieved. A sterile ring tourniquet (Tournicot) or Esmarch band provides adequate haemostasis. Exsanguination should take place from the distal to the proximal end of the toe. Tourniquets should be retained for a minimum period, ideally under 30 minutes to avoid congestion and swelling later.

Non-invasive

Total nail removal. Total nail ablation requires separation of the hyponychial edge. An elevator is pushed under the plate, thus breaking the bond between the villus-like connection, known as the onychodermal band (Fig. 6.13), and is then pushed proximally under the plate until all resistance ceases. The eponychial fold is freed to prevent tearing. A mosquito or Spencer-Wells forceps is clamped either side of the nail plate; a strong pair of forceps is recommended. The forceps are twisted to the centreline of the plate. The nail usually comes away in one piece. The nail bed is cleaned and dried. The practitioner must make sure that no small nail segments or loose pieces of skin remain.

Partial nail removal. Wedge or partial resection

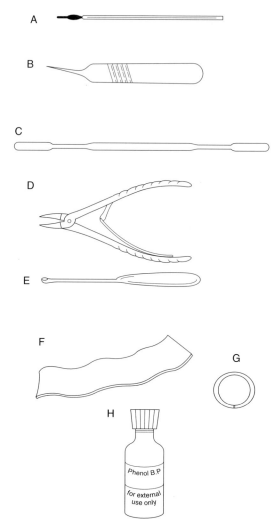

Figure 6.12 A basic set of instruments used for nail surgery comprises: A, small probe (phenol application); B, nail splitter; C, nail elevator; D, straight forceps (Stamms shown); E, curette; F, Esmarch tourniquet; G, tournicot; H, correctly labelled phenol for external use only. The instrumentation also includes two Spencer-Wells forceps and a scalpel as shown in Figure 6.1.

should ideally only remove 25–30% of the plate. The reason for this lies in the need to preserve some sensible cosmetic appearance (Fig. 6.14). If a greater proportion of nail is removed, the nail plate might just as well be removed in one piece. Once the tight adhesion of the most lateral side of the eponychial fold is released, by positioning an elevator to separate the two, a pair of fine, straight-sided nippers can be used to cut down the nail. The nippers are pushed firmly down the length of the nail plate until a point

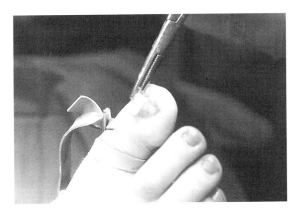

Figure 6.13 Nail ablation is achieved by manual separation of the nail plate from the nail bed, working from the hyponychial (distal or free edge) border. The plate will separate easily once the onychodermal band has been freed.

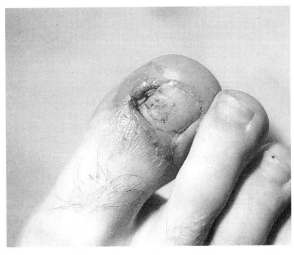

Figure 6.14 The partial nail ablation (PNA) is designed to remove up to 30% of the nail permanently when the matrix is destroyed. The illustration shows a PNA at first dressing. A small amount of inflammation is present around the base of the toe and on the medial side.

is reached when they either meet resistance or cannot progress further. If needed, a Beaver with a 61 blade (chisel-shaped) or nail splitter can be used to cut the remaining nail edge. The nail will give at the most proximal point. It must be appreciated that the most proximal limit of resistance is against the distal phalanx, which lies close to the interphalangeal joint. The risk of infection is greatest at this point. Forceps should grasp the spicule, rotating the piece towards the midline. It is incumbent upon the practitioner

to check down the open sulcus and feel for deep fibrous attachments and broken nail; leaving a loose piece of nail in the sulcus will promote infection.

Destruction of the matrix. Chemical and thermal treatments have been used to destroy the nail matrix. The following methods have been used:

- phenol (carbolic acid)
- sodium hydroxide
- trichloroacetic acid
- nitrous oxide
- carbon dioxide
- negative galvanism
- silver nitrate stick.

Phenol is by far the most popular method and is a powerful steriliser, a point well established by Lister in 1865. Exsanguination (removal of blood) is essential, as blood will dilute the phenol as it coagulates protein on contact. Diluted phenol will effectively reduce the success of the operation. Phenol can be used at 80% strength or as a saturated solution. Eighty per cent phenol appears to be as effective as the saturated solution and may reduce the number of phenol burns.

There has been much speculation about the best way to apply phenol. Originally, three separate 1 minute times were used. Phenol has a continuous action and is therefore probably not sensitive to time alone. Tissue uptake is likely to be more relevant. Fragile older tissues need less time than young healthy tissue. The change from pink to dirty brown-white is a useful indication. Moist (hyperhidrotic) tissues may need longer.

The type of phenol is also important. Phenol should be fresh and have no pink tinge. This can best be achieved by throwing small bottles of liquid or crystals away after each use.

One of the problems associated with nail ablation techniques is regrowth. Andrew & Wallace (1979) found that, out of 107 patients treated by phenolic destruction of the matrix, only 6% required further treatment, compared to 18% who needed further treatment following surgical excision. Ramsey & Caldwell (1985) provided evidence of only 3% of regrowth in 1013 cases. Chemical preparations, such as 10% sodium hydroxide and trichloroacetic acid, have also been used with success.

Freezing with gases such as nitrous oxide was reported by Tollafield (unpublished work, 1980). Healing appeared to be better than with phenol, but the apparatus to procure a freeze was expensive and needed specialist probes. In a small research project of seven cases, patients experienced greater postoperative pain from nitrous oxide than phenol. In 1983, Apfelberg (see Apfelberg 1987) described the use of carbon dioxide for nail ablation.

Polokoff described the use of negative galvanism in 1961 (see Polokoff 1987). This is an electrical technique which produces sodium hydroxide at the site of the active (cathode) electrode with a direct current, as opposed to an alternating current. Negative galvanism is performed without a tourniquet. Technically, this is not a popular technique, in that it is time-consuming and produces a slight electrical hazard for patients with metal implants and pacemakers. Cautery loops have been used. Thin metal wires become heated with a small current, offering another form of thermal destruction.

Invasive

Zadik. Zadik (1950) described the procedure of surgical ablation by dissecting the matrix away. This is a difficult procedure and should be reserved for experienced specialists, as partial regrowth is common. The process requires active debridement of the bone, peeling away the matrix carefully. The lines of incision must be carried on down the lateral sides of the nail apparatus to avoid spicular regrowth (Fig. 6.15A).

Winograd. Winograd described the partial matricectomy in 1929 (see Winograd 1987; Fig. 6.15B). The

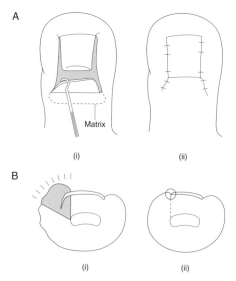

Figure 6.15 Various types of surgical nail ablation can be achieved by excising the matrices. A: Zadik's operation for total nail bed excision: (i) incision lines, (ii) sutured flaps. B: Cross-sections through Winograd procedure for extensive paronychial tissue excision.

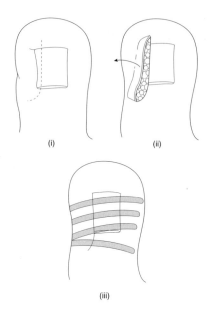

Figure 6.16 Partial matricectomy (Steindler or Frost) for minimal exposure matrix excision (i, ii). Sterile tapes (Steristrips) have been used to close the wound (iii).

excised tissue is sutured afterwards. Any cells left behind commonly produce new nail growth. This tends to occur in partial cases of removal at the proximal edge of the sulcus. The appearance is that of a little horn. If this occurs following healing, a small amount of liquid phenol can be placed on the site once the nail spicule has been ablated.

Partial matricectomies (Frost and Steindler). These two techniques differ from the Winograd procedure in that a flap of periungual tissue is raised (Fig. 6.16). Sutures or sterile tapes can be used after deep dissection has been completed to secure the wound. Necrosis of flaps can occur if the skin is cut too thinly without regard for the blood supply. Postoperative healing is rapid (Fig. 6.17).

MANAGEMENT FOLLOWING NAIL SURGERY

There are a great number of ideas in the literature, ranging from packing the sulcus at the time of surgery, to keeping the initial dressing on for 7 days before redressing. Some advocate bathing through the dressing by immersing toe and bandage in saline. Removal of the dressing after 24 hours is also practised. Daily bathing in a footbath is also common.

Packing the sulci after surgery, often with a paraffin tulle, results in the dressing becoming hard and may cause discomfort, especially when attempts are made

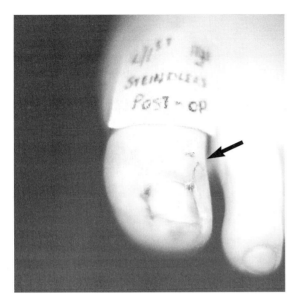

Figure 6.17 Non-phenol technique—postoperative view of Steindler procedure closed with Steristrip sutures.

to remove it. Some practitioners dislike the use of packing as they consider drainage may be prevented, particularly as phenol intentionally causes a discharge. There is no evidence to suggest that packing helps healing. Patients who keep their dressing on for 7 days may find that they develop a pungent odour, the dressing becomes discoloured and, in some cases, where there has been a discharge, strike-through occurs. Immersion in a salt footbath with the dressing on does not appear to have any advantage over bathing with the dressing off, as long as a new dressing is reapplied. A suitable environment needs to be created for healing. The oedema and resultant exudate which may occur postsurgically may well reduce the rapidity of such a process. In most cases, postoperative resolution is achieved by simple cleansing and good hygiene. However, where the nail bed becomes macerated or a sulcus becomes particularly inflamed, an antiseptic should be used. Fucidin and cicatrin (topical antibiotic agents) are no more beneficial, and may cause a risk of skin sensitivity. Creams such as Ponoxylan (now more difficult to purchase) have an anti-inflammatory effect, which is thought to be highly beneficial in drying the nail bed following surgery.

Altman et al (1990) considered other products applied topically after nail surgery. A control, silver sulphadiazine, and hydrocortisone 1% creams were used separately and in combination. Criteria used to judge success revolved around reduction of pain, discharge, inflammation and drainage. The combintional product was slightly more effective in reducing the four associated criteria. The control did surprisingly well. Altman et al were able to show that using hydrocortisone did not impair healing and can be helpful in postoperative nail surgery care. Silver sulphadiazine is a topical medicament useful in the management of burns.

Complications arising from non-invasive nail ablation

Complications are not uncommon with nail surgery. Four weak links exist and give rise to problems in any surgical situation. These include the operator, the technique used, the environment and the patient.

Infection. Phenol procedures have a slightly higher chance of becoming infected than do others. The reason for this lies in the resultant oedema in digital tissue, the open nature of the wound and damaged tissue which is devitalised by the effects of the caustic.

Infection should be treated with antiseptics in the early stages and by copious daily bathing, depending upon the patient's own capability and mobility. Antibiotics should be reserved for the occasion when the wound fails to respond to antiseptics, or where culture and sensitivity shows a positive infection. If poor healing (without proven infection) continues for several weeks, antibiotics appear to improve the situation. Tollafield & Parmar (1994) noted in a 5-year surgical audit that antibiotics often fail to give adequate relief unless the course is extended to 10–14 days for foot infections. *Staphylococcus aureus* is the most common infective agent and flucloxacillin is the drug of choice, at a dose of 250 mg (adult) q.d.s. Allergies and sensitivities are not uncommon to this effective group of antibiotics, and erythromycin may be given as an alternative, at a dose of 250 mg every 6 hours.

Phenol burns. Phenol techniques may appear easy to use, but they should not be employed by the inexperienced practitioner who cannot appreciate the care required in applying an invisible caustic. The chemical often does not show its most potent effects for several hours, after the toe has lost its anaesthetic effect. Phenol spillage should be avoided as it provokes a pernicious response and may take many weeks to heal, even on healthy skin (Fig. 6.18). Burns due to phenol spillage on the skin must be protected from infection and the patient must be warned about such a risk and told how to minimise the problem. Most toes heal in the end. Patience is more likely if the patient knows the risks from nail surgery in advance.

Delayed healing. Healing is sometimes slow, and can

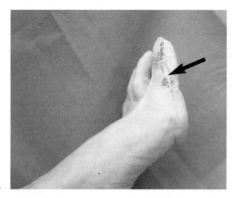 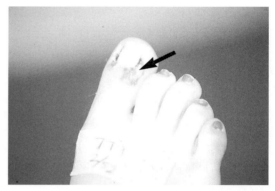

A   B

Figure 6.18   Phenol can leave considerable tissue damage if care is not taken. This burn took many weeks to recover despite the phenol only remaining on the skin briefly. A: Spillage down the side of the toe. B: Over-zealous phenolisation around the base of the hallux.

last from 1 week to 5 months. Drainage is common for 3–4 weeks, but does not always sustain significant cultures. The larger the surface area phenolised, the more likely it is that a patient will heal slowly. However, it has been found that total ablations do not necessarily always follow this trend, because nails that have undergone this technique drain better than those that have undergone partial ablations. Likewise, age and tissue quality appear to have some bearing upon healing. The older skin tends to be weaker to the effects of phenol and may take longer to heal.

Periostitis. Periostitis may occur as a result of phenolisation techniques, although it is rarely documented. Gilles et al (1986) reported the case of a 29-year-old woman who had a positive culture recorded with a pyrexic state of 98.6°F. Periosteal elevation, seen on X-ray, is less evident in the absence of pus. X-rays are important for ruling out osteomyelitis, which is indicated in the phalanges by radiolucency. Periosteal elevation is less likely unless there is sufficient pus. If periostitis is suspected and the presence of infection has been ruled out, a Sher injection should be administered; this technique involves placing 0.1–0.2 ml of corticosteroid into the epidermal edge under a ring block of anaesthesia. The injection should be performed at 90° to the surface, to avoid damaging the dermal blood supply.

Hypergranulation (Fig. 6.10B). Hypergranulation may be detrimental if left. The excessive vascular tissue can distort the toe and, if abundant, can recreate the problem, as seen in Fig. 6.10A. Small amounts of pink tissue can be left without too much concern. The easiest technique for removing tissue is to cut it away with nippers (Stamm bone nippers) or to dissect it with an elliptical cut. The deeper and wider the cut, the more difficult it will be to close the wound. Larger

sections of hypergranulation may need to be curetted when trimmed, in order to leave a clean granulating base. Phenol should not be allowed to seep into this part of the wound.

Postoperative pain. Pain that does not respond to basic analgesics such as paracetamol compounds should be carefully examined to rule out reflex sympathetic dystrophy (RSD). Radiographic features (Sudek's atrophy) may take several weeks to show. Vasomotor changes cause alarming colour patterns, such as hot flushed to a mottled cyanosed effect, either at the site or over the whole foot. The condition is poorly understood and pain is triggered by inconsequential trauma (Tollafield 1991). If pain cannot be alleviated within 4 weeks and there are no signs of infection, a pain clinic should be consulted.

Regrowth. Regrowth of nails following surgery is an accepted hazard. Practitioners will accept this inevitability at some time in their careers, but should take all steps to minimise its occurrence. Patients must be warned that not every case is successful and that re-phenolisation may be necessary; this can be achieved by dropping some phenol down the nail groove, once the spicule has been removed under local analgesia, if required.

Complications arising from invasive techniques

Sutures have been found to increase postoperative pain (Tollafield 1994). The preferred method of closure is surgical taping for 2 weeks. Regrowth of nails following invasive surgery described above is higher than from phenolisation by 30–40%. The infection rate seems no higher than that resulting from phenol techniques; it may even be a little lower. There are no risks from burns, but inclusion cysts do occur where nail cells become incorporated into the wound at the proximal edge.

INCISIONAL APPROACHES TO SURGERY

Indications

There are a number of reasons for incising the skin on the foot, and these fall into four categories:

1. to gain access to perform a surgical procedure to correct or ameliorate a problem that lies deep to the skin (Ch. 7)
2. to release a deep-seated abscess from pressure of exudate and pus, to remove an old suture or to remove a foreign body, e.g. an inclusion cyst
3. to remove a verruca that does not respond to conservative treatment
4. to remove a section of a lesion for histological investigation when its precise nature is unclear.

Each of the above examples results in the need for a surgical operation which will require anaesthesia, haemostasis and appropriate postsurgical care. The instruments used will vary according to personal preference. Such instruments should ideally be pre-packed and sterilised by a licensed department together with drapes and dressings. The majority of techniques described in this chapter use instruments which can be packed in small pre-sterilised bags. Surgery performed to a depth greater than that of the subcutaneous layers requires specialised instruments. The description and discussion of the various uses of such instruments is left to other texts.

Techniques

Principles of incision

The following discussion concerns the general principles behind skin incisions. All operative techniques should be planned to provide the best result possible. The site and direction of the incision are important considerations. An incision should be long enough to gain access to the anatomy. It may be easily lengthened but should not be stretched so that blood vessels near the surface are damaged. Linear (straight) incisions are easier to close (with suture repair) than tortuous or lacerated wounds. The blade which cuts through the epidermis must do so vertically to avoid stripping the delicate neurovascular supply between the dermis and epidermis. Careful tissue handling

is imperative in order to avoid large contusions (bruises) below the surface and trauma that might create necrosis. Such problems will lead to sloughing and raise the risks of infection and hypertrophic scarring. The epidermal skin must not be squeezed tightly or pulled under tension needlessly with forcep-type instruments.

For many years, the plantar surface of the foot has been considered as a 'no go' area. However, some operations do require access through this surface. Where possible, the skin should be incised to one side of the metatarsal in order to prevent scarring over a load-bearing surface. Extrusion of plantar fat from a weight-bearing area is a sure way to invite a corn or intractable plantar keratoma.

Linear incisions should never be made across a joint. Cicatrisation or scarring may limit movement and cause contraction. Examples of these areas include the dorsal metatarsophalangeal surface and the anterior surface of the ankle. The incision should curve so that potential contraction is spread in more than one direction. Known anatomical structures should be avoided.

There are parts of the foot where incision lines must be made in specific directions. If a round-bodied instrument, such as an awl, is inserted about 2.5 cm into the skin of these parts, the wound lengthens rather than showing up as a round hole. This phenomenon was identified by Dupuytren in 1834, and expounded by Langer in 1861—hence the term Langer lines. When sufficient holes were made in a cadaver, they formed the pattern of these lines. Langer found that the connective tissue attached to muscle underlying the skin was disturbed and affected the constant tension within the skin. Such lines run perpendicular to the action of muscles and may or may not coincide with wrinkle lines. Scars made along the Langer lines are considered to interfere less with body dynamics when placed transversely (perpendicular to the action) across muscles and joints. Testing for these lines can give rise to variance, as found by Cox in 1941 (McGlamry 1987). Pinching the skin deeply, to take in underlying tissues, shows resistance in one direction. By pinching in a direction perpendicular to this, the skin is picked up more easily. If the skin is squeezed too superficially, it will be difficult to differentiate the line of relaxed tension. The use of tension can assist in a simple skin biopsy.

Planning surgery in advance

Once an excisional wound has been created, the surgeon cannot always rely upon closure from double ellipse incision. Faced with a gap, two alternatives arise. The gap can be left—if it is closed, the blood supply will be compromised due to the tension of the skin—or the skin can be incised in such a way as to allow the defect (or gap) to be repaired as well. Naturally there are situations where skin autografts are required, e.g. where the defect is large. Surgery that may lead to possible unpredictable problems must be performed by trained surgeons in the correct theatre setting, where equipment and hospital can provide adequate support for any unexpected needs.

Curettage

This means literally 'to clear out'. Verrucae with well defined circumscribed outlines respond well to this technique; however, other, non-surgical treatments do exist and will be described in Chapter 15. Curettage is also a valuable technique for scraping the base of wounds such as ulcers, hypergranulation, pyogenic granuloma and the base of excised verrucae. Curettage is often performed with electrocautery, which offers haemostasis. This technique should only be used for small lesions which will not produce extensive scarring on healing. Larger lesions are better dealt with by incision and suturing in order that healing can occur by primary intention.

The force required to curette a lesion within the epidermis is significant. In order to reduce the size of this force, the lesion should initially be incised in a circular manner, using a scalpel to the level of dermis. The sharp edge of the curette is then inserted into the incision. Curettage is not the method of choice for producing histology samples, as too much cellular damage may occur.

Biopsy techniques

Biopsy involves the removal of a part, or all, of a lesion for histopathological testing. Three techniques can be used: excisional, shave or puncture biopsy. Excisional biopsy has the advantage of providing a tissue sample and treatment at the same time. The excisional biopsy technique comprises a double ellipse incision around the skin lesion. The length needs to be four times the width, in order to achieve adequate closure of the wound. The shave biopsy is achieved by pinching up the skin and slicing the lesion across; this allows fat and dermis to remain. The main difficulty with this technique lies in the need to ensure that all cells are adequately biopsied, reducing the need for further tissue samples. This technique is rarely used on the foot.

A punch biopsy can be used to provide a sample from a large lesion but brings with it the disadvantage that a further operation may be needed later.

Wound closure

Having incised the skin, it is essential that the appropriate environment is created to ensure that healing takes place. The principles of repair are as follows:

- control haemorrhage
- provide good tissue apposition
- enhance repair
- minimise scarring
- restore function.

Suture materials. The following materials can be used for sutures (*sutura*—Lat. 'seam'):

- adhesive surgical tape (various sizes)
- synthetic braided threads
- synthetic monofilament threads, e.g. nylon, polypropylene
- natural materials, e.g. silk, cotton.

Sutures are either absorbable or non-absorbable. Absorbable sutures are subject to degradation within human tissue. Suture strength is determined by the type of material and size and by the suture technique used. As a rule, this strength is measured in days. Catgut (collagen from the intestines of sheep) lasts about 1 week before it loses its strength. It is highly reactive and not used in the foot very often. Chroming the catgut (tanning) will increase the strength to 3 weeks. Common absorbable sutures used are polyglactin 910 or polyglycolic acid (PGA), and these can retain their strength for 40–60 days.

Non-absorbable sutures are derived from modern plastics, although cotton, silk and steel wire are still available. The two most commonly used sutures are polypropylene and polyethylene. Such materials are hypoallergenic and therefore relatively inert.

The size of a suture is determined by its gauge. '000' or '3/0' lies in the middle of the range of common surgical sutures. 1/0 is large and thick, while 6/0 is small and fine.

Needles. Each suture is suaged to a needle. This means that the small attachment of suture to needle does not result in skin being stretched at the point of skin exit, as there is no 'eye' spreading out behind the needle.

Needles come in all shapes. The curved shape allows the needle to be recovered easily from the opposing side of the wound. Larger sutures and their needles tend to have larger curvatures. Quarter circles of

A

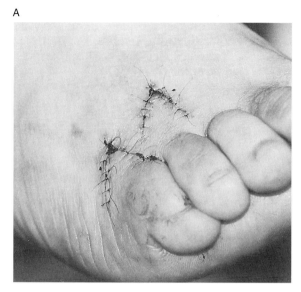

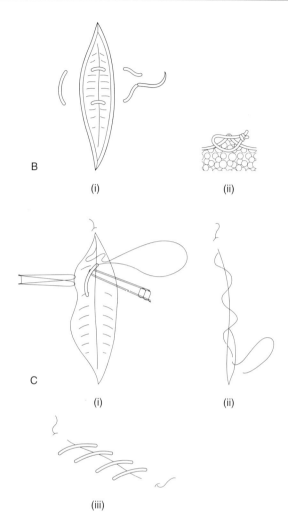

Figure 6.19 Methods of suturing (adapted from Mercado 1976) A: Simple suture. This is formed from a single loop of thread which is tied off as a reef knot. The advantage lies in the fact that it is easy to perform and the wound has an even spread of tension along its length, as long as the sutures are spaced evenly. If an infection arises, one or more sutures can be removed without compromising the wound. The patient in this figure has been incised with two V-Y flaps to reduce the fourth and fifth toes. 5/0 sutures of polypropylene have been used to minimise damage to the sensitive blood supply under the skin. B: Horizontal mattress. This type of suture offers two main advantages. Firstly, the suture is made up of two loops, and thus closure is faster than with the simple suture (i). This suture is also harder to remove than the simple suture. Secondly, the wound haemostasis is improved because the skin is compressed (ii). C: Subcuticular suture. This is chosen for its cosmetic postsurgical results. It cannot be placed in a wound where tension is required. The suture is placed through the skin below the dermal-epidermal junction (i). By pulling on both ends, the wound pulls together (ii). Absorbable sutures do need to be bridged. Sterile tape is often used to support the wound after closure (iii).

19–20 mm are the commonest size for foot surgery. The length of needle represents its length before curvature. Half-circle needles are useful for deep wounds.

The cross-section of the needle is important for its function. A rounded cross-section might be fine for fat or mucous tissues, but epidermis is tough and will bend the needle quickly. A triangular cross-section with a trocar point offers strength and ease of application. Cutting and reverse-cutting needles are popular for use in the tough tissues of the foot.

Suture techniques. The techniques used to close wounds must ensure that the skin edges are brought together and not buried, otherwise an epidermoid cyst could result. Three common techniques are shown in Figure 6.19, although there are many other variations which can be found in surgical texts.

General considerations when suturing
- Wounds should never be closed in the presence of infection
- Sutures should never be placed under tension
- Sutures in the foot should be removed between 10 and 21 days; plantar repair requires 21 days
- Stitch abscesses can occur due to intra-epidermal irritation from buried suture ends.

SUMMARY

This chapter has covered the range of basic operative

techniques which can be used to treat lesions affecting the epidermis and dermis, including the nail apparatus.

A range of examples have been illustrated to demonstrate the breadth of clinical skills required. The general considerations and complications which may occur have been discussed, together with their management. The chapter has provided a broad overview but does not purport to provide sufficient depth for all types of foot surgery. It is essential that the reader consults more detailed texts.

REFERENCES

Altman M I, Sulensky C, De Lisle R, De Velasco M, 1990 Silver sulfadiazine and hydrocortisone cream in the management of phenol matricectomy. Journal of American Podiatric Medical Association 80(10): 545–547

Andrew T, Wallace W A 1979 Nail bed ablation—excise or cauterise? A controlled study. British Medical Journal 9: 1539

Apfelberg D B 1987 In: McGlamry E D (ed) Comprehensive textbook of foot surgery. Williams and Wilkins, Baltimore, vol 1: 24

Gilles G A, Dennis K J, Harkless L B 1986 Periostitis associated with phenol matrictomies. Journal of the American Podiatric Medical Association 76(8): 469–471

McGlamry E D (ed) Comprehensive textbook of foot surgery. Williams and Wilkins, Baltimore, vol 2: 685–688

Mercado O A 1976 Podiatric surgical dissection. Fundamental skills. Corolando Education Materials for Podiatric Medicine, Illinois, p 20–23

Polokoff M 1987 In: McGlamry E D (ed) Comprehensive textbook of foot surgery. Williams and Wilkins, Baltimore, vol 1: 23

Ramsey G, Caldwell 1985 Phenol cauterization for ingrown toenails—unreviewed reports. British Medical Journal 291: 110

Tollafield D R 1991 Reflex sympathetic dystrophy in day case foot surgery. British Journal of Podiatric Medicine & Surgery 3(1): 2–6

Tollafield D R, Parmar D G 1994 Setting standards for day care foot surgery. A quinquennial review. British Journal of Podiatric Medicine & Surgery 6(1): 7–20

Winograd A M In: McGlamry E D (ed) Comprehensive textbook of foot surgery. Williams and Wilkins, Baltimore, vol 1: 19

Zadik F R 1950 Obliteration of the nail bed of the great toe without shortening the terminal phalanx. Journal of Bone and Joint Surgery 32-B(1): 66–67

7

Surgery and the foot

D. R. Tollafield

INTRODUCTION

No book written about the foot and its treatment would be complete without some reference to surgery. Much of the content of this chapter is intended for reference. The unpretentious examples provided here relate to patients seeking elective (voluntary) rather than emergency surgery. Surgery can be undertaken in a hospital or in a surgical day centre. The decision to initiate surgery often lies with the non-surgical practitioner. Specific details on foot surgery and further details of anaesthetic management can be found in specialised texts.

Surgery plays an important role in the management of foot problems. While the most desirable form of treatment is conservative care, surgery must be used on occasions when deformity, trauma and infection arise. The practitioner's role, in addition to considering the merits of surgical intervention, is to advise patients of the pitfalls of, and likely benefits from, such an intervention. Some knowledge of surgery is particularly helpful when providing patients with advice following previous episodes of foot surgery. Either way, the quality of advice offered by practitioners is closely allied to their understanding of surgical principles. The practitioner is responsible initially for generating a referral; in so doing, he or she must understand that, even in the hands of a meticulous surgeon, surgery is not without complication. The implications of failure must be included in any advice given to the patient, ideally before referral.

The practitioner must consider each patient's personal and social background as much as their medical welfare when selecting a surgical option. It is assumed in this chapter that a patient's medical health has already satisfied the requirements for safe admission, either as a day patient or as an in-patient.

SELECTING PATIENTS FOR SURGERY

Failure to make an appropriate referral to the surgeon (podiatric or orthopaedic) will waste time, lead to dissatisfaction from all parties and engender a loss of faith in the system. Furthermore, the cost in wasted time affects patients in a variety of different ways, e.g. through loss of earnings, travel difficulties (relying on fellow neighbours or family) or taking an existing patient's position in the appointment system away from them.

The case history in Box 7.1 attempts to illustrate the tripartite nature of the decision-making process—the practitioner, the patient and the surgeon will each have a different set of criteria that will influence the acceptability of surgical intervention.

The practitioner will need to answer a number of questions before deciding to refer a patient for surgery:

- Is surgery applicable?
- Will surgery ameliorate the problem efficiently, with little disruption to the patient's lifestyle or occupation?
- Can surgery be undertaken effectively at reasonable cost without
  (i) affecting the patient's income adversely, or
  (ii) incurring unreasonable overheads if the outcome is unpredictable?
- Will surgery place the patient's health at risk?
- Can surgery prevent the problem from deteriorating?

Box 7.1   Case history: the tripartite nature of the decision-making process

A 54-year-old company manager was referred to a podiatrist by his family GP. The complaint was a fixed flexion deformity associated with the proximal interphalangeal joint of the second toe. The patient was suited to surgery because permanent relief of his symptoms could be achieved, but he declined surgical intervention.

The patient sought his GP's view regarding the complaint. Referral to the podiatrist was considered reasonable in light of the patient having no existing medical problems. Having assessed the patient's complaint, the podiatrist concluded that conservative treatment was less likely to result in a satisfactory outcome than surgical intervention. Taking account of patient motivation, medical welfare, home support and the ability to manage after surgery, the podiatrist was satisfied that surgery was in the patient's best interest.

The patient was fully informed and provided with a description of the surgical process. As part of the information, he was sent an informed consent by post, in advance of surgery. The patient read the consent and declined surgery because he felt that the stated risks were unreasonable and because a period of immobility was recommended. The risks highlighted on the consent form included possible infection, swelling and pain; it was also stated that there was a need to rest the foot for several weeks before returning to work.

Comment

Hospital consent forms rarely describe specific risks— such risks as are applicable are often left to a personal discussion before the operation. More often than not, consent forms are signed by the patient on the day of admission.

The GP, the podiatric surgeon and the patient each had their own criteria preset for the treatment involved. The referral was correct, the procedure selected carried the likelihood of a successful outcome, but the patient

believed that the risks stated on his consent sheet outweighed the benefits offered by surgery. Additionally, the patient felt that he could not take the recommended period of time off work.

As part of the process of acceptance, all parties should agree that the referral and treatment are appropriate; only two agreed in this case. If all consents were provided in advance in detail (as opposed to on the day), would the number of elective surgical cases decrease? This raises possible problems with the process of consent. Do patients feel any pressure to consent when confronted with a form on admission? In the case of day surgery, where admission and treatment are undertaken on the same day, do patients feel pressure not to proceed? Such pressure may arise when, after a lengthy wait, the need for surgery is doubted.

The correct and most satisfactory resolution to these potential problems lies in the patient having adequate counselling before admission and being given an explanation of all the attendant risks. By the time that a consent requires signing, there should be no room for doubt.

In reality, practitioners believe that the patient understands the implications of treatment and risks after the consulting session. Audit has shown that many patients in fact have not understood the implications of surgery. A podiatric study showed that only 89% of 175 patients surveyed felt that proposed surgical treatment had been explained (Tollafield & Parmar 1994). Only 91% of patients agreed that complications had been explained. These results are useful when we find that 3% of patients did not want to know such details! The only way to improve patient understanding is to reinforce any information given by asking the patient to repeat it—in many cases this remains impractical. Additional written information can assist with verbal reinforcement. Consent and informed consent is also considered in Chapter 3.

- Can the patient's quality of life be improved by surgery?
- Will such intervention extend the patient's life span? (Refer to 'Qualys', Ch. 2, p. 30. This question should also consider longer term success expected from surgery.)

Health status

A full medical assessment should be undertaken to avoid any known existing disorders that could place the patient at risk.

Many patients fail to see the risks that might arise from treatment. The desire to be cured may suppress the reality that a procedure can make some patients worse. Personal and social factors can have a greater impact on success from surgical management than health welfare alone. The decision to operate must take into consideration a variety of factors not related to health:

- support at home (social)
- occupation (financial)
- mobility (after surgery)
- accepted risk (complications)
- chances of success (rated outcome)
- patient motivation and attitude
- age.

Social circumstances

Patients should not be left alone following their discharge from the hospital or surgical centre. They should have a telephone in case of problems, and should be able to reach the hospital or surgical centre easily to attend follow-up appointments. The patient's lifestyle and home support can make a considerable difference, particularly where the patient has a dependent (children/parents). The patient's partner has to assume many of the patient's responsibilities, and tension can rise, particularly where recovery may be prolonged.

Occupation

Some employers provide few benefits for those in lower paid jobs. Examination of the patient's occupational circumstances is essential before agreeing to an operative solution, unless of course the operation is essential or is likely to have minimal effects on mobility. Prolonged periods off work are particularly hard for single parent families, those without a partner's support and those in demanding positions at work.

Mobility

The effect of surgery on feet clearly has a marked impact on the ability to walk and carry out normal ambulatory functions, such as climbing stairs, driving, shopping, going to work and undertaking hobbies. While surgery performed on both feet at the same time may not be, proportionally, twice as painful, and the cost to the service may appear less, the resultant immobility can have a marked effect on ambulation. The postoperative requirements of bilateral surgery must be discussed to ensure that the patient fully understands the likely limitations. Prolonged bed rest poses a risk of deep vein thrombosis (DVT) and pulmonary thrombosis.

Risk

Infection, swelling and pain are commonplace in foot surgery. In some cases, it may not be possible to wear shoes for anything from 6 weeks to 6 months. Such conditions need to be discussed with the patient, in terms of how long each phase will last and what steps will be taken to ameliorate the problem.

Dysfunction, loss of sensation, poor tissue healing and hyperaesthesia form a second, albeit lower, risk. Nonetheless, if a patient should have any of the second series of problems, resolution may take much longer. Complications arising from surgery are discussed later on in this chapter.

Success

Successful treatment can never be guaranteed. Careful audit of treatment provides an indication of the likely outcome. Patients will want to know how successful a particular procedure will be. Audit should be incorporated into the practitioner's routine, so that outcome can be expressed in terms of a percentage success rate. In each case, likely success and shortfall should be discussed with the patient in an unbiased manner. The final decision should be taken by the patient, based on the evidence presented. This activity, together with the risk element, forms the basis of obtaining informed consent.

Motivation

Expected patient compliance is an important part of planned management. A patient who fails to understand or even agree with the suggested surgery may spell disaster. Well-informed patients recover more quickly and generally do better than those who remain ignorant.

Age

While age should be considered, age as a sole factor should not preclude a patient from surgery. On the contrary, many older people fair better than younger patients, despite the fact that youth suggests better health and quicker healing. The truth is that each age group presents the practitioner with different problems.

PRINCIPLES OF FOOT SURGERY

Surgery aims to reduce deformity, restore function and ameliorate pain—in some cases all three aims will be achieved. Building evidence from blood tests, biopsy, imaging studies, neurological function tests and good clinical judgement will guide referral. In some cases, however, these tests should be carried out by the surgeon involved. Early communication between practitioner and surgeon may help to ensure that tests are undertaken at the most appropriate time, thus avoiding repetition and unnecessary costs.

The methods available for surgical management of the foot can be summarised in terms of their individual principles and their perceived indications and limitations. The advent of new technology and ideas supported by research studies have allowed many fundamental techniques to be modified. Increasingly, simple carpentry tools such as chisels and hammers are being replaced by precision power tools which function with greater speed and accuracy. Biocompatible products, such as absorbable rods and screws, promise to minimise the need for removal later on. Nine fundamental techniques associated with foot surgery are considered here:

- excision
- excisional arthroplasty
- replacement arthroplasty
- arthrodesis
- osteotomy
- soft tissue surgery
- tissue replacement
- amputation
- fixation.

Excision

The removal of tissue is the common method for dealing with swelling or prominences. Soft tissue is excised when it is thought to be malignant, or to cause infection or pain. Bone is excised when it is found to create pressure between bone and skin, and skin and footwear. Excision can be performed by

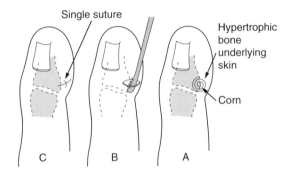

Figure 7.1 A–C: Osteotripsy. An example of minimal incisory surgery is associated with the fifth toe. An interdigital corn due to a hypertrophic phalanx is reduced using a percutaneous incisory technique. Before the wound is closed with a single suture, bone paste from the process of rasping is flushed out with saline.

minimal incisional exposure surgery or by full (open) surgical exposure.

Percutaneous excision of bone, for example, provides entry by a small incision in the skin. The additional term 'keyhole surgery', for percutaneous surgery, has been popularised in some circles. However, this has received poor press, particularly where a complicated procedure has been attempted without the benefit of a clear operative view – obscurity resulting in damage is hard to repair. *Osteotripsy* is synonymous with the percutaneous technique to reduce bony prominences. A manual rasp or power burr is introduced through the incisional aperture to reduce overlying bony projections (Fig. 7.1). The advantage of minimal incisional techniques is that they permit rapid recovery with minimal exposure of tissue; however, the risks associated with infection may still arise.

Arthroscopy is an ideal way of inspecting joint surfaces and offers the option to biopsy and excise tissue at the same time. The arthroscopic technique has been included in this section because, unlike the case of blind percutaneous surgery, it is a very accurate method of undertaking excision. The arthroscope provides an instant visual diagnosis using an optic camera through a small hole in the skin (Fig. 7.2). Investigative surgery associated with small foot joints and structures (e.g. metatarsophalangeal [MTP] joints, subtalar [ST] joints, fascia and nerve releases) has been developed as the heads of optic cameras and adjunctive equipment have become smaller and more refined.

Two portals of entry are required to provide a clear picture. One portal conveys water to insufflate the joint space, while the other maximises the optical position of the camera. The range of arthroscopy

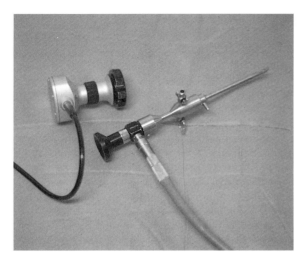

Figure 7.2 An arthroscope allows percutaneous diagnostic examination of a joint. The surgeon may have the option to perform either excisional or osteotripsy surgery. Defects in cartilage can be curetted and abnormal synovial debris removed. The camera attachment (shorter body) fits into the optical probe (longer body). The lenses are designed at different angles to provide the best visibility.

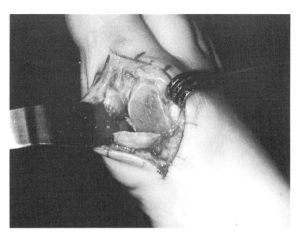

Figure 7.3 Exostectomy—bony prominences can be removed to prevent underlying tissue and skin irritation. The procedure essentially offers 'salvage' in situations that may not be suited to extensive surgery, e.g. the elderly and infirm and those at higher risk of infection. A medial first metatarsal exostosis is illustrated; the exostosis fragment has been displaced medially, showing a smooth cancellous bone surface.

instrumentation is wide and consists of grasping forceps, burrs, probes and suction systems. Laser has recently been introduced into arthroscopy and promises controlled, precise destruction of inflamed tissue and other defects, offering faster recovery than from manual/power equipment.

Older patients presenting with areas of ulceration and breakdown over common sites, such as the medial first metatarsal, may benefit from an exostectomy. This procedure is an example of the full, or open, exposure technique, often requiring redundant skin to be trimmed after the bony eminence has been removed. No corrective benefit is achieved where a concomitant hallux valgus deformity coexists (Fig. 7.3). The tissue will heal quickly and provide relief of symptoms. This is particularly beneficial for the patient, reducing the risk of recurrent infections from intractable pressure.

Cheilectomy is the excision by open surgery of small portions of bone formed by osteophytes. Osteophytic degeneration associated with osteoarthritis distorts skin and reduces joint spaces. Cheilectomy is useful where joint replacement may not be appropriate. The metatarsal can be trimmed so that skin is not distorted and damaged, and any irritation of the synovial lining is minimised—synovitis can cause greater discomfort than a stiff joint.

Excisional arthroplasty

An arthroplasty may involve the removal of either one or both sides of a joint surface. The extent of excision is dependent upon the type of operation. The term arthroplasty is misleading in that a new joint is not really formed. The gaps created by excising joints fill in with scar tissue (see Fig. 7.5A). Lesser toes and interphalangeal (IP) joints remain stiff after such surgery and may swell. Larger toe joints, such as the first MTP joint, may appear more mobile, but such flexibility will depend upon the extent of bone removed.

Degenerative joints with synovitis can be relieved by excisional arthroplasty. Deformity may be reduced but not always corrected. The procedure is destructive, and careful biomechanical consideration should be included in any assessment. In the case of *Keller's excisional arthroplasty* for hallux valgus, the toe position may be improved but the deformity can recur (Fig. 7.4). The foot may experience a transfer of pressure over lesser metatarsal heads as load shifts laterally. This arises because the hallux is shortened during surgery and has less purchase on the ground (Henry & Waugh 1975). While arthroplasties are often considered more appropriate in older patients, younger patients may well benefit from excisional arthroplasty however, the surgeon should not wantonly destroy the biomechanics of the first ray. Other options

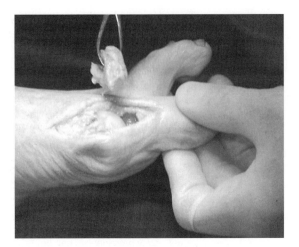

Figure 7.4 Keller's excisional arthroplasty consists of removing the base of the proximal phalanx and exostosis (see Fig. 7.3). The reason for the higher failure rate of this otherwise successful procedure is associated with too much bone being excised. The illustration shows removal prior to a first toe implant and therefore a slightly shorter length than usual is removed. One-third of the length of phalanx provides sufficient correction and moderate shortening without the toe becoming frail. The procedure can be combined with osteotomies.

should be considered to preserve the joint in the younger patient.

Excisional arthroplasty is commonly used for problems associated with MTP and IP joints. The use of arthroplasty in the lesser MTP joints is less common than in the first MTP joint. The bases of proximal phalanges are trimmed in severe lesser toe deformities, but in most cases an arthroplasty technique will cause toe shortening—something the patient should be aware of beforehand. The *panmetatarsal head* excision is an arthroplasty technique reserved for multiple toe deformity and pressure over the metatarsal heads. Panmetatarsal head excision has many names and tends to be reserved for rheumatoid and psoriatic arthritis. This procedure offers the patient a highly effective, although seemingly destructive, operation to manage pain associated with synovitis, deformity from deranged MTP joints and poor tissue viability. The resultant effect leaves the foot remarkably more functional than if it were left untreated.

Replacement arthroplasty

A new joint is usually referred to as a replacement arthroplasty. In some cases, namely first MTP joints, lesser MTP joints and IP joints, silastic or dual metal–polypropylene implants can be used to replace the

joint completely. Replacement of large joints in the foot, such as the ankle, appear to do less well than those of the hip and knee.

Replacement joints (prosthetic implants) can only be used in cases where there is no infection and where the bone substance has adequate quality. Selection of implants is currently based upon the extent of joint damage and age. An older patient is likely to be less active than a younger patient, and therefore lower loads are experienced—wear and tear occurs more slowly. Conversely, younger patients have better 'bone stock' for receiving implants, as compared with older bones with poor mineralisation. Older patients have fewer expectations of postoperative joint motion and will demand less, physically, of their new joint. Revision is necessary where patients expose the replaced joint to too much stress.

The silastic 'spacer' implant has a hinged concept (Swanson et al 1991). Figures 7.5A–C illustrate the silastic implant without metal grommets and in position after surgery, as seen by X-ray. Metal grommets (square washers), when used, may well improve the longevity of the implant. The grommet allows the metal, rather than the bone, to take the load from pistoning forces that build up. Silastic implants are soft and can tear and even pop out of the reamed square holes in which the two stems sit. Single-stem implants have fallen from favour at present, even though the hinged implant offers less freedom of movement and is restricted to sagittal plane motion.

Newer replacement joints made of two components, metal titanium and plastic, have recently been introduced into foot surgery. Technically, the prosthesis is harder to use and special reaming guides are required. There have been insufficient longitudinal studies to predict the success of the two-component joint system to date. However, the ball and socket component replicates the mechanical function of the actual MTP joint more closely than does the hinge system.

A successful joint replacement will allow the patient to bear weight within a week of surgery. Acute pain from the diseased joint should recede during this same postoperative period. Joint replacement requires extensive tissue handling and postoperative pain will be marked. Prophylactic broad-spectrum antibiotics are used by many surgeons for implant surgery, but this protocol is by no means mandatory.

The most common joint replaced in the foot is the first MTP joint, as illustrated in Figure 7.5B. The patient should be aware that movement expected from the joint after surgery can vary. Fibrotic infill along the hinge in the silastic implant can build up

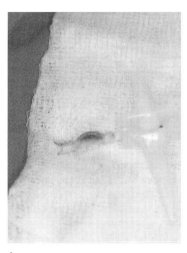
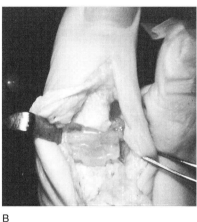
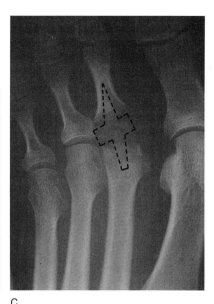

A   B   C

Figure 7.5   Replacement arthroplasty. A: The implant made of silastic material (Swanson design), having been removed from a foot, shows the fibrotic plug along the implant. The fibrous material prevents hinge movement unless the patient rehabilitates early. B: The implant in place without grommets. C: Weight-bearing X-ray showing a lesser metatarsal phalangeal joint with implant as part of salvage for old Freiberg's disease.

quickly from an initial haematoma—early mobility is preferred for this reason.

Complications from silastic implants have been noted and patients need to be advised of these. While problems are rare, bone abnormalities include fibrous hyperplasia, bone cysts and degenerative erosion. Potential problems associated with the implant material include foreign body granuloma and reactive synovitis from silicone. Fracture of the material may arise due to fatigue; accidental damage from sharp instruments during surgery can sometimes contribute to this.

Arthrodesis

In arthrodesis, all cartilage covering the bone ends must be completely removed and the denuded surfaces apposed and allowed to fuse together. The patient must understand that restriction of movement is permanent. Fixation can be achieved by autogenous materials, i.e. bone from the body itself, or exogenous materials from other species. Material from other species may be rejected depending upon the tissue used. Metal fixation materials come in the form of screws, wires, plates and pins.

Arthrodesis not only corrects the primary deformity but will improve the function of weaker muscles and tendons that pass around the joint and adjacent bones. In the case of paralysis or congenital instability, a healthy muscle/tendon can be transferred. The arthrodesed joint will provide a stronger mechanical beam and thereby restore foot stability. Further description of tendon transfers is given later (p. 115). The ends of bones can be reshaped to correct moderate deformity as well as to reduce joint pain.

Arthrodesis has become popular for flexed deformities of the lesser toes because each toe is turned into a rigid lever. Patients should be aware not only that IP joint movement will be lost as a result of surgery, but also that, because failure of fusion can arise, toes can swell. Lack of fusion results from too much fibrous replacement, with poor phalangeal compression in the presence of movement in the toe.

Where an arthrodesis is used in the foot, compensation may develop in distal or proximal joints to account for deficient movement; for example, an ankle arthrodesis can lead to greater subtalar and midtarsal joint movement. As a consequence, pain can arise in these otherwise normal joints where function has had to change. Recalcitrant painful flat foot problems may require surgery to fuse the medial border of the foot, raising the arch and improving tibialis anterior and posterior muscle function. The foot may adopt severe subtalar joint (STJ) pronation, causing disability with

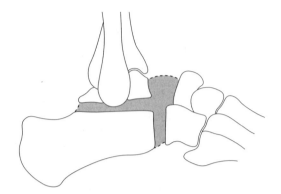

Figure 7.6 Arthrodesis. The triple arthrodesis shown is for stabilising the hindfoot at the talocalcaneal joint, the calcaneocuboid joint and the talonavicular joint. The technique allows for the surfaces (shaded) to be refashioned to change the relationship of any deformity present.

gait problems. The STJ arthrodesis is effective for recalcitrant pain in the hindfoot with severe deformity. The calcaneus is fused to the talus to limit pain, prevent further deformity and stabilise the hindfoot. The calcaneus may be fused to the talus, the talus fused to the navicular and the calcaneus fused to the cuboid bones collectively (Fig. 7.6). Where all three articulations are fused, the procedure is known as a triple STJ arthrodesis. This procedure is usually regarded as the most extensive form of arthrodesis in the foot. In many cases, single or double arthrodeses affecting one or two of the aforementioned joints will suffice.

Supinated foot deformity as in the case of pes cavus, presenting with a marked forefoot equinus, may also benefit from arthrodesis. The navicular can be morticed or cut back into the talus, thus lifting the forefoot up. The articular surfaces can be fashioned to alter the position of the deformity. Many modifications of hindfoot arthrodesis have been developed; bone is trimmed to produce the correction desired— each modification might be named after the author. The abundance of named procedures today can easily cause confusion.

Cutting bone with recesses, holes and pegs provides a superior form of fixation. The surgeon will make use of shortening bone to correct deformity by also relaxing contracted tissue around joints. The most effective arthrodesis ensures that bone-to-bone contact is well apposed, using screws, staples and plates to achieve adequate compression. When a patient is advised that surgery can assist with the foot condition, the practitioner must discuss the use of 'hardware', a colloquial term for any internal fixation. It usually makes sense to suggest to the patient that all hardware will require removing eventually.

Osteotomy

Bone deformity can be corrected by arthrodesis, but the resulting stiffness across joints causes compensation, as movement must develop from other joints. When an arthrodesis associated with the first MTP joint is used, the type of footwear and heel height may be restricted. An osteotomy is carried out by surgically dividing the bone away from the joint. Not only will deformity be corrected, but joints can be spared surgical fusion.

Osteotomies in the foot are reserved for pain and deformity, but the end result will hopefully increase the life of a joint before degeneration becomes symptomatic. Where cartilage is thinned out, shear stress increases (Radin et al 1992). The bone should have adequate mineral density (bone stock) to accept surgical fixation across the surgical division.

After division, the abnormal bone position can be realigned to improve the biomechanics of the joint. Once decompression has been achieved, any inflammatory changes associated with synovitis may settle. Propagating cracks known as fibrillation will be prevented if abnormal stresses across the surface can be dissipated by improving the cartilage surface relationship. Carrying out an osteotomy in the case of an arthritic condition is based on the hope that such surgery will create a remission of symptoms and pathology. If adverse joint changes can be resolved, the use of other destructive surgical techniques may be averted.

Sliding, rotational, closing and opening wedge osteotomies are the principal types of osteotomy performed. While the principle of this surgical technique is directed at changing bone alignment, bone can also be lengthened or shortened; this is explained below. Careful preservation of neurovascular tissues is required in lengthening procedures.

A sliding/displacement osteotomy is shown in Figure 7.7 and illustrates how hallux valgus can be corrected with lateral capital displacement. The MTP joint space is increased, that is to say, decompressed and shortened by surgery. While release of the adductor hallucis and lateral capsule may be necessary, the shortening of the metatarsal often relaxes tissues, saving unnecessary dissection.

Rotational osteotomies correct torsion in bone, and are more commonly performed in the tibia and femur than in the foot. A closing wedge osteotomy is performed by removing a triangular section of bone;

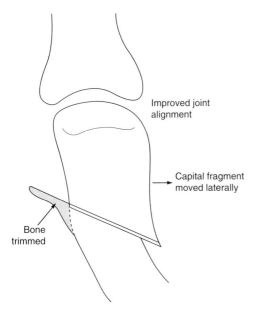

Figure 7.7   Displacement osteotomy. The illustration shows a single oblique cut made after the medial eminence has been removed. Few capital osteotomies are undertaken in adult patients without trimming the medial eminence first. The hallux valgus is corrected by a capital osteotomy. The metatarsal length is shortened to decompress the joint and to move the capital fragment laterally.

one or two planes of deformity can be corrected simultaneously. In the case of a hallux valgus deformity, with an abnormal proximal articular set angle (PASA), both the cartilage surface and the distal metatarsal position can be influenced (Fig. 7.8). The metatarsal is shortened but the cartilage surface is preserved after the joint space has been increased. The hallux valgus is improved as the distal head of the metatarsal is displaced laterally (not shown in the illustrations). By combining different types of osteotomy, correction can be influenced in more than one plane. While a fuller description would not be appropriate in a general text such as this, most osteotomies, except for the open wedge type, can affect the length of a metatarsal. The surgeon must guard against removing too much bone in the first metatarsal, to avoid increasing mechanical stress over the second or third metatarsals. Usually the effects of such shortening are to cause callus or increased shaft thickness of the metatarsal seen on X-ray. Pre-surgical judgement should take account of the corresponding second and first metatarsal lengths. The opening wedge osteotomy uses autogenous bone or bone from other sources, such as attenuated bovine bone, to lengthen one side. The wedge osteotomy avoids problems associated with shortening, but technically the procedure is more

A

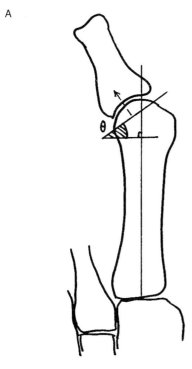

B

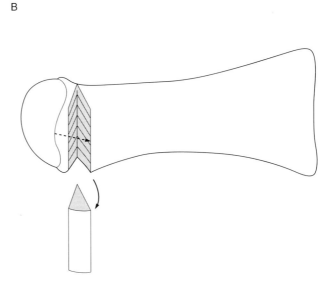

Figure 7.8   Closing wedge osteotomy—single plane correction. A: The proximal articular set angle (PASA) is shown influencing the direction of hallux deformity. B: A wedge is removed to correct the articular alignment and decompress the joint.

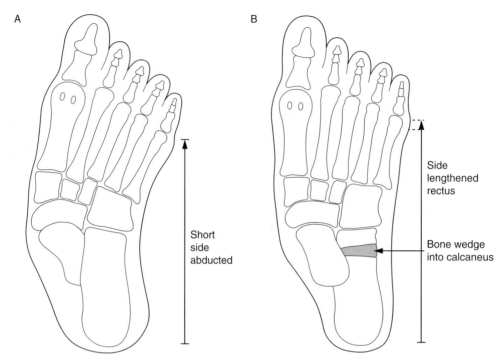

Figure 7.9 Opening wedge osteotomy. A: The lateral side is shortened by the abduction associated with foot pronation. B: Bone graft inserted into the calcaneus will lengthen the lateral side of the foot. This simplified illustration does not indicate the potential surgery required on the medial side.

difficult and problems can arise with normal bony union. Wherever possible, autogenous (homogeneous) bone from the patient should be used as this is less likely to be rejected.

The osteotomy principle can be used anywhere in the foot. Flexible flat foot with a pronated shorter lateral border (without metatarsus adductus) can be treated by an open wedge osteotomy to lengthen the lateral border (Fig. 7.9). The medial border is stabilised simultaneously by fusing the navicular and cuneiform bones together. Pes cavus associated with a high inclination angle of the calcaneus can be improved by a dorsal displacement osteotomy as illustrated in Figure 7.10.

Soft tissue surgery

Some deformities are caused by soft tissue rather than by bone alone. Tendons and capsules contract, maintaining deformity. Simple surgery may release these tissues but unfortunately often fails unless the patient is young. A large number of terms exist for operating on soft tissue—the use of a prefix (asso-

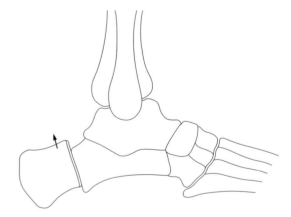

Figure 7.10 Calcaneal displacement osteotomy for pes cavus foot with a high inclination angle associated with the hindfoot.

ciated with the anatomical structure) is followed by *-otomy* or *-desis*. The suffix will mean to incise, to divide or to limit movement. To add confusion to surgical terminology, some surgical techniques may have more than one form of nomenclature. *Capsulotomy* and *arthrotomy* involve an incision into a joint. As most joint surgery involves incising all the structures affecting a joint, the descriptors tend to refer to the general method employed, e.g. arthroscopy of the ankle, arthrodesis with capsulotomy of the MTP joint.

Where bones remain relatively soft (compared to tendons and capsule), and have not as yet been irreversibly affected by ankylosis (fibrous fusion) and torsion (permanent twisting of bone), surgery is indicated. If a deformity is left, the potential for successful restoration by division or incision reduces proportionally with age. As the patient ages, the adaptation by bone and soft tissue requires attention together, because the latter tissue will atrophy and contract. The child with club foot (congenital talipes equinovarus, CTEV) therefore responds better to early surgical intervention because most of the deformity is associated with tendons contracting abnormally during foot development.

Tenotomy is a technique involving transection of a tendon. A digital deformity in an 8-year-old will benefit from this quick, minimal exposure procedure. The flexor tendons can be transected through a small percutaneous incision; the toes can be splinted with soft Betadine soaks without sutures and the child can return to walking immediately. The toes can then be splinted for 6 months with silicone orthodigita to ensure that constant tension allows the flexor tendons to retain their length as they heal. If surgery is delayed beyond adolescence, then the deformity associated with flexion of the IP joints leads to ankylosis, necessitating an arthrodesis. Early intervention is successful and causes little stress to children, although a short general anaesthetic may be preferred.

Tendon transfers are indicated where muscle function needs to be re-established. Miller (1992) identified the goals of tendon transfer, as follows:

- to improve motor function
- to eliminate deforming forces
- to restore loss of power
- to improve muscle balance
- to eliminate the need for bracing
- to improve foot appearance.

When a transfer is considered, joints should have minimal disease and have free mobility on clinical examination. Surgery should ensure that the biomechanics associated with transfer maintains the joint axis as close to perpendicular as possible with the new insertion. Faulty muscles attached to bone through their tendons may require detaching and moving proximally. The case of the triggered hallux associated

with pes cavus in Charcot-Marie-Tooth is well documented (McGlamry et al 1992, Mann & Coughlin 1993). The flexible hallux at the MTP joint is stabilised once the long extensor tendon is moved from its insertion to a new point through the metatarsal neck. The IP joint must be turned into a rigid beam by an arthrodesis, otherwise propulsion would be affected. The newly positioned tendon lifts the first metatarsal, reducing the effect of plantarflexion which maintains the hallux in retraction.

Split tendon transfers may be used to divide the power of tendons where spasticity causes an overpull. The tibialis anterior provides a good example in cerebral palsy. The forefoot inverts with spasticity. The split anterior tibial tendon transfer (SPLATT) reduces the inversion power by transferring the moment of force to the lateral side of the foot. The site of insertion may involve either the peroneus tertius tendon or the cuboid bone.

A tendon may be transferred or split in order to route it to another site to enhance foot function. Abnormally tight tendons such as the tendo Achilles must be lengthened to avoid problems with inefficient heel contact. The foot adapts to ankle equinus through the midtarsal or subtalar joints. The efficiency of midfoot tendon transfers will be severely affected if the tendo Achilles is not attended to at the same time.

There are many examples of tendon transfer techniques. Research using electromyographic (EMG) studies should ideally be used before surgery is attempted, to analyse the effect of such surgery. Foot pressure analysis with Harris ink mats and pedobarographs (PBG), for example, will allow the surgeon to evaluate successful weight-bearing changes after surgery. Many more examples of measuring foot pressure are available but the two methods mentioned have been in practice the longest.

Soft tissue surgery may involve dividing ligaments, tendons and capsular structures. An adductovarus fifth toe position may improve after a simple capsulotomy with tenotomy, or an adjunctive skin lengthening may also be required. One of the problems affecting toes following minimal surgery relates to scar tissue forming around MTP joints. The toe becomes dorsiflexed after a short period of success. The toe gradually lifts with contracture, particularly where the short and long extensor tendons fuse together forming a thick knot. Transfer of small tendons, such as the toe extensors, can be routed into metatarsal heads. Alternatively, a portion of tendon can be removed; this procedure, known as a *tenectomy*, may prevent some recurrence of the contracture. Established contracture around the MTP joint will require

A

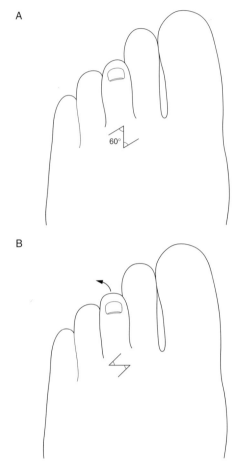

B

Figure 7.11 A, B: A Z-skin plasty is a popular method of rotating skin to a new position with the effect of increasing length. The central line represents the direction in which the scar has been moved, so that less contracture is placed proximal to the digit.

removal of bone, such as the base of the phalanx, and an osteotomy if the deformity cannot be corrected or improved.

Skin incisions used to correct deformity should be planned carefully to take advantage of potential lengthening. The use of a Z-plasty will allow scar tissue to be sited to a different position, minimising recurrence of the contracture (Fig. 7.11). Care in relation to skin incisions is described in Chapter 6 (p. 101).

Tendons and ligaments may be shortened or lengthened. Shortening, or *plication*, is not very common although it may be beneficial in conditions such as congenital convex pes planus (CCPP). In CCPP, the head of the talus sits in a vertical position and stretches the tibialis posterior and short/long flexor tendons, together with the medial deltoid ligament.

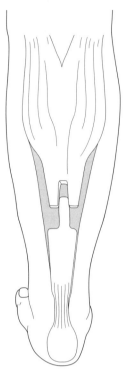

Figure 7.12 Soft tissue surgery—gastrocnemius recession for ankle equinus position. (Adapted from Downey 1992.)

As the calcaneus everts, the ligaments of the lateral side of the ankle shorten. The medial side is plicated and the lateral side is divided prior to holding the foot in a leg cast. As with CTEV, CCPP must be corrected shortly after birth to offer the best prognosis.

Tendons are lengthened not only to reduce deformity but also to improve the biomechanics of the foot. The tendo Achilles is perhaps the most common musculotendon group to be operated on. Ankle equinus is responsible for maintaining a flexible flat foot deformity in both normal and spastic patients. Too much lengthening will weaken the tendo Achilles. A Z-plasty is applied to the tendon in a different manner to that described for skin (Fig. 7.12). Downey (1992) describes lengthening of the tendo Achilles by distal recession. It is reasoned that, by only lengthening the gastrocnemius component, recovery from surgery is improved. Full-thickness lengthening is commonly described in surgical texts. Smaller tendons can be lengthened by exactly the same technique, although repairing the paratenon is much more difficult. The paratenon is the very thin diaphanous membrane that surrounds the tendon and carries the fine vascular supply (Fig. 7.13).

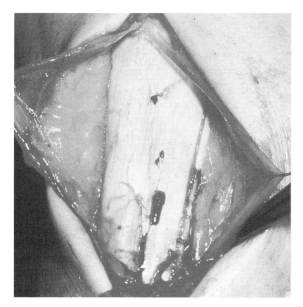

Figure 7.13 The thin membrane surrounding the tendo Achilles should be carefully preserved because of the vascular network. (Reproduced with permission from the Courtesy Fifth Avenue Hospital, Seattle.)

Tissue replacement

Tissue from sources other than humans can be implanted into the foot. Specialised bone from bovine sources (Xenograft) or from other humans (Allograft) can be used as a matrix into which new bone cells will migrate (Fig. 7.14). Bone grafts may come from the iliac crest, tibia, fibula or calcaneus. Homogenous (autograft) bone is preferred—the donor site is usually from the iliac crest where the graft yields three sides of strong cortex (Fig. 7.15). Grafts include small cancellous chips, slivers of cancellous bone and slab grafts. Bone grafts can be used to assist heal delayed fractures and bone defects, can act as a fixation component for arthrodesis and can repair congenital defects.

Skin from sources such as porcine graft is less readily accepted than skin from human sources and it may only act as a temporary cover to be replaced later by homogenous skin from the thigh. The thigh provides a wide expanse of skin from which a graft large enough for the foot is available (Fig. 7.16). The donor site may be more painful than the recipient site, since

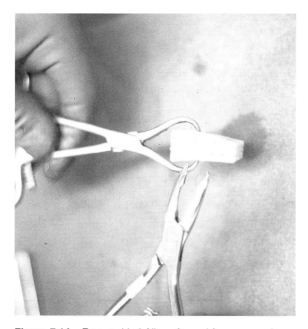

Figure 7.14 Freeze dried Allograft used for open wedge osteotomy. Human donated bone is specially prepared and treated according to standards laid down by statutory bodies such as the Centre for Disease Control in the USA.

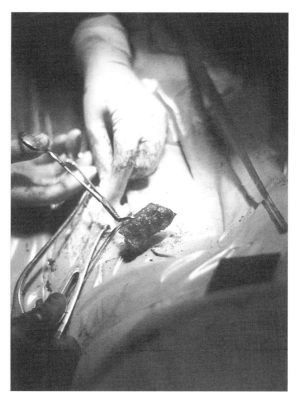

Figure 7.15 Bone taken from the iliac crest for implantation into the foot of the same patient. This is known as homogenous or autografted bone.

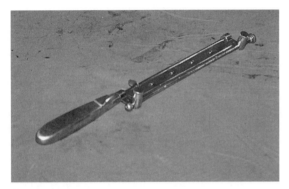

A

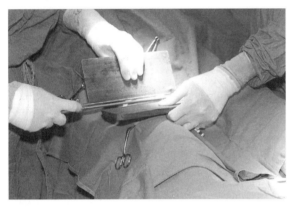

B

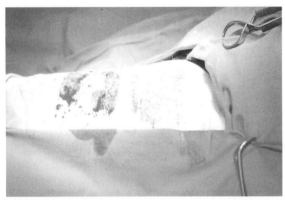

C

Figure 7.16 A: A Humby knife is used to remove a fine layer of skin. A number of systems, including electric roller/cutters, are available. B: The skin is kept taught using two slabs of wood as shown. The skin is rolled up and kept moist before being carefully unravelled over the recipient site. C: Three areas of skin have been removed from the thigh (donor site). (Reproduced with permission from Mr J. D. Bromage, Kettering General Hospital.)

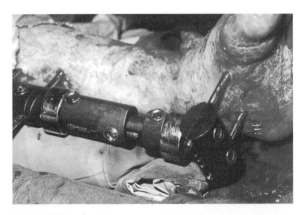

Figure 7.17 Myocutaneous graft used to cover bone and defects where little blood supply would allow a skin graft to take. A fixator is valuable when the wound is infected and the tissue cannot be closed. Bone can still be immobilised and grafting can be undertaken later on. (Reproduced with permission from Dr Ira Fox, Atlantic City, USA.)

the thickness of the graft usually exposes fine nerve endings, as shown in Figure 7.16B. Thinner grafts heal more quickly than thicker ones and can be perforated to stretch further and prevent build-up of exudate and haematoma. In the latter case, the graft might perish causing an infection to set in.

Where tissues are devitalised, as in the case of diabetics, specialist centres can offer myocutaneous flaps to cover larger avascular defects. The concept behind these flaps is to allow a large blood supply to be transposed with muscle. The muscle, with its rich supply, will provide nutrient and bulky covering to the skin (Fig. 7.17).

Skin grafting can be used after trauma in the case of chemical and physical burns, or after surgery where tissue has been sacrificed. This latter indication might include neoplasia, as illustrated by the case history in Box 7.2.

Tissue replacement with internal prostheses has been successful elsewhere in the human body: Dacron for blood vessels, heart valve replacement, and metal prostheses following removal of bone tumours. The foot has to withstand remarkable loads and the types of prosthesis used most frequently are associated with smaller joints. The most common joints include the ankle, and the IP and MTP joints. The subtalar arthro-eresis peg (STA peg) is unique to the foot. Made of silicone, the peg fits under the lateral side of the talus body and reduces the influence of pronation during development. The STA peg is later removed and orthoses may still be required to maintain the corrected position. The STA peg is not yet widely used in the UK.

Box 7.2   Case history: skin graft after malignant melanoma excision

A 74-year-old male was referred by his general physician with a wart under the right first metatarsal head. The patient's history was complicated by respiratory disease and psoriasis. The GP had used the usual preparations on the lesion which covered the metatarsal head. Upon admission to the day surgery unit, a dark pigmented nodular lesion was identified. The borders were irregular and the lesion was bleeding. The appearance was complicated by the use of keratolytics. A large excisional biopsy was taken under regional ankle block and the lesion was found to penetrate to, and include, the capsule of the first MTP joint. An underlying sesamoid was trimmed and the skin sample sent to histopathology. Two days later, preliminary stains strongly suggested a malignant melanoma, which was subsequently diagnosed as an acral lentiginous melanoma. Good closure was affected, but the lesion required further excision, necessitating a split skin graft (Fig. 7.18) rather than a full ray excision.

Comment

Despite some doubts about the skin graft failing, the lesion covered the defect without any Koebner phenomenon from psoriasis. The use of skin grafting provided an alternative form of management to loss of part of the first ray in a patient already ill with respiratory disease. The poor long-term prognosis expected with the malignancy of the acral lentiginous melanoma was accompanied by an adjunctive medical condition. Skin grafts can be successfully used on the plantar surface of the foot.

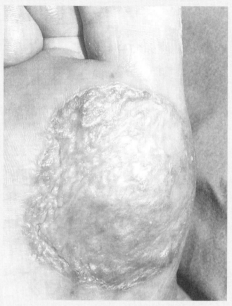

Figure 7.18   Skin graft used to cover a defect following surgical excision of a positive biopsy for malignant melanoma. (Reproduced with permission from Manor Hospital, Medical Photography Department, Walsall.)

Amputation

While the practitioner strives to maintain tissue viability and function wherever possible, amputation has a place in surgical management. The indications for amputation are:

- recalcitrant pain
- gross deformity
- necrotic change
  —thermal damage
  —vascular impairment
- expansile neoplastic change
- severe disabling injury
- failed surgery.

When planning an amputation, the practitioner should be sensitive in the care taken with the patient. In most cases, patients understand the need for surgery but are less able to comprehend the effects that an amputation can have on their lives—e.g. psychological effects, dysfunction and, later, the need for a prosthesis.

Following amputation, symptoms would be expected to resolve. The loss of part, even an extensive part, of the foot will leave some reduced function. Most patients accept the loss of a lesser toe well (Fig. 7.19). The practitioner must point out that the gap may fill in with a drifting toe, as in the case of

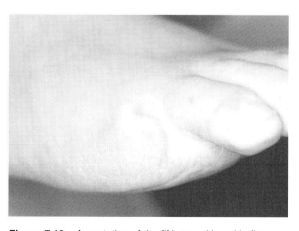

Figure 7.19   Amputation of the fifth toe with a skin flap fashioned to retain underlying fat and a healthy blood supply.

hallux valgus, but otherwise no functional disruption should arise. In fact, of all the toes, only the first toe will cause problems with balance. Any deficit of first ray or hallux function can be successfully compensated by a prosthesis (Ch. 12). The patient should be aware that hammer toes may arise following first toe amputation. Toes are occasionally removed to replace lost thumbs in order to retain the pincer effect with the index finger.

Multiple toe amputations will cause a rise in vertical contact forces and pressure under the metatarsals. Ideally, the patient will be fitted with an insole or forefoot extension prosthesis to assist the shortened foot fit in a regular shoe.

Midfoot or transmetatarsal amputations (Fig. 7.20), ray excisions and those through the midtarsal joint will seriously affect biomechanical function. Tendons from the leg should ideally be inserted into remaining bone to maintain some function. The fascia should be retained wherever possible to support weight-bearing

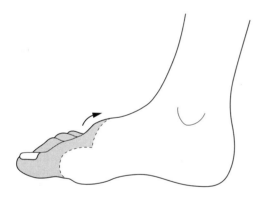

Figure 7.20 Lateral view of transmetatarsal amputation for the forefoot. A plantar flap is created and brought onto the dorsum.

heel stumps. Skin flaps that bear weight should have as much deep soft tissue transposed at the time of surgery as possible, otherwise nerve ending and scar line corns will form—increasing pain and patient distress. While the retention of the talus and calcaneus together is better if a full foot prosthesis is required (Choparts's amputation), the calcaneus and talus can be removed if the underlying fat pad is large enough and viable to sustain weight-bearing. The traditional Syme's amputation, named after the Edinburgh surgeon, Sir James Syme, in 1843, not only successfully removed the talus but also trimmed the malleoli (Fig. 7.21).

The use of amputation for the dysvascular foot, particularly in diabetic patients, is somewhat controversial. The common difficulty lies with wound healing and closure—if the wound were to become infected, it could lead to a below-knee amputation. Earlier intervention with a below-knee amputation may forestall many of the problems encountered by failed local amputations, metatarsal ray, or transmetatarsal surgery. While the surgeon ideally wishes to maintain as much of the original structure as possible, unless the timing of surgical intervention is appropriate, the foot may have deteriorated too far. Below-knee amputations are therefore often performed at the outset of deterioration. In the case of the diabetic or vascular patient, the main aim is to keep the patient alive—the fewer operations required, the more likely it is that this objective will be achieved.

Fixation

In much the same way that skin can be held together by sutures, bone can be sutured with fine gauge wire. Malleable surgical stainless steel wire can be placed through drill holes and twisted to bring the ends

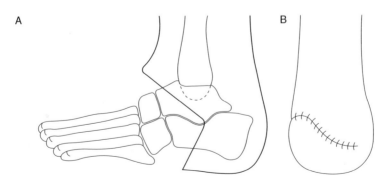

Figure 7.21 A, B: Syme's whole foot amputation. A moccasin prosthesis would be required.

together. This technique, known as *cerclage wire*, is still in common practice, but is probably used less frequently now with the advent of AO (ASIF) fixation. The Association of the Study of Internal Fixation (ASIF), developed in Switzerland in 1958, led to the formation of the study group which heralded AO (*Arbeitgemeinschaft für osteosythesisfragen*) fixation methods.

Internal fixation

Osteotomies or fractures heal best when well apposed and compressed at the ends. In the UK, as in the USA, the podiatric view that bone should be fixed by some mechanism is based on the premise that bone ends can move and thus delay union. As bones in the foot take, on average, 12 weeks to unite adequately, weight-bearing is limited following surgery. The use of casting is helpful, but very restrictive, and can create an element of demineralisation within the bone. Early ambulation following surgery is ideal, as the constant weight-bearing will increase new bone formation and not only reduce potential cast disease (pain with demineralised bone and tissue swelling), but also limit the risk of DVT and reflex sympathetic dystrophy through postoperative disuse.

There is a wide variety of fixation hardware: pins, screws, staples and plates. New designs of screws have flooded the surgical market, many bearing similarities to the AO system. Designs include self-tapping and cannulated screws, which reduce the need to systematically tap the drill hole each time. The cannulated screw system makes use of a hollow shaft. The screw fits over a pin called a Kirschner wire (K-wire). The K-wire keeps the screw in correct line and reduces the need for some of the usual AO overdrilling as well as tapping. A clamp is used to ensure that the bone ends do not move as the screw is inserted into the pre-drilled hole. The lag effect is used by ensuring that the furthermost hole is tighter. In this way, the pitch of the screw can bite into the bone substance drawing the ends closely together.

Plates are used when screws alone will not provide the stability required (Fig. 7.22). Access to some fracture sites is considerably limited. The plate is usually pre-stressed and has screw holes drilled eccentrically away from the fracture line. As the tapered screw heads make contact with the plate holes, the fragments are compressed together (Corey & Ruch 1992).

Pins are commonly used to achieve the same result as screws, but their compression ability is poor. Pin thickness varies from 1.25 to 1.6 mm, although smaller and thicker wires are available. These wires are used

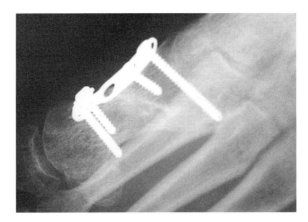

Figure 7.22 A plate with four AO screws is illustrated after an osteotomy of the first metatarsal failed to heal adequately at 6 weeks.

for stabilising small bones as in the case of toes (arthrodesis) and metatarsal osteotomies. Pins may be smooth or threaded. Threaded pins tend to act like small screws because the thread turns in one direction, biting bone as it pierces the cortex. The advantage of such a product lies in its purchase and in the fact that it moves less frequently than the smooth version. No special equipment is necessary and the introduction is quick and efficient. Premature removal is most difficult because, unlike screws, no head exists into which a screwdriver will fit. Pins have to be over-drilled out. Percutaneous positioning works less well, as the thread wraps around soft tissue causing damage.

In the hindfoot, particularly the calcaneus, thicker *Steinman* pins are used, because they can carry greater loads than Kirschner wires. Pins are generally designed to stabilise bones rather than take the load of weight-bearing.

Staples have always been used, but from time to time they become unpopular. With the advent of power-driven staples, a quick system is now available to secure clean bone division. New technology has recently produced a metal staple sensitive to heat. Once the staple has been inserted, the body heat causes the metal to contract, forcing the two fracture ends closer together.

Absorbable fixation. The technology used in biodegradable sutures is now being applied to rods and screws. One of the first designs, Orthosorb (Johnson & Johnson), has been used by orthopaedic and podiatric surgeons in the UK. The rod works on the basis that it locates the bone in its ideal position. Based on polyglycolic acid (PGA), the rod swells, making the alignment firmer. Osteotomies are not compressed, but nor would they be with smooth K-wires. Current research looks encouraging and side-effects are minimal, although additional swelling in toes has been noted.

Polymers of lactide and glycolide have been used to develop a range of screws. Development of this new product has been undertaken in the USA, but it awaits approval by the Medical Devices Agency in the UK. The screw, made of poly-L-lactide, promises to carry the load for fracture fixation but then disappear after the bone has regained its strength. The makers of SmartScrew (Bionix) offer a wide range of screw diameters. Lengths can be cut to suit the depth required. This means that less equipment (and a smaller range of stock) is required, and surgical removal is obviated, both providing resource savings which would look attractive to any surgical department.

External fixation

Although internal fixation provides the patient with an invisible reduction device, a place does exist for external fixation, mainly in trauma. Pins can be introduced through undisplaced bone using an image intensifier. The main advantage in having a wire externally sited lies in the minimal surgical exposure required and the ease of removal. Pins can be easily removed from bone, providing that insertion is not too deep. In this case, local anaesthetic is advised to remove firmer pins. Sharp ends of pins should be protected by some cover, such as a 'Jurgan ball' (Fig. 7.23; Tollafield 1995). The risk of infection and loosening should be discussed with the patient.

External fixation can be achieved using a fixator (Figs 7.17 and 7.24). This is a larger version of the type of device that can be used in smaller, metatarsal and tarsal bones. Several large pins are inserted through bone and plates are bolted on externally to the ends to maintain traction and stability. While a minimal amount of motion will speed up osteogenic activity, too much movement and displacement will cause bone healing to fail. The primary aim in any bone healing process is to maintain good compression and reduction of bone fragments. The external applicator is beneficial where an open wound needs constant care or is awaiting skin grafting, because this can be done without affecting bone repair. Because external fixation devices impede walking, internal fixation systems are more popular.

COMPLICATIONS ASSOCIATED WITH FOOT SURGERY

Earlier in this chapter, the risks associated with sur-

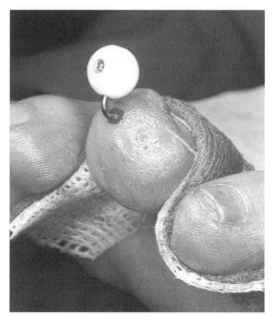

Figure 7.23 Jurgan ball (RFO Medical) placed on the end of the Kirschner wire to protect the point. The balls can be adjusted by a small grub screw and tightened against the wire. While corks and other methods are not recyclable, Jurgans balls withstand sterilising through an approved HSDU/CSSD. The procedure shown is an arthrodesis of a third clawed toe.

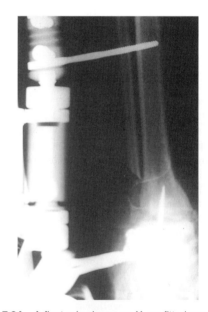

Figure 7.24 A fixator is shown on X-ray fitted proximally through the tibia and distally through the foot. A ball and socket joint at each end allows accurate placement and fit. (Reproduced with permission from Dr Ira Fox, Atlantic City, USA.)

gery were highlighted. The practitioner will ideally select the surgeon best capable of dealing with a specific foot problem. However, no matter how experienced the surgeon, problems will arise. For the most part, problems will relate to minor inconveniences; however, the practitioner must always bear in mind that a minor inconvenience may be perceived by the patient as a major difficulty.

Many problems that beset patients following surgical intervention arise because they become impatient and attempt to undertake more than is wise during the postoperative period of recovery. The referring practitioner expects the dutiful surgeon to provide sufficient information to limit misunderstanding and prepare the patient for aftercare. No less care should be envisaged with this part of surgery—the time spent dealing with a problem and resources required following surgery can increase out of all proportion to the cost of the actual surgery performed.

The role that practitioners play in surgery will vary from advice to acting upon a problem. Specific areas of activity include:

- preparing a patient for surgery
- undertaking re-dressings
- diagnosing a latent complication
- advising on appropriate salvage of a problem with further surgery.

Swelling

The extent of the inflammatory process varies between patients and surgical procedures. Certain parts of the foot, such as the toes, have a greater tendency to swell than others. Toes probably suffer most, as the return of fluid is least efficient here as swelling blocks natural drainage.

Heat, particularly during the hotter times of the year, too much standing, and insufficient daily rest can lead to localised swelling. Healing of skin in healthy patients will only take 2–3 weeks, at which time sutures are normally removed. The non-compliant patient can burst stitches and any residual swelling that develops may place abnormal pressure on the wound. In this case, the sutures will need to be released immediately to safeguard the local tissue. Feet rarely stay swollen for long—if they do, the practitioner must suspect infection, DVT, non-union of bone or overuse (by the patient).

Management of swelling can be achieved with physical therapy such as the cryogenic boot (Aircast; Fig. 7.25). Simple home remedies can also be used and should include raising the leg above the heart. The

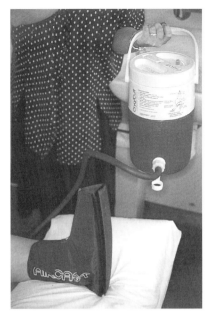

Figure 7.25 An Aircast cryogenic boot will allow iced water to recirculate in a closed system. The effects of the coldness and compression can last for many hours before a change of water is necessary. Patients should not attempt to fall asleep with the device attached, in order to avoid adverse effects of cold on the tissues. Recyling of the iced water is achieved by elevating the reservoir above the body.

knee should be slightly flexed to prevent tension on the sciatic nerve. Ice, crushed in plastic bags, or frozen peas wrapped around the ankle can be applied for 20–30 minutes every few hours, provided that the patient does not fall asleep—ice can cause ischaemia.

Walking aids such as crutches should limit the weight taken by the foot for the advised period of non-weight-bearing. Dressings should be firm and should compress the wound evenly. They should be carefully placed to avoid nerve pressure.

Recalcitrant swelling in toes after surgery may be treated, provided that infection is not present, with a single injection of corticosteroid with local anaesthetic. The patient should be told that toes can remain swollen for many months as a matter of course. Swelling associated with congenital lymphatic disorders, inguinal tumours, dependent oedema from heart failure and varicose veins will inevitably add to the problem. Diuretics to reduce retained interstitial oedema must be used with some caution, because the patient will need to go to the toilet more frequently. Previous trauma around the ankle will also encourage swelling. Both feet should always be compared and more serious problems ruled out.

Deep vein thrombosis

DVT can arise following foot surgery, although this should only account for a small percentage of patients with this condition. DVT has already been discussed in Chapter 4.

Prevention

Those at risk from DVT should be given prophylactic heparin before surgery. The risk of venous stasis increases with bed rest. DVT is inevitably reduced if patients can walk early and exercise their calf muscles. While the patient has to rest, hourly exercise should be undertaken using knee movement. Younger females taking the pill are at risk, as much as older females, from the effects of DVT. Any decision to stop contraception should be discussed with the patient's physician as a matter of course. The view upheld by the medical profession to cease contraceptive therapy before surgery is less than clear for elective minor surgery. Major surgery tends to be viewed differently, especially if a period of stasis arises.

DVT presents with alarming calf pain. The foot and leg may be very swollen and colour changes may be noted. The sudden hardness to palpation provides a strong clue. On examination, pressure should not be applied to the deep tibial vein in case an embolus arises. The circumference should be noted as soon as possible to monitor deterioration or improvement. The next stage of treatment may require a venogram if the condition is thought to be progressive. Admission to hospital allows the patient to be monitored. The silent DVT occurs without warning. Chest pain with shortness of breath indicates a pulmonary embolus. The patient will be in extreme distress, requiring pain control and thrombolysing with the hospital's standard protocol, e.g. streptokinase, alteplase and anistreplase.

In both DVT and pulmonary thrombosis, a team approach is essential. Both problems are uncommon in practice and are not necessarily associated with major surgery. If patients have not had a DVT before, then postoperative risk can only be suspected. Blood-clotting screens may help raise a concern but cannot be used to provide a definitive confirmation of the risk. The best standard blood assay in patients unknown to have a DVT propensity is still the platelet count as it is sensible and cost-effective. The problem of DVT is more likely to arise in females, long surgeries and where periods of immobility are prolonged. DVT symptoms can arise within a few days to several weeks. The practitioner should explain such risks with a view to educating the patient to call for assistance as a matter of urgency.

Infection

The foot is more commonly infected following surgery than many other sites on the body. Audited data seem to suggest that some 2% of podiatry operations may lead to infection (Tollafield & Parmar 1994). Infection is associated with swelling and the patient is in discomfort more often than not. Signs of cellulitis are identified as a demarcation of colour, the skin is tense and may be shiny. Lymphangitis and lymphadenitis may be present. Pyrexic change suggests serious levels of toxicity. Blood assay should include FBC and ESR, as well as a white cell count to establish the severity of any infection and monitor improvement.

Infection is likely to arise after 24–72 hours. Infection should be suspected if pain is difficult to control after the immediate postoperative period. Early antibiosis is likely to provide a favourable reduction in symptoms within 48 hours. Most infections affecting the foot following surgery are associated with *Staphylococcus aureus* unless contracted from within a hospital (nosocomial infection).

Oral antibiosis is usually satisfactory although an initial double dose as a bolus may help to increase the blood level of antibiotic. All the principles of ice, rest and elevation should be applied and the patient should refrain from walking—full rest with elevation is the key to the best resolution.

Where infection does not resolve, pus may be in evidence, causing a rise in pressure at the site of the wound. The wound dehisces, exposing the area to further infection. Necrotic tissue should be debrided until healthy bleeding is visible. The wound is laid open to drain and then packed. The course of management in complicated infections is described in the case history in Box 7.3 and illustrated in Figure 7.26.

Osteomyelitis imposes a protracted period of care. Long-term antibiotics should be used as a dual drug therapy, e.g. flucloxacillin with fusidic acid. In severe cases, admission to hospital for i.v. drug administration may be necessary. Surgical debridement of bone is advocated where sequestrae are identified and where blood tests remain high despite adequate antibiotic levels. In all cases of infection, the patient can expect to remain off work for three times the normal expected period.

> **Box 7.3**   Case history: postsurgical infection
>
> A 48-year-old female had a base wedge osteotomy performed to correct her hallux valgus. Surgery was unremarkable but 1 week later the foot swelled and an infection was noted. The wound burst and oral antibiotics failed to contain the bacteria (*S. aureus*). The internally placed screw loosened and backed out of the bone, revealing the head of the screw in the wound. The patient was readmitted to theatre and the hardware removed and deep infection thoroughly lavaged. Infection had produced a papery separation between the skin and the superficial fascia. Exudate had pushed under the skin causing it to separate. The wound was extensively debrided and the antibiotic strength was doubled and extended for 3 weeks. The wound was left open to drain and packed; dressings were changed three times a week. The wound took 3 months to settle and the bone required the use of an 'Aircast' to maintain fracture site stability.
>
> *Comment*
>
> This case was unusual in that the patient had complied with her postoperative instructions. The summer temperature had reached 32°C (90°F) and the patient had been unable to cope with it. The inflammatory response and infection had loosened the well-positioned screw as the bone dimensions had expanded slightly. The main concern lay in retaining good bone alignment and preventing an osteomyelitis from developing. The whole episode delayed the patient's recovery by 5 months, when 1 month was the anticipated recovery period. The end result was greater scarring with some loss of underlying tissue, causing a dented appearance. This settled in time, giving a flat scar line.

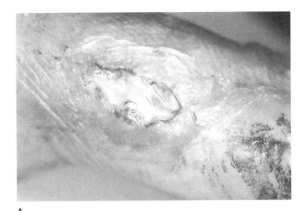

A

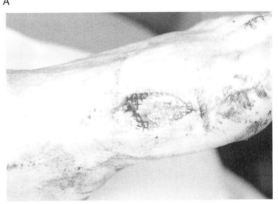

B

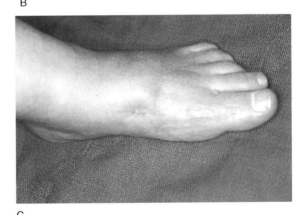

C

Figure 7.26   A: A screw is seen in the wound in the presence of dehiscence and cellulitis. B: At 1 week after surgery, the screw has been removed and debridement has created a new bed of healing following drainage. C: At 12 weeks, the skin has healed by secondary intention.

Pain

Patients respond to pain in different ways. The elderly are often stoic and may need encouraging to take pain medication. Patients who are sensitive to pain can often be identified by asking about their analgesic medications used at home. Those patients who have no drugs in their house probably cope better than those who constantly use analgesics and become tolerant to the lower strength paracetamol/codeine compounds.

Unremitting pain through inadequate control is not acceptable—the cause must be identified. Suppression of pain should be achieved, after considering the patient's medical history, with appropriate drug therapy. In particular, the health of the gastro-intestinal tract should be considered, as many drugs can irritate the lining. Hiatus hernia, ulcers and gastric reflux are common ailments which will be irritated by NSAIDs (non-specific anti-inflammatory drugs).

The patient should be provided with pre-emptive pain control suited to the type of operation. The main objective of pain control is to prevent the patient from becoming anxious, crying or losing sleep. The operative site may throb and be generally sore, but should be controlled at a level commensurate with the patient being able to hold a conversation, and to eat and drink as part of coping psychologically. The pain regimen should last for the shortest period at the lowest dose able to bring relief. Nausea and vomiting complicate pain control and analgesics can be injected intramuscularly (i.m.) or used per rectum (p.r.) if this is a cause of stomach irritation. Anti-emetics may be required if marked nausea and vomiting arises.

Local anaesthetic blockades are invaluable and work as well as morphine without causing hallucinogenic side-effects. The source of pain should always be identified and managed before increasing the level of pain medication. Ice and elevation are essential components of good analgesic postoperative pain management. Patients should know that pain normally lasts for only a short period and should be expected. Pre-operative discussion of pain levels should always be undertaken. Overstating the anticipated pain level is far better than understating the problem—such psychoanalysis works wonders! The two most common problems to arise following surgery relate to pain medication not given early enough (and then only on demand), and to too weak a dose being given when pain control is provided.

Transcutaneous nerve stimulators (TNS) have a role in pain management. They should be placed above the ankle along the nerve routes. New products for pain management reach the health market constantly, although many appeal to the psychologically sensitive by autosuggestion rather than providing direct scientific benefit. Rest, ice and elevation provide important supportive strategies to analgesia which should not be underestimated.

Scar lines

All operations have scars; some patients are lucky enough to have only faint lines. The scar line starts off as vascular for some months. The incision line swells and then regresses slowly, appearing soft and flat. The surgeon normally elects to keep scar lines away from the surfaces most exposed to pressure; these include plantar metatarsals primarily, and skin over the heel, which may come into contact with the heel counter of the shoe. Incision lines over joints may thicken, especially those just over tendon routes.

Both white and black skins can suffer from hypertrophic (thickened) scarring. Careful questioning before surgery should include discussion about the effects of previous surgery. Examination of previous scars should be carried out and noted in the records under the plan of care. Corticosteroid medication should be infiltrated under the sutured incision line to prevent unwarranted hypertrophy at surgery. Hypertrophy is a minor complication which may not cause any discomfort, but it can result in severe elevation around lesser toes. A Z-plasty may be required to deal with contracture, but only after a period of at least 2 years, as scars slowly regress with time. Keloid is a condition where the wound heals outside the normal boundary expected. The scar is raised and has an irregular edge which can spread widely. Surgical revision is fraught with recurrence and the opinion of a plastic surgeon should be sought before further surgery is anticipated.

Ultrasound and vitamin A/E cream and other softening emollients should be used after steroid injections. The scar line should be compressed with silicone gel pads for as many months as appears beneficial. Both practitioner and patient must adopt patience. Scars may take 2 years before they show any noticeable improvement (Fig. 7.27).

Necrosis

During the healing process, some swelling and colour change are normal and should cause little concern. Dressings should ideally be changed early to assess deterioration. Patients who seem not to understand instructions well must be reviewed early. Colour changes are associated with oxygenation and perfusion, swelling and skin tension. Dark mauve colours indicate severe trauma—with rest, the tissue recovers. High red areas are due to pre-ulcerative change. Monitoring such changes is essential every few days. Skin with darkened edges usually means that the tissue edges have been traumatised or that the skin was handled roughly during surgery. Local sloughing is of little consequence, but will result in healing by secondary intention. Distal darkening, red to black, is of greater concern, particularly if the area is extensive. The skin will slough, leaving a healthy pink underlayer. During the rather alarming postoperative period of change, the patient should have the wound dressed and kept clean. Antibiotic cover should be used if the wound weeps or appears fragile. The attraction of anaerobes is as unwelcome as aerobes at this point. Vascular studies, e.g. Doppler or heat thermography, may help to determine blood flow. Any tight sutures should be removed immediately—resuturing should never be attempted.

If the patient looses tissue or the tissue ulcerates, a split thickness skin graft can be used after the base has healed. If the circulation is compromised, the

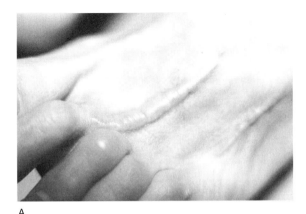

A

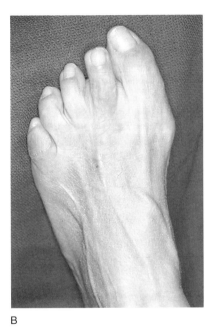

B

Figure 7.27 Hypertrophic scarring has arisen over the dorsum of the foot in a white 57-year-old female. A: After surgery. B: Two years later the scar has settled over the second metatarsal. At no time was the scar painful, merely unsightly.

part will have to be debrided until healthy circulation can be established. The patient will need to be protected by i.v./oral antibiotics.

Loss of sensation

Localised sensory loss is common after surgery. Small nerve fibres become damaged during surgical dissection. The permanency of this damage depends upon the site and the type of destruction imposed. Regene-

ration may take 9 months; after this period of time any areas of sensory loss will most likely be permanent.

In hallux valgus surgery, the medial branch of the superficial peroneal nerve is commonly transected. The medial skin of the great toe may become insensate. Most patients tend to recover after 2 months. Ankle (arthroscopy) surgery and surgery using percutaneous techniques can inadvertently damage both nerve and blood vessels.

Repair of damaged nerves should be referred to a neurosurgeon only where the function of the foot and quality of life is affected. Damage to the plantar surface, for example, could lead to pressure ulcers as a result of an iatrogenic neuropathy. Nerve conduction studies may provide assistance in determining early damage, but the distal nerves in the foot are difficult to monitor accurately. Postsurgical compartment syndrome will require a fasciotomy to be performed as a matter of urgency. Increased interstitial fluid builds up under tension and can cause the circulation to become compromised.

Increased sensation and dysfunction

While surgery can damage nerves, reducing their ability to transmit signals, nerves can be affected by increased sensitivity—hyperaesthesia. Entrapment neuromata arise within scar tissue between tissue layers or within the skin. A sensitive scar line may have to be re-excised if it does not settle within 3 months. Postneurectomy pain may trouble patients following Morton's neuroma resection. A stump forms in the intermetatarsal tissue and is actively excited as it becomes irritated. The surgeon may have correctly biopsied the nerve tissue, confirming the original diagnosis, but revision can still be required. Plantar surface exposure identifies amputated nerve endings which can become surprisingly thickened. Patients with recurrent symptoms may require an MRI or ultrasound scan to show the presence of the nerve. A high suspicion warrants surgery and this should be offered after 3 months if conservative injections fail to assist improvement.

Hyperaesthesia is a highly sensitive response even to light touch. Two forms are described. The first, causalgia, may result in burning pain along a specific peripheral nerve route, but this usually follows a known injury. Nerves should be identified and the appropriate speciality consulted. The second, reflex sympathetic dystrophy syndrome (RSDS), provides the most alarming and serious side-effect seen after surgery, particularly associated with hands or feet. RSDS is not exclusive to surgical trauma. While minor injury can cause the problem, the reaction to such minimal injury is highly aggressive. Known RSDS patients or even those suspected as presenting with RSDS should be evaluated by a pain specialist before surgery is attempted. The cardinal signs of RSDS include vasomotor colour changes, hyperalgesia, bone atrophy, known as Sudek's atrophy, and stiffness. A psychological diathesis may well be associated with the type of person likely to suffer; another theory behind the cause relates to a hypersympathetic reaction, similar to the Raynaud's sufferer.

Whether temperament or autonomic control forms the basis for RSDS, the normal inflammatory response fails to turn off the pain transmitters, histamine, bradykinin and substance P. RSDS can deteriorate, causing gross disability and dependency on crutches or a wheel chair, and can affect the contralateral side. Patients soon become labelled, and in children the condition can affect the stability of the family unit.

Treatment is poorly defined. If the signs and symptoms can be recognised early—within weeks—mobility can be improved with spinal blocks of guanethidine or local anaesthetic. Sympathectomy is used and has some success, but no treatment offers a definitive outcome. The earlier that mobility can be restored, the faster the pain cycle is broken and vasomotor control settles. This condition is one where, after a while, the patient is often driven to seek legal resolve.

Bone union

While power instrumentation improves the surgeon's efficiency, the rapid oscillation of saw blades can burn the ends of bone, causing necrosis.

Most problems with a delayed union result in too much movement across the fracture site. Well-positioned fixation can limit this problem. Non-union arises after 9 months, when radiographic evidence suggests that the bone has atrophied (demineralised) and the ends have failed to develop callus. In cases of delayed union, there are no signs of new bone formation at around 6–8 weeks. Bone reduced with screws may show little activity and should not be confused with a delay in union; furthermore, the area around the screw may show signs of osteopaenia.

If bone union problems occur, the first stage in treatment is immobilisation in a cast for 6 weeks. A walker cast can be used for a further 6 weeks until radiographic evidence supports improvement. Where the bone shows no signs of healing, revision surgery in which a plate is used to reduce the fracture site may be required. The ends of the bone should be cleared

of fibrous material to allow new bleeding and osteoblastic activity to develop. Electrical bone stimulators have been used to improve bone activity by piezoelectric effect of calcium hydroxyapatite crystals. Vitamin D/calciferol and calcium supplements can be given, and there is a role for hormonal replacement therapy in postmenopausal women; supplements of this nature, can support new bony mineralisation if the patient is likely to have some immobility.

Pain may result from poor union, but once the correct diagnosis has been made, treatment is usually effective. The patient should know that postsurgical recovery can be delayed for up to 6–12 months.

ANAESTHETIC TECHNIQUES FOR FOOT SURGERY

The practitioner may be asked questions by the patient concerning the most suitable anaesthetic technique for surgery. A variety of anaesthetic methods are available for surgery on the foot. All the techniques described should be performed in a hospital. The exception to this rule is local anaesthetic infiltration for short day-case surgery, but all units should have provision for basic resuscitation, which ideally includes oxygen and an approved defibrillator with heart monitor.

General anaesthetic (GA)

The patient is unconscious during the operation, having been sedated initially (PO), anaesthetised and provided with an intra-operative analgesic. Full patient monitoring is essential throughout. Gas inhalation is commonly used to maintain the level of anaesthesia (Fig. 7.28). Modern anaesthetic techniques

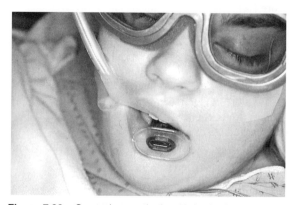

Figure 7.28 General anaesthetic with intubation and gas inhalation. A small Guedel oropharyngeal tube has been used to ensure that the teeth are protected.

are safe and newer anaesthetic agents are easier to recover from than was previously the case. The ideal anaesthetic does not result in postoperative nausea and vomiting (PONV), and recovery is rapid.

The *advantages* of general anaesthetic are rapid induction, elimination of anxiety and improved case load efficiency, as anaesthesia is predictable when compared with local anaesthetic. Longer surgical operations may be easier under GA, where patients would find the duration difficult to tolerate under local anaesthetic (LA). Children and uncooperative patients may best be referred for general anaesthetic for this reason.

The *disadvantages* of GA are associated with cost. An anaesthetist and recovery team are required. Patients may have to be admitted overnight if PONV is uncontrolled or any side-effects arise, such as low or high blood pressure. Procedures over 1 hour are more likely to require admission into hospital. Many drugs used in GA upset the hormone and biochemistry balance. The risks from cardiac arrest, anaphylaxis and malignant hyperthermia are rare but fatal. Aspiration of stomach contents poses another problem. Vomit and productive phlegm has to be managed by careful suction removal during recovery, to prevent asphyxiation or postoperative respiratory problems. Prolonged operations may result in pressure sores where theatre staff are inattentive to tissue over prominences and correct turning procedure.

Local anaesthetic (LA)

Locally injected anaesthetic agents can be contrasted to GA for a range of surgical techniques. In minor biopsy surgery, for example, the anaesthetic can be infiltrated under the lesion, with or without adrenaline. Analgesia, rather than true anaesthesia, is achieved—while pain, temperature and sharp/deep pressure are removed, consciousness remains.

Ring blocks around toes allow access for nail ablations and IP joint arthrodesis. A Mayo block (Fig. 7.29) is suitable for surgery around the first metatarsal head and great toe. Regional blocks are favoured by podiatrists because higher volume anaesthetics are kept away from the surgical site and are less painful to administer. A good block can effectively anaesthetise the foot, allowing most distal ankle surgery to be performed safely and effectively.

The *advantages* of LA are to do with the reduced cost of the procedure. An anaesthetist is not required and the postoperative care team is replaced by an intensive in-theatre care team, which consists of a person caring for the patient who remains awake

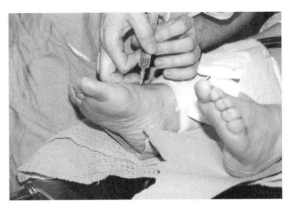

Figure 7.29 The Mayo block for the distal first metatarsal segment is quick and easy to perform along the lines of the digital ring block. Skilled podiatrists find this relatively uncomfortable for patients and will use regional ankle blocks in preference.

throughout. The patient does not require any recovery, does not suffer from PONV and rarely requires admission. The patient management is probably slightly more predictable than under GA. LA can be used in selected patients with high blood pressure, kidney and liver disease, and disturbs controlled diabetics less than GA. Patients do not have to fast and must be reminded to eat before surgery to avoid low blood sugar which can lead to unexpected syncope. However, longer cases under planned LA may need to fast, if the option to convert to GA is available. Such conversion is prevented if food has been recently ingested.

The *disadvantages* of LA lie in the delay associated with regional blocks. Some blocks can take 60 minutes to perform satisfactorily. Anxious patients are difficult to manage in this situation—in rare cases, practitioners may find that anaesthesia is impossible to achieve, despite flooding the area locally. While problems associated with LA are rare, all such drugs should be used in volumes that are within the optimum dose recommended by the manufacturer. Too great a volume of anaesthetic can cause ischaemia, even without the use of vasoconstrictors. Side-effects can arise, causing serious CNS and cardiovascular depression, e.g. CNS fitting and CVS hypotension and cardiac arrest.

Sedation anaesthesia

This is another form of GA. Drugs used to provide sedation include benzodiazepines such as diazepam and midazolam. In small doses, the patient may remain awake, while in larger doses sleep will be produced but arousal is possible. Many i.v. and i.m. drugs produce a range of effects that can give rise to different levels of anaesthesia. Propofol (Diprivan, Zeneca) is another useful drug, which, when combined with midazolam, allows the anaesthetist to control the patient's level of consciousness. Local anaesthetic must be given for pain control. This technique avoids problems associated with alfentanil, fentanyl and other intra-operative opioid analgesics causing potential respiratory depression.

Sedation anaesthesia has the *advantage* of providing the patient with the benefits of both LA and GA. PONV is very much less common and the patient's recovery is very quick, although drowsiness can last for an hour afterwards. The *disadvantages* are minimal in the hands of an experienced anaesthetist.

Intravascular block

The Biers block uses low strength local anaesthetic, such as 0.5% plain xylocaine or prilocaine, infused into a vein below an ankle cuff. The cuff is double-chambered and monitored by the anaesthetist (Fig. 7.30). Intravascular leakage above the cuff can affect the brain and heart, given the high volumes

(20–40 ml) required, and poses a greater risk than that from local anaesthetic infiltrated around specific nerves. Intraosseous absorption can still arise despite the use of a tourniquet.

The *advantages* lie in a quick perfusion technique which seeps into bone and soft tissue. *Disadvantages* lie in the high risk of fits from early release of the cuff or leaky cuffs. A full system of monitoring should be instituted and an i.v. cannula should be in place before any drug is administered. Surgery must last at least 30 minutes to allow absorption into the tissues before safely deflating the cuff. Biers block cannot be used for short cases.

TNS—regional blocks

Recent advances with nerve stimulators (TNS) have allowed accurate placement of regional blocks at the level of the sciatic nerve, but it can also be used at the level of common peroneal or tibial nerves (Fig. 7.31).

The main *advantage* lies in a long-acting block used proximally, keeping anaesthesia away from the surgical site. The only nerve in the foot which must be separately infiltrated is the saphenous nerve. *Disadvantages* include failure—Dryden et al (1993) reported the need for general anaesthetic in 10% of cases where the sciatic block failed. The patient cannot ambulate easily for several hours following surgery.

Spinal/epidural anaesthesia

This provides an additional method for anaesthetising the foot. Spinal and epidural anaesthesia have similar points of insertion and contrasting effects. In the case of spinal analgesia, a fine needle is advanced until

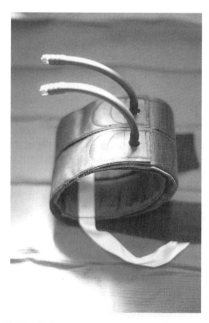

Figure 7.30 A double-cuffed chamber placed around the ankle in a Bier block. This provides an essential safety requirement to prevent premature vascular leakage affecting the heart or CNS.

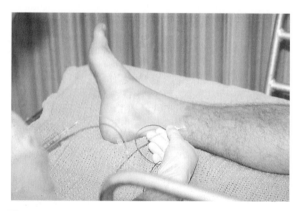

Figure 7.31 A nerve stimulator needle (stimulator not shown) is used with a tibial regional nerve block to effect plantar analgesia (Braun Medical, Aylesbury, UK).

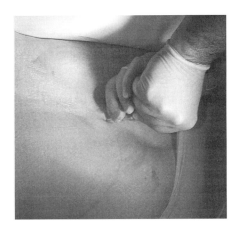

Figure 7.32 Spinal/epidural anaesthesia is popular in many centres, particularly where patients are at risk. One of the main complications is associated with a dramatic fall in blood pressure (see text).

the subarachnoid space can be infiltrated (Fig. 7.32). In epidural analgesia, a thicker needle is used and the subarachnoid space is not breached. The main *advantage* lies in managing patients who might not be suited to general anaesthetic.

There are several *disadvantages*. Both lower limbs are affected. Obese patients are difficult to inject, although it is the case that the obese patient will make anaesthetic more difficult in most operative procedures. As with most regional blocks, this technique is slower

than GA and affects a great deal more than just the foot. Postoperative problems include induced hypotension following sympathetic paralysis and dilatation, anaphylaxis, local infection, backache, headaches and urinary retention. A skilled anaesthetist is also required.

SUMMARY

The principles of surgical management, their complications and methods of anaesthesia have been briefly outlined in this chapter.

In all cases of referral, the practitioner should ask four important questions:

- does the patient require surgery?
- will the patient be made better by surgery instead of other methods of management?
- is the surgery cost effective?
- will surgery create unwanted side-effects that can be avoided by using conservative care instead?

Referral of patients who are unsuitable for surgery creates unnecessary anxiety for those who might already fear such intervention.

Much of the preparation for surgical referral can be achieved by good initial patient advice. As with all types of management, the practitioner must bear in mind that successful surgery relates to a partnership between the patient, the person undertaking the referral and the person undertaking treatment.

REFERENCES

Corey S V, Ruch J A 1992 Principles of internal fixation. In: McGlamry E D, Banks A S & Downey M S (eds) Comprehensive textbook of foot surgery. Williams & Wilkins, Baltimore, p 141

Downey M S 1992 Ankle equinus. In: McGlamry E D, Banks A S & Downey M S (eds) Comprehensive textbook of foot surgery. Williams & Wilkins, Baltimore, p 710–711

Dryden C M, Lloyd S M, Todd J G 1993 Sciatic nerve block as anaesthesia for foot surgery and the effect of preservatives in local anaesthetic solutions on the characteristic nerve block. The Foot 3: 184–186

Henry A P J, Waugh W 1975 The use of footprints in assessing the results of operations for hallux valgus. A comparison of Keller's operation with arthrodesis. Journal of Bone and Joint Surgery 57-B: 478–481

McGlamry E D, Banks A S, Downey M S 1992 Comprehensive textbook of foot surgery, 2nd edn. Williams & Wilkins, Baltimore, vols 1 & 2

Mann R A, Coughlin M J 1993 Surgery of the foot and ankle. Mosby, St Louis, vols 1 & 2

Miller S 1992 Principles of muscle tendon surgery and tendon transfers. In: McGlamry E D, Banks A S & Downey M S (eds) Comprehensive textbook of foot surgery. Williams & Wilkins, Baltimore, p 1306

Radin E L, Rose R M, Blaha J D, Litsky A S 1992 Practical biomechanics for the orthopaedic surgeon. Churchill Livingstone, New York, p 139–140

Swanson A B, de Groot Swanson G, Maupin B K, Shi S 1991 The use of a grommet bone liner for flexible hinge implant arthroplasty of the great toe. Foot & Ankle 12(3): 149–155

Tollafield D R, Parmar D G 1994 Setting standards for day care foot surgery. A quinquennial review. British Journal of Podiatric Medicine 6(1): 7–20

Tollafield D R 1995 Protecting Kirschner wires postoperatively. British Journal of Podiatric Medicine 7(4): 71

FURTHER READING

Cracchiolo A, III 1993 The rheumatoid foot and ankle: pathology and treatment. The Foot 3: 126–134

Lunn J N 1991 Lecture notes on anaesthetics. Blackwell Scientific Publications, London

Paton R W, Galsko C S B 1991 Accurate structural assessment of idiopathic CTEV. The Foot 2: 71–73

Rosen J S, Grady J F 1986 Neuritic bunion syndrome. Journal of American Podiatric Medical Association 76(11): 641–644

Saxby T, Myerson M, Schon L 1993 Compartment syndrome of the foot following calcaneus fracture. The Foot 2: 157–161

Swanson A B , de Groot Swanson G, Mayhew D E, Khan A N 1987 Flexible hinged results in implant arthroplasty of the great toe. Rheumatology 11: 136–152

8

Pharmacology

J. Carpenter
L. M. Merriman

INTRODUCTION

There is a range of prescription-only and over-the-counter drugs which contribute to the management of foot problems. The majority of these pharmacological preparations reduce and control the symptoms of the condition rather than address the underlying cause. Antibiotics are the exception to this. In the management of foot problems, pharmacological treatments are often combined with non-pharmacological strategies in order to bring about the best therapeutic effect.

Drugs used in the management of foot problems are usually administered topically. Other routes, such as oral, subcutaneous and intra-articular, are also used, but to a lesser extent.

It is important that practitioners have a good working knowledge of the properties, actions and contraindications associated with drugs they may use in the treatment of foot problems. Practitioners must undertake a thorough assessment of the patient's medical history and be aware of past and current drug therapy for other health-related problems prior to prescribing pharmacological preparations. There are a whole range of contraindications associated with the use of drugs and these must be taken into account for each patient before a clinical decision is reached about whether pharmacological preparations should be used.

This chapter describes ways in which drugs can be administered and goes on to explore the following therapeutic drug groups used in the management of foot problems:

- analgesics
- anhidrotics
- anti-inflammatories (non-steroidal and steroidal)
- antimicrobials
- antipuritics
- caustics

- counter-irritants
- emollients.

Dressings and desloughing agents, as they are applicable to ulcer management, are addressed in Chapter 18.

TERMINOLOGY

In its widest sense, a *drug* is any substance which modifies normal physiological function. Normal hormones and neurotransmitters, such as hydrocortisone and adrenaline, must be considered to be drugs, especially if they are used medicinally. A *medicine* is a preparation which contains one or more drugs made up in such a way that it is convenient to administer and from which the drugs can be absorbed efficiently.

All proprietary drugs have at least three names. The first of these is its *full chemical name*, for example (±)-1-isopropylamino-3-(naphthyloxy) propan-2-ol hydrochloride. For obvious reasons this name is seldom used, and never in clinical practice. The second name is the drug's *non-proprietary (official, approved, or generic) name*. For the chemical described above, this is propranolol. Note that the non-proprietary name is not spelled with a capital letter. Any company with rights to manufacture and sell a drug can use this non-proprietary name, and since each drug has only one of these, drugs mentioned in this chapter are always referred to by their non-proprietary names. Drugs listed in the British National Formulary are arranged in therapeutic groups in the alphabetical order of their non-proprietary names (except for important drugs typical of their type which are sometimes listed first and out of alphabetic order). The third name is the *proprietary (trade) name*. In fact, one drug can have many proprietary names. Propranolol is sold under the names Inderal, Bedranol, Efektol, Pylapron, Tesnol, and about 38 more. Note that proprietary names are always spelled with a capital letter. Proprietary names are the properties of individual companies and cannot be used by other companies without a contractual agreement between them.

The term 'generic' is often used instead of 'non-proprietary name', which is unfortunate because it means that there is no useful word to describe drugs belonging to a particular group or class. For example, 'barbiturate' and 'sulphonamide' are true generic names, embracing classes of drug, whereas the non-proprietary names of the individual barbiturates or sulphonamides are not truly generic—they are specific.

Most multiple-ingredient, fixed-dose formulations have only a proprietary name, although a few such medicines are recognised as being particularly worthy of recognition and are given non-proprietary names, e.g. co-trimoxazole (a mixture of trimethoprim and sulphamethoxazole in the proportions of 1 part to 5 parts) and co-proxamol tablets (dextropropoxyphene hydrochloride 32.5 mg plus paracetamol 325 mg per tablet).

Non-proprietary names are generally designed to indicate the class to which the drug belongs. For example, all cephalosporin and cephalomycin antibiotics have 'cef' or 'ceph' in their non-proprietary names: cefaclor, cefadroxil, cefixime, cefodizime. Unfortunately, this standardisation is only quite recent and older drugs may have non-proprietary names quite unrelated to other drugs with the same mechanism of action in the same therapeutic class, e.g. buprenorphine, codeine, dextromoramide, dipipanone, meptazinol, pentazocine, and pethidine are all opioid analgesics.

MODE OF ADMINISTRATION

Before a drug can produce its effects, it must reach its site of action. The majority of drugs are not administered directly to the site of drug action, so that molecules of the drug must move from the site of administration to the site of action (Fig. 8.1). The exception to this is the topical application of drugs directly to a site and the injection of a drug into a joint.

In order to cross 'barriers' in the body, a drug must be able to cross cell membranes, which are largely composed of lipid. To cross such membranes, drug molecules must be *lipid-soluble*. This is a confusing term because many lipid-soluble drugs dissolve readily in water. When a drug is described as lipid-soluble, it means that, when exposed to both a lipid or oil and water, the drug will dissolve preferentially in the oily layer. Alternatively, if the drug is already dissolved in water then it will tend to move out of water (aqueous phase) into surrounding cell membranes (lipid phase). 'Lipid-soluble' is thus a jargon short-hand term meaning 'High oil:water partition coefficient'.

Sites of administration

Oral. This is the most convenient form of drug administration. It is only effective for drugs that are lipid-soluble, resistant to the acid environment of the stomach, and not rapidly broken down by hepatic enzymes. The time to maximal plasma concentration after oral administration is considerably greater than

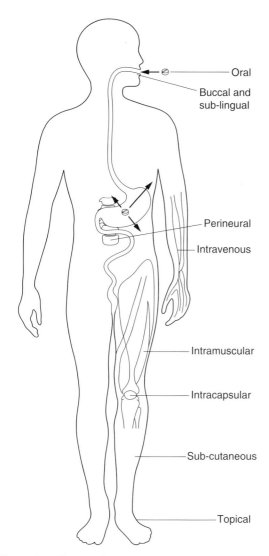

Figure 8.1 Routes of administration of drugs.

Buccal and sublingual. The mucous membrane of the mouth is very thin and richly supplied with blood vessels. Consequently, lipid-soluble drugs are readily absorbed from the lining of the mouth. This is the preferred route for drugs that are susceptible to hepatic *first-pass metabolism*, such as glyceryl trinitrate. This is because the venous drainage of the mucous lining of the mouth is not part of the hepatic portal system and thus the drug enters the systemic circulation without passing through the liver.

Intravenous. Drugs administered directly into a vein reach their peak plasma concentration instantaneously. Plasma concentrations then fall continuously (Fig. 8.2). Intravenous injection is the preferred route when therapeutic concentrations must be achieved rapidly, for example in life-threatening infections, or if the drug is too highly water-soluble to be absorbed from the gastrointestinal tract or too irritant to be given by any other route.

Intramuscular. Skeletal muscle (gluteus, deltoid) is richly supplied with blood vessels, so that a drug injected into muscle will readily enter the systemic blood supply. Peak plasma concentrations are reached more slowly than they are after intravenous injection, but more quickly than after subcutaneous injection (Fig. 8.2). This is the preferred route of injection as it does not involve the same level of skills as intravenous injection and is suitable for most water-soluble drugs that are not irritant.

Subcutaneous. There is a thin layer of fatty tissue, immediately under the skin, supported with a poor blood supply. Drugs injected into this layer will therefore be absorbed quite slowly. After subcutaneous injection, the peak plasma concentration is reached more slowly than after either intramuscular (i.m.)

after parenteral administration (by injection). Formulations for oral administration include liquids (often syrups or suspensions), capsules and tablets. Tablets are sometimes specially coated to protect the drug they contain from the activity of gastric acid and enzymes. Such tablets are known as enteric coated tablets. Capsules are usually made of gelatin, which dissolves in the stomach releasing the active drug. There are also several other formulations designed to release the drug slowly over prolonged periods in order to extend the duration of action of the drug. These are known as sustained-release (or controlled-release) formulations.

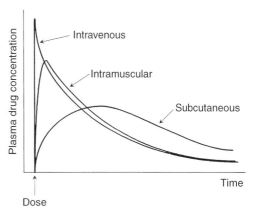

Figure 8.2 Plasma drug concentration levels for intravenous, intramuscular and subcutaneous injections.

or intravenous (i.v.) injection (Fig. 8.2). Subcutaneous injection into the thigh or abdomen is the preferred route of injection for non-irritant, water-soluble drugs when a more sustained action is required than can be achieved by other routes, e.g. insulin.

Intracapsular. Injection of a drug directly into a synovial cavity bypasses the diffusion barrier presented by the thick synovial membrane and allows therapeutic concentrations to be reached rapidly. Moreover, the membrane also slows diffusion of drug out of the capsule so that the systemic concentration of the drug will be much lower than that inside the capsule. This is important for drugs that have a marked systemic effect, e.g. corticosteroids.

Perineural. There are several ways in which drugs, e.g. local anaesthetics, can be injected so that they remain at high concentration around a nerve trunk. The principle is that because the blood supply to the area is so poor, the drug diffuses away slowly. When local anaesthetics are administered by infiltration, a vasoconstrictor drug is sometimes used to prolong the drug's action by reducing the local blood flow. In spinal and epidural anaesthesia, the local anaesthetic is injected either into the cerebrospinal fluid (CSF) of the spinal cord or into the epidural space surrounding a particular nerve root.

Topical. Normally, the skin presents a more or less impermeable barrier to water-soluble drugs. Consequently, application of such drugs to the skin allows high concentrations to be achieved on the outer surface of the skin, with little if any absorption into the rest of the body. This enables systemically toxic drugs to be used against, for example, fungal infections of the skin. However, if the integrity of the skin is broken, for example by abrasions or as a result of burns, appreciable absorption can occur, leading to systemic toxicity. Similarly, if the skin becomes indurated with water, as under an occlusive dressing, water-soluble drugs can be absorbed.

For lipid-soluble drugs, appreciable absorption will occur across the skin. This can be made use of in two ways. Firstly, application to the skin is a convenient way of administering lipid-soluble drugs when prolonged action is required. Skin patches which deliver nicotine (for withdrawal from smoking), glyceryl trinitrate (for angina), oestrogen (for hormone replacement therapy) or hyoscine (for travel sickness) are now widely used. Secondly, by applying a high concentration of a lipid-soluble drug to a limited area of skin, relatively high concentrations will be achieved in the tissues underlying the area of application. If such administration is prolonged, the systemic concentration will eventually rise sufficiently for systemic rather than local effects to be produced. This will happen more readily if the area of application is large, if the drug is very lipid-soluble, or if the skin integrity is reduced. It should be borne in mind that the surface/body mass ratio is much higher in children than in adults, so that topical administration to children is more likely to lead to significant systemic concentrations of drug.

THERAPEUTIC DRUG GROUPS USED IN THE MANAGEMENT OF FOOT PROBLEMS

ANALGESICS

Analgesics are drugs which relieve pain. There are two main types, opioids which stimulate the body's *opioid* (or *narcotic*) receptors, and those that work as anti-inflammatories (prevent prostaglandin synthesis). The latter are known as *antipyretic analgesics*.

Analgesics have a number of uses in the management of foot pain. They can be used:

- pre-operatively to reduce postoperative pain
- to prevent pain during an operation (local anaesthetics)
- postoperatively to reduce pain
- to manage acute, non-surgically derived pain
- to manage chronic, non-surgically derived pain.

They can be administered orally, intravenously, intramuscularly and topically. The oral, intramuscular and topical routes are the most favoured.

The management of foot pain is complex. Every effort should be made to identify the cause of the pain and reduce or remove its effects. Analgesics are a form of pharmacological treatment which have an important role to play in the management of pain alongside non-pharmacological strategies. If analgesics are to be used, it is essential that a thorough patient history has been taken to exclude the presence of allergies, gastrointestinal ulcers or gastric reflux, all of which contraindicate the use of antipyretic analgesics. A wide range of analgesics are available over the counter. Patients require good advice as to which analgesics are appropriate for their pain, and should be made well aware of the unwanted effects which may arise.

The following analgesics are discussed in the remainder of this section:

- opioid
- antipyretic

- local anaesthetics
- topical anaesthetics.

Opioid analgesics

Indications

The maximal degree of analgesia that is attainable with opioid analgesics varies. Morphine and diamorphine ('heroin') have the highest ceiling effects, with pethidine rather less. Dihydrocodeine and codeine have intermediate and low ceiling effects, with dextropropoxyphene the least.

Although all the drugs described above are active after oral administration, diamorphine and morphine are not absorbed very rapidly, and consequently are usually administered by injection. Codeine, dihydrocodeine and dextropropoxyphene are well absorbed from the gastrointestinal tract.

Smaller doses of opioid analgesics are needed to *prevent* pain than are necessary to abolish pain once it is present. Consequently, opioids are very helpful when repeated small doses are taken prior to elective surgery, as they prevent the onset of postoperative pain.

Mechanism of action

These drugs have the same mechanism of analgesic action as the active ingredients of opium, the dried latex of the opium poppy. The principal ingredient of opium is morphine. The term narcotic is sometimes used because in high doses these drugs cause stupor and unconsciousness. Opioid analgesics produce their effects by interacting with receptors for enkephalins, endorphins and dynorphins, which are natural peptide transmitters involved in controlling our perception of pain and well-being.

Analgesia results from interference with both transmission of the pain signal up the spinal cord and its interpretation by the limbic system in the brain. Opioids are more effective against constant, general pain than against sharp pain, although they do help sharp pain. In addition to an analgesic action, most of the useful opioids cause some *euphoria*. This may contribute to the analgesic action by making the pain more bearable.

Unwanted effects

The most troubling unwanted effect for patients treated with opioid analgesics is constipation. The most dangerous adverse effect is respiratory depression, and this is the usual cause of death from overdose. However, the respiratory depression is not accompanied by general cardiovascular depression, unlike most sedative/hypnotic/anxiolytics. Allied to respiratory depression is the ability these drugs have to suppress cough—an *antitussive* action. Codeine is a common ingredient of cough linctuses, as is pholcodeine. All the opioid analgesics suppress cough at subanalgesic doses.

Extended use of opioids results in *tolerance* and *physical dependence*; the patient needs progressively more of the drug to achieve the same degree of pain relief (tolerance), and withholding the drug causes the patient to suffer a *withdrawal* (or *abstinence*) *syndrome*. Withdrawal syndromes result when the body has adjusted to the presence of a drug so that normal function is disturbed when the drug is suddenly removed. As the body readjusts to the absence of the drug, the severity of the withdrawal syndrome declines. The signs and symptoms of withdrawal syndromes are generally the opposite of the actions of the drug. For the opioid analgesics, withdrawal of the drug from a dependent patient results in a sense of extreme discomfort (*dysphoria*), pain from normally non-painful stimuli, such as the touch of clothing (*hyperalgesia*), diarrhoea, dilated pupils (*mydriasis*), lack of sleep (*insomnia*) and hyperventilation. These are usually accompanied by a craving for the drug. The withdrawal syndrome can be abruptly terminated by giving an opioid; all of the opioid analgesics (with the exception of the partial agonists) will substitute for one another in supporting a physical dependence.

The more rapidly the blood concentration of the drug falls, the more severe will be the syndrome. Hence the short-acting opioids (diamorphine and morphine) produce more severe withdrawal syndromes than the more slowly eliminated drugs, such as dihydrocodeine or methadone. It is most unlikely that a patient will become physically dependent on an opioid during treatment for acute pain.

Antipyretic analgesics

Indications

These drugs are so named because they combine an analgesic action with the ability to lower body temperature in fever (*pyrexia*). In fact, most drugs in this group combine analgesic and antipyretic properties with anti-inflammatory properties. All of the non-steroidal anti-inflammatory drugs (NSAIDs) are antipyretic analgesics (see section on anti-inflammatories, p. 142). *Paracetamol* is atypical in that it is not a potent anti-inflammatory drug in peripheral tissue, which is why it is usually classed as an antipyretic analgesic as opposed to a NSAID. Paracetamol is a widely available pain-relieving drug. It may be combined with NSAIDs, such as aspirin, or opioids, such as codeine, thus complementing its action with either an anti-inflammatory effect in peripheral tissues or improving its pain-relieving capacity.

Mechanism of action

In fever and headache, antipyretic analgesics are effective because they inhibit the production of prostaglandins in the brain. Fever has been shown to result from the central production of prostaglandins in response to toxic substances (pyrogens) produced by foreign organisms, such as bacteria. Paracetamol selectively inhibits cyclo-oxygenase in the brain; it has a much lower activity against cyclo-oxygenase in peripheral tissues.

Unwanted effects

In quite small overdose (2–3 times the maximal therapeutic dose), paracetamol can produce serious, potentially fatal, adverse effects. When the liver enzymes responsible for the normal phase II metabolism of paracetamol become saturated, metabolism of paracetamol continues by phase I oxidation. However, this produces a toxic metabolite. At first this toxic metabolite is inactivated by phase II conjugation with glutathione. Unfortunately, stores of glutathione in the liver are limited, and once these stores are used up, conjugation of the toxic metabolite ceases and the metabolite accumulates. This causes necrosis of liver and kidney cells, which typically begins 1 or 2 days after the overdose. Patients should be warned of the small margin of safety with paracetamol.

Patients suspected of taking a paracetamol overdose should be urgently admitted to hospital, even if they show no signs of poisoning. The effective antidote to paracetamol overdose is *acetylcysteine* or *methionine*, used to increase the production of glutathione. Treatment must be started within a few hours of the overdose (6–8 hours), otherwise too much damage to the liver will have occurred.

Local anaesthesia

Indications

Local anaesthetics are primarily used to remove pain during a surgical procedure. They are increasingly

---

> **Box 8.1** Advantages of local anaesthetics (Scott 1991)
>
> - Reduction in psychological stress
> - Patient conscious
> - Reduced costs
> - Fewer fatalities
> - Do not require anaesthetists to administer

being used for this purpose as they have a number of distinct advantages over general anaesthetics (Box 8.1). Local anaesthetics have non-surgical uses; they can be very effective, as a short term measure, in reducing acute pain.

Most local anaesthetics are either *esters*, e.g. amethocaine, benzocaine, or *amides*, e.g. lignocaine, prilocaine, bupivacaine. Although some metabolism of the ester local anaesthetics occurs in the tissue into which they are injected, termination of local anaesthesia depends mainly upon the drug being carried away from the tissue in the blood. Local anaesthesia prevents transmission in sympathetic vasoconstrictor fibres so that blood flow in anaesthetised tissues usually increases. Prilocaine is unusual in that it does not cause vasodilatation. The most commonly used local anaesthetics are lignocaine, bupivacaine and prilocaine.

When using local anaesthetics, it is important that the optimum safe dosage is not exceeded.

Mechanism of action

Local anaesthetics (Gr. *an*, without; *aesthesia*, sensation) interfere with the development and transmission of nerve action potentials. They do not distinguish between sensory or motor nerves, somatic or autonomic nerves. As a result, local anaesthetics do not just lead to the loss of pain sensation but also to reduction or loss of other sensations and loss of function.

The small diameter nerve fibres are anaesthetised faster than large diameter fibres. Type C nerve fibres are the most sensitive, whereas type A α (motor) fibres are the least sensitive. This is simply because the former fibres have a greater surface area/volume ratio, so more of the drug enters the nerve fibre in unit time (Fick's law of diffusion). In addition, non-myelinated fibres become anaesthetised before myelinated fibres because the myelin sheath presents a diffusion barrier that the drug must penetrate before acting on the nerve itself.

It is only necessary for a short length of nerve to be anaesthetised for transmission to fail at that point.

If a bundle of fibres is anaesthetised, the whole of the region of the body supplied by (or supplying) the nerves in the bundle will be paralysed or will become anaesthetic.

Normal activity in nerves depends upon transmission of action potentials. Action potentials are self-propagating waves of electrical activity which rely upon the electrical potential energy stored in the nerve fibre by virtue of its resting membrane potential. The membrane of excitable cells (mainly skeletal muscle and nerves fibres) is selectively permeable. It is moderately permeable to K^+ ions, but highly impermeable to Na^+ ions. Furthermore, there is a high concentration of K^+ and a low concentration of Na^+ inside cells. Extracellular fluid is conversely rich in Na^+ but poor in K^+. As a result, K^+ ions tend to leak out of the cell down the K^+ concentration gradient. As most of the negative charge inside cells is carried on proteins, which are too large to pass across the membrane, the leak of K^+ carries a net flux of positive charge out of the cell. The inside of the cell becomes progressively more negatively charged relative to the outside. As this negative charge builds up, it acts to oppose the leak of K^+ ions, because these cations are attracted back into the cell by the intracellular negative charge. Consequently, there are two forces at work in opposition: a concentration gradient for K^+ directed out of the cell and an electrical gradient for K^+ directed into the cell. Eventually these two forces are equal and the rate at which K^+ ions leave the cell under the concentration gradient exactly equals the rate at which other K^+ ions enter the cell under the electrical gradient. This electrical gradient is known as the *equilibrium potential* for potassium.

For this system to work the cell has to be able to keep the intracellular concentration of K^+ ions high and the intracellular concentration of Na^+ ions low. This is achieved by a biochemical pump (*Na^+/K^+-ATPase*) that uses the energy provided by ATP (adenosine triphosphate) to pump Na^+ ions out of the cell in exchange for K^+ ions, which it pumps into the cell. The biochemical energy provided by the operation of the Na^+/K^+ pump running continuously is in the end responsible for the potential energy stored in the nerve fibre in the form of electrical potential—the *membrane potential*. In some ways, the nerve fibre can be viewed as an electrical accumulator which is constantly 'trickle charged' by the Na^+/K^+ pump.

During the transmission of an action potential, the electrical potential across the membrane falls, i.e. the inside becomes less negative. When this happens, the membrane changes its properties. Embedded in the nerve membrane, there are millions of specialised cylindrical protein structures which pass right through from the cytoplasmic side of the membrane to the extracellular surface. These have the ability to change their conformation and allow the passage of Na^+ ions. These so-called 'Na^+ channels' have what amounts to two 'gates' which can open or close the central pore of the channel. These gates are known as the 'm' gate and the 'h' gate (Fig. 8.3A). At normal resting membrane potentials (typically −120 mV), it is thought that the 'm' gates are closed and the 'h' gates open. When the membrane potential falls to a threshold level, the 'm' gates open quickly (*channel activation*), allowing Na^+ ions to enter the cell, carrying positive charge. This causes depolarisation, i.e. the inside of the cell becomes less negative relative to the outside. This depolarisation causes the 'h' gates to close, but they do this moderately slowly. Thus the Na^+ channels close (*inactivate*), stopping the fall in membrane potential. The depolarisation also stimulates K^+ channels to open, and an efflux of K^+ through these channels helps the cell to repolarise quickly. Once the critical membrane potential is reached, the 'm' gates close rapidly and the 'h' gates slowly open again. Until the 'h' gates are open, another action potential is impossible; the fibre is said to be *refractory*. As one part of the membrane depolarises, it activates the sodium channels in the adjacent piece of membrane so that the action potential is propagated along the fibre rather like fire down a trail of gunpowder; the heat of burning grains of gunpowder sets fire to adjacent grains of gunpowder which set fire to adjacent grains, and so on.

Local anaesthetics block the movement of Na^+ ions through these channels, thereby preventing the depolarisation that is necessary for an action potential to be transmitted along the fibre (Fig. 8.3B). Local anaesthetics do this in two ways. Firstly, they are believed to dissolve in the nerve membrane, changing its physicochemical properties so that the protein of the Na^+ channels becomes distorted and less able to function. Secondly, some, if not all, of the local anaesthetics are believed to interact with a specific receptor site located inside the channel pore, near the intracellular end of the sodium channel. When a molecule of local anaesthetic is bound to this receptor, Na^+ ions cannot pass through the channel. Local anaesthetics do this by causing the 'h' gate to close. However, these receptor sites are not accessible to local anaesthetic molecules from the extracellular fluid. Local anaesthetic molecules can only bind to these receptor sites in the pore if they approach from the cytoplasm. This means that the drug must be able to enter the cytoplasm before it can exert this action.

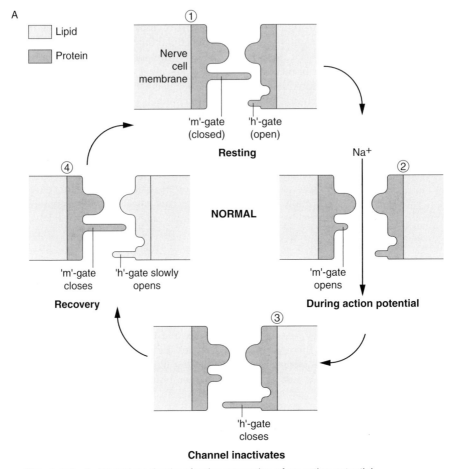

Figure 8.3 A: Normal mechanism for the generation of an action potential.

To gain access to the cytoplasm, the drug must first pass through the cell membrane; only lipid-soluble forms of local anaesthetic molecules can do this. At pH 7.4 (tissue pH), local anaesthetics are partially ionised. Local anaesthetics are weak bases, and so the ionised form is a cation. Although only the non-ionised form diffuses across nerve cell membranes, it is the cationic form that combines with the receptor. Once the non-ionised form has crossed the membrane, it partially dissociates again (typically 80% exists in the ionised form at pH 7.4).

To prolong the duration of anaesthesia, some local anaesthetic preparations contain a vasoconstrictor to prevent vasodilatation. Two vasoconstrictors are available: *adrenaline* and *felypressin*. Adrenaline acts on α_1-adrenoceptors, much like noradrenaline released as a result of activity in sympathetic nerves. Felypressin is a peptide analogue of antidiuretic hormone (ADH, also known as vasopressin). Felypressin stimulates vasopressin receptors to cause vasoconstriction and is preferred if there is a risk that adrenaline may not be tolerated.

Unwanted effects

The main problems which may arise with the use of local anaesthetics are type 1 hypersensitivity reactions (anaphylaxis) and toxic reactions. Anaphylaxis is more common with the ester-type local anaesthetics. Toxic reactions occur in the presence of high plasma concentrations of the local anaesthetic. This initially leads to stimulation of the central nervous system (excitement, nausea, euphoria), followed by dizziness, shivering and drowsiness. In severe cases, the patient may have convulsions. These events are followed by depression of CNS activity, which may affect the cardiovascular system and can lead to circulatory collapse.

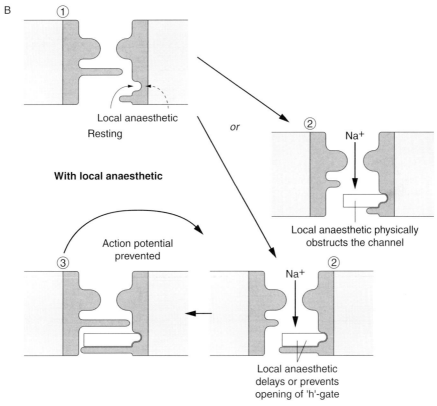

B

Local anaesthetic
Resting

or

② Na+

Local anaesthetic physically
obstructs the channel

With local anaesthetic

Action potential
prevented
③

② Na+

Local anaesthetic
delays or prevents
opening of 'h'-gate

Figure 8.3 B: Mechanism of action of local anaesthetics. By physically obstructing the Na+ channel or by interfering with the opening of the 'h' gate, local anaesthetics prevent Na+ entry into the nerve. As a result, action potential generation is prevented.

Local effects, which may occur as a result of injecting anaesthetics, are irritation and inflammation. If the local effects are severe, this may result in tissue damage and necrosis. The use of local anaesthetics combined with adrenaline or felypressin may lead to prolonged vasoconstriction. This may have irreversible effects in digits, which have a large surface area to volume ratio. Ischaemic changes which lead to gangrene may ensue.

Tricyclic antidepressants act, at least in part, by reducing inactivation by uptake into nerve endings of adrenaline and noradrenaline. There is therefore a risk that patients taking tricyclic antidepressants may develop excessive vasoconstriction in response to adrenaline. Sometimes patients are given monoamine oxidase inhibitors to treat depression. These drugs inhibit the metabolism of adrenaline and there is a small risk of excessive vasoconstriction if adrenaline-containing local anaesthetic is used. Felypressin is not potentiated by either tricyclic antidepressants or

monoamine oxidase inhibitors and therefore may be preferred to adrenaline.

Topical anaesthetics

Indications

Various preparations are used for topical anaesthesia: salicylates, benzocaine, amethocaine, lignocaine and prilocaine. These preparations may be combined, as in EMLA cream, which contains 2.5% lignocaine plus 2.5% prilocaine. The effectiveness of topical anaesthetics is questionable. Their use is often confined to analgesia of the skin prior to the administration of an injection. Additionally they may be incorporated into antipruritics.

Topical anaesthetics may be presented in lotions, creams, ointments, sprays or skin patches. Up to 10% of the free base in an oily vehicle has been found to be effective in achieving a small localised area of skin anaesthesia.

Mechanism of action

Local anaesthetics such as benzocaine and lignocaine produce analgesia when applied to mucous membranes and broken skin. Their action on intact skin is debatable. If applied to intact skin they must be applied for at least an hour, under occlusion, in order to penetrate the skin barrier and have any noticeable effects.

Salicylates, when administered orally, inhibit prostaglandin synthesis. It is known that salicylates are absorbed percutaneously, and therefore it is postulated that topical application of salicylates prevents the local synthesis of prostaglandins. As salicylates also have a known hyperaemic effect, it is also thought that their counter-irritant effect aids analgesia. It is believed that topical analgesics containing salicylates are best applied by massage; the action of massage is considered to aid rapid clearance of locally-produced pain-inducing substances.

ANHIDROTICS

Indications

Anhidrotics are useful in the treatment of hyperhidrosis. The main anhidrotics are the aldehydes and aluminum salts. The aldehydes, e.g. glutaraldehyde and formaldehyde, can be very effective topically, especially in concentrations of 10%. Preparations based on the aluminum salts are the most popular and appear to be the most effective, e.g. 20% aluminum chloride hexahydrate and 19% aluminum hydroxychloride.

Mechanism of action

Most anhidrotics have a drying effect on the skin. This effect may be brought about by reversible damage to the eccrine glands, e.g. by reducing the size of the lumen, so that the production of sweat is reduced. Some astringents appear to act by producing a physical blockage of the sweat duct. Aluminum hydroxide is deposited within the distal intra-epidermal portion of the eccrine duct and forms a plug.

Unwanted effects

There are no major unwanted effects. Care should be exercised with the use of aldehydes as sensitisation can occur and the skin may also be stained brown when glutaraldehyde is used.

ANTI-INFLAMMATORIES

Inflammation is part of the body's defensive response to injury, caused by trauma or invading organisms. Classical inflammation involves a local increase in blood flow (causing redness and heat), swelling, pain and impaired function. There are many chemical mediators of inflammation, but one particularly important group is the *prostaglandins*. Prostaglandins are 20-carbon fatty acids produced from the precursor arachidonic acid by a cascade of enzymes, the most important of which is *cyclo-oxygenase* (Fig. 8.4). The prostaglandins are largely responsible for the swell-

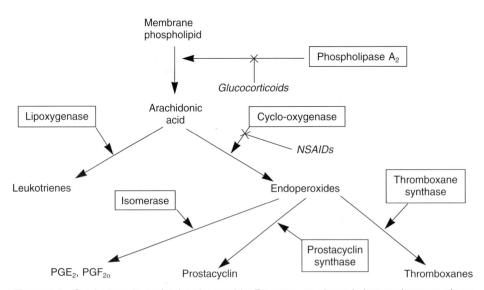

Figure 8.4 Synthetic pathway for the eicosanoids. Enzymes are shown in boxes; drugs are shown in italics.

ing, vasodilation and pain that develops after the first 2 or 3 hours of an inflammatory response. The pain results not from direct activation of pain fibres by prostaglandins, but from *sensitisation* of pain receptors by prostaglandins, so that previously non-painful stimuli are felt as pain.

Anti-inflammatories are widely used in the pharmacological management of inflammation in the foot. There is also a range of non-pharmacological strategies which can be very useful in the treatment of inflammation (see Ch. 9). Because of their effect on prostaglandin synthesis, some anti-inflammatory drugs are also effective analgesics and may be used because of this combined effect. Many factors can cause acute and chronic inflammation in the foot. Sudden or repeated trauma or invasion by pathogenic micro-organisms are the most likely causes. The other prime cause is the local or systemic effect of hypersensitivity and autoimmune reactions; examples are contact dermatitis (local) and rheumatoid arthritis (systemic). The majority of dermatological conditions also invoke an inflammatory reaction, e.g. psoriasis, eczema, lichen planus.

Anti-inflammatory drugs can be conveniently classified by their action, diclofenac sodium that is non-steroidal or steroidal. They are effective if administered orally, via intracapsular injections or topically. The two types of anti-inflammatory drugs are considered below, followed by a discussion of the administration of anti-inflammatories parenterally and topically.

Non-steroidal anti-inflammatory drugs (NSAIDs)

Indications

The main non-steroidal anti-inflammatory drugs are aspirin, ibuprofen, diclofenac sodium, indomethacin and mefenamic acid. Although these drugs reduce pain, swelling and redness, and improve function, they have no effect on the underlying disease process.

Mechanism of action

NSAIDs act by inhibiting cyclo-oxygenase so that fewer prostaglandins are produced (Fig. 8.4). This reduces local vasodilatation, swelling and pain. All the useful NSAIDs are quite well absorbed after oral administration.

Unwanted effects

Nearly all NSAIDs are weak acids that bind strongly to plasma proteins, which can lead to interactions with other drugs. By binding avidly to plasma proteins, NSAIDs can displace molecules of other drugs which were previously bound. This raises the free plasma concentration of the other, previously bound drug, so that the patient is effectively overdosed. All cause some degree of gastric bleeding by interfering with the production of the protective layer of mucus by the stomach lining, as production of this protective layer of mucus involves the local release of prostaglandins. This is a dose-dependent effect and is worse if the drug is chemically irritant, e.g. aspirin. Aspirin, being a weak acid, also tends to accumulate within cells lining the stomach, including the mucus-producing cells. This is because the acid environment causes the aspirin to be non-ionised, and therefore more lipid-soluble, so that it enters cells readily. Inside the cells, however, the pH is less acid (approximately 7.4), and a considerable proportion of the aspirin molecules dissociate, thereby becoming more water-soluble and unable to diffuse out of the cells. This process is known as 'trapping'. Coating tablets so that they pass through the stomach without disintegrating can reduce the risk of gastric bleeding because the local concentration of drug in the stomach mucosa is reduced.

In patients with asthma, NSAIDs can precipitate asthmatic attacks, possibly by diverting the arachidonic acid pathway to produce bronchoconstrictor mediators, e.g. leukotrienes (Fig. 8.4).

Inhibition of prostaglandin synthesis in the kidney can lead to disturbed kidney function, so that salt and water are retained. This can be particularly troublesome in patients with heart failure, as it can worsen the condition. Aspirin, but not other members of the group, also inhibits the renal excretion of uric acid. Aspirin is therefore contraindicated in gout.

Corticosteroids

Indications

The prime use of corticosteroids in the managment of foot problems is to suppress inflammation. They may be administered orally for systemic problems; for example, the symptoms of rheumatoid arthritis are suppressed by glucocorticoids. They may be injected subcutaneously to suppress symptoms from a localised condition such as enthesopathy or plantar digital neuritis. Intracapsular injections may be used for acute arthritis. Topical anti-inflammatories may be used to reduce inflammation of the skin associated with dermatological conditions such as psoriasis.

If used topically when infection is present, they can mask the features of infection.

The corticosteroids (natural and artificial) are highly lipid-soluble which means that they are rapidly absorbed by all routes, even after topical administration. The most important synthetic corticosteroids can be classified as follows:

- *mainly glucocorticoid* but with appreciable mineralocorticoid activity, e.g. prednisolone
- *highly selective glucocorticoid activity*, e.g. betamethasone, beclomethasone, dexamethasone, fluocinolone
- *highly selective mineralocorticoid activity*, e.g. fludrocortisone.

Mechanism of action

The adrenal cortex synthesises and releases several closely related hormones, the corticosteroids. Most have very short half-lives once released from the adrenal cortex, whereas synthetic derivatives of the natural hormones have durations of action long enough to make them therapeutically useful.

The effects of the natural corticosteroids have been classified largely into two groups—glucocorticoid and mineralocorticoid actions. The major physiological mineralocorticoid is *aldosterone*, which has hardly any glucocorticoid activity. The major physiological corticosteroids are *hydrocortisone* (*cortisol*) and *cortisone*, both of which have some mineralocorticoid activity. Most useful synthetic corticosteroids are selective for either mineralocorticoid actions or glucocorticoid actions (Table 8.1).

The anti-inflammatory and immunosuppressant actions of the corticosteroids are mediated through the production of *lipocortins*, small messenger proteins. These lipocortins inhibit phopholipase A_2, the enzyme that begins the prostaglandin/leukotriene synthesis cascade (Fig. 8.4).

Table 8.1 Effects of corticosteroids

Mineralocorticoid	Glucocorticoid
Na^+ retention by kidney	Mobilisation of peripheral amino acids
K^+ loss by kidney	Decreased glucose uptake Increased gluconeogensis Mobilisation of fatty acids from fat stores Suppression of inflammation Suppression of the immune system

Unwanted effects

Prolonged high doses produce a set of effects that resemble adrenal hyperactivity (Cushing's syndrome). These include salt and water retention, muscle wasting, osteoporosis, deposition of fat on the face ('moon face') and between the shoulder blades ('buffalo hump'), diabetes, susceptibility to infections and psychosis. Other effects include peptic ulceration, cataract and glaucoma.

After prolonged treatment, the adrenal cortex atrophies as a result of feedback inhibition of the release of adrenocorticotrophic hormone (ACTH) from the pituitary gland. When the exogenous corticosteroid is stopped, it takes time (months) for the atrophied adrenal cortex to start producing endogenous adrenocortical hormones, even though ACTH levels rise almost immediately. During this time the patient will show severe adrenocortical insufficiency. Corticosteroids should therefore be withdrawn slowly over a period of months to allow the hitherto involuted adrenal cortex to recover.

Injectable anti-inflammatories

Indications

Corticosteroids, often combined with analgesics, may be used for injection into joints or subcutaneous tissues. Two main types of corticosteroids are used (all are more potent than hydrocortisone):

- methylprednisolone acetate
- fluorinated hydrocortisone, e.g. betamethasone, dexamethasone, triamcinolone.

Methylprednisolone acetate (MPA) has approximately five times the glucocorticoid action of hydrocortisone and is 1.25–1.5 times stronger than prednisolone. Betamethasone is 8–10 times more potent than prednisolone. MPA can be used in all joints of the foot and plantar fascia. Table 8.2 provides a summary of the indications for MPA and betamethasone (Tollafield & Williams 1996).

Injectable corticosteroids do not offer a panacea—as with all pharmacological preparations, they should be used with care. A thorough assessment to identify the underlying cause and the use of non-pharmacological strategies is necessary.

Greenfield et al (1984) found that patients with plantar digital neuritis preferred the use of injectable corticosteroids (with 1% lignocaine) to conservative treatment involving orthotic prescription and/or modification of footwear. In a retrospective study of 65 patients, Greenfield et al (1984) found that a

Table 8.2 Indications for the use of methylprednisolone and betamethasone (Tollafield & Williams 1996)

Methylprednisolone	Betamethasone
Rheumatoid arthritis	Capsulitis
Keloid	Heel pain
Granuloma annulare	Postoperative swelling
Synovitis	Neuroma
Tenosynovitis	Bursitis
Plantar fasciitis	
Bursitis	

mean of three injections per patient was administered and that 50% of the patients experienced temporary relief. Total relief was recorded in 14% of patients after one injection.

Corticosteroids should neither be injected into an infected joint nor used in immunocompromised patients.

Mechanism of action

The anti-inflammatory effect of injecting corticosteroids into joints is thought to involve:

- inhibition of chemotactic migration of white blood cells
- reduction in the permeability of the synovial membrane
- stabilisation of leucocytic lysosomal membranes which in turn prevents the release of cytotoxic enzymes
- inhibition of the formation of inflammatory prostaglandins through an inhibition of phospholipase A_2.

Unwanted reactions

MPA has been implicated as having a deleterious effect on cartilage. Hydroxyapatite crystal deposition following steroid injection has been found in experimental animals and this is thought to increase the effects of osteoarthritis (Ohira et al 1986). Loss of matrix glycosaminoglycans can lead to replacement with collagen, causing a reduction in the flexibility and resilience of cartilage. However, the overall effect on cartilage may not be completely detrimental, as decreased swelling protects synovial vessels and stabilises chondroblasts and intimal cells of the synovium (Shoemaker et al 1992).

Corticosteroids can enter the circulation after injection into joints. Absorption from the joint cavity is affected by the lipid solubility of the drug, the dose and the surface area. Clinical problems with the use of injectable corticosteroids are rare. Greenfield et al

(1984) and Tollafield & Williams (1996) reported 'steroid flares'.

Topical corticosteroids

Indications

Corticosteroids are the most potent and effective topical anti-inflammatories. As they also have the ability to inhibit cell division, they are useful in the treatment of conditions such as psoriasis, which is characterised by a rapid epidermal cell transit time.

The effectiveness of topical corticosteroids is related to their potency and rate of absorption through the skin; the potency of topical steroids varies. Corticosteroids can be presented in a variety of vehicles: creams, ointments, sprays or gels. In general, ointments are better tolerated than creams or gels.

Betamethasone sodium phosphate may be injected in small amounts into the lesion; this may be helpful in cases of mucoid cysts, keloids or psoriatic plaques. Corticosteroids may also be incorporated with other topical preparations such as antifungals, e.g. miconazole, or keratoplastics, e.g. urea and lactic acid. It should be noted that the combined use of corticosteroids and antibacterial or antifungal preparations may mask the features of spreading infection.

Mechanism of action

There are marked regional variations in the percutaneous absorption of topical steroids; absorption through scrotal skin is much quicker than through the skin of the sole of the foot. Hydration of the skin markedly improves percutaneous absorption (increases four- to five-fold). If applied under an occlusive dressing, absorption may increase 100-fold. Topical steroids are far more easily absorbed through broken skin than through intact skin.

It is difficult to ascertain the optimal dose of topical steroids. Patients vary in the amount they apply and the frequency of application. On account of their side-effects, all topical steroids should be used sparingly.

Unwanted effects

Topical corticosteroids may lead to atrophy of the skin, telangiectasia, folliculitis and striae. If used over a prolonged period of time systemic side effects may occur as a result of topical absorption.

ANTIMICROBIAL

There is no simple term which covers all the pathogenic organisms with which the body can be infected. The term 'microbe' probably comes closest to this and it is used here to refer to any foreign organism responsible for infection. Such organisms include bacteria, fungi, viruses, protozoa and metazoa. Drugs which are useful for dealing with invading organisms are different from most other drugs because they offer the prospect of a true cure for a disease, rather than modification of a disease process or a symptomatic treatment. These drugs achieve this by being toxic to the invading organism but not to the host.

Antibacterial drugs

Indications

At one time, the term 'antibiotic' was applied only to those antibacterial drugs extracted from biological sources, such as fungi or other bacteria. As many of these antibiotics can now be synthesised chemically, or are subjected to heavy chemical modification, this distinction is no longer sensible or workable. It is therefore unreasonable to deny the term to drugs such as the sulphonamides, which are totally synthetic. However, the term 'antibacterial' is used in this section to avoid this still somewhat contentious issue.

Bacterial infections occurring in the foot are usually due to *Staphylococcus aureus*, although culture often reveals the presence of Gram-negative bacilli such as *Pseudomonas aeruginosa*. These Gram-negative bacilli are found as commensals of the gut. Their presence in the foot is usually a result of poor personal hygiene or contamination of antiseptics, in particular cetrimide, and medical equipment such as air hoses. Streptoccal infections are not common but, when present in the foot, can have major deleterious effects due to their rapid spread across and through tissues.

Most antibiotics are prescribed once infection has become established in the foot. Prophylactic antibiotics are increasingly being used pre-operatively to prevent infection from becoming established. The use of pre-operative antibiotics is indicated for patients who:

- are receiving implant surgery
- already have a surgical implant or prosthesis
- have a history of rheumatic fever or heart valve defect
- have previously been shown to be at risk of postoperative infection
- are about to undergo major surgery to the foot.

Mechanism of action

Antibacterial drugs are either *bacteriostatic*, i.e. they

act by arresting the growth of the organism, or *bactericidal*, i.e. they kill the organism. Bacteriostatic drugs rely upon the body's immune system to destroy the organism once its multiplication has been stopped. Consequently, such drugs are ineffective in patients with impaired immune systems, whether this be because of disease, such as AIDS, or whether it be drug-induced, for example by immunosuppressants used to prevent transplant rejection, or steroids for asthma or arthritis. Sometimes it is necessary to combine drugs to achieve effective treatment of infection. However, bacteriostatic and bactericidal drugs should not be combined, because each is likely markedly to reduce the efficacy of the other. This is because bactericidal drugs are usually most effective on bacteria which are actively growing or dividing. Bacteriostatic drugs therefore protect bacteria from bactericidal drugs.

Unwanted reactions

One of the major problems with antibacterial drugs is the emergence of resistant bacterial strains. It is important therefore that the practitioner uses antibacterial drugs in the manner least likely to encourage the development of resistance. Resistance to antibacterial drugs is acquired in several ways. In a population of bacteria of any one species, some will be naturally more resistant than others. These will be the last organisms to die when exposed to an antibacterial drug. Inadequate treatment will therefore leave the patient with an infection composed of the most drug-resistant strains of the organism.

In any population of bacteria, naturally more resistant strains are constantly evolving by spontaneous mutation. Only when non-resistant strains are killed by drugs are these resistant strains selected. The problem of resistance is further complicated by the ability of many bacteria to transmit genetic material to other bacteria, even to bacteria of different families. The genetic material comprises *plasmids*, strands of DNA-containing genes which encode enzymes that convey resistance. Another way in which genetic material can be transmitted is through viruses which infect bacteria (*bacteriophages*). A good example of transmission of resistance can be found in the enzyme beta-lactamase which inactivates penicillins and cephalosporins. This has appeared in many strains of bacteria which did not originally possess the gene for the enzyme. The risk of encouraging resistance can be minimised if some basic rules are followed (Box 8.2).

Box 8.2   Factors to be addressed in order to prevent the development of resistant bacterial strains

- Do not use an antibacterial drug unless it is really necessary. Chronic infections may not need chemotherapy, whereas most acute infections do

- Make the most precise diagnosis that the signs and symptoms allow. This will narrow the choice of drug by identifying the most likely organism. Samples for laboratory testing should be taken before treatment is started, but treatment should not be delayed until a bacteriology laboratory report is received, as this may take a day or more

- Avoid the indiscriminate use of broad-spectrum drugs. Before the infecting organism has been identified by culture, there is a great temptation to use the broadest spectrum drug available to cover all eventualities. Only if precise identification of the organism is impossible should broad-spectrum drugs be used, and then it is best to avoid using the drugs with the broadest spectrum; these should be reserved for the most problematic infections

- Give the drug for long enough to enable all organisms to be eliminated. This usually means at least 5 days, although disappearance of symptoms does not mean that all organisms have been eliminated

- Use combination therapy when resistant strains are known to be responsible for the infection. The probability of an organism being resistant to two drugs is four times less than the probability of its being resistant to either one of the two drugs alone

- Ensure that you have up-to-date knowledge of local resistance patterns. By being aware of local resistance patterns, the practitioner is less likely to use a drug that will encourage resistance to develop

- Abide by agreements about reserving drugs for particular conditions. Most microbiologists and practitioners agree that new antibacterial drugs should not be used widely as long as older drugs still work. Some drugs are 'reserved' for treating infections with organisms which cause serious, life-threatening infections. If these drugs are used to treat trivial infections, resistance may develop and this resistance could be acquired by the organism responsible for the serious infection, thereby rendering the drug ineffective

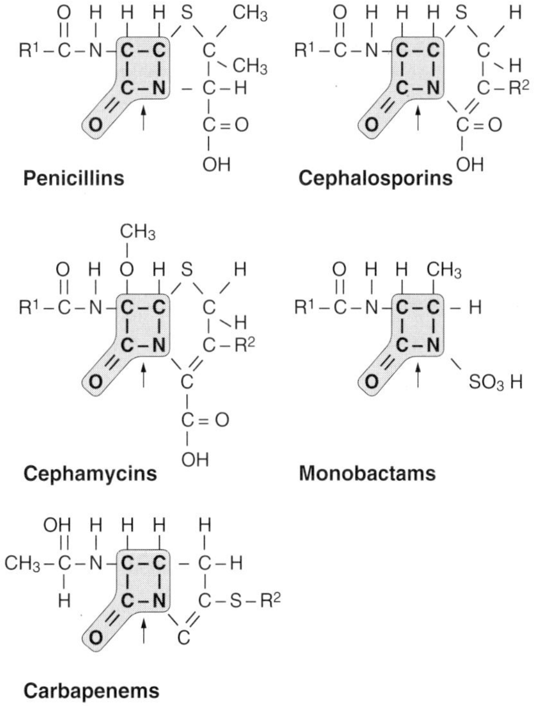

Figure 8.5   Beta-lactam antibacterials. The lactam ring is shown bold. The arrow indicates the site of the action of inactivating beta-lactamases.

Classes of antibacterial drugs

Beta-lactams. These are antibacterials which have a beta-lactam ring as the central feature of their structure (Fig. 8.5). The group includes the natural and semi-synthetic penicillins, the cephalosporins, cepha-

mycins, carbapenems and the monobactams. They are among the most highly selective and least toxic of all drugs, which means that very high plasma concentrations can be achieved, giving high kill-rates with a low incidence of adverse effects. These drugs interfere with the synthesis of the peptidoglycan layer of the bacterial cell wall. As a result, the cell swells as water enters by osmosis and eventually bursts. Beta-lactams are therefore bactericidal. They owe their high selectivity firstly to the fact that mammalian cells do not have cell walls, and secondly to their being structural analogues of d-alanyl-d-alanine, a precursor of the peptidoglycan; mammalian cells do not have the capacity to use d-isomers of amino acids.

The spectrum of activity is similar for all the beta-lactams, all Gram-positive bacteria and Gram-negative cocci, although some of the newer drugs have a wider spectrum of activity than this. The chief reason for bacterial resistance to beta-lactams, among normally sensitive species, is the possession by the organism of an enzyme (beta-lactamase; penicillinase) capable of hydrolysing the lactam ring, thereby inactivating the drug. Most staphylococci are now resistant to beta-lactamase-sensitive antibacterials.

Although rare, some patients become hypersensitive to penicillin so that an anaphylactic reaction develops on subsequent exposure. A high proportion of such patients will also be allergic to cephalosporins.

Penicillins. Penicillins are highly water-soluble and so penetrate the blood–brain barrier poorly. Some penicillins have enough lipid solubility to be absorbed after oral administration, but the original penicillin (benzylpenicillin) must be injected, partly because it is water-soluble and partly because it is broken down by the acid in the stomach. The penicillins are weak acids and are actively secreted by the kidney tubule so that the clearance of penicillin is very high (most of the penicillin entering the kidney is excreted in the urine). Probenecid interferes with the pump responsible for secreting penicillins from the kidney tubules and consequently extends the duration of action of the penicillin.

Benzylpenicillin (penicillin V) is susceptible to beta-lactamases, but remains the drug of choice for streptococcal, pneumococcal, gonococcal and meningococcal infections. It is also recommended for anthrax, diphtheria, gas-gangrene, leptospirosis, syphilis, tetanus, yaws and Lyme disease in children.

Procaine penicillin is an almost insoluble salt of benzylpenicillin which is suitable for intramuscular injection as a 'depot'. Penicillin is released slowly from the depot over a long period so that bactericidal tissue concentrations are maintained for at least 24 hours after a single injection.

Phenoxymethylpenicillin (penicillin V) is less potent than benzylpenicillin but has essentially the same spectrum. Unlike benzylpenicillin, it is resistant to gastric acid and is therefore suitable for oral administration, although absorption is erratic because the drug is so water-soluble.

Cloxacillin and flucloxacillin are resistant to beta-lactamase and so are active against staphylococci that are resistant to the older penicillins. Flucloxacillin is more lipid-soluble than cloxacillin and so is better absorbed after oral administration.

Ampicillin has a broader spectrum of action than the penicillins listed above, as it is active against some Gram-positive species as well as Gram-negative organisms, although it is sensitive to beta-lactamase. Most staphylococci, 50% of *Escherichia coli* and 15% of *Haemophilus influenzae* strains are now resistant to ampicillin. Absorption of ampicillin from the gut is poor and is further hampered by food.

Amoxycillin has almost the same spectrum of activity as ampicillin but it is much better absorbed, so that adequate bactericidal concentrations can be easily achieved with oral dosing. Other orally active wide-spectrum penicillins include bacampicillin and pivampicillin.

Clavulanic acid is structurally related to penicillin and like the penicillins is produced by a fungus. Its value is that it inhibits bacterial beta-lactamase. Consequently a mixture of clavulanic acid and an otherwise beta-lactamase-susceptible penicillin will be active against beta-lactamase-producing organisms. Clavulanic acid is available in a fixed-dose combination with amoxycillin called co-amoxyclav.

Carbenicillin and *ticarcillin* (carboxypenicillins) are broad-spectrum penicillins which are active against *Pseudomonas aeruginosa*. Ticarcillin is also active against *Proteus* species and *Bacteriodes fragilis*. Azlocillin and piperacillin have a spectrum of activity similar to ticarcillin. Tazobactam, like clavulanic acid, is a beta-lactamase inhibitor and is available in combination with piperacillin.

Cephalosporins, cephamycins and other beta-lactams. Cephalosporins have very similar properties to the broad-spectrum penicillins and share their dispositional characteristics. In addition, about 10% of patients who are allergic to penicillins will be allergic to cephalosporins.

Cephradine and cephazolin are 'first generation' cephalosporins, which have been superseded by 'second' and 'third generation' agents. Second generation cephalosporins, such as cefuroxime and cephamandole, have more resistance to beta-lactamase than the older drugs. This gives them activity against *H. influenzae* and *Neisseria gonorrhoeae*. Cephalexin, cephradine and cefadroxil are orally active first generation drugs. Cefaclor is an orally active second generation cephalosporin.

Third generation cephalosporins tend to be more active than second generation drugs against Gram-negative organisms, but less active against Gram-positive organisms. The third generation cephalosporins are cefotaxime, ceftazidime, ceftoxime and cefodizime. Ceftriaxone has a very long half-life and is suitable for once-daily administration. *Pseudomonas* is susceptible to cefsulodin and ceftazidime, for which they should be reserved. Cefixime is the longest-acting orally active cephalosporin, and has recently received a licence for use in acute infections.

Cefoxitin is a cephamycin which has been found to be particularly useful in treating peritonitis because it is active against organisms found in the bowel. Aztreonam (a 'monobactam') is active only against Gram-negative aerobes and should therefore only be used when the infecting organism has been positively identified. Imipenem is a carbapenem which has a broad spectrum of activity, including aerobic and anaerobic Gram-positive and Gram-negative organisms. It is available in combination with cilastatin, an enzyme inhibitor which prevents the enzymic breakdown of imipenem in the kidney.

Macrolides. The macrolides, like the beta-lactams, inhibit bacterial cell wall synthesis, but have a slightly different site of action. Consequently their spectrum of activity is similar to the beta-lactams and they are often suitable alternatives for use in patients with penicillin (or cephalosporin) allergy. Erythromycin is indicated for respiratory infections in children, whooping cough, legionnaires' disease and enteritis caused by *Campylobacter*. Some of the macrolides are usually active against *Chlamydia* and *Mycoplasma*. Azithromycin and clarithromycin are concentrated in tissues and so achieve higher antibacterial concentrations with long tissue half-lives.

Tetracyclines. These broad-spectrum antibacterials prevent protein synthesis by binding to aminoacyl-tRNA, which prevents the ribosome from translocating along the mRNA template. The selectivity of tetracyclines for microorganisms is due to the selective accumulation of these drugs by the organisms by virtue of an ATP-driven active transport system. The tetracyclines bind avidly to metal ions such as calcium, aluminium, magnesium and iron (*chelation*), and consequently are poorly absorbed from the gastro-intestinal tract if they are taken with, shortly before or after milk, antacids, iron-containing 'tonics' and haematinics, and calcium supplements. Tetracyclines also chelate with calcium in developing teeth and growing bones, causing unsightly staining of the teeth, and as a result they should not be given to children with developing teeth (under 12 years) or to pregnant women.

Although resistance to tetracyclines has been developing (largely by selection of strains which lack the accumulation system), tetracyclines are of vital importance in the treatment of infections with *Chlamydia*, *Rickettsia*, *Mycoplasma*, *Brucella*, and Lyme disease. The spectrum of activity of all tetracyclines is similar, except that minocycline has activity against *Neisseria meningitidis*. The principal tetracyclines are tetracycline itself, doxycycline, demeclocycline, lymecycline and oxytetracycline.

Aminoglycosides. The aminoglycoside antibacterials, e.g. gentamicin, inhibit protein synthesis in bacteria by binding irreversibly to part of the ribosome (the 30S subunit). This prevents aminoacyl-tRNA from binding to the acceptor site, and elaboration of the peptide chain ceases. Aminoglycosides selectively inhibit bacterial protein synthesis. Nevertheless, aminoglycoside antibiotics have only a narrow therapeutic window. They all cause permanent damage to the hair cells of the inner ear causing deafness (ototoxicity) if the plasma concentration rises only a little above the effective bactericidal concentration.

Aminoglycosides are active against some Gram-positive and many Gram-negative organisms. Some (amikacin, gentamicin, tobramycin) are also active against *P. aeruginosa*. Streptomycin is active against *Mycobacterium tuberculosis* and should be reserved for treating tuberculosis.

All the aminoglycosides are highly water-soluble and are therefore not absorbed after oral dosing. Their high water solubility also means that they are eliminated by filtration at the kidney, with a clearance that approximates to the glomerular filtration rate (approximately 100–120 ml/min). Injections are therefore usually given every 2–3 hours to maintain the narrow therapeutic range of plasma concentration needed to kill bacteria without causing ototoxicity. In patients with impaired kidney function, dosage adjustment is essential. An indication of impaired kidney function is provided by measurement of the plasma creatinine concentration. A raised concentration suggests that kidney function is impaired and that a careful evaluation of the dosage regime is needed. This may include a full creatinine clearance assessment. Neomycin is too toxic for systemic use and can therefore only be used to treat skin and mucous membrane infections.

Sulphonamides, dapsone and trimethoprim. The sulphonamides were the first safe and effective antibacterial drugs to be developed. They came about because of Paul Ehrlich's observation that many bacteria could be selectively stained by certain synthetic dyes. He argued that it ought to be possible to attach a toxic group to the molecule and thus deliver a lethal message selectively to bacteria that took up the dye. Eventually a red dye (prontosil) was found which inhibited the growth of bacteria in culture and cured mice of otherwise lethal infection. It was first given to humans in the late 1920s and early 1930s. It was soon realised, however, that the effect of prontosil was due to a metabolite which was a sulphonamide. In the 1930s, the mechanism of action was worked out and a number of potent and effective sulphonamides were in production by the 1940s.

Sulphonamides are structural analogues of para-aminobenzoate, which is used by bacteria to synthesise dihydrofolate, an intermediate in the synthesis of the purine and pyrimidine bases needed during the manufacture of nucleic acids (Fig. 8.6). Mammals do not need to synthesise dihydrofolate (folic acid) because mammalian cells are permeable to it. Bacterial cell membranes/cell walls are impermeant to folic

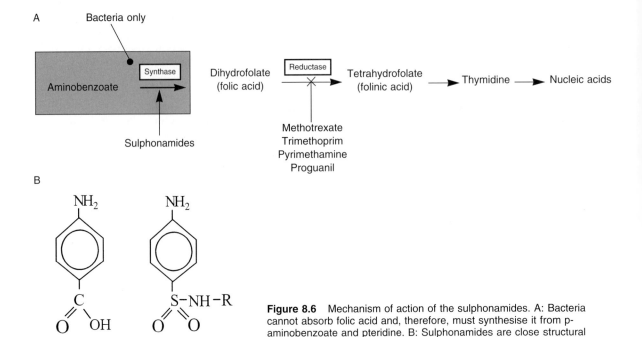

Figure 8.6 Mechanism of action of the sulphonamides. A: Bacteria cannot absorb folic acid and, therefore, must synthesise it from p-aminobenzoate and pteridine. B: Sulphonamides are close structural analogues of p-aminobenzoate.

acid. Sulphonamides are so similar in structure to para-aminobenzoate that they can react with the enzyme dihydropteroate synthetase in its place, but the complex does not dissociate readily and so the enzyme is inhibited. Sulphonamides are therefore bacteriostatic as they prevent cell division by limiting the availability of nucleic acids. However, most bacterial cells have reserves of dihydrofolate and tetrahydrofolate, so that there is usually a time lag between inhibition of dihydropteroate synthetase and the stopping of bacterial cell division.

Sulphonamides are limited in value because many sulphonamide-resistant strains have appeared. The main value of sulphonamides (e.g. sulphadimidine) is in the treatment of urinary tract infections and meningococcal meningitis. *Dapsone* is a close chemical relative of the sulphonamides and is invaluable in the treatment of leprosy.

Trimethoprim is not a sulphonamide but, like the sulphonamides, it inhibits nucleic acid synthesis. It does this by interfering with the enzyme dihydrofolate reductase. This enzyme takes as its substrate the dihydrofolate made by dihydropteroate synthetase and turns it into tetrahydrofolate. Although trimethoprim is used on its own, it is also available in combination with the sulphonamide sulphamethoxazole (the mixture is called co-trimoxazole). By interfering

with nucleic acid synthesis, by stopping two adjacent steps in the synthesis pathway, co-trimoxazole is less likely to produce resistant strains than either constituent drug given alone.

The 4-quinolones. The 4-quinolones (e.g. ciproflaxin and nalidixic acid) inhibit the enzyme DNA gyrase (also known as topoisomerase II). This enzyme is normally responsible for winding the DNA helix into a so-called 'supercoiled' form. The drugs are selective for bacteria because the enzyme in bacteria is structurally different from that in mammals.

Ciproflaxin is effective against Gram-negative bacteria such as *Salmonella*, *Shigella*, *Campylobacter*, *Neisseria* and *Pseudomonas*. It has some activity against Gram-positive bacteria such as *Streptococcus pneumoniae* and *Strep. faecalis*. Ciproflaxin is also active against *Chlamydia* and some mycobacteria, but is inactive against most anaerobes. The main use for ciproflaxin is the treatment of respiratory and urinary tract infections, although it is not effective against pneumococcal pneumonia. Nalidixic acid is used almost exclusively for uncomplicated urinary tract infections.

The 4-quinolones are secreted into the urine, where they reach high concentrations and can crystallise unless adequate water intake is maintained. A potentially serious adverse effect of this group of antibacterials is that they can precipitate convulsions in susceptible patients, particularly in patients with a history of epilepsy.

Nitroimidazoles. The mechanism of action of the nitroimidazoles (metronidazole and tinidazole) is uncertain, but it may be that the drugs or, more likely, their metabolites cause breaks in the DNA of parasites. The selectivity is thought to be due to the selective appearance of these metabolites within parasites. Metronidazole was developed as an amoebicide, but in addition to activity against *Entamoeba histolytica* and *Giardia lamblia*, it is very effective against many anaerobes. It is therefore useful for surgical and gynaecological sepsis, especially infections with colonic anaerobes such as *Bacteroides fragilis*. Both metronidazole and tinidazole are well absorbed after oral administration, but tinidazole has a longer duration of action. Although most of a dose of metronidazole is excreted unchanged in the urine, some metabolism may occur and as the metabolites are strongly coloured this gives the urine a dark brown colour.

The nitroimidazoles interfere with the enzyme aldehyde dehydrogenase, the enzyme responsible for the second step in the metabolism of ethanol. This leads to an accumulation of acetaldehyde (ethanal) after the consumption of ethanol, which causes marked vasodilatation, headache, nausea, vomiting and a general feeling of malaise. Patients taking these drugs should not drink alcohol during treatment and for several days after stopping the drug.

Miscellaneous antibacterials. Fusidic acid salts are extremely narrow-spectrum antibacterials. They inhibit protein synthesis by preventing translocation of the ribosome along the mRNA chain of codons. Sodium fusidate is well absorbed after oral administration and is particularly useful because it penetrates and accumulates in bone. However, its narrow spectrum of action requires that it be used with another antistaphylococcal antibiotic, usually flucloxacillin or erythromycin, to limit the emergence of resistant strains.

Chloramphenicol is an extremely potent and valuable broad-spectrum antibacterial, the usefulness of which is limited by its propensity to cause fatal aplastic anaemia. The incidence of this adverse effect is about 1 in 50 000–100 000. Consequently chloramphenicol is reserved for dealing with life-threatening infections, such as typhoid fever and *H. influenzae* septicaemia. Chloramphenicol inhibits protein synthesis by preventing the growth of the chain of amino acids as the ribosome moves along the mRNA molecule.

The polymyxins (colistin and polymyxin-B) are cationic detergents composed of peptide chains with hydrophilic and lipophilic amino acids. They have some selectivity for those bacterial cell membranes which are more susceptible to damage than mammalian cell membranes. They are bactericidal by disrupting the phospholipids of the membrane. These antibiotics are not absorbed after oral administration and so colistin can be used to 'sterilise' the gut (usually in conjunction with an antifungal agent such as nystatin). Both colistin and polymyxin-B are generally considered to be too toxic for systemic use, although colistin is available in a form suitable for injection. They are both active against Gram-negative organisms, including *P. aeruginosa*.

Topical antibacterials

Topical antibacterials are traditionally termed antiseptics. Antiseptics are defined as substances applied to living tissues to destroy or inhibit the reproduction or metabolic activity of microorganisms. The term 'disinfectant' is reserved for the use of such substances on non-living material. In general, antiseptics are sensitive to their local environment, and hence their action may be impeded by the presence of tissue debris, blood or pus. Antiseptics are not usually effective against spores.

Some of the antibiotics discussed in the previous section can be used topically, e.g. neomycin. However, their popularity has reduced over the years, due to the problems associated with resistance. It is difficult to control how much is used and where it is used, especially if the patient is self-applying the antibiotic. Unlike oral preparations, which are dispensed in carefully metered doses, topical antibiotics come in powder or cream form, the amount of which used can vary with each application.

Antifungal drugs

Indications

Antifungal drugs are usually administered either orally or topically. There have, in the past, been a number of unwanted effects associated with the oral antifungals, which have restricted their use to severe infections. This situation is now being reversed due to the arrival on the market of oral antifungal drugs with fewer unwanted effects. However, it is still primarily the topical antifungal preparations that are used.

There are a wide variety of over-the-counter preparations which come in a range of formulations—creams, ointments, sprays, paints and lotions. These preparations may be combined with 1% hydrocortisone, as fungal infection of the skin is often accompanied by an inflammatory response and pruritus. Penetration of topical agents to the site of infection in the treatment of onychomycosis may be problematic, which is why systemic therapy is considered to have a more beneficial effect.

When using topical antifungal preparations, it is important that their use is continued for up to 3 months after the signs and symptoms have resolved. This is because of spore formation—most topical antifungals are not particularly effective against spores. With infected nails, treatment must continue until a new nail has grown (6 months for fingernails, 12 months for toenails). The treatment of fungal infection of the nails can be speeded up by the surgical or chemical (urea cream) removal of the nail prior to the application of the antifungal preparation. If this is not feasible, reduction of the nail with a nail drill will facilitate penetration of the antifungal agent into the nail.

Mechanism of action

As with antibacterial drugs, antifungals may either be fungistatic (prevent growth) or fungicidal (kill). The classes of antifungals, their specific mechanism of action, adverse effects and mode of administration are considered below.

Polyenes. Nystatin and amphotericin bind to ergosterol in the membrane of fungal cells and form channels through which the important intracellular components can diffuse, causing the cells to effectively starve to death. The polyenes are selective for fungal and yeast cells because mammalian cell membranes do not have ergosterol. Nystatin is too toxic for systemic use, but is so water-soluble that it is not absorbed from the gut after oral administration and so can be effectively used to rid the gastrointestinal tract of candidal infection (thrush). It is commonly used in topical preparations.

Amphotericin is less toxic than nystatin, but is also highly water-soluble, and hence for systemic treatment it must be injected. However, it is still quite toxic, causing primarily renal damage, which may be permanent, and loss of potassium, which may be severe enough for the patient to require potassium supplements.

Imidazoles. These agents kill a wide range of fungi and yeasts. They act by preventing the synthesis of ergosterol. Miconazole is highly effective as a topical agent for some forms of ringworm. Other imidazole antifungals available in creams for topical use include econazole, sulconazole and clotrimazole.

Miconazole can be used orally to eliminate gastrointestinal fungal or yeast infection as it is highly water-soluble and therefore poorly absorbed. It can also be injected for systemic infection, e.g. aspergillosis, candidiasis and cryptococcosis. Ketoconazole is absorbed moderately well after oral administration but has been reported to cause liver damage which can be fatal. Fluconazole and itraconazole are safer alternatives, although the use of itraconazole in patients with significant liver disease is undesirable. Fluconazole, although water-soluble, reaches antifungal concentrations in the CSF, whereas itraconazole does not penetrate the blood–brain barrier as effectively. Triazoles are the most recent azole derivatives.

Allylamines. These act by inhibiting squalene epoxidase, an enzyme which is required for fungal cell biosynthesis. The resulting build-up of squalene in the fungal cells kills the organism. Terbinafine and amorolfine are new antifungal agents available for systemic and topical application for use against tinea and candidiasis of the skin. Amorolfine is also available as a lacquer for use against onychomycosis.

Undecanoates. Undecanoates, e.g. zinc undecanoate, were at one time the mainstay of topical treatments for fungal infection of the foot. They have been largely replaced by the imidazoles, e.g. clotrimazole and miconazole. These substances also tend to be effective against yeasts. Tolnaftate is only available for topical application for dermatophytes such as tinea pedis but is not effective against *Candida*.

Miscellaneous antifungal agents. Griseofulvin is a narrow-spectrum antifungal agent isolated from the mould *Penicillium griseofulvum* in 1939. It acts by interfering with microtubule function and is fungistatic rather than fungicidal. Consequently, it must be given for long periods of time, otherwise regrowth and re-infection from the remaining inhibited, but not killed, fungal hyphae will occur. After oral administration it is not particularly well absorbed, but it is particularly useful against tinea infection of the skin and nails because it is selectively accumulated in these tissues as it binds to newly formed keratin. Treatment should continue until the infected keratin has been shed—perhaps a year or more for tinea infection of the toe nails.

Flucytosine is active orally. It is converted in tissues into 5-fluorouracil, which blocks DNA synthesis by inhibiting thymidylate synthetase. Fungal cells convert flucytosine to 5-fluorouracil much more rapidly than do mammalian cells. The drug is well tolerated, with mild toxic effects such as gastrointestinal disturbances, although alopecia and neutropenia have been reported.

Antiviral agents

At present, antiviral drugs are in their infancy. The only truly effective antiviral drugs, acyclovir, gangcyclovir and idoxuridine, are only effective against certain herpes viruses and closely related DNA viruses. Zidovudine delays the onset of full-blown AIDS in patients infected with the retrovirus HIV, but does not cure the disease. Amantadine has some prophylactic value against influenza. There are currently no antiviral drugs for the treatment of verrucae pedis.

ANTIPURITICS

Indication

Pruritus may be due to systemic or local causes. It is a symptom of an underlying condition, e.g. fungal infection. In many instances, treatment of the underlying cause, where known, will reduce the symptom. This is fortunate as there is no really effective antipruritic drug. A variety of preparations have some antipruritic effect.

Calamine, either in lotion, cream or oily form, has been traditionally associated with the relief of pruritus, although its mechanism of action is unclear. Antihistamines, oral and topical, are considered to be useful where the underlying cause is an allergic reaction. Counter-irritants may also be used for pruritus; vasodilation is thought to 'block' the pruritic effect. As dry skin is associated with pruritus, emollients may also reduce the effects.

CAUSTICS

A caustic is defined as any substance that is destructive to living tissue. The following caustics are primarily used to treat corns and verrucae.

Salicylic acid. This is caustic in concentrations greater than 6%. It acts by solubilising the intercellular cement in the stratum corneum. Once this impermeable barrier has been damaged, water accumulates in the lower layers of the epidermis leading to maceration. Due to the maceration, salicylic acid is able to permeate into the lower layers of the epidermis where it has a necrotic effect on cells undergoing keratinisation. Salicylic acid is said to have a cumulative action and this, consequently, is why return periods should be relatively short (2–7 days) and why all affected skin should be debrided at subsequent visits. Salicylic acid is a common component of many proprietary preparations for corns and callus. Unfortunately, if the manufacturer's instructions are not

followed carefully, unwanted side-effects, such as ulceration and infection, may occur.

Silver nitrate. This is usually used in the form of a toughened stick produced by fusing silver salt with sodium chloride. Unlike salicylic acid, it has a superficial effect, forming a black eschar on the skin surface. This is due to a chemical action between silver nitrate and the constituents of sweat. On denuded skin such as hypergranulation tissue, it leads to shrinkage of the tissues. Silver nitrate should not be used on sensitive skin and should be avoided interdigitally unless used in lower strengths.

Mono-, di- and trichloroacetic acids. These act by precipitating and coagulating skin proteins. They are effective local cauterising agents most commonly used in the treatment of verrucae. Monochloroacetic acid is more destructive than trichloroacetic acid, and is therefore a more useful preparation. Monochloroacetic acid combined with salicylic acid is a popular treatment for verrucae pedis.

COUNTER-IRRITANTS

Counter-irritants result in vasodilation, which aids the removal of metabolites and promotes resolution of lesions. Topical vasodilators are mainly the nicotinates (methyl, ethyl, phenethyl and thuryl) and essential oils such as turpentine, cajuput and capsicum. The massaging action used in applying these preparations is considered to play an adjunct role in promoting vasodilation. There are many proprietary products on the market, all of which can be purchased without a prescription.

EMOLLIENTS

Indications

The normal water content of the skin is 10%. In patients with dry skin, the water content is much less. Dry skin may be a condition in itself or a complication of a local or systemic pathology, e.g. ischaemia. Patients with dry skin appear to be more prone to developing a range of dermatological conditions such as hyperkeratosis, seed corns or fissures. It is important that the water content of the skin is maintained in order to prevent these complications from occurring.

Mechanism of action

Water is the most important plasticiser of the epidermis. The application of an emollient increases the amount of water in the epidermis (Schwartz & Murray

1991, Loden 1992). In vitro, the stratum corneum can absorb as much as five times its own weight of water and can increase its volume up to three times when soaked in water.

Emollients achieve their effect by one or both of the following mechanisms:

- addition of water to the skin
- retention of water in the skin.

Addition of water is primarily achieved by the application of a water-based cream. Patients prefer this type of emollient as it is readily absorbed and does not leave a greasy film on the skin. Retention of water is achieved by the application of an oily based preparation, e.g. ointment, water in oil preparation or silicone. These preparations leave an oily base and, depending on the base, may not be so user-friendly. Some preparations achieve both of the above, adding water to the skin and keeping it there with a hydrophobic substance.

Urea-containing creams, especially those containing alpha-hydroxy acids such as lactic acid, produce prolonged hydration and help remove scales and crusts. The active ingredients are hydrophilic and act by enhancing the ability of the stratum corneum to hold water, and thus counteract the tendency of the skin to dry out. These preparations are referred to as keratoplastics because of their effect on the epidermis.

Salicylic acid at concentrations between 3 and 6% is keratoplastic as it causes softening of the horny layers and shedding of scales. It facilitates desquamation by solibulising the intercellular cement and enhances the shedding of corneocytes by decreasing cell-to-cell adhesion.

Emollients have a very short life span as the epidermis is constantly desquamating. Therefore, they need to be applied on a regular basis, once or twice a day, to have any therapeutic effect.

PREMEDICATION PRIOR TO SURGERY

Some patients may be fearful or apprehensive of a surgical procedure undertaken under local anaesthesia. In such circumstances, it may be necessary to use drugs to assist the patient in coping with surgery.

Benzodiazepines

These are useful because they allay the apprehension many patients have before surgery. The dose is chosen so as to produce light sedation. The shorter-acting benzodiazepines are more logical choices than the longer-acting drugs. In addition to sedation, benzo-

diazepines can induce a period of amnesia. If the dose is timed properly (perhaps 30–60 minutes before surgery), the patient may well have no memory of the stressful part of the procedure. For surgery carried out under local anaesthesia, this amnesic action of benzodiazepines can be very useful.

Benzodiazepines act mainly by increasing the effect of gamma-amino butyric acid (GABA), the most abundant inhibitory neurotransmitter in the brain. Benzodiazepines also have a small, non-specific depressant effect on nerve cells in general by virtue of their lipid-soluble nature. None of the benzodiazepines have any antidepressant or antipsychotic properties. The anxiolytic action of the benzodiazepines is mediated through their action on GABAergic transmission in the limbic system. This is achieved at doses that are not sedative. All the benzodiazepines can cause dependence on prolonged use. The withdrawal syndrome is unlikely to be a problem if a patient has taken a long-acting benzodiazepine for less than 3 weeks, but can develop within days for short-acting drugs. The withdrawal syndrome is characterised by effects that are the opposite of those of the drug. Consequently, if the drug has been prescribed to treat anxiety, stopping the drug may be associated with a return or worsening of the anxiety as a withdrawal effect. This can prompt a new prescription unless it is recognised as part of the withdrawal syndrome. The common benzodiazepines, their duration of action and common uses are given in Table 8.3.

The shorter-acting benzodiazepines, e.g. midazolam and temazepam, are useful as anaesthetic premedication agents, as they allay fears and produce a period of amnesia. Diazepam is sometimes also used to produce sedation and amnesia for unpleasant procedures. The patient will be sedated or drowsy for some time and a second phase of sleep 4–6 hours after the dose is not uncommon. This is thought to be due to the appearance of its active metabolite, nordiazepam.

Like all depressant drugs, benzodiazepines have an additive effect with other depressants, including alcohol and antihistamines. Consequently, patients must be warned that they should not take other depressant drugs. Those benzodiazepines with very long half-lives ($t_{1/2}$) also accumulate when taken over a prolonged period of time. For a drug with a $t_{1/2}$ of 80 hours, e.g. diazepam plus its active metabolites, the time taken to reach a steady-state blood level will be at least 3 weeks. Similarly, when the drug is stopped, it will take 3 or more weeks to be eliminated. Benzodiazepines also interfere with the performance

Table 8.3 Properties of common benzodiazepines

Drug	Plasma $t_{1/2}$ (hours)	$t_{1/2}$ of active metabolites (hours)	Uses
Chlordiazepoxide	20	30–200	anxiety
Clobazam	35	40	anxiety, epilepsy
Clonazepam	25	–	epilepsy
Diazepam	30	30–200	anxiety, epilepsy
Flurazepam	inactive (prodrug)	30–200	anxiety
Ketazolam	inactive (prodrug)	30–200	anxiety
Lorazepam	20	inactive	anxiety, insomnia
Medazepam	inactive (prodrug)	30–200	anxiety
Midazolam	3	inactive	insomnia, premedication
Nitrazepam	30	inactive	insomnia*
Oxazepam	7	inactive	anxiety
Temazepam	13	inactive	insomnia, premedication

* Although nitrazepam has a long half-life, it was promoted as a hypnotic. Its use in this role has been superseded by drugs with shorter half-lives.

of tasks requiring vigilance and rapid reactions, such as driving or operating machinery. With long-acting benzodiazepines, a person may be unfit to drive the day after taking the drug.

Diazepam is active after oral administration, and has a very long $t_{1/2}$ (diazepam + active metabolites, $t_{1/2}$ = approximately 30–200 hours). This means that the drug can be given a considerable time before surgery. It also means that the patient is likely to suffer from a 'hangover' for some time after dosing. Temazepam has a much shorter duration of action than diazepam ($t_{1/2}$ = 8 hours) and is so lipid-soluble that it is absorbed rapidly and completely from the gastrointestinal tract. Sedation and anxiolysis last for about 1–2 hours, after which the patient will be alert but drowsy. Lorazepam has a slightly longer duration of action ($t_{1/2}$ = 12 hours). Nitrazepam, which is promoted as an aid to sleep, nevertheless has a very long duration of action ($t_{1/2}$ = 28 hours). Patients are more likely to suffer from the after-effects of the drug the next day, i.e. persistent sedation and drowsiness, than with short-acting drugs. Midazolam is similar in duration to the action of temazepam but is injected intramuscularly or intravenously rather than taken orally.

SUMMARY

Pharmacological preparations have a valuable role to play in the management of foot problems. As highlighted in the introduction, they are used, in many instances, to control and reduce symptoms rather than cure the underlying cause. Any pharmacological preparation should be used with care. It is essential that the practitioner, before deciding to use such a preparation, has undertaken a full assessment and is aware of the patient's current and previous medication, as well as the likelihood of any contraindications or adverse reactions.

REFERENCES

Greenfield J, Rea J, Ilfield F 1984 Morton's interdigital neuroma: indications for treatment by local injections versus surgery. Clin Orthop Rel Res 142–144

Loden M 1992 The increase in skin hydration after application of emollients with different amounts of lipids. Acta Dermato-Venereologica 72(5): 327–330

Miller S 1992 Morton's neuroma. A syndrome. In: McGlamry E D, Banks A S, Downey M S (eds) Comprehensive textbook of foot surgery. Williams & Wilkins, Baltimore, p 310

Ohira T, Ishikawa K, Kumato S 1986 Hydroxyapatite deposition in articular cartilage by intra-articular injections of methylprednisolone. Journal of Bone & Joint Surgery 68-A(4): 509–510

Schwartz S, Murray R 1991 Assessment of epithelial thickness by ultrasonic imaging. Decubitus 4(4): 29–30

Scott N 1991 In: McClure J, Widlsmith J (eds) Mechanisms and management of conduction blockade for post operative analgesia. Edward Arnold, London

Shoemaker R S, Bertone A L, Martin G S, Mellwraith C W, Roberts E D, Pechman R, Keaney M T 1992 Effects of intra-articular administration of methylprednisolone acetate on normal articular cartilage and on healing of experimentally induced osteochondral defects in horses. American Journal of Veterinary Research 53(8): 1446–1453

Tollafield D R, Williams H A 1996 The use of two injectable corticosteroid preparations used in the management of foot problems—a clinic audit report. British Journal of Podiatric Medicine 51(12) 171–174

FURTHER READING

British National Formulary (BNF) British Medical Association and the Royal Pharmaceutical Society of Great Britain *Updated and published twice a year (March and September)*

Foster R W 1996 Basic pharmacology, 4th edn. Butterworth's, London

Laurence D R, Bennett P N 1992 Clinical pharmacology, 7th edn. Churchill Livingstone, Edinburgh

Laurence D R, Carpenter J R 1994 A dictionary of pharmacology and clinical drug evaluation. UCL Press, London

Rang H P, Dale M M 1991 Pharmacology, 2nd edn. Churchill Livingstone, Edinburgh

9

Physical therapy

S. J. Avil
W. Turner
A. Hinde

INTRODUCTION

Physical therapy can be used to treat feet thera-peutically without the need for pharmacological preparations or invasive methods. The conjoint use of mechanical therapy will assist many foot problems after physical therapy has achieved the desirable effects of reversing, or at least stabilising, any inflammatory process. Physical therapy will therefore generally employ heat and cold in the treatment of musculoskeletal conditions, injury or insult; indeed, heat and cold are the most common first line treatments associated with this type of therapy. Electrical methods offer more sophisticated systems, producing similar results to thermal methods. The properties of enhancing the vascular system to local anatomy, as well as diminishing pain sensation, confer some of the essential benefits to the patient using a range of different physical modalities.

COLD AND HEAT

Cold and heat have been used in the management of trauma since as far back as 400 BC. The physiological effects of heat and cold help many of the local adverse pathological changes associated with tissue trauma. Pain may be reduced, healing aided and rehabilitation time improved.

The effects of thermal treatment on tissue response are compared and contrasted in Table 9.1.

Physiology of cold and heat

Cold

The topical application of cold causes excitation of sympathetic adrenergic nerve fibres, which causes constriction of arterioles and venules resulting in

Table 9.1 Effects of thermal treatment on tissue response

Cold	Heat
Vasoconstriction	Vasodilation
Decreased pain	Decreased pain
Decreased muscle spasm	Decreased muscle spasm
Decreased vascular permeability	Increased vascular permeability
Decreased metabolism	Increased metabolism
Reduced swelling/oedema	

vasoconstriction. The direct effect of cold on the tissues is to reduce the metabolic rate, thus reducing the effect of chemical mediators associated with the inflammatory process. The demand for oxygen and nutrients will also be reduced and the inflammatory process can be minimised. A decrease in vascular permeability arises with an increase in the viscosity of blood as the vessel walls constrict. Reduction of leakage of transudate from vessels will slow the acute inflammatory response and reduce the amount of swelling.

Heat

Conversely, the application of heat will cause a rise in the superficial skin temperature, resulting in *vasodilation.* Temperature elevation increases the demand for oxygen and nutrients. This demand is met by increased blood flow from stimulated vasodilation. *Vascular permeability* arises with the release of chemical mediators, allowing leakage from the blood vessels. The resultant cellular activity will remove harmful substances, although inevitably this creates some of the problems that physical therapy is attempting to minimise. Therefore, the objective behind heat application is to encourage defence and repair. Heat should not be used where the circulation to the area is poor. Any increased metabolic effect will be deleterious to the local anatomy, causing the surrounding tissues to break down and ulcerate.

Heat will beneficially affect nerve conduction velocity, lowering pain perception; this in turn reduces muscle tone. Joint motion may be limited by spasm caused by tonic contraction. While spasm is protective, it nevertheless prevents the joint from functioning normally. In the foot, common joints affected by tonic spasm include the subtalar joint (peroneal muscle) and the first metatarsophalangeal (MTP) joint (short flexor hallucis spasm). Heat will increase the extensibility of collagen and can be used to reduce scar tissue, particularly around joints (Fig. 7.5B). Initially, cold is used to minimise swelling and exudate, to reduce haematoma and to slow down the process

producing scar tissue. Once the joint is stable, and adjacent soft tissues have been identified as not being torn and not requiring surgical repair, heat can be used to build up motion, muscle strength and flexibility. Joints kept immobilised for long periods become stiff and may have to be manipulated under anaesthetic (MUA). Early gentle movement and heat therapy will be used by the practitioner to ensure that immature scar tissue is stretched and mobilised. Intracapsular adhesions are therefore discouraged before they become a problem.

CRYOTHERAPY

Cryotherapy is the therapeutic application of cold. The methods employed range from the simple application of ice to more sophisticated and destructive systems, such as those used in the treatment of skin lesions (Fig. 15.21). Cold is an ideal treatment for limiting the tissue response provoked by inflammation. Cryotherapy may be used until 48 hours later after the initial injury.

The physiological effects of ice have been described above and in Table 9.1. All of these effects slow down the initial vascular response to trauma, assisting early rehabilitation by controlling some of the inflammatory mediators. Cold can be used in a number of forms:

- ice cube/frozen peas
- crushed ice in towels or cloths
- frozen gel packs
- cold or cooling sprays
- iced water or bowls of ice cubes
- cryogenic cuff.

Clinical indications

Ice. Ice is readily available and cheap. Ice cubes wrapped in hand towels or water frozen in yoghurt pots supported by wooden spatulae may be massaged over injury sites. Massage may be continued for approximately 15 minutes at a time and may be repeated after an equal period of rest from the ice. Ice can be crushed in a strong plastic bag and wrapped in a soft towel or cloth. Frozen peas or sweet corn are as beneficial as crushed ice, conforming equally well to the uneven foot contours.

Ice packs. These may be commercially purchased. The reagents, when crushed, create a temporary cooling effect due to the chemical reaction evoked. Commercial products such as Koolpack (Williams Medical Supplies) have the advantage of easy storage over a system where ice has to be produced first. Practitioners treating sportspersons in the field can carry the dry packs around safely, so that they are instantly ready for use on an acute foot injury.

Gel packs have been available for many years. These products (Fig. 9.1) can be either frozen in a refrigerator or heated to deliver the appropriate temperature to the affected part. The problem with most ice delivery is that the beneficial coolant effect is eventually lost. A new cryogenic system is available (Aircast), however, comprising a zip-up boot that fits over the foot, with a tube containing a one-way valve delivering iced water from a reservoir held above foot/ankle level (Fig. 7.25). This method of delivery offers a controllable dry cold application with an effective compression around the foot due to the head of pressure. New iced water can be introduced by altering the pressure valve on the reservoir every 10–15 minutes.

Cold footbath immersion. Cold therapy can also be achieved by immersing the foot into a bucket, or bowl of ice cubes, crushed ice, ice cubes in cold water or just cold water. Although cold water may not contain ice, the patient may not be able initially to tolerate the sensation. The short-term use of this system is to effect immediate analgesia. Immersion methods require the patient to submerge the foot below the level of liquid/crushed ice for approximately 3 minutes, or for as long as can be tolerated, up to 6 minutes. This may be repeated three or four times a day and is a useful home therapy.

Cold sprays. The main use of cold sprays (Fig. 9.1) is in the acute phase of injury. The sprays are used in short blasts of 5–10 seconds, three or four times over a period of 2 minutes. These are more commonly seen in use on a sports field. The value of such sprays prior to cutaneous injection of local anaesthetic is variable because the temperature at the nozzle end is dependent upon the chlorofluorocarbon (CFC) content. In the UK, CFCs are banned and therefore the environment takes precedence over the effectiveness of this type of coolant spray. The same problems of accessibility are not yet evident in the USA, where CFCs are still used in such sprays. The skin is cooled rapidly by the evaporation of the spray when it contacts the skin, producing the effects required to reduce pain, swelling and muscle spasm.

Contraindications

Cryotherapy should be avoided in patients with poor tissue viability. Impaired circulation will intensify the effect of the therapy, and ischaemia affecting the skin can arise, as well as ice burns and cold hypersensitivity. The practitioner should be aware of the sudden effect on the heart of immersion therapies, particularly on the elderly patient or those with a history of heart problems.

HEAT THERAPY

Infrared (IR) forms part of the electromagnetic spectrum. The wavelength is longer than visible light and so cannot be seen. All 'hot bodies' are sources of IR radiation. Infrared radiation is produced using a lamp that is either luminous or non-luminous. The terminology is self-explanatory, in that one form of IR can be seen while the other cannot.

Physical effects

The IR radiation emitted is absorbed into the body and converted into heat energy and can be applied to the chosen treatment site. *Non-luminous* forms penetrate to the epidermis, while *luminous* forms will penetrate to the dermis and the superficial fascia.

Method of application

All manufacturer's instructions should be carefully read when dealing with any equipment requiring or releasing energy. The lamp should be switched on and set up before the patient arrives. IR is directed (at a distance recommended by the manufacturer) at the uncovered site associated with the problem. Once the lamp has been heated up prior to treatment, it may be positioned at right angles to the surface of the

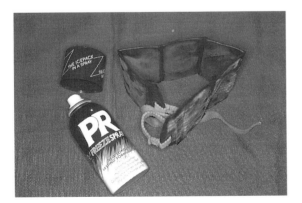

Figure 9.1 Cold can be applied as a spray from a pressurised canister. The cold spray acts momentarily, unlike gel pads which can be pre-frozen and applied as cold packs for 10–20 minutes, or alternatively as heated packs if required.

skin. The skin should be monitored periodically to ensure that the response is normal and no blistering has arisen. The epidermis and dermis may be heated by gentle heat which stimulates the free nerve endings, producing some pain relief. A gentle hyperaemia should be apparent. The duration of each treatment should be no longer than 15–20 minutes. This may be repeated daily.

Clinical indications

IR can be used on chronic musculoskeletal and traumatic non-acute conditions; these may include sprains, strains, affections of joints, tendons, plantar fasciitis and conditions associated with non-infected arthritides.

Contraindications

The greatest danger lies in the possibility of thermal damage from burns where the lamp has been placed too close to the patient. Dressings and clothing over the site of treatment must be removed first to avoid blocking the IR radiation. The fibres found in these materials will retain heat, perpetuating the problem of skin burns. Any oil or embrocation must be removed first, as this may also enhance the heating effect. Large areas of skin should not be exposed to IR radiation, in order to avoid the possibility of hypotension if the patient rises quickly following treatment.

ULTRASOUND

Ultrasound is a mechanical vibration (longitudinal wave) produced by the piezo-electric deformation of a crystal when subjected to a high frequency (0.75–3 MHz) of alternating electric current. The energy of the longitudinal wave will produce the mechanical effects of compression/rarefaction in the tissues through which it passes. The mechanical energy is dissipated due to frictional losses at tissue interfaces. The dissipation is described in terms of the residual energy per unit distance from the site of application and is known as the 'half-value distance'. This distance is typically 5 cm for a 1 MHz output, the half-value reducing as the output frequency rises.

Physical properties

The physical effects on biological tissues are a result of the compression/rarefaction phases. Fluid is moved away from the treatment face of the equipment in a process called *acoustic streaming*. The mechanical

energy frictional losses convert into thermal gains, increasing the temperature at the tissue interfaces. The beneficial physiological effects are associated with the result of acoustic streaming, which increases the tissue fluid flow rates at the site of application.

The compression/rarefaction wave action results in the following changes:

- increased capillary and cell permeability
- breakdown of complex biochemically active molecules
- decreased ground–substance viscosity.

The thermal gain results in all the normal changes brought about by heating tissues:

- rise in tissue temperature
- increased cell metabolic rate
- vasodilation.

Methods of application

Ultrasound is applied either directly or indirectly (Fig. 9.2):

- *directly*—when the treatment face of the equipment is in contact with the skin via a coupling medium
- *indirectly*—when the part to be treated is immersed in water. The treatment face does not contact the skin directly because the water medium acts as the conductor.

It is essential to maintain continuous contact between the whole of the treatment face and the skin, if damage to the equipment or tissues is to be avoided (direct method). Some manufacturers of ultrasonic equipment supply a number of treatment heads, to enable the practitioner to select the most appropriate diameter. Where the curvature of the part to be treated prevents complete contact being made, the immersion (indirect) technique is safer and more efficient. This applies to most of the foot and ankle region of the lower limb.

Once the absence of contraindications has been confirmed and the dangers noted, indirect treatment may commence. The following points should be noted:

- the part should be immersed in water
- air bubbles should be brushed from the skin and treatment face
- the dosage should be selected and applied
- the treatment face should be continually moved to direct the energy over the area
- the part should be dried and inspected.

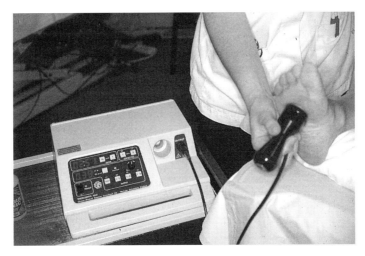

Figure 9.2 Ultrasound therapy uses high-frequency compression waves, offering a wide range of indications for foot problems: oedema, spasm of muscle, calcified tendinitis, synovitis and fasciitis.

As with all treatment, any values should be recorded in the patient's notes—dose, frequency, mode, time of application, plus follow-up instructions given to the patient.

When ultrasound is applied in the *continuous mode*, the thermal and mechanical effects are produced in the tissues through which the energy travels. When applied in the *pulsed mode,* the mechanical effects predominate. This is because the length of time during which the mechanical energy is produced is very short (typically 2 ms) and the resting phase is relatively long (typically 8 ms). The thermal gain is therefore limited and there is a period of heat dissipation before the next period of thermal gain. Manufacturers of ultrasound equipment sometimes offer the facility to adjust the pulsing ratios.

Clinical indications

The main indications for therapeutic ultrasound are listed in Table 9.2. Ultrasound waves will accelerate any active biological process at the time of application.

Dosage

For acute conditions, thermal effects should be avoided if further pain and tissue damage are to be avoided. The 'pulsed' mode should be chosen, with settings which give minimal energy input:

- low intensity output settings (<0.75 W/cm2)
- short time setting (<3 minutes).

As the condition improves, either or both of these parameters may be increased, so as to increase the energy input to the tissues.

As the acute inflammatory response reduces, the intensity and time settings may both be increased, gradually introducing thermal effects. Where chronic oedema is present, with adhesion formation, high energy input is normally chosen:

Table 9.2 Indications for therapeutic ultrasound

Reduction of oedema	Reduction of pain	Mobilisation of collagen
Acoustic streaming	Reducing the volume of any oedema	Depolymerisation of the proteins, thus lowering the elastic modulus to allow stretching at lower forces
Increasing capillary permeability	Removal of the pain-stimulating chemicals released by trauma to the cells	
Increasing blood flow through the area	Reduction of relative ischaemia by increasing blood flow through the area	

- 'continuous' mode
- higher intensity output (>0.75 W/cm^2)
- longer time settings (>5 minutes).

The patient should always be warned that symptoms may increase 6–8 hours after treatment but should settle again 12 hours after treatment. This effect often results from the relatively arbitrary nature of deciding the dose to be applied, and may be taken as an indication for the progression of the treatment:

- if post-treatment discomfort is great, reduce or repeat the settings at the next visit
- if no post-treatment discomfort has been felt, repeat or increase the settings at the next visit.

Contraindications

The use of ultrasound is contraindicated when:

- there is an infection in the area
- there is a deep vein thrombosis or arterial disease
- tumours or TB are present
- the patient has haemophilia
- the patient is receiving radiation therapy.

Furthermore, caution must be exercised when:

- an area of skin is anaesthetised
- the underlying bone surface is concave
- there may be metal in the tissues
- there may be air-filled cavities in the area
- there is a suspected fracture (see diagnosis of stress fracture, Ch. 16, p. 353).

Many of the dangers come from the possibility that energy reflected from the surface of bone, metal and air-filled cavities may create a point of high intensity in the tissues.

The waves of compression/rarefaction may cause cavitation in the tissues under treatment. This effect can be prevented by ensuring that the treatment face is always moving over the skin and that light, even pressure is applied. When the immersion technique is used, cavitation is less likely to occur, but movement should still be carried out. Air bubbles form on the treatment face and skin. These should be removed by brushing during the treatment, or the ultrasound will be attenuated before reaching the patient.

RADIOFREQUENCY HEATING

Radiofrequency heating is a general term covering those techniques which use the short-wave band (short-wave diathermy, SWD) or the microwave band (microwave diathermy, MWD). Both forms of diathermy involve the generation of electrostatic or electromagnetic fields and are associated with the electromagnetic spectrum. SWD treatment is usually at the frequency of 27.12 MHz (wavelength 11 m), and MWD treatment is usually at the frequency of 2450 MHz (wavelength 122.5 mm). Technological advances in equipment generating radiofrequency have resulted in a wider range of frequencies than those above being utilised. The output from the generator may be continuous or pulsed.

The physical consequence of the electrostatic or electromagnetic fields is to create heat in the tissues, as well as exerting a number of electrophysical field effects:

- the rotation of dipole molecules
- the distortion of non-polar molecules
- the vibration of ions
- the production of eddy current fields.

The fields created by the generators will tend to concentrate in those materials of low dielectric constant, e.g. blood and muscle, in preference to those of high dielectric constant, e.g. air and bone. Tissues with high fluid content will therefore be preferentially heated by using these techniques.

The physiological effects of applying radiofrequency heating result from the responses of tissues to heating as listed in Table 9.1 and additionally include:

- reduction of muscle tone
- reduction in blood pressure
- rise in body temperature with time.

Method of application

The manufacturers of these heat sources supply a number of applicators to fit their machines. For SWD, there are a number of differently sized 'plates', either rigid and enclosed in plastic or glass holders or flexible and enclosed in rubber sheaths (Fig. 9.3). These produce their effects by creating electrostatic fields in the tissues. There may be a long cable enclosed in a rubber sheath. For MWD, there are usually a number of applicators, used singly, which are of different sizes to correspond with different body areas. The therapeutic effect is achieved by creating electromagnetic fields in the tissues.

The applicators are not placed in contact with the patient's skin but must always be separated by an air space or by dry padding. The size of the applicators must correspond to the size of the body part being treated (Fig. 9.3)—too large an applicator will result in excess heating of the superficial tissues parallel with the field lines, while too small an applicator

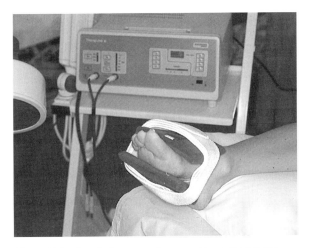

Figure 9.3   An electromagnetic current is applied to the right foot as short-wave diathermy. This type of physical therapy offers the deepest form of heat available to the practitioner/physiotherapist. Its uses for feet include degenerative joint disease, tenosynovitis/synovitis and haematoma.

will result in field concentration in the tissues adjacent to the applicator and, consequently, excessive heating.

When selecting the applicator to be used for SWD, the choice of size or type will depend on the following points:

• For electrostatic fields, two plate electrodes are used, one for either side of the area to be treated. The plates should be slightly larger than the area—one may be flexible and one may be rigid, if necessary.

• For electromagnetic fields, the cable enclosed in a rubber sheath is used.

The choice of applicator for MWD will be based on the size of the area to be treated and the range of applicators supplied with the generator. The sizes of the applicator and the area to be treated should be similar. For circular applicators, the maximum heating effect is around the outside of the field.

When using the cable, a choice of arrangement is available depending on the technique of heating required. If an electromagnetic field is desired, the centre of the cable is wound around the part to be treated, whereas an electrostatic field is produced by using the ends of the cable. The continuous modes of application are predominantly used for the thermal effects they produce, while in the pulsed mode there is a thermal effect during the 'on' phase, but the heat created will be dissipated during the 'off' phase. Manufacturers offer various pulsing ratios to allow

the practitioner to select the appropriate thermal/non-thermal effects for the patient.

Many practitioners using SWD will select the cable technique and wind it around the calf and foot with approximately 2 cm of towelling between the patient and the cable as padding, or, alternatively, they will place two small applicators, separated with an air spacing, on either side of the area so that the field passes through the foot from the plantar to the dorsal aspects. If MWD is used, the smallest applicator is placed (with an air spacing) over the part to be treated.

The therapeutic benefits from radiofrequency heating are those which result from the thermal effects. In the pulsed mode, these thermal effects last for much shorter periods than in the continuous mode, typically 0.4 ms, and may be summarised as follows:

• an increase in the blood flow through the site
• stimulation of cell activity, e.g. skin growth in wounds
• a decrease in muscle tone
• a decrease in pain perception.

When the continuous mode is used, there will be a gradual increase in temperature of blood returning to the core. This will bring about a whole-body reflex vasodilation in an attempt to control the body temperature, an effect which is called *reflex heating*. This vasodilation results in a reduction in peripheral resistance, and will therefore be accompanied by a reduction in blood pressure. Time must be allowed for the blood pressure to rise naturally before any exercise is commenced following treatment. A medical opinion may need to be sought before exposing patients with cardiac disorders to the demands imposed by radiofrequency treatment. Good communication and rapport with medical physicians will avoid placing patients at unnecessary risk.

Heating another site on the body, at a different location (with a healthy blood supply), will still cause a reflex vasodilation at the impaired site. In this situation, the increased cellular metabolism created is less likely to create a deleterious problem than if applied directly to the impaired site.

When acute inflammatory conditions are being treated, low energy levels should be applied. This may be achieved by using the pulsed mode at low intensity, or, where the continuous mode is the only one available, by adjusting the output to a subthermal level, where no heat is perceived by the patient. As the acute response reduces, the thermal effects may gradually be introduced.

When there are chronic changes at the site to be treated, the generator is altered to produce different thermal effects best suited to deal with this level of pathology. Treatment may progress in the following way:

- if, following treatment, intolerable discomfort arises, reduce or repeat the settings
- if no discomfort arises after treatment, repeat or increase the settings.

Contraindications

The electromagnetic and electrostatic fields generated by the equipment may affect subjects other than the patients being treated. For this reason, departments using such generators must display signs at their entrances informing *all* people who intend to enter of the presence of the generators. Anyone who has a cardiac pacemaker must report the fact to the practitioner because its function may be affected by an external electrical field. Similar dangers exist for hearing aids. Any practitioner intending to switch on a radiofrequency generator must first check that no other patient in the room has a cardiac pacemaker.

The use of radiofrequency heating is contraindicated in the following cases:

- when *malignancies* are known or suspected to be in the treatment fields
- if *circulatory changes* are likely in the limb, such as those found in ischaemic conditions, thrombosis or phlebitis
- when *cardiovascular* pathologies are present, as they may be exacerbated by the increased circulation caused by treatment imposing an effect on blood pressure variation
- if there are metal or plastic *implants*, e.g. intrauterine contraceptive devices, in the treatment field, as they may be affected by radiofrequency heating
- if there is *infection* present, as it is exacerbated by the radiofrequency-generated treatment field
- excessive *fluid* in the treatment fields should be avoided; this could include non-inflammatory oedema, external wet dressings or even excessive perspiration on the skin
- if there is *haemorrhage* or if haemorrhage may be caused, as in the case of haemophilia
- where there is *impaired thermal sensation*, either hypo- or hypersensitivity, in which case the control settings should be reduced
- when patients are unable to understand the instructions concerning the treatment, in which case the practitioner may prefer to use a safer source of therapy.

Application of radiofrequencies to most parts of the calf and foot can be undertaken. The practitioner will choose the size and type of applicator to be used according to the patient's medical history and tissue sensitivity. In order to prevent an electric shock, the patient must not touch the generator or any other metal fittings. The part to be treated may therefore require supporting in order to mobilise the foot and limb safely. If toes are included in the treatment field, the spaces between the toes should be padded with small quantities of cotton wool to help prevent any build-up of perspiration and therefore the possibility of burns.

The practitioner needs to monitor the part being treated frequently. The level of heat applied should be no more than 'mild gentle heat' and should be applied for no longer than 20 minutes. On completion of the treatment, the patient's blood pressure should be given time to rise before the patient stands or begins to exercise.

HYDROTHERAPY

This therapy involves the use of a water medium in which the patient may perform movements against the water's resistance. Foot and leg hydrotherapy baths may include a spa effect which can have additional benefits.

Therapeutic effects

By immersing either the body or the limb in water, the reduced effect of weight-bearing and gravity will lower the stresses at the affected site while strengthening muscles and mobilising joints. Rehabilitation is brought about by limiting pain while allowing active strengthening of damaged tissues. Mobility is increased and stiffness discouraged by limiting adhesion formation. The water is usually heated and may have jets of air/water directed to provide massage at the same time. Pain-free movements can improve blood flow so as to stimulate tissue repair.

Method of application

This will depend on the particular requirement but can range from directed exercises utilising the non-weight-bearing state the patient can attain in the pool, with or without resistance to massage, to a simple application of heat. The body will need to be immersed in a pool to cover the injured site, with the patient either sitting or being supported while performing exercises.

Clinical indications

Hydrotherapy may be used as a method of upgrading fitness, strength, flexibility and cardiovascular fitness. Specific active or passive exercises with movements may help to relieve muscle spasm, produce relaxation and restoration of joint motions, increase muscle strengths, and enhance power and endurance. If used for patients with overuse injuries, hydrotherapy offers a medium in which training can be continued while limiting the effects of gravity yet maintaining muscle bulk and fitness.

It may be used for acute and chronic conditions associated with musculoskeletal or articular complaints.

Contraindications

Constant supervision should be arranged where whole body immersion is used to avoid accidental drowning. Wounds should be protected to avoid excessive maceration, contamination of the water or further infection. Infected wounds should not be immersed.

Footbaths

Therapeutic heat or cold sources can be used in a variety of media, ranging from water to wax or mud. If required, medicaments may be added to the water baths for skin complaints or wounds. Warm saline baths may be used as a postoperative measure for phenolisation treatments or following acid therapies as an attempt to neutralise too severe an action.

Methods of application

Hot footbaths. The temperature of warm water should be 5–10°C above body temperature. The foot should be immersed in a bowl of the water for 15–20 minutes. This may be repeated two or three times per day. For cold footbaths, see cryotherapy (p. 159).

Contrast footbaths. This type of therapy utilises the physiological effects of cold and heat on the body (see Table 9.1). One hot footbath (40–50°C) and one cold (tap water) footbath are prepared. Colder mixtures may be used by adding ice cubes. The foot is placed into the cold footbath for 2 minutes and then into the hot footbath for the same length of time. This process is repeated, ending with a dip into the cold bath.

Wax footbaths. Heated baths of paraffin wax are set at approximately 50°C. The patient's foot is immersed or dipped into the wax and then lifted out of it. A period of 15–20 seconds is allowed for this first coat

to form on the skin before re-immersing. The process is repeated approximately six times so that a good coating of wax provides a strong envelope around the foot and retains heat. The foot is then wrapped in a plastic bag or plastic sheet and further wrapped in a blanket. The patient is then left to relax for 20–30 minutes. This process produces a comforting heat, ideal for arthritic complaints and chronic musculoskeletal injuries.

Contraindications

Footbaths should be avoided when skin wounds are open, except where antiseptic is added intentionally to assist with drainage for infections and ulcers. Hypersensitivity to hot and cold will adversely affect conditions such as reflex sympathetic dystrophy.

MISCELLANEOUS APPLICATIONS

MUSCLE STIMULATION

Interrupted direct current applied to nerve and muscle will produce a contraction of the muscle. Faradic-type currents are used on normally innervated muscle to produce a contraction (Fig. 9.4). The pulse duration is usually selected to be between 0.02 and 1 ms. A depolarised pulse is used to prevent electrolytic burns. The output must be surged to produce a tetanic-like response from the stimulated muscle. The contraction of the muscle itself will produce a number

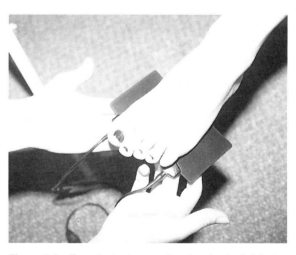

Figure 9.4 Two electrodes are placed under the left foot for muscle stimulation.

of physiological effects. Direct stimulation of motor neurones will produce a contraction in innervated muscle.

Therapeutic effects

Stimulation of muscle will invoke two effects. The stimulation of muscle tissue will raise its metabolic level, creating a reactive vasodilation. Circulation must be adequate to cope with the required venous return. Fibrous adhesions may be stretched, especially where the stimulation is preceded by a thermal treatment. The increased tone of muscle may well assist in reducing muscle discomfort and dynamic function.

Method of application

The output of the Faradic-type current is applied directly to the patient through metal (Zinc) electrodes (Fig. 9.4). The electrodes can be covered with a wetted cloth and strapped onto the treatment site. Alternatively, the electrodes may be placed in a shallow water bath in which the foot is immersed so that the current may act over the treatment site. Both methods can be combined.

Muscles may be stimulated individually or in groups, depending on the specific aim of the treatment. The most efficient points for electrode location are on the peripheral nerve supplying the muscle and on the motor point of the muscle. The motor point of a skeletal muscle is that point where there is greater concentration of motor end plates. The position is typically at the junction of upper and middle thirds of the muscle belly.

In order to reduce the intensity of the sensory stimulus and at the same time produce an efficient contraction with the minimum current, it is advisable to wash the sites thoroughly for electrode placement. Soaking the calf and foot in hot water for approximately 10 minutes before treatment helps to reduce skin resistance, and makes the treatment more comfortable for the patient. During this time the equipment may be prepared.

One electrode is placed on the peripheral nerve supplying the muscles. If treating a single muscle, e.g. abductor hallucis, the other electrode is placed over the motor point of the muscle. The water bath method will usually be more efficient when treating an intrinsic muscle group. A shallow plastic tray is filled with water and the foot is placed into it. Electrodes are placed at each end of the tray in line with the muscles to be stimulated. When the current is flowing, the muscle will contract. The practitioner must regu-

late the frequency and intensity of the flow to bring about a painless contraction. The patient can augment contraction by voluntarily activating the muscle (although this is difficult with intrinsic foot muscles).

During treatment, the intensity of the current is reduced. The muscle should be placed in its shortest position and the patient encouraged to maintain the strength of contraction. Once voluntary contraction can be maintained without the current being used, the electrodes can be removed. The skin should be dried and inspected for rashes brought about by chemical irritation at the electrode sites.

Clinical indications

Faradic-type stimulation is applied to muscle to improve contraction where the muscle is weak or has suffered some recent paralysis associated with deficient motor innervation. Once a popular method employed for all forms of flat foot pathology, this technique is reserved for specific conditions and provides adjunctive rather than primary therapy, i.e.:

- postsurgical-related pain inhibition preventing muscle function
- education of muscles after tendon transplantation (Ch. 7)
- to improve recent rather than long-standing muscle atrophy.

Secondary effects associated with stimulating muscle tissue improve tissue blood flow and venous/lymphatic drainage from the area.

Contraindications

Electrical stimulation should not be used in the following circumstances:

- on skin with loss of sensation
- over skin lesions, malignant or otherwise
- in the presence of infections
- where there is a presence of metal
- where there is ischaemia or abnormal local circulatory status
- where the patient may not be able to comprehend clinical instructions.

TRANSCUTANEOUS NERVE STIMULATORS

Transcutaneous electrical nerve stimulation (TNS) is another electrically modified method similar to Faradism, but rather than working to increase muscle tone, the small unit acts on nerve pathways to reduce pain via contact electrodes. A direct current is produced across the skin and deeper tissue. Non-thermal micro-massage and some motor stimulation are produced (with lower current (mA) levels and frequency).

Therapeutic effects

The precise mechanism associated with TNS therapy is still poorly understood. Much of the theory initially postulated was based upon Melzack & Wall's (1966) pain gate theory which has now fallen out of favour. In this theory, an applied electrical current was thought to interfere with the transference of impulses along the nerve fibres, diminishing pain response. Large afferent nerves are particularly affected. The TNS system increases cell permeability and stimulates natural endogenous opiates associated with pain relief.

Method of application

Transducers are coated in a lubricating gel which forms a contact medium. The transducer pads (Fig. 9.5) are fastened over the painful area or nerve route using hypoallergenic tape. The intensity of the current is increased to obtain a tingling effect. The current can then be adjusted after 2–3 minutes to maintain analgesia. The sensation should be pleasant. Too high a current will cause unpleasant muscle contractions. The treatment is designed to be used continuously and is powered by a portable battery unit. Therapy is set at the lowest level to confer analgesia. Many

of these units are now economical enough for patients to purchase, although they are very basic. The unit shown in Figure 9.5 can utilise four electrode pads. The pulsing effect can be altered by altering the frequency and current (mA), offering greater flexibility.

Clinical indications

Painful problems can be assisted with TNS, offering an alternative to analgesic drug therapy. The use of TNS units in feet has not been as well documented as has their use with labour pain.

Another popular method of providing TNS therapy is via an acupuncture needle. The current is directed at the entry site rather than using a conducting pad.

Contraindications

TNS units may interfere with cardiac pacemakers. Where pain may be diminished following an application of TNS, the patient must not overuse the part to avoid further injury due to desensitisation.

MANUAL THERAPY

Massage, manipulation and mobilisation to assist in the recovery from injury and disease were used by ancient civilisations over 5000 years ago. More recently, there has been a resurgence in the use of hand massage and manipulation in the management of musculoskeletal disorders. While the foot and ankle offer a small area to work on, manual techniques used elsewhere on the body can still be used on the foot.

Massage

Soft tissue can be manipulated by effleurage (stroking), petrissage (deep friction) and kneading movements. The energy generated by the fingers creates the same beneficial effects as seen in previous methods using heat and electrical stimulation. Little clinical research has been offered to support the science of massage. However, the physical effects of touch produce relaxation and a feeling of well-being.

The therapeutic effects associated with stimulating local circulation with massage bring about inflammatory mediators. Effleurage is used to push the circulatory volume towards the heart with the palms of the hand or pulpy tips of the fingers. Drainage is stimulated especially with movements along the long

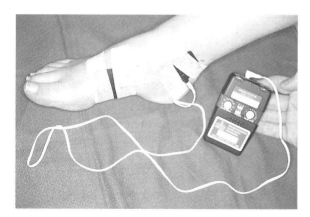

Figure 9.5 A portable transcutaneous nerve stimulator provides two (to four) electrodes applied along the medial plantar nerve branch as it passes through the ankle into the sole of the foot. TNS provides an alternative form of analgesia.

arch and calf muscles. Effleurage is ideally performed prior to other manipulations.

Petrissage is applied by direct pressure to the area of chronic injury or damage with the tips of the fingers. Interfibril adhesions and scarring can be immobilised. This technique is useful on muscles, tendons and ligaments. Tissue compression and nerve excitation provide additional pain relief.

Kneading will enhance the analgesic effect and again can be used on the arch and calf areas. Soft tissue can be picked up and squeezed with a rolling manoeuvre against harder tissue. Collagen fibres that form abnormal cross-linkages can be mobilised by kneading. These areas of tissue may be palpated as 'masses' and 'knots'. The function of kneading will assist the reabsorption of these abnormal areas and create greater flexibility.

Contraindications

Massage should not be undertaken when infection is present. Apart from the additional pain created, infection could be forced further through the tissues. Phlebitis and thrombosis could be made worse by massage. Essentially, any undefined or unrecognisable inflammatory process or mass should be avoided.

Mobilisation and manipulation

Method of application

Movements are performed with sudden thrusts at high speed. This technique should not be performed where joint motion is likely to be inhibited by a synostosis (bone bar). Mobilisations are passive movements aimed at restoring motion to stiff and painful joints. An oscillatory movement is performed on the patient within the joint's accepted anatomical range. Patients may perform some of these manoeuvres themselves.

Manipulation differs from mobilisation in that it is a movement or thrust performed at high speed to a joint at the end of its range of motion. In these circumstances, the patient has little control of the movement and is not able to prevent it. Once again, the reason for the success of these techniques is poorly understood. The joint is taken through a range of motion and then stressed at the end of its range of excursion. Physiological function may be improved by actively stimulating the controlling mechanisms such as the mechanoreceptors within the joint capsule. Manipulative stimulation can help to reduce pain. If the joint is too painful to move, traction may be applied for up to 20 seconds, or the joint may be compressed without movement.

Clinical indications

Mobilisations may be used for any joint where there is stiffness and reduction of normal range of motion with pain. Manipulations are used on stiff, pain-free joints, or on acute, locked joints following mobilisation.

Contraindications

Contraindications to mobilisation and manipulation are:

- bone disease/malignancy
- central nervous disease
- infection
- neoplasia
- acute nerve route compression
- spondylolisthesis
- gross joint instability
- inflammatory bone disorders
- fractures
- epiphyseal plate lesions.

LASERS

Lasers have become a popular addition to physical therapy. Laser is an acronym for 'Light Amplification by Stimulated Emission of Radiation'. Initially, lasers used in medicine were high-powered devices, such as the carbon dioxide laser. These were used for tissue destruction by carbonisation, vaporisation and burn-off. These lasers are still commonly used in surgery, dermatology, gynaecology and ophthalmology, and are being used in arthroscopic surgery (Ch. 7).

Early research demonstrated that surgical wounds created by laser healed faster than wounds created by scalpel. This has led to much research into the effects of laser on tissue healing. Lasers operating at very low power outputs were found to alter the rate of healing in experimentally induced wounds. Low level (power) lasers have subsequently been developed to achieve this therapeutic objective, and can significantly increase the rate of wound healing.

Physical properties

Lasers have several important characteristics: they are well collimated, wavelength-specific, they exhibit energy uniformity and are coherent.

Light emitted from a laser source will travel in a

straight line, with relatively little divergence of the beam. The light is therefore said to be *collimated*. However, with most commercially available laser probes, some degree of divergence will be inevitable, making close contact between the probe and the skin essential.

Light emitted from a single laser probe will all be at the same wavelength. This has led some to term low level laser therapy as 'pure light' therapy. Wavelengths used in low level laser therapy are usually in the range 660–950 nm, and are found in the visible and infrared parts of the electromagnetic spectrum.

Energy delivered by laser is consistent, owing to the fact that each photon of light 'carries' the same amount of energy. This *energy uniformity* is an important characteristic of laser.

Coherence of a laser is said to occur when all waves of light are in phase or 'in step' with one another. This property is not thought to be clinically important. Laser probes which produce coherent light are much more expensive than probes which produce incoherent light, however, the value of coherence has not been established.

Laser energy is released on interaction with tissue, producing either a thermal effect or a photochemical effect, or both. It has been proposed that low level laser therapy (LLLT) produces a photochemical effect, causing molecular changes to occur within cells, thus leading to metabolic changes. The effects of LLLT on tissue can be summarised as follows:

- increased ATP synthesis
- increased macrophage activity and phagocytosis
- increased fibroblast proliferation and collagen synthesis
- increased lymphocyte proliferation
- increased vasodilation
- increased vascular permeability and mast cell degranulation.

Clinically, these effects are useful for treating a wide range of lower limb pathologies. The vascular and cellular effects augment cell-mediated immunity, making LLLT suitable as a therapy for verrucae. Increased collagen production and keratinocyte proliferation encourage wound granulation and re-epithelialisation. Sports and soft-tissue injuries respond well to LLLT, and relief from pain is achieved in conditions like rheumatoid arthritis.

Clinical indications

Low level laser therapy can result in improved local cell-mediated response and wound healing, and can reduce pain.

Wavelength, pulse frequency and energy density are important factors to consider before starting a course of laser treatment. The most effective wavelengths for podiatric purposes are 660 and 820 nm; a 915 nm super-pulse probe may be indicated for the treatment of bone lesions. A 660 nm probe will act fairly superficially and activate macrophages and fibroblasts and cause mast cell degranulation. The 660 nm probe is therefore appropriate for the treatment of verrucae and fungal infections, but may also be used to encourage wound healing. An 820 nm probe has a deeper penetration and will also stimulate macrophage and fibroblast proliferation, but it also appears to be more effective in the management of pain. The 820 nm probe is therefore appropriate for the treatment of chronic pain (as in rheumatoid arthritis) and deeper soft-tissue injuries.

Pulse frequency is also important. Most conditions will respond favourably to a frequency of 20 Hz, but frequencies between 10 and 20 kHz may be chosen. Stimulation of fibroblasts is most effective at 700 Hz, and infected conditions will respond best to frequencies between 1 and 20 kHz. If a condition fails to respond following a reasonable number of irradiations, changing the pulse frequency may be all that is necessary to bring about improvement.

Energy density is also an important consideration, since therapeutic effects are energy-dependent. Too low or too high an energy density could result in negative effects. As a rule, energy densities between 3 and 7 J/cm^2 are the most widely used and effective, with 4 J/cm^2 appearing to be particularly beneficial. The energy density may be calculated from the following formula:

$$\frac{\text{Energy}}{\text{density}} = \frac{\text{probe power (W)} \times \text{irradiation time (s)}}{\text{area of irradiation (spot size, cm)}}$$

Close contact between the probe and the skin is important, and it is essential to keep the probe at 90° to the skin surface. For wounds and verrucae, irradiation around the perimeter of the lesion at 2 cm intervals is recommended, together with irradiation of the central lesion. For large wounds, irradiation of the central wound area may be better achieved with a multidiode cluster probe. Some suggested treatment protocols are given in Table 9.3.

Contraindications

There are fewer contraindications associated with laser therapy than with many other physical therapies. To avoid eye injury, laser operators, patients and

Table 9.3 Suggested irradiation protocols (Omega)

Condition	Wavelength	Energy density and pulse frequency	Frequency of treatment
Verrucae	660 nm followed by cluster	$4J/cm^2$ 20 Hz	Twice weekly
Wound healing	660 nm followed by cluster	4–6 J/cm^2 20 Hz–10 kHz 700 Hz (higher if infection present)	Weekly to twice weekly
Pain and injury	820 nm	4–7 J/cm^2 20 Hz–10 kHz	Weekly if chronic; as much as daily if acute

any observers must wear goggles *appropriate to the wavelength of light* emitted by the device.

Lasers should not be used on pregnant mothers or patients with cancer. Lasers should not be used over an area which has recently (within the previous week) received a corticosteroid injection. Epileptic patients may receive laser therapy, providing the probe is shielded from the patient's view, using a towel or a sheet. Koebner's phenomenon at the site of laser irradiation in patients with psoriasis has been reported. Caution should be taken in the case of photosensitive individuals and in patients with porphyria.

A notice warning that a laser is in use and restricting access to the room should be placed on the door of the clinic before the beam is switched on. The room should contain no highly reflective surfaces, so as to reduce risk of laser reflection.

SUMMARY

Physical therapy uses heat and cold to modify inflammation and pain. There are many more methods to generate heat than there are to generate cold. Both approaches are used at specific points during the inflammatory phase—cold is applied during the early stages of trauma, while heat is usually applied later than cold and is predominantly used to promote early repair and to support analgesic care. Equipment has become more sophisticated, safer and more user-friendly over the years. Contraindications exist and the method used should take account of the patient's health and conditions which can be directly affected by vasomotor and electrical changes. Physical therapy often produces beneficial responses without the need for other interventions described in this book; however, adjuvant therapy can often help to make physical therapy more effective.

FURTHER READING

Low J, Reed A 1990 Electrotherapy explained: principles and practice.

Wadsworth H, Chanmugam A P P 1988 Electrophysical agents in physiotherapy, 2nd edn. Science Press, Marrickville NSW

10

An introduction to mechanical therapeutics

D. J. Pratt
D. R. Tollafield

INTRODUCTION

Mechanical therapy is a very broad subject. It is sometimes called biomechanics, but this is not particularly accurate since the term mechanical therapy is used to represent any treatment that influences foot function, and includes relatively minor solutions, such as limiting pressure over the skin, as well as more major interventions such as altering the load within joints. The type of therapy therefore varies widely, from simple dressings and taping to more complex made-to-measure devices. Biomechanics, on the other hand, refers to the response by living tissue to physical forces. Mechanical therapy will therefore influence biomechanics.

There are a number of texts already in existence which deal in depth with the subject of biomechanics, and thus only those fundamental elements of biomechanical principles and material science that are important to practitioners are presented here.

In this chapter and Chapters 11 and 12, the role played by mechanical therapy in alleviating foot pathology is discussed. Each chapter deals with different approaches to managing foot pathology, based on improving foot alignment. Chapter 11 concentrates on clinically based skills and products that can be dispensed without the use of expensive facilities. Chapter 12 focuses on orthoses that result from prescriptions and casts produced by a well-equipped orthotic laboratory.

In this chapter, the purpose of mechanical therapy is discussed and the concept of orthoses is introduced. A foot orthosis is an orthopaedic device that is used to support, to absorb shock, to correct a deformity, to relieve pressure or to improve the intrinsic function of the foot or of the whole body interfacing with the lower limb. Inlays, insoles, orthodigita and prostheses all have an orthotic function, and orthoses therefore act as conduits for mechanical therapy.

Also in this chapter, the types of materials that are available in modern therapy, many of which are based on plastics technology, are described. Knowledge of these materials and mechanical principles (stresses and strains) forms the basis of an accurate laboratory prescription.

Mechanical therapy improves a patient's mobility by reducing the pain experienced during motion. It also offers an alternative to other treatments which may be less suitable for the patient. In particular, the patient may be averse to the idea of surgery or may not wish to depend on adhesive dressings and padding. A single treatment strategy will always appeal to patients; orthoses may often satisfy this need. The ultimate objective of mechanical therapy is a complete discharge from the clinic; if this is not possible, one would aim at least to reduce the frequency of visits to the clinic, and in this context a patient must be made aware that while treatment is designed to alter the function of the foot, a complete cure is not always possible. It is in this latter case that the provision of orthoses is considered more beneficial than other techniques described in this book.

As there are many approaches to treating problems of the foot, a practitioner may find it desirable to combine mechanical therapy with other methods of management.

PRINCIPLES OF ORTHOTIC MANAGEMENT

Orthoses can be used to control the foot. Control involves stabilising abnormal pronation, reducing shock against the foot and minimising skin wear. In all cases, the aim of treatment is to reduce pain and inflammation in the anatomical structures. The presence of disease will offer greater challenges to the practitioner and in many cases a compromise may be required. The objectives of orthotic therapy are summarised in Box 10.1.

There are three types of foot pathology:

- foot instability or deformity due to muscle (or neuromuscular) weakness or imbalance
- foot instability or deformity due to structural malalignment
- deformity arising from a loss of structural integrity within the foot.

In practice, two laws are used to describe the way in which tissues adapt to external stresses—Davis's law

---

Box 10.1 Objectives of orthotic therapy

- *Redistribution*—relief of pressure from localised areas of stress such as debrided keratoses, infected or ulcerated lesions, or from prominent structures subject to trauma from shoe pressure
- *Accommodation*—rigid deformities cause pressure points which need containing. Better achieved by prescription orthoses or soft Plastazote inlays
- *Stabilisation*—realignment of bony structures (joints) in an attempt to improve function and improve soft tissue function
- *Compensation*—use of cushioning or shock attenuation supplement to repeatedly traumatised areas, in some cases serving to augment areas of natural fibro-fatty padding which have undergone atrophy or pathological displacement
- *Rest*—reduction of the effects of excessive friction on the skin
- *Immobilisation*—inhibiting movement of a part by applying force to overcome motor power
- *Containment*—a means of controlling the application of medicaments so that only the required site is subjected to the desired action

---

and Wolff's law. The former is used in relation to soft tissue, while the latter is used for bony tissue. Davis's law is more applicable to young feet prior to maturation, as developing collagenous structures are influenced more readily. Bone does not adapt as well to externally applied forces as it does to those internal forces applied through plates and pins, and yet the biological control mechanisms that produce the effects described in Wolff's law are still poorly understood (Burnstein & Wright 1994). Davis's law is described later in this book in direct relation to orthodigital function (Ch. 15).

In addition to managing soft tissue such as ligaments and bone around joints, the therapeutic objective must consider the protection of superficial (skin) lesions. In the following, some basic orthotic principles are discussed, and are used to show that forces can improve foot function.

Stabilisation

No matter what the underlying cause of the foot pathology, its orthotic management is always governed by the same principles (Pratt et al 1993). Many foot orthoses work by realigning the force between the foot and the ground (ground reaction force) in such a way as to reduce or counteract a deforming moment. However, this type of correction is usually temporary, lasting only for the duration that the orthosis is applied to the foot. On the other hand, the symptoms associated with the deformity or dysfunction can be ameliorated for much longer periods, since the aim is to reverse the effects of the pathology. In this case, a patient may well become dependent on an orthosis, once it has been found to be beneficial.

A simple example of this is the way in which a shoe can be modified to help correct a pronated foot. With an unmodified shoe, the line of action of the ground reaction force will be lateral to the line of action of the weight (force) at heel strike, thus producing a valgus moment, which forces the subtalar joint into further pronation. This can be avoided by moving the point of initial contact medially so that the ground reaction force now produces a correcting varus moment. This can be achieved by flaring the heel of the shoe medially, as shown in Figure 10.1. Such a flare will not, however, have any effect upon the final position of the calcaneus relative to the ground, and this is required if pronation is to be controlled. The simplest way to adjust the position of the calcaneus would be to use a heel wedge either placed in the heel of the shoe or, more effectively, built into an in-shoe orthosis (Fig. 10.2).

Wedging, also known as posting, is one of the principles used in functional foot orthoses; the exact angle at which the rearfoot is canted forms part of the assessment of the patient. This approach can also be used for a supinated foot, with the wedges and flares applied in the opposite sense.

Three-point force systems are often used in the design

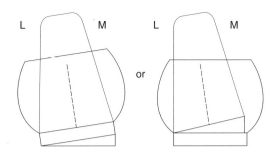

Figure 10.2 The principle of a rearfoot post on the resting calcaneal position.

of orthoses, for example in the management of hallux abductovalgus (HAV). This deformity comprises an abducted hallux at the metatarsophalangeal joint. The hallux may well deform the second toe and subsequent lateral toes. The metatarsal is adducted and, in severe cases, the medial side of the metatarsal becomes prominent with a bursal sac (bunion). Orthotic management of this deformity requires that the hallux be adducted and the first metatarsal shaft be abducted (Fig. 10.3). Two three-point force systems

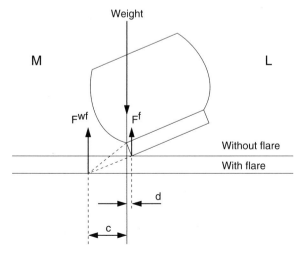

Figure 10.1 The effect of a flare on the heel designed to convert a deforming valgus ($F^f \times d$) moment to a correcting varus moment ($F^{wf} \times c$).

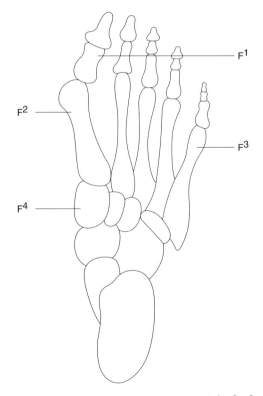

Figure 10.3 Two three-point force systems, (F^1, F^2, F^3) and (F^2, F^3, F^4), being used to correct an HAV deformity.

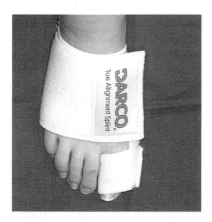

Figure 10.4 A Darco day splint for hallux valgus provides a simple example of the three-point force system.

are used, with F^1, F^2 and F^3 correcting the hallux, and F^2, F^3 and F^4 correcting the first ray. Unfortunately, this can result in a very bulky device, although some orthoses, such as the Darco splint, are designed for daytime (Fig. 10.4). To keep the corrective forces small, they are applied as far from the joint centres as possible and the pressures are reduced by spreading the forces over large areas.

Redistribution

Often, pressures are increased to painful and damaging levels under fixed or depressed metatarsal heads. The therapeutic aim is either to move the metatarsal shaft back into alignment with the others or to redistribute the load under the fixed metatarsal head. In the former case, a pad is used to push the shaft dorsally and thus realign it. If the deformity is only partially correctable or not correctable at all, then the area of increased pressure should be relieved (Fig. 10.5). To do this, the area under the plantarflexed head is excavated relative to the other heads, so that pressure is reduced and spread more evenly over each head (Whitney & Whitney 1990). This is a sim-

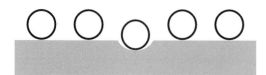

Figure 10.5 The principle of pressure reduction by spreading the forefoot load over as large an area as possible, instead of concentrating it on, in this case, the third metatarsal head.

plification since in fact there are often multiple sites requiring relief, and the tissue viability of the skin and underlying structures may be poor, preventing the redistribution of pressure where it should ideally be placed.

Compensation

While redistribution forms the principal approach in managing symptoms, several other approaches may need to be dovetailed into orthotic management. In many cases, pain is due to an excessive shock transmission through the joints during walking or running, as a result of a loss of the natural shock-attenuating properties of the foot, particularly at the heel. Such excess shock can be harmful as well as painful and should be treated seriously (Collins & Whittle 1989). Simply replacing the lost shock attenuation property of the foot with a tissue-equivalent material is often sufficient to relieve the symptoms. This approach of increasing the attenuation of shock is known as compensation for loss of fibro-fatty (adipose) tissue, which is common with old age and certain disease processes. When selecting the material to be used, one must take account of various factors, such as the weight of the patient, the location of the pain, the conditions producing the discomfort, and the general health and activity of the patient. No one material can satisfy all of these constraints, but studies have been carried out on a range of materials and so there is much information available to help the practitioner to arrive at the most suitable selection (Campbell et al 1984, Oakley & Pratt 1988, Pratt 1990). Compensation is used in cases where a limb has been shortened or where a part of the anatomy has been lost altogether. The loss is made up using additional material directly under the heel or on the outer sole. In cases of severe pain, load has to be taken off the foot by using devices such as patella-tendon-bearing ankle foot orthoses (AFOs) (McIlmurray & Greenbaum 1958). Detailed discussion of this type of device is outside the scope of this text, although AFOs are considered further in Chapter 12.

Accommodation

Accommodative orthoses primarily accommodate fixed deformities and are valuable in patients who are particularly 'at risk' from the effects of poor tissue viability (Janisse 1993). Casted orthoses are prescription orthoses prepared on positive moulds of the foot. They may conform to feet purely with the primary objective of moulding around lesions, offering compensation as well as redistribution from specific points affected by high load.

In conclusion, it should be noted that, sometimes, the therapeutic objectives outlined in Box 10.1 will overlap. For example, rest and immobilisation might well be by-products of redistribution, stabilisation or compensation.

The influence of the foot on the proximal skeletal structures, and vice versa, has been recognised as a significant component of gait. As such, this relationship must be assessed (Tollafield & Merriman 1995) and considered when taking the decision to use foot orthoses. No foot treatment should be considered without careful regard to proximal joint problems at the level of the knee, hip or back. The need to make adjustments must always be borne in mind, as the effect of torque forces will add to, rather than ameliorate, pathology.

MECHANICAL PRINCIPLES

In order for mechanical therapy to be effective, the practitioner will need to able to select materials from a large range of products. In this next section, we will consider properties of the foundation materials (Material Science) of some common products described in this book, which are also widely advertised in journals.

Basic physics

The effects of forces on an object are often poorly understood, and the foot is no exception. Suffice it to say that forces generated by activities such as walking or standing cause stresses and strains in the foot which need to be taken into account when designing orthoses. It is equally important to be aware of the stresses and strains generated in the materials designed to assist the foot, as this will affect their choice.

In order to understand the effects of forces and levers on the skeletal structure when considering orthotic function, familiarity with a number of physics and mechanics principles is required. Without this knowledge, and also an appreciation of the properties of materials used to produce an orthosis, mistakes are likely to be made when fitting and dispensing. Physical principles are used in the design of orthoses, and some practical examples are used here to illustrate some of the general points. A more detailed description can be found in Chapter 12.

Units

The SI system of units will be used throughout for all mechanical units. In everyday practice the principles of biomechanics are increasingly encountered. Before specific quantities and principles are described, it is worth mentioning that there are two types of quantity—*scalars* and *vectors*. Scalar quantities are those that need only a magnitude to describe them fully, such as temperature, whereas vectors comprise both a magnitude and a direction. Examples of vectors include force and velocity and these are discussed later. This difference in the way quantities are specified also means that the ways in which they are added together, i.e. vector addition and scalar addition, are different. These two methods of addition are described below.

Displacement, velocity and acceleration

If an object is moved from one position to another then it has been displaced. Hence, the distance it has moved is its displacement. In order to specify its new position, however, it is not sufficient to say that the displacement is 5 metres (m), because the direction in which it has been moved is also required (thus this term is a vector). The direction is usually referred to a set of three mutually orthogonal axes (x, y, z). This enables a complete description of the object's starting and finishing positions. The rate of change of displacement with time (t) is called velocity (v), and is measured in metres per second (m/s or m s^{-1}). It is sometimes written as ds/dt, which represents the change in s divided by the change in t. Velocity is therefore also a vector, since both the magnitude and direction of motion are required to describe how it is moving. Speed, on the other hand, is a scalar. When we say a car is moving at a speed of 30 mph, we do not need to specify the direction of motion; you *cannot* say that a car has a velocity of 30 mph unless you specify a direction—it is meaningless! The rate of change of velocity with time is called acceleration (a) and is measured in metres per second squared (m/s/s, m/s^2 or m s^{-2}). It is sometimes written as dv/dt. Again, this is a vector quantity.

Force

A force (F), measured in newtons (N), is defined as any action which produces, or tends to produce, acceleration of an object on which it acts. For example, if you push a wheelchair containing a patient, it will start to accelerate. Once moving, if there was no frictional force, it would continue to move at a uniform velocity until another force acted upon it. However, friction is present and therefore a small force input is required to keep the chair moving, although this is less than the initial force required to start the chair moving. If there was a heavier patient in the chair, the forces required to achieve the same velocity would be greater. The amount of matter that makes up an object, in this case the wheelchair and the patient, is called mass (m) with units of kilograms (kg). The force required to accelerate the wheelchair is given by

$$F = m \times a \ (N)$$

This too is a vector quantity, requiring both magnitude and direction to describe it fully. At this point, we should note that weight is also a force and that it is the product of the mass of an object and the gravitational acceleration (g). In order to define weight force fully, its point of application on the object has to be defined. This is called the centre of gravity and is, in effect, the same as centre of mass. It is the point at which the mass of the object may be considered as being concentrated.

As mentioned earlier, the addition of vectors is different from the addition of scalars. With scalars, the addition is simply the sum of the two numbers, but with vectors we need to use vector addition. This requires the use of vector diagrams.

Vector addition

Figure 10.6 shows two people pushing a bed, each with a different force (F^1 and F^2) and in a different direction. To find the total force acting on the bed and its direction of motion, we need to redraw the diagram as shown in Figure 10.7. Here the two forces are represented by arrows. The length of each indicates the magnitude of the force, and the angle indicates the direction, or line of action. The lines are drawn parallel to their actual positions. F^2 follows from the end of F^1 and, if there were more forces

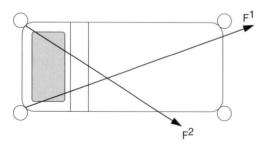

Figure 10.6   Diagram of two people pushing a bed with forces F^1 and F^2.

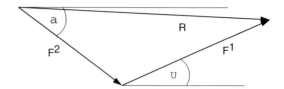

Figure 10.7   The principle of adding two forces, F^1 and F^2, vectorially to give a single resultant force.

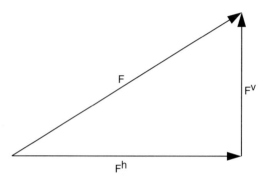

Figure 10.8   Resolution of the force F into two components, F^v vertically and F^h horizontally.

involved, they could be added to the end of the last arrow in any sequence. This results in a line of arrows with a start and a finish. The sum effect of all the forces is found by joining the two free ends with a new arrow to give a new force (R). The length denotes its magnitude and the angle gives its direction. This new force is called the resultant force.

This process is often used in reverse to produce two forces acting along specific axes from a single one. This may seem like a pointless activity, but it is helpful when adding the effects of forces. This is called 'resolution of forces' and Figure 10.8 shows how this is done. The force F has been resolved into two component forces, F^v vertically and F^h horizontally. These component forces are given in terms of the original force by

$$F^h = F \cos \theta \ (N)$$
$$F^v = F \sin \theta \ (N)$$

Resolving forces is very useful; vertical and horizontal component forces can be simply added. These two final components can be added vectorially, as described above, to give the overall effect of all the forces; this simplifies the mathematics considerably.

Moments of force

The moment of any force about a point is the product

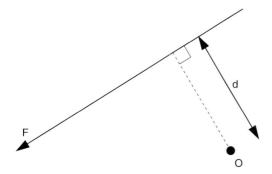

Figure 10.9 The moment of the force F about point O is related to the perpendicular distance between the line of action of F and O.

of the magnitude of the force and the perpendicular distance between the point and the line of action of the force (the moment arm). Thus, in Figure 10.9, the moment of F, measured in newton metres (Nm), is given by

Moment = F × d (Nm)

Moments can be used to find muscle and joint forces when used in conjunction with the concept of equilibrium. This concept states that when an object is at rest or moving with a uniform velocity, it is in equilibrium. Thus, in this state, the net sum of all the forces and their moments about any point must be equal to zero.

Figure 10.10 shows a highly simplified schematic

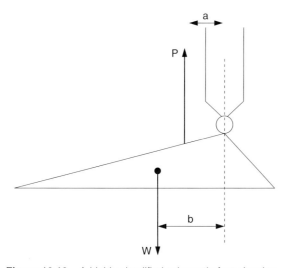

Figure 10.10 A highly simplified schematic foot showing the forces in the muscle (P) and that due to the weight of the foot (W) in equilibrium. To balance the plantarflexion moment of W × b, the muscle needs to apply a dorsiflexion moment of P × a.

foot being held at 90° to the tibia by the action of the muscle force (P). In this simplified case, the muscle force is only required to resist the weight of the foot (W). Both of these forces are assumed to act vertically at distances a and b, respectively, from the point of rotation (the ankle joint centre). As this foot is at rest, it is in equilibrium, and hence all the forces and moments are equal. So we have a basic equation, Pa = Wb. If W can be measured, or calculated, and a and b are measured, then P can be found from P = Wb/a. In fact, in this case, as there are no other forces, one could simply say that W = P. In reality, however, the picture is more complicated than this, with many more forces acting at varying angles to each other in all three planes. In these circumstances, both force resolution and equilibration of moments are needed.

Pressure

Pressure and force should not be confused. They are different, although they are related by a single quantity—area. Pressure, measured in newtons per square metre (N/m^2) or pascals (Pa), is the force per unit area (F/A). So, if a force of, say, 100 N acts on two surfaces, one with an area of 10 square metres and the other with an area of 20 square metres, the pressures will be 10 Pa (100/10) and 5 Pa (100/20), respectively. Thus, the pressure resulting from a force can be reduced by increasing the area over which it is applied. (Note: in many medical texts, millimetres of mercury (mmHg) are used as units for pressure; 1 mmHg = 133.322 Pa).

Whilst it may seem of little practical value to know about force, it does have some very practical applications. For example, orthoses function by applying forces to the body as a way of influencing the skeletal structure. The interface between the orthosis and the skin needs to be protected from forces which could damage the skin (Pratt 1994), and a few simple rules based on the above are invaluable.

The way in which the imposed force is distributed throughout the material is called stress. Stress (σ) is the force (F) divided by the cross-sectional area of the object at the point of interest (A). (Note—stress has the same units as pressure). Stress is thus given by

σ = F/A (Pa)

There are three types of stress—tensile, compressive and shear—usually acting together at any point in an object (Fig. 10.11).

Strain arises when a force is applied to any structure, whether it be an organic or inorganic material.

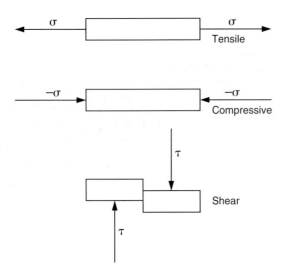

Figure 10.11 The three types of stress: tensile, compressive and shear.

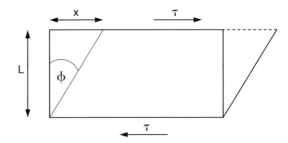

Figure 10.12 The effect of shear force on a rectangular object.

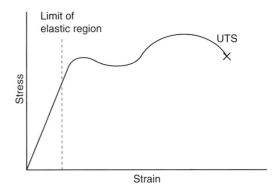

Figure 10.13 A typical stress–strain curve showing the limit of elasticity and the ultimate tensile strength (UTS).

Strain is related to compression or tension and has no units as it is the ratio of the change in length to the original length. Pathology may well arise when there is no recovery in the length (of, for example, a ligament) after a force has been applied. Body tissues such as ligaments and tendons normally provide an element of recovery in length once the force (stress) applied has ceased. In the case of Davis's law, mentioned earlier, treatment may include the maintenance of externally applied stress to bring about a permanent change in length.

Compressive or tensile strain (ε) is given by

ε = change in length/original length

i.e.

$$\varepsilon = \delta l / l$$

Another quantity of interest is shear stress (τ). This type of stress is more complicated to define but Figure 10.12 shows its effect on an object where it causes the material to deform by a distance x on one surface, corresponding to an angular deformation ϕ. This angular deformation is called the shear strain (measured in radians) and is given by

$$\phi = x / L$$

The ratio of the shear stress to shear strain is called the modulus of rigidity (G) and is measured in N/m. Thus

$$G = \tau / \phi$$

If a piece of inorganic material such as metal is

stressed, the strain increases linearly up to a point called the elastic limit (Fig. 10.13). If the stress is removed at any point up to this limit, the material will return to its original length. The slope of the line up to this limit is called the modulus of elasticity, or Young's modulus (E), and is a measure of the stiffness of a material. It is thus defined as

$$E = \sigma / \varepsilon$$

Young's modulus has the same units as stress (N/m^2). After the elastic limit has been reached, the relationship between stress and strain is no longer linear and the material enters a plastic region where permanent deformation takes place. At some point the material will fail, usually at a point lower than its maximum strength, which is called its ultimate tensile strength (UTS).

Ductility and *brittleness* are terms that are often used to describe the performance of materials. A ductile material has the ability to demonstrate 'plasticity' over very large increases in stress before failing, whereas a brittle material undergoes little or no plastic deformation. In general, ductile materials are tougher, i.e. they are more able to withstand impact loads. Toughness is a measure of the energy needed to fracture a piece of material, and this is a function of ductility. Thus, ductile materials are more suitable for use in orthotics or prosthetics, as their impending failure is signalled by the plastic deformation taking place. A brittle failure gives no advance warning and as such can be dangerous for someone who is relying on the support that the device is providing. Furthermore, brittle materials that fracture sometimes leave sharp fragments which can lacerate the skin, e.g. unmodified plastics. Certain types of plastics, e.g. polythenes, are ductile and offer the ideal properties for many orthoses. The material will allow some structural change or 'give' without losing its shape. The resilience of plastic, while offering such ideal physical properties, will inevitably vary between products due to the different polymeric structures used with chemical production techniques.

Let us now consider how these aspects of materials and mechanics can be used to establish principles that are useful for orthotic management and material selection. The subject of *orthopaedic biomechanics* is extensive and the detail is beyond the scope of this book. The interested reader is directed to the section on further reading.

MATERIAL PROPERTIES

There is a constant influx of new materials onto the market, and the large number of materials to choose from can easily confuse the practitioner. While it is unnecessary for the practitioner to acquire the same knowledge as a chemist, a working knowledge of some of the newer technologies can help to differentiate those materials ideally suited to the situation at hand from those that are not. A keen practitioner who fails to be well informed will experience personal disappointment and patient dissatisfaction.

Foundation materials

Basic chemistry

Many of the materials used today are plastics, and these can be broadly divided into two categories, *thermoplastic* and *thermosetting*. The first of these, the thermoplastics, which include common plastics such as polystyrene, polyvinylchloride (PVC) and polyethylene, are materials which can be softened by heating, formed into a new shape and then allowed to harden by cooling. This process of softening and hardening can be repeated many times with no degradation to the plastic. Thermosetting materials, on the other hand, first soften on heating and then, with

further heating, set hard and cannot be altered again by heating. An example of this is the old 'Bakelite' type of plastic used for door handles and old radio cabinets. These different behaviours are a result of chemical differences.

Plastics are materials with long chains of molecules called polymer chains. In thermoplastic materials, these long molecules are separate from each other. In thermosetting materials, heating or chemical reaction causes strong chemical links between chains to be formed (cross-links), thus linking them firmly together.

The term polymer has been used above and it is worthwhile describing the polymer molecule. Much of chemistry is concerned with molecules of between 2 and 50 atoms which exist as solids, liquids and gases. However, there are many molecules which cannot be classified conveniently into these three types: fibres such as wool or nylon, thermoplastics which soften on heating to form thick viscous fluids instead of mobile liquids, and rubbers.

All these substances consist of collections of large polymeric molecules joined together. The polyethylene (often called polythene) molecule, for example, has typically 1000 (CH_2CH_2) units linked end to end. The bulk thermoplastic has thousands of these chains packed together, sometimes regularly, sometimes tangled.

There is no precise point at which a line can be drawn between large and small molecules, but a molecule may be considered as large when it gives rise to substances which possess resinous, rubbery or fibre-like properties.

There are two basic chemical reactions by which long chain molecules are formed: condensation and addition polymerisation.

Condensation polymerisation. In this process a small molecule (usually water, ammonia or hydrochloric acid) is eliminated when an organic base, e.g. ethyl alcohol, condenses with an organic acid like acetic acid. Thus

$$C_2H_5.OH + CH_3COOH = C_2H_5.O.CO.CH_3 + H_2O$$

If the base possesses two hydroxyl groups (OH) and the acid possesses two carboxyl groups (COOH), condensation produces an ester with a basic and an acidic group which can condense further with another ester molecule. An example of this is polyethylene terephthalate (PET or Terylene):

$$HOOC.C_6H_4.COOH + HO.CH_2CH_2.OH =$$
$$HOOC.C_6H_4.CO.O.CH_2CH_2.OH +$$
terephthalic   ethylene H_2O
acid   glycol   +
$$HOOC.C_6H_4.CO.O.CH_2CH_2.OH$$

$HOOC.C_6H_4.CO.O.CH_2CH_2.O.CO.C_6H_4.CO.O.CH_2.$
$CH_2.OH + H_2O$
diester

Further condensation produces the general form

$H(O.OC.C_6H_4.CO.O.CH_2CH_2)nOH + nH_2O$
polyester (Terylene)

The nylons are another product of this type of reaction.

Addition polymerisation. Usually this form of polymerisation involves carbon–carbon double bonds. This process occurs in three steps:

1. Initiation

$IN^* + C_2H_4 \rightarrow IN.CH_2CH_2^*$

The initiator (IN^*) may be an ion, resulting in ionic polymerisation, or a free radical, resulting in a radical polymerisation.

2. Propagation

$IN.CH_2CH_2^* + C_2H_4 \rightarrow IN.CH_2CH_2CH_2CH_2^*$
$IN.CH_2CH_2CH_2CH_2^* + C_2H_4 \rightarrow$
$IN.CH_2CH_2CH_2CH_2CH_2CH_2^*$ etc.....

The chain grows rapidly with the evolution of heat until a termination stage is reached.

3. Termination. This involves the loss of a proton from the chain end:

$IN.(CH_2)nCH_2CH_2^+ \rightarrow IN.(CH_2)nCH = CH_2^+ H^+$
(solvated)

In polyethylene, n is of the order of 1000. Examples of this type of plastic are polyvinyl chloride, polypropylene and polystyrene.

The repeating unit of a polymer (a monomer) can be either a straight chain molecule (aliphatic) or in the form of rings (aromatic). The aliphatic molecules have three divisions based upon the nature of the hydrocarbon bonds. Alkanes have a single bond, e.g.

$$
\begin{array}{ccc}
 & H & H \\
 & | & | \\
H - & C - & C - H \quad \text{(ethane)} \\
 & | & | \\
 & H & H
\end{array}
$$

Alkenes have unsaturated hydrocarbon bonds in the form

$$
\begin{array}{cc}
H & H \\
| & | \\
C = & C \quad \text{(ethylene)} \\
| & | \\
H & H
\end{array}
$$

Alkynes have even more unsaturated bonds, such as

$$H - C \equiv C - H \quad \text{(ethyne)}$$

Monomers can be combined either as the same unit repeated (a homopolymer) or using different units (a copolymer), and the chains can be linear or branched and may be cross-linked.

Having outlined some of the structural and chemical principles on polymers, some of the many different types of polymer can now be described and their uses in mechanical therapy presented. It is not the intention here to list all possible polymers, as only those of value to mechanical therapy are relevant.

Polycarbonates

A polycarbonate is a thermoplastic polymer with linear polyesters of a carbonic acid with diphenylpropanol. Carbonic chloride is reacted with these with pyridine to form the polymer sheet. Polycarbonates are hygroscopic, i.e. they absorb water into the chemical structure. Before heat processing they need to be thoroughly dried out, otherwise water bubbles form in the bulk of the material, causing a loss of mechanical strength. This drying takes about 24 hours at an elevated temperature which is below the material's moulding temperature. Polycarbonates can be used for manufacturing orthotic plates (the basic shell vacuformed around a cast). During heat processing, care must be taken because overheating can result in the release of benzene gas, which is hazardous. Polycarbonates provide a high strength, but they are expensive and are therefore not often used in foot orthoses.

Polyvinyl chloride (PVC)

PVC is a thermoplastic polymer to which plasticisers may be added. These are materials that improve the elasticity of the polymer. They are used in sheet form to make rigid foot orthoses, although they are valuable as a cover material with or without a foam backing. PVC can be modified by adding cross-linkages and co-polymerised to form an impact-modified PVC. If overheated, it also gives off benzene, phthalic anhydride and hydrogen chloride, all of which are hazardous.

The general form of PVC is

$$
\left[CH_2 - \underset{\underset{Cl}{|}}{CH} \right]_n
$$

Trade names are Pacton and Darvic (ICI Plastics).

Polyethylene (polythene)

This plastic is a thermoplastic polymer formed by addition polymerisation. The properties that are most suitable for orthoses are found in the high molecular weight versions of polyethylene. These materials are ideal for use in semi-rigid (SR) orthoses, which have some flexibility while still possessing the controlling, non-deforming properties offered by acrylic, polycarbonate, polyester and high-impact PVC (trade name, ICI), materials used in rigid orthoses.

The general form is

$$\left[CH = CH \right]_n$$

The main advantage offered by this material is that there are few real dangers in the heat processing stages, although acrid fumes are produced if it burns. Trade names are Ortholen and sub-Ortholen (Teufel).

This material can be foamed to produce closed cell foams. Foamed materials provide a matrix of individual bubbles or cells unconnected to their neighbours. In the foam form, it is used as a soft padding for insoles or, in the more rigid foam formulations, as a very light raise to compensate for leg length discrepancy. It does, however, suffer badly from compression set. This is when permanent collapse of the foam occurs under repeated loading (Pratt 1990). The trade names of this foamed version are Plastazote (BXL) and Evazote (BP Plastics).

Polypropylene

This is the most commonly used plastic for orthoses, being suitable for UCBL (University of California biomechanics laboratory) orthoses and AFOs (ankle foot orthoses), as well as many other bespoke (made-to-measure) applications.

Polypropylene is a thermoplastic polymer made by addition and has many isomeric forms (an isomer is a different structural arrangement of the same monomeric units, often with very different physical and chemical properties). The general form of this polymer is

$$\left[CH_2 - CH \atop | \atop CH_3 \right]_n$$

The three isomeric forms of significance are the isotactic, syndiotactic and atactic forms, which relate to the arrangement of the CH groups on the helical polymer chain. If all of these are on the same side of the chain, the isotactic isomer is formed, whereas if they alternate between sides then the isomer is in the syndiotactic form. The atactic form is more random, with areas where the groups are on the same side followed by alternating sections. This form is also non-crystalline and has a low softening temperature and poor mechanical properties.

Because of the excellent moulding properties of polypropylene and its resistance to mechanical failure, it is widely used in orthotics. It is found either as a homopolymer, which is comparatively brittle, or as a copolymer, the latter being the material of choice.

Dangers during processing include the release of toxic fumes if overheated, with a great deal of black smoke.

The trade name is Propylex (Courtalds).

Polymethyl methacrylate (PMMA)

This has both thermoplastic and thermosetting polymerplastic properties, depending upon the form in which it is used. PMMA has been modified by cross-linkages and copolymerisation to give improved mechanical properties in the sheet form, and is very useful for rigid foot orthoses. It is available in a variety of thicknesses and colours.

The general form of this polymer is

$$\left[CH_2 - \overset{\displaystyle CH_3}{\underset{\displaystyle \underset{\displaystyle OCH_3}{C = O}}{\overset{|}{\underset{|}{C}}}} \right]_n$$

In powder form, when mixed with a polymerising agent, PMMA is used to form rigid posts in functional foot orthoses. It is also sold as dental acrylic for the repair of dentures. In this form the material has thermosetting properties.

The trade names are Perspex (ICI) as unmodified sheet, Novaplast (Kraemer) as modified sheet, and Orthoresin (DeTrey) as a powder for posting orthoses.

The dangers of using this product depend upon the form being processed. If it is overheated during processing, small quantities of cyanide fumes can be released. In the two-part system the liquid is very flammable, with a flash point of only 13°C. In recent years, the form known as Rohadur or Plexidur O has been withdrawn from production for environmental reasons.

Polyurethane

Polyurethanes have a complex structure and tend to

be mixtures of crystalline and non-crystalline polymers that phase separately. There are two different types—polyether urethanes and polyester urethanes. They are all characterised by the urethane linkage (–NH–CO.O–) and exist in many forms too numerous to list here.

These polymers can be produced in sheets or as foam. The sheets are dense polymers which can be used to replace the loss of shock attenuation in the foot. However, many of these shock-attenuating properties can be found in polyurethane foam, which is produced by adding water during production. This produces carbon dioxide and hence foaming (Pratt 1988).

Trade names for the sheet form are Viscolas (Cabot) and Sorbothane (IEM Orthopaedics), while those for the foamed product are PPT (Langer Biomechanics), Poron (Rogers Corporation) and Cleron (Seaton and Price).

The dangers associated with use of this material depend upon how it is supplied. If supplied as a sheet, there are no specific dangers unless the product is burned. If supplied as two parts of the foam product to be mixed in situ, the liquid methylene di-isocyanate can be a respiratory irritant.

Silicones (siloxanes)

These are thermosetting inorganic polymers with rubber-like properties. They are formed by a condensation reaction to give a polymer of the general form

$$HO \left[\begin{array}{c} R \\ | \\ Si - O \\ | \\ R \end{array} \right]_n H$$

(where R is any of a range of organic groups).

Silicones can be produced in a gum form (e.g. bathroom sealants) and can then be used to make insoles (Pratt et al 1984). However, the preservative agent, acetic acid, makes this form rather noxious to use. In addition, silicones can be used in a two-part mix—gum with catalyst—to form protectors for the digits in situ. These can be used, for example, to protect toes from high pressures (Whitney & Whitney 1990). There are many silicone gums available and, combined with a catalyst as a paste or liquid, they will cure quickly (within 2 minutes), allowing the practitioner to dispense the plastic orthodigital device during the consultation. Otoform, a silicone introduced originally for hearing aid impressions, has remained popular for over a decade. Further applications of this substance are discussed in Chapter 11.

Trade names are Podiaform (Footman), Otoform (Dreve), Verone and KE20.

Table 10.1 outlines the comparative properties of most of the commonly used polymers in orthotic manufacture, together with some other potentially useful products. For full details of the dangers of processing plastics, the reader is referred to a publication by the Health and Safety Executive (1990). Practitioners directing or carrying out any form of manufacture with plastics must be aware of all the necessary safety precautions concerning respiration, and eye and ear protection, as well as ensuring that reasonable safety and guard protection are applied to moving parts.

Composite materials

A group of materials comprising both a plastic matrix and a reinforcing fibre are emerging as a useful addition to the field of orthotic application (Bader 1993). There are certain products on the market, based

Table 10.1 The comparative properties of most of the commonly used polymers in orthotic manufacture

Polymer	Density (Kg/m^3)	Yield stress (MPa)	Modulus (GPa)	Impact strength (J/m)	Fatigue stress (MPa)	Maximum service temperature (°C)	Coefficient of friction	Relative flammability
Polycarbonate	1200	60	2.5	700	7	120	0.2	26
Polyvinyl chloride	1500	45	2.5	300	15	70	0.4	45
Polyethylene (Low density)	930	12	0.3	–	15	70	0.6	17
Polyethylene (High density)	960	27	0.7	800	15	80	0.25	17
Polypropylene	1120	85	5.0	100	20	110	–	16
Polymethylmethacrylate	–	150	12.0	–	–	200	–	16
Polyurethane								
Moulded	1100	22	0.3	–	–	120	–	–
Foamed	500	15	–	–	–	90	–	–

on carbon fibre, that are used primarily for selective strengthening of orthoses; these are moulded at the same time as the main plastic (Compcore, Becker Orthopaedic). Composite materials which offer a superior strength-to-weight ratio compared with conventional polymers (TL2100, Medical Materials Corp) are also available for the production of rigid foot orthoses. The dangers of these materials are those associated with the matrix plastic, as outlined above, as well as those associated with the the reinforcing fibre. The latter dangers are chiefly related to the production of small particles of fine fibres during the finishing process which can act as respiratory irritants. As yet, carbonised orthoses are still in their infancy, although they are gaining in popularity.

Impression materials

Casting materials are important for taking impressions and replicating models from the foot and lower leg with varying degrees of accuracy. Further details of how these impressions are referred to professional laboratories, with a specific prescription format, will be provided in Chapter 12. The end product of this procedure is a bespoke orthosis. A number of these casting materials also play a role in limiting motion or acting to redistribute load from a central area of pathology, such as an ulcer. In this respect, casting has two main functions: impression taking and therapeutic function.

Traditionally, casts were made of Plaster of Paris (calcium sulphate dihydrate). This material, while still useful, has been superseded for therapeutic use by mixtures of polymers, including composites, often used together with inorganic compounds. As this field is changing rapidly, it is only sensible to outline the general properties and leave specifics to the current journal publications.

Several studies have been carried out on these new materials, with a view to providing comparative data on their performance. Despite the number of newer materials, Plaster of Paris is still used for many orthotic impressions, because it rapidly sets to give a good pattern of the limb segment, is easily moulded around the limb, and is still cheap. Furthermore, many of the newer products offer improved mechanical performance but are much more expensive and less easily conformable. These latter problems are still being tackled by the producers. Rowley & Pratt (1986) examined most of the products available at that time and produced a comparative table (Table 10.2).

Alginates were originally used for taking dental impressions. This rubbery material is based upon alginic acid extracted from brown seaweed. Alginic acid comprises two stereoisomers, guluronic acid and mannuronic acid, and forms the basis of alginate. When combined, in powder form, with water, alginate creates cross-linking to produce insoluble calcium alginate from sodium alginate and calcium ions. The process of cross-linking is common to many thermosets, including polyurethane and polyester casts which form by the same principle, whereby a soft material cures to a state in which it has greater strength.

Clinical materials

Many materials originally used for treating foot complaints have now been replaced by plastic products. There is little value in describing all the potential products, as new materials are introduced frequently and can be found in many journals that carry advertisements. Therapeutic selection will be better assisted with some fundamental knowledge of the types of material suited to foot management. Materials such as felt, foam rubber and strapping will be adhered to the foot or combined with ready-made products. Chiropody treatment was founded on such materials, but many have become obscured by the advent

Table 10.2 Comparison of casting materials available in 1986 (Rowley & Pratt 1986)

Casting material	Density (Kg/m^3)	Yield strength (MPa)	Flexural modulus (GPa)	Fatigue life cycles	X-ray absorption coefficient (mm^{-1})	Exotherm (°C)
Gypsona	740–810	1.53–2.62	0.642–0.828	13	0.18	27
Cellona	–	2.87	1.11	15	0.17	–
Zoroc	920	3.14	0.840	70	0.19	28
Crystona	950	1.36	0.227	60	0.13	29.3
Scotchcast	680	39.97	0.340	24 200	0.08	26.8
Scotchflex	380	13.70	0.133	18 500	0.05	25.3
Baycast +	410	7.86	0.660	3200	0.01	25.6
Dynacast	–	36.30	0.690	30 000	0.07	–
Hexcelite	490	3.76	0.031–0.066	39 700	0.02	35–38

of easily dispensed, ready-made pads and insoles. It is incumbent on the modern practitioner to make the appropriate selection of these useful adhesive products, particularly for short-term use.

Foot padding materials

Strapping and tapes are used in a variety of ways, either to limit motion or to allow adherence of dressings to the foot (Ch. 11).

Felt. This is made up by layering wool, compressing and steaming it under rollers. Because felt is expensive, mixtures of synthetic material such as nylon reduce the wool content. Unfortunately, the market has been flooded with low durometer, high synthetic content materials, which are not of the same quality as wool felts. In this respect, over-the-counter products, while expensive, have less resilient properties than felt purchased from main supply houses. It is common practice to describe felt as compressed or semi-compressed, although a durometer or hardness measurement, usually between 9 and 65 on a scale 0–100, is sometimes specified. Recent changes in the UK market have affected the quality of felt.

Rubber. This product has many applications in treating the foot. Rubber latex sheeting can be used for toe and tarsal loops as replaceable padding. An older but still occasionally practised technique uses liquid latex that cures as it dries. This is preserved in ammonia. Hallux and digital shields can be made by immersing plaster models of toes in dipping latex. Padding in foam latex is sandwiched between layers of dipping latex. Natural rubbers may be combined with synthetic rubbers to achieve the same physical properties as the original rubber, while offering greater shear strength; for example, isobutene and isoprene are combined to produce butyl rubber. A very common rubber is neoprene (2-chlorobutadiene, Du Pont), which is synthetic.

Spenco is still one of the most widely used of synthetic rubbers (a neoprene). It is used for insoles and foam pads. Rubbers are also mixed with plastics, such as styrene butadiene rubber (SBR). These synthetic rubbers are less likely to perish with age, but do not have the softness needed for clinical application. They can be used in compound manufacture, where a mixture of different products are selected for their combined physical properties. Ethyl vinyl acetate (EVA), used in running shoes, is very popular as a wedging material or as a whole orthosis.

Foams have been discussed earlier as being produced by a chemical process that causes plastics to expand. Rubber latex (natural isoprene rubber) is useful, although granular in nature, as a foam. When covered with a fabric, the material is less compressible and is remarkably long-lasting.

PVC foams may be available as strips, very similar to tapes on a roll. They can be adhered over joints to prevent shear forces creating blisters. Fleece web and moleskin, not surprisingly, do not arise from either sheep or moles. Both are thin synthetic materials and are indicated for patients whose shoes cannot accommodate thicker materials. Fleece web has greater elasticity than moleskin, but only in one direction. Both are covering materials and are useful for binding foams together or for binding foams onto card insocks as a temporary measure. Fleece web can tether the epidermis down, preventing deep shear stress or surface friction using the feature of one-directional stretch. Any form of tensionable strapping will offer varying degrees of therapeutic immobilisation.

Adhesives

Felts and foams adhered to the foot tend to be affected by water and salts associated with sweat. Adhered materials were formerly made from a thin rubber backing on the desired material. Natural rubber made up the main base and was mixed with a resin known as colophony or one from a synthesised hydrocarbon. Plasticisers, such as lanolin or liquid paraffin, were added for flexibility. A filler, usually zinc oxide (ZO), was used to give the backing strength. This type of skin tactifier is no longer used, because, whether it was used for strapping or for padding to the sole of the foot or toes, it would store poorly, become brittle and lose its stickiness, causing the padding to be less resilient. Clinically, many patients were recorded as having a ZO allergy. In fact, the zinc oxide was rarely the allergen, the cause of the problem usually being the rubber or other preservatives. Many shoe components still create the same problems because of the wide use of rubber products and preservatives, dyes and allergenic linings.

Hypoallergenic taping

A wide range of low allergy tapes are now available. The adhesives are made from methylmethacrylate as a polymerised monomer, or from other plastics such as polythene and PVC. The adhesives themselves are water-based or solvent-based (Micropore, 3M).

Apart from the fact that hypoallergenic tapes have a greater tolerance, the acrylic adhesives are light and can be applied very thinly, resulting in thinner tapes which are more easily accommodated in shoewear than ZO-based tapes. These tapes are primarily used for binding dressings and the aforementioned range of padded dressings to the foot. However, hypoallergenic tapes are generally less suitable for strapping injuries and preventing motion around joints because they are light in composition and offer less strength. This problem has been addressed in newer products, which have elastic properties and offer an alternative to ZO tapes. ZO tapes deteriorate much more quickly in storage and have less water resistance when applied to the skin surface. Modern tapes are dispensed on a roll or with a peelable backing to the desired length. The wide availability of plastic polymers means that the practitioner has an ever-increasing range of adhesives to choose from.

Cement is a broad term often used interchangeably with the term adhesive. Both are synthetic chemicals based on hydrocarbons. Glue, on the other hand, has its roots in animal by-products such as bone and hooves.

When manufacturing orthoses, the adhesive needs to run freely to prevent hard lumps forming. The appropriate viscosity should be selected. The drying rate will be influenced by the rate at which the solvent evaporates. 'Tack life' is a term used to describe the period of time after application during which there is still a possibility of making a good bond. The 'green strength' is the strength of the adhesive after making the bond. Again, given the range of materials now available, it is not good enough to rely on one adhesive for bonding all products.

The manufacturer's information must be followed to ensure that the material being used is bonded with the most appropriate adhesive. The effects of shear force upon materials, mentioned at the beginning of this chapter, can be observed in weak bonds, when the adhesive might behave in a brittle manner. Adhesives have to resist multidirectional forces, as well as the effects of varying pH within sweat.

Neoprenes (polychloroprene), polyurethane, epoxy resins and rubber solutions are four groups of adhesive that are used in different situations. *Primers* are often recommended for improving the bonding ability of adhesives. They have the effect of softening the surface, making the adhesive easier to attach, particularly to an asperitous surface. Some adhesives respond to reheating, allowing surfaces to rebond after being separated. This is known as reactivation.

Cohesive bonding

This is possible with materials such as polymethylmethacrylate (PMMA) and polyethylenes. This action occurs when similar molecules are bonded together. PMMA bonds as a resin, while polyethylene is heated so that the chains of molecules can recombine together, forming a very strong bond indeed. Plastic welding rods are available to enhance this process, as well as filling in any gaps between the parent material and the additional material being combined.

Safety

Adhesives are inflammable, and health and safety aspects are paramount in regard to their storage and fire prevention. Solvents can cause respiratory difficulties and depress the central nervous system, causing drowsiness. Good air circulation and venting is essential.

SUMMARY

In this chapter a wide range of principles has been covered, highlighting the types of problems likely to influence the effectiveness of orthoses.

Modern materials have the advantage of being light-weight while still offering strong mechanical properties, but even these have difficulty in overcoming the triplanar effects of movement of the body over the foot. Successful management with orthoses depends upon a healthy marriage between shoes, the type of orthosis prescribed and the patient's ultimate requirements.

REFERENCES

Bader D L 1993 The potential of advanced composites in orthotic applications. Journal of Orthotics and Prosthetics 1: 33–41

Brown R N, Byers-Hinkley K, Logan L 1987 The talus control ankle foot orthosis. Orthotics & Prosthetics 41: 22–31

Burnstein A H, Wright T M 1994 Fundamentals of orthopaedic biomechanics. Williams & Wilkins, Baltimore, p 200

Campbell G J, McLure A, Newell E N 1984 Compressive behaviour after simulated service conditions of some foamed materials intended as orthotic insoles. Journal of Rehabilitation Research and Development 21: 57–65

Collins J J, Whittle M W 1989 Impulsive forces during walking and their clinical implications. Clinical Biomechanics 4: 179–187

Health and Safety Executive 1990 The application of COSHH to plastics processing. HMSO, London

Janisse D J 1993 A scientific approach to insole design for the diabetic foot. The Foot 3: 105–108

McIllmurray W J, Greenbaum W 1958 A below-knee weight-bearing brace. Orthotics and Prosthetics Journal 12: 81–82

Oakley T, Pratt D J 1988 Skeletal transients during heel and toe strike running and the effectiveness of some materials in their attenuation. Clinical Biomechanics 3: 159–165

Pratt D J 1988 Polyurethanes in orthotics and orthopaedics. Cellular Polymers 7: 151–164

Pratt D J 1990 Long term comparison of some shock attenuating insoles. Prosthetics and Orthotics International 12: 59–62

Pratt D J 1994 Some aspects of modern orthotics. Physiological Measurement 15: 1–27

Pratt D J, Rees P H, Butterworth R H 1984 RTV silicone insoles. Prosthetics and Orthotics International 8: 54–55

Pratt D J, Tollafield D R, Johnson G R, Peacock C 1993 Foot orthosis. In: Bowker P M, Condie D N, Bader D L, Pratt D J (eds) Biomechanical basic for orthoses. Butterworths, London, p 72–98

Rowley D I, Pratt D J 1986 Orthopaedic bandage form splinting materials. Clinical Materials 1:1–8

Tollafield D R, Merriman L M 1995 Assessment of the locomotor system. In: Merriman L M, Tollafield D R (eds) Assessment of the lower limb. Churchill Livingstone, Edinburgh, p 146–147

Whitney A K, Whitney K A 1990 Padding and taping therapy. In: Levy L A, Hetherington V J (eds) Principles and practice of podiatric medicine. Churchill Livingstone, Edinburgh, ch 28

FURTHER READING

Bates B T, Osternig L R, Mason B et al 1979 Foot orthotic devices to modify selected aspects of lower extremity mechanics. American Journal of Sports Medicine 7: 338–342

Bowker P 1993 An update in essential mechanics. In: Bowker P, Bader D L, Pratt D J, Condie D N, Wallace W A (eds) The biomechanical basis of orthotic management. Butterworth Heinemann, Oxford, ch 2

Radin E L, Rose R M, Blaha J D, Litsky A S 1992 Practical biomechanics for the orthopaedic surgeon, 2nd edn.

Churchill Livingstone, New York

Robins R H C 1959 The ankle joint in relation to arthrodesis of the foot in poliomyelitis. Journal of Bone and Joint Surgery 41B: 337–341

Tollafield D R 1985 Mechanical therapeutic coursework, Nene College

Wright D G, Desai S M, Henderson W H 1964 Action of the subtalar and ankle joint complex during the stance phase of gait. Journal of Bone and Joint Surgery 46A: 361–382

11

Mechanical therapeutics in the clinic

R. Goslin
D. R. Tollafield
K. Rome

INTRODUCTION

This chapter concerns foot problems that can be managed either wholly or in part by orthotic control at the time of consultation. Broadly, the philosophy of orthotic care provision is that a programme of temporary management be followed until a 'stock' or 'prescription orthosis' is considered more appropriate. The term 'stock' is used in this chapter to refer to ready-prepared orthoses. These are often pre-packaged, such as Frelon, AOL and Tuli heel cups, and many are now available over the pharmacy counter.

There are certain criteria which should be considered when deciding whether to use mechanical therapy, and these have been summarised in Box 11.1. Alongside the use of orthoses, there is also a role to be played by dressings and other more substantial materials, and this role is discussed below. These materials can provide considerable mechanical therapeutic benefit, even though traditionally they are not considered to be orthoses themselves.

Mechanical therapy can be provided without laboratory prescription in one of five ways:

- dressings and bandages
- clinical padded dressings
- limiting foot and ankle movement
- replaceable orthoses
- moulded thermosetting and thermoplastic orthoses.

Each of these five will be discussed in turn, and for each technique, the function and method of application will be considered, highlighting its advantages and disadvantages.

The main objective of mechanical therapy is to resolve a problem as quickly as possible using physics and material science as the bases of treatment. Most orthotic management, whether it uses a simple dressing or a manufactured prescription (Ch. 12), is carried

Box 11.1 Criteria used in considering mechanical therapy

- *Will the patient benefit from mechanical therapy?*
  Is mechanical therapy likely to succeed for the condition being treated, e.g. skin lesions versus joint lesions?

- *Will adjunctive therapy be required?*
  Success may be improved by implementing more than one therapy; e.g. heel pain—use of heat, NSAIDs, injectable steroid and a combination of mechanical modalities

- *What is the prognosis from applying such therapy?*
  e.g. will a fixed toe deformity be corrected or interdigital neuroma be relieved by orthoses rather than surgery?

- *What is the patient's expectation?*
  Does the patient understand what an orthosis is and what it can achieve? Does the patient realise the limitations imposed by orthoses used in more than one pair of shoes?

- *Is the patient's footwear suitable?*
  Can the patient fit the ideal orthosis into a shoe—if not, will successful treatment be thwarted and the patient become frustrated or even feel cheated?

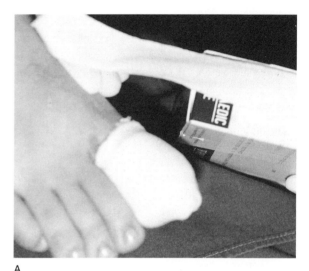

A

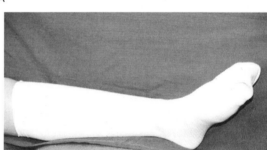

B

Figure 11.1 Examples of tubular dressings which offer the advantage of easy application during consultation (applicator not shown). A: Tubegauz 12. B: Tubigrip E.

out with the aim of achieving one or more of the objectives described previously in Box 10.1.

DRESSINGS AND BANDAGES

Over the last 20 years, there has been a considerable increase in the number of dressing materials available on the market, and to discuss all of them in detail would fill a chapter all by itself. Besides, all too frequently information such as this rapidly becomes out of date. However, the practitioner should be aware of the main products on offer.

It is worth mentioning the simple tubular bandage, however, which has revolutionised the speed at which dressings can be applied to digits, and which offers much greater security to the digit than previous methods (Fig. 11.1A). Gauze and adhesive dressings (formerly 'Bandaids' and 'sticky plasters') have also simplified the approach to dressing wounds.

In addition to the improvement in dressing materials, there have been a number of accompanying innovations (see Table 11.1). The application of tubular bandages, for example, has been greatly eased with the introduction of various applicator aids. Some of these applicators look like badminton shuttlecocks, while others resemble wire cages. The advantage of using an applicator is that there is minimal distur-

bance of the gauze dressing under the bandage, and also the likelihood of compression causing a patient discomfort is reduced. Applicators are designed to slide dressings over toes, as well as over the whole limb.

There are two types of environment that may be provided by dressings and bandages—dry and moist. Moist bandages, which are used in cases of varicose ulcers and ankle eczema, are not discussed in this book, but it should be borne in mind that they do have a part to play in skin rehabilitation. Joint movement can be deliberately impaired by bandages impregnated with zinc and ichthammol paste, while soothing irritated skin. Dry bandages, on the other hand, offer the foot restriction without the need for messy ointments, are less expensive and are easier to handle.

Indications

Dressings fulfil a number of broad objectives. They

Table 11.1 Bandage category of dressings

Non-tubular	
Open weave	Dressing lesions, e.g. K band, Kling
Crepe	BPC dressing for lesions and light support
Adherent	Rubberised elastic bandage, stretches, good antislip, highly compressive, e.g. Coban, 3M
Elastic material	Support ankles/knees
Wool 5–10 cm	Cast lining and thick dressing padding, e.g. Velband (Rayon, cotton wool bandage)
Polyurethane foam (PF)	e.g. Deltatape—again, used for lining casts and bandages, partial water repellency
Animal wool	Lambswool used largely for insulation properties within tubular bandages
Polymer bandage	See below, e.g. Silopad—compression and emollient properties
Tubular non-elastic	Dressing lesions and supporting gauze against skin, e.g. Tubigauz (Scholl), Tubinette (Seton)
Sizes 01,12	Digits, hallux
34	Forefoot
56	Whole foot
78	Lower limb
Elasticated	Supporting joints, dressings, reducing oedema and haematoma, increasing shock absorption, lining casts. Water-repellent properties available, e.g. Tubiton (Seton)
Elastic net	A wide gauge net, offers good ventilation, good ability to stretch (Nylon)
Elastic interwoven	Bandage with coloured lines: whole foot and foot/leg for cast lining—red (small, 3.2 cm), green (5 cm) and blue (8 cm)
Stockinette	e.g. Tubigrip (Seton), sizes increase alphabetically in variable incremental size increases—A (4.20 cm), C (6.75 cm), D (7.50 cm), E (8.75 cm), F (10 cm) and G (12 cm)
Open-cell foam bonded to bandage	Polyurethane (PU) padded on Tubigrip small (7 cm), medium (8 cm) and large (10 cm)
Foam-lined digital bandage	Single- or double-rolled (X) PU foam—A (15 mm) to D (25 mm), or AX to DX for digits
Non-foamed polymer	Digital, forefoot and heel bandages with pads incorporated within thin bandage, e.g. Silipos gel, Silopad
Heel anklet bandages	Heavy-duty bandages pre-formed to fit a variety of circumferences. Incorporation of silicone pads, e.g. Bauerfeind

protect a wound, allow the absorption of exudate, prevent infection from external sources and stimulate healing.

A dressing can assist with the restoration of limb function, even though its main objective is to reduce pain. An adhesive padded dressing prevents shear over the skin, as well as preventing the exposure of fine nerve endings to the outside environment. The ability to select dressings correctly comes both with the experience gained by 'doing it yourself' and from watching other practitioners.

Bandages are used to support feet and are available in a number of widths, usually between 5 and 10 cm, although 15 cm bandages can be obtained for use with larger feet. They are used to hold gauze dressings in place, and are also valuable in the case of strains and sprains, where movement needs to be restricted. Elastication provides compression and prevents slip-

page, as in the case of 'Tubigrip' bandages (Fig. 11.1B), and this means that oedema is likely to be reduced, thus limiting chronic inflammatory changes. The ankle joint benefits best from this type of wraparound bandage. Generally, the heavier the material, the stronger the action. The life span of the material also tends to increase with weight, and thus the heavier designs can usually be washed and reused.

A conforming or compression bandage can create skin abrasion and can even limit circulatory flow. Patients should be made aware of complications such as numbness, tingling and cyanotic or white colour changes around their digits, signifying impairment. Older patients, and those with weaker skin, can develop blisters between the toes if rubbing from dressings ensues.

Adhesive techniques are commonly used with all types of foot dressing, and the problem of skin damage must be considered before application. All forms of dressings, plasters or bandages can result in varying degrees of cutaneous moisture; an increase in the number of microbial flora under adhesive dressings can increase the mechanical damage resulting from long-term use.

Discussion

Dressings offer a quick method to secure and support the area in question, and usually allow a temporary programme of rest during which the lesion, open or otherwise, resolves. Some of the more heavy-duty products available as stock items are designed to last and may incorporate component padding which in itself can offer emollient benefits.

Open lesions or lesions that have an inflammatory base are the most likely candidates for a dressing. Clinical padding may be incorporated within elasticated forms of bandages to enhance protection.

CLINICAL PADDED DRESSINGS

Padded dressings play a large part in conservative foot management. The many designs available have traditionally been taped to the foot with adhesive

Table 11.2 Clinical padding materials

Material	Description
Felt	
Semi-compressed	Plain (no adhesive) 2, 5, 7 mm Hypoallergenic 5, 7 mm. Membrane adhesives (thinner) 5, 7 mm *Properties:* hygroscopic (absorbs perspiration)
Compressed Newer felts	Hypoallergenic 2, 5, 7 mm 30% viscose added. Semi-compressed only. Also available as 10 mm. Otherwise as above
Foams	Polyurethane (PU open-cell foam) with cover or without. Thin cover provides greater strength, e.g. Fleece foam, Dalzofoam, Elite 5, 7 and 10 mm. Latex (rubber, closed-cell foamed) 4.5, 5 and 7 mm depending upon backing— Swanfoam, Molefoam have fabric covers to improve recovery upon foot loading as PU above Adhesives vary as with felt
Fine coverings	Carded cotton, stretch two directions, e.g. Fleecy web Thinnest single stretch covering Moleskin or Stockinette

strapping. Used in this way, they provide a first line method of treatment for both acute and chronic problems.

As a group, padded dressings include foamed pads, felt pads and thin coverings such as moleskin and fleece web. Each material is characterised by different physical properties. Felt is used in conforming dressings, offering resilience sufficient to reduce pressure. Felt is frequently used with cut-outs and cavitations to limit pressure over the load-bearing parts of the foot with most symptoms. Foam has the elastic properties offered by synthetic plastic, acting as 'rubber'. Foam lasts surprisingly long compared to felt, which has the disadvantage of absorbing moisture more readily. Cavities in foam are less effective than those in felt and are only necessary to improve foot–skin contour. The thin covering pads limit surface shear and can anchor skin when it is placed under tension.

Indications

The main advantage offered by adhesive dressings lies in the fact that there is an element of some bulk positioned next to the lesion. Such dressings tend not to move once they are placed, although you should remember that patients do remove dressings and often replace them incorrectly. Nowadays, hypoallergenic adhesive backing is more common in clinical adhesive products than rubber-based zinc oxide and so allergic reactions are few and far between. The movement of adhesive attachments, however, does sometimes causes sensitive skin to mimic allergy. Note that in this case there is usually an absence of blistering or of a red outline around the pad. True allergies can only be properly ascertained with a patch test, when a piece of the offensive material shows positive.

Adhesive padding offers selective immobilisation by limiting tissue movement; herein lies the success of thin dressings which cover the skin and prevent frictional rub. Additionally, these thin materials take up little room in the shoe.

The practitioner is cautioned against allowing patients to become dependent upon the common padded dressing, because many of the benefits, while effective, are only temporary.

A list indicating some of the diverse uses of these dressings to ameliorate pain in the foot is provided in Box 11.2.

The mechanical basis of selection

When deciding which dressing to use in treatment and how to use that dressing, two questions need to

---

Box 11.2   Indications for the use of padded dressings

- Corns (IPK)—redistribution (plantar/dorsal/apical/interdigital)
- Ulcers—protection by redistribution (as for corns plus malleoli)
- Bony alignment protection—prominences associated with HV, exostoses and Tailor's bunion
- Increased alignment and loading of dysfunctioning metatarsals
- Heel pad shock attenuation—posterior or plantar foam pad in 3–6 mm thicknesses
- Digital deformity alignment—props under toes
- Arch discomfort—infills (valgus pads for fascia strain)
- Elevation of part of the foot—for tendo Achilles pain, limb length discrepancy
- Inflammation and blistering—cutaneous or deeper trauma, skin movement limited
- Tongue pads and heel protection—for shoes (see Ch. 13)

be answered: what is the desired objective and what is the most appropriate material to use in achieving that? Below, we discuss this question of selection in terms of the objectives of orthotic management described in Box 10.1.

Redistribution. In order to reduce pressure, one must decrease the influencing force or increase the area over which that force acts. When an intermittent force is applied to a relatively small, localised area of the foot, adhesive padding can provide the increased surface area needed to dissipate that force.

The pad must be large enough to provide sufficient surface area to achieve the desired reduction in pressure; it must consist of a material that will resist compression; it must be positioned so as to achieve maximal protection without actually encroaching on the site; and its thickness must be such that it can be accommodated in the shoe. A successful result will not be achieved unless:

- the cause of the pressure is correctly diagnosed
- the direction of the pressure is correctly gauged
- an evaluation is made of the area to which pressure is to be redistributed.

Generally, the adhesive material used for the purposes of redistribution is semi-compressed felt. No scientific evidence supports such a selection and, as previously mentioned, foamed pads can offer equal benefit. Cavitations and cut-outs using felt probably

work better than those in foam, but the reason for selecting felt is probably historical and based on the ease of handling such materials with scissors.

Compensation. The objective of compensation is shock attenuation, that is, to decrease the velocity of impact of the force causing the undesirable stress. A material placed over the area that is being stressed does this. The material needs to be sufficiently dense to be truly effective. Foams offer satisfactory resilience because of the cells created during the foaming process. The material acts as a pneumatic cushion; with foot–ground pressure, the foam deforms and air is expelled. When the pressure is released, air re-enters the matrix, returning the pad to its original shape. Effective new materials such as Sorbothane (Viscolas) and Silopad (Silipos) are reducing the popularity of adhesive cushioning.

Rest. Surface friction is often generated between the foot and the shoe. When this force becomes excessive, blisters form which can lead to callosity. A thin material placed between the two surfaces will reduce tissue movement, as well as friction and shear stresses, the material itself absorbing the forces and the heat that is generated. The most widely used anti-frictional material is a fleecy web and this consists of loosely knitted wool fibres on which an adhesive is spread. It is easily stretched and consequently conforms to the contours of the foot. Skin movement into the toe sulcus can be temporarily prevented by applying tension proximally with a fleece cover anchored just beneath the toes.

Stabilisation. The temporary realignment of bony structures occurs when the force, and hence the weight, borne by an otherwise non-weight-bearing part is increased. This may occur, for instance, at the second metatarsal head, which, if the first metatarsal does not contact the ground efficiently, becomes overloaded; the manifestation of this extra load is usually seen as a callus. In this case, a pad is required to withstand compression. Compressed felt is preferred but is often too hard to adhere to the surface of the foot. It is used more frequently on insole bases.

Containment. Application of medication, such as emollients, keratolytics and caustics, within firm dressings is most effective when the medication is confined to a precisely defined area. This containment of medicaments is achieved by using a variety of shapes of dressing, e.g. crescents, cavities or complete apertures in the pad (Fig. 11.2).

Application of padded dressings

Individual dressing pads have evolved over time

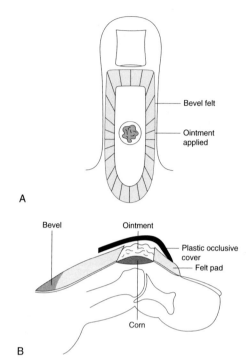

A

B

Figure 11.2 A: The dorsal cover provides greater deflection of load over the IPJ of the digit, as well as providing a cavity or aperture through which medication can be introduced. B: A thin cover, cut from a plastic bag or sheet, will prevent any undue leakage of the medication.

and there are now many variations in design. The discussion of various pads that follows does not purport to be a definitive one, but merely aims to describe those that are most commonly used.

This group of firm dressings is almost always secured with strapping, and as such this means of holding pads in place will be considered first. (The term 'taping' is synonymous with 'strapping'; however, in the context of this book, taping has been used to describe a therapeutic technique (see later) and strapping is used to describe the securing of padded dressings.)

Strapping. Strapping can be used in many different ways. Whatever method is employed, the dressing should achieve the following: it should conform to the foot, provide the patient with comfort, have good adhesion, and maintain the correct position against the foot.

Avoiding problems. In order to achieve the above aims, one should ensure that the strapping does not create wrinkles in the skin which can cause discomfort, that all edges of the padding are covered, and that the edges of the strapping are rounded so

Box 11.3 Summary of points to consider when applying padded dressings

- The shape of the pad should conform to the size and natural contours of the individual foot
- The perimeter should be bevelled gradually to avoid bulky and uncomfortable ridges. The bulk of any pad should lie in the natural hollows of the anatomy and posterior to the structures to be protected
- Bevels are angled cuts made on the top surface (top-bevelled) or undersurface—adhesive side (underbevelled). The straight bevel can be cut along the edge or a pie crust bevel can be selected perpendicular to the edge, allowing the pad to curve. A double bevel is created by two parallel bevels made along the edge, thus widening the bevel
- Cavities within the pad should be half the thickness of the material used and of sufficient depth to accommodate dressings and protuberances
- Cavities and apertures may be optionally bevelled slightly on the adhesive side to aid conformity to tissue contours

as to reduce the chances of it peeling away from the skin and taking the padding with it.

Particular care should be taken when strapping a digit—one should ensure that the digital circulation is not constricted. Modern elastic-type strapping is ideal for digits as it conforms neatly to contours and will stretch if for any reason the digit should swell. Tubular toe bandages such as 'Tubegauz' are popular in securing digital pads.

Padding. The basic concept of a pad or firm dressing as described in this chapter should be modified to the requirements of the presenting problem. However, certain principles of construction should always be followed; these are described in Box 11.3.

Design of padded dressings

Digital padding

The digital pads described below are usually constructed from semi-compressed felt. Single, and in some cases multiple, pads are secured with 01/12 Tubegauz. Shaped adhesive strapping is used to ensure that there is no movement from the pad/dressing against the skin.

Dorsal digital cover. The thickness of the dorsal digital cover lies on the dorsum of the toe and extends its complete length from the base of the nail. The distal border is slightly shaped to follow the base of the nail, the proximal border is slightly rounded, and both sides run longitudinally straight down the toe without extending down from the dorsum. The pad has a top bevel on all sides and a cavity on its adhesive aspect, or aperture, usually at the level of the proximal interphalangeal joint (PIPJ). The indication for use is where redistribution of pressure from the PIPJ is required, and so the material of choice is felt (Fig. 11.2).

The *dorsal digital crescent* is a modification of the dorsal cover and may be employed where less bulk is required within the shoe. The distal border lies proximal to the joint or lesion to be protected and is underbevelled. A further modification involves the extension to a double or multiple crescent which serves adjoining toes (Fig. 11.3).

Horseshoe pad. This pad offers redistribution of pressure over a greater area than does the dorsal digital cover and offers a means of protecting a dorsal

digital lesion that allows dressings to be changed without disturbing the pad. As the name suggests, the pad is roughly the shape of a horseshoe, with two longitudinal arms which may lie, for instance, on the dorsum of toes 2 and 4, and is continuous with a central crescentic section which sits immediately behind a lesion on toe 3 (Fig. 11.4). The pad is top-bevelled around its outer margin. Underbevelling in the crescentic area proximal to the lesion is optional. A cavity or aperture in one of the longitudinal arms can be adapted to accommodate a second lesion on an adjacent toe.

Apical crescent. This pad is designed to redistribute pressure from a lesion at the apex of the toe. The pad sits around the pulp of the digit and is bevelled by small vertical cuts (pie crusting), allowing the pad to be shaped around the end of the digit (Fig. 11.5). The pad is commonly used where there is a degree of rigidity in the toe and straightening is not practical, and where lesions constantly develop on the tip or around the nail edge.

Digital prop and long prop. The prop is designed to have an extension effect on the clawed toe, thus assisting with ground purchase. In the case of fixed toe deformities, it offers protection and redistribution of high loads. In this latter respect there is some similarity to the apical crescent. The adhesive side is bevelled to fit into the toe crease and, where the toe is

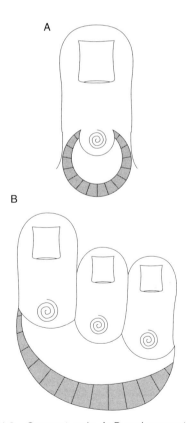

Figure 11.3 Crescent pads. A: Dorsal crescent used to create less bulk than dorsal cover; this is not as effective for holding medicaments. B: Multiple crescents for more than one toe, e.g. retracted toes with dorsal lesions. The bulk of this padded dressing can sit in the space created by the drawn back toes.

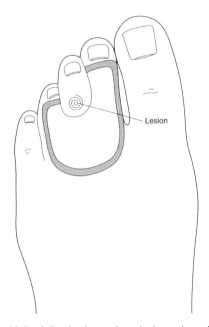

Figure 11.4 Adhesive horseshoe design—shaped to spread load across adjacent digits with bevel indicated. Excellent for assisting healing ulceration over IP joints.

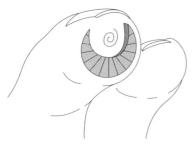

Figure 11.5 Apical crescent is best pie crust bevelled. This technique allows better conformation around the end of the toe and can then be secured with 01 or 12 Tubegauz.

sufficiently flexible, to extend the distal IPJ forwards. The side bevels fit against the lateral toes as shown in Figure 11.6. In its adhesive form the pad is only suitable for short periods. It is usual to progress to silicone moulds or to a replaceable orthodigital device. The long prop is a modification of the single prop, and is applied in cases where additional toes need supporting; often, the three central toes need to be supported together. The prop can be secured with 1.25 cm wide tape.

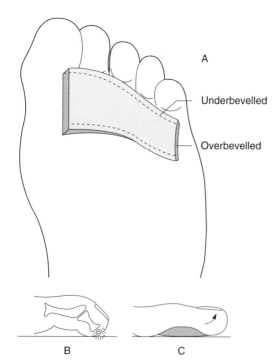

A

Underbevelled

Overbevelled

B   C

Figure 11.6 Props. A–C: The long prop shown is an extension of the single prop affecting the apex of toes—protective and partially corrective in function.

Interdigital wedge (IDW)/dumb-bell pad. This is a protective dressing which separates adjoining toes, reducing the shear stresses. The IDW is shaped to fit the side of the toe; the underbevelled base is shaped to fit the webbing, and the top-bevelled sides follow the shape of the toe distally and extend slightly in the dorsal and plantar directions. The distal border is either crescented to fit proximal to the lesion or extends almost the full length of the toe, in which case the pad will contain a cavity if redistribution of pressure is the aim. Some practitioners prefer to strip the adhesive backing from the foam material, as the toes can hold the IDW with stockings adequately (Fig. 11.7A). This technique offers a non-adhesive removeable pad.

The dumb-bell pad is so called because of its shape. The central stem of the dumb-bell is underbevelled to strip away its adhesive and placed interdigitally at the base of the cleft. The two bulbous ends are top-bevelled and adhered to the foot on the dorsal and plantar aspects. The use of these pads has been largely superseded by silicone devices. The dumb-bell's main function is to spread two toes, particularly toes 4 and 5, the cleft of which is a common site for soft corns. The pad is palliative and will rarely eradicate the problem and so is used for short periods to reduce symptoms (Figs 11.7B and C). Adhesive tape is the preferred means of attaching the dorsal and plantar 'bulbous' ends to the skin.

Plantar phalangeal pad for hallux. This pad is used almost exclusively for the hallux but is occasionally used for a lesser toe. It offers protection from a plantar lesion over the IPJ either by redistribution or by cushioning, depending upon the material used. Short-term alleviation from the symptoms of corns (IPK), cysts and bursae can be obtained. The dressing is shaped to resemble the plantar surface of the toe. The base is underbevelled and follows the line of the toe as it joins the webbing. The top-bevelled sides follow the line of the toe distally and the distal border is rounded to the end of the toe. A cavity or aperture may be employed where necessary (Fig. 11.8).

Plantar padded dressings

In this section, four main plantar padded dressing techniques are described, each offering a different function. Unfortunately, few studies have been conducted into their effectiveness despite the use of pressure and force plate techniques to analyse load deflection. Plantar dressings of this nature often seem to work empirically in reducing foot pain. The practitioner is advised, as with many of these padding

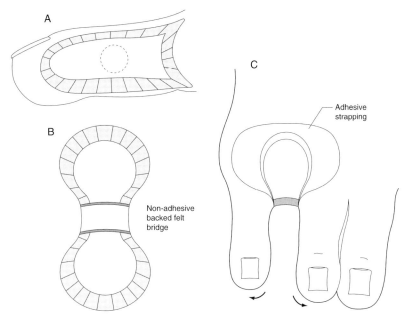

Figure 11.7   A–C: Interdigital dressings. A short-term alternative to silicones. The dressing in (A) provides a small degree of separation and uses a cavity. That in (C) spreads two toes where the lesion lies at the base of the cleft, commonly digits 4–5.

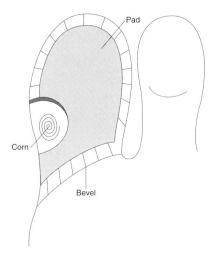

Figure 11.8   Plantar phalangeal pad used most commonly for the hallux.

strategies, to prescribe the metatarsal pads on a short-term basis (i.e. 5–7 days) and then to consider conversion to an insole or alternative design should management appear successful. These padded dressings are strapped into place, overlapping the edges 50:50. The methods used to secure the pad vary: 'goal post' (boxing the pad in) and 'church door' (formation of an 'A' around the pad) strapping have in most cases been replaced by the overlapping horizontal method, which starts at the base of the pad, ending with the distal tape trimmed to conform to the plantar skin without reaching into the sulcus.

Plantar cover. Lesions commonly arise under the metatarsal heads and an adhesive plantar cover is used in order to provide redistribution of pressure, shock attenuation (cushioning), or friction reduction depending on the material used.

The shape in foam rubber provides full thickness of material over metatarsal heads 1–5. The top-bevelled distal border follows the metatarsal formula (anterior metatarsal order of length), allowing space between its termination and the webbing area for the application of strapping.

The sides, also top-bevelled, pass proximally in line with the foot, covering the full plantar metatarsal surface without extending towards the dorsum; the bevel allows the pad to curve along the side of the foot at the extreme plantar edge. All borders are singly top-bevelled, except for the proximal edge which uses a double bevel. The plantar cover extends proximally 1.25–2.5 cm distal to the styloid process of the fifth metatarsal.

The felt material version of the plantar cover is designed to have an aperture or modification to its shape; this may take the form of a 'wing' for metatarsal head areas 1 or 5, or a 'U' for areas 2–4. When redistribution is to be combined with cushioning, the 'winged' or 'U-shaped' area may be filled with foam rubber. The same principle may employ a cushioning button within a complete aperture in the felt. An aperture lies over the lesion, thus affording protection from mechanical stress. The use of semi-compressed felt without some aperture is generally considered to be undesirable as it has no benefit to the patient. In the case where a full, non-apertured dressing pad is used, foam is preferable, at least for its shock-attenuating properties (Fig. 11.9A).

Metatarsal bar. The metatarsal bar differs from the plantar cover in that the main bulk of the material lies behind the metatarsals. This design takes up less shoe room as well as redistributing load from the metatarsal heads proximally.

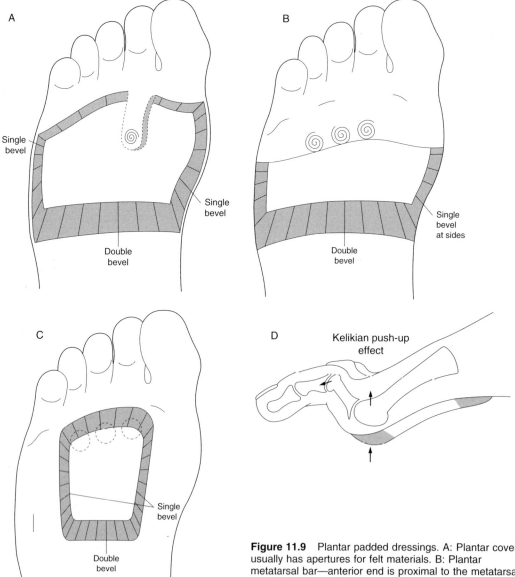

Figure 11.9 Plantar padded dressings. A: Plantar cover—usually has apertures for felt materials. B: Plantar metatarsal bar—anterior end is proximal to the metatarsal heads. C: Plantar metatarsal pad—the distal bevel elevates and appears to influence the metatarsal alignment at the metatarsal head level (this influence shown in D).

The pad is shaped and bevelled similarly to the plantar cover but does not extend as far distally. The distal border follows the metatarsal formula but has its full thickness lying behind the metatarsal heads. Some use a bevel, while others prefer the full pad thickness without a bevel to allow maximum load distribution from the metatarsal heads to the shafts. A modification to the pad uses a foam apron to cushion a traumatised metatarsal head region (Fig. 11.9B).

Plantar metatarsal pad (PMP). This is a traditional pad and it provides a different function to those described above. The PMP, often confused with the plantar cover, has been used to elevate metatarsal heads sufficiently to extend the proximal phalanges at the metatarsophalangeal joint (MTPJ). The effectiveness of this technique as long-term correction is questionable. In flexible deformities it can be argued that contractures are dissuaded at the MTPJ. The use as a metatarsal brace or for metatarsal alignment does seem to have value with some forms of metatarsalgia and indeed there is some degree of success in treating Morton's plantar digital neuroma in its early stages (Figs 11.9C and D).

The PMP is made from felt. The distal edge follows the metatarsal formulae with the width spanning between metatarsals 1–2 and 4–5, the extent of its lateral top bevels. The proximal end is placed, as with other metatarsal pads, 1.25–2.5 cm distal to the styloid process, and the distal top bevel must have its greatest thickness over the metatarsal heads to provide some lever function.

Shaft pad. An unmodified shaft pad attracts a high proportion of load-bearing to the underlying metatarsal and therefore alters the amount of pressure sustained by the remaining metatarsals. The pad may either elevate the metatarsal or be used to protect it.

The distal edge of the pad, constructed in felt, is rounded and extends over the MTPJ. The sides follow the edges of the metatarsal, the whole width of the bone being covered, and extend its full length. The proximal border is cut squarely across the foot with the edges being top-bevelled. The area covering the metatarsal head may be cavitied or crescented as required (Figs 11.10A and B).

Another modification may be employed when there is pain in the first MTPJ. An extended shaft which passes distally to the IPJ of the hallux serves as a splint to the MTP joint, reducing the capacity for dorsiflexion and, therefore, pain associated with movement. Alternatively, this same pad may be used to redistribute pressure from an IPJ lesion.

L pad. This pad is a variation on the shaft pad and combines the effect of an extended shaft with a metatarsal bar into one pad. It is usefully employed when significant lesions are present over several metatarsal heads and the IPJ of the hallux. The pad follows the same specifications as the extended shaft, except that it also extends laterally into the described shape of the metatarsal bar, thus appearing like the letter 'L'. If a lesion is present under the first metatarsal head, this may be protected by means of a cavity (Fig. 11.10C).

Padded dressings for the rearfoot

Plantar calcaneal pad. The design of this pad follows the shape of the plantar aspect of the heel to the anterior of the calcaneus, where it is cut straight across and proximal to the styloid process by 2.5 cm. A single top bevel is employed all around to ensure good contact upon strapping into place, except at the anterior border where a double bevel is used. A felt pad may be cavitied or apertured to redistribute pressure from lesions or to contain ointment using the model already illustrated for the digital pad in Figure 11.2. Unmodified, and in sufficient thickness, it may raise the heel slightly in the shoe and give a degree of rest to a strained Achilles tendon. Foam material in various thicknesses may be applied for shock attenuation in a traumatised heel.

Retrocalcaneal pad. Used for redistribution of pressure away from a lesion at the posterior of the heel, this pad always contains a cavity or an aperture. A pie crust (vertical bevel) all around ensures good conformation around the lesion. The base of the pad follows the line of the weight-bearing aspect of the posterior of the heel, while the vertically ascending sides curve inwards and complete the shape at the top of the posterior of the heel. In order to achieve comfort and ensure retention, it is essential that the sides of the pad fully embrace the contour of the heel and do not terminate prematurely forming a prominence (Fig. 11.11).

Miscellaneous dressings

Valgus pad. The valgus pad is essentially a space filler and is valuable in a cavus-type foot and in pronated feet experiencing discomfort from fascial strain. In the high arch foot, tension is removed from the tightly strung fascia, giving some temporary relief.

Sometimes promoted as an antipronatory device, it is unlikely to fulfil this function, particularly in an adhesive form which has relatively low bulk. However, it does reduce deformation of the foot under load, and as such imparts a certain amount of rest

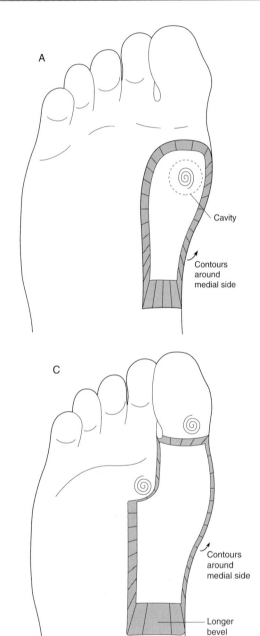

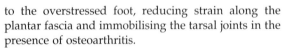

Figure 11.10 Variants on the plantar pad. A: Shaft pad over the first metatarsal. B: An extended first ray shaft is used to completely immobilise the first MTP joint. C: The L-shaped pad functions to protect a distal lesion over the plantar hallux as well as over the second metatarsal head.

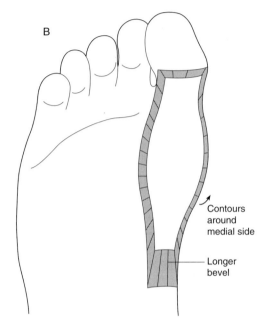

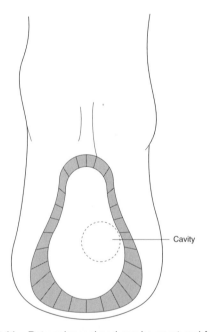

to the overstressed foot, reducing strain along the plantar fascia and immobilising the tarsal joints in the presence of osteoarthritis.

The anterior border of the pad sits just behind the first and second metatarsal heads. From the medial aspect, the pad passes backwards to the tuberosity of the navicular and from there to the medial edge of the weight-bearing aspect of the heel as a cut-away.

Figure 11.11 Retrocalcaneal pad can be apertured for bursae or painful spurs created by Haglund's deformity, or where tissue overlying the heel has become inflamed or sensitive, e.g. perniosis, heel neuroma.

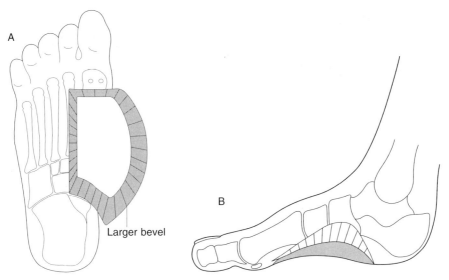

Figure 11.12   A, B: Valgus pad. Adhesive pads are shaped somewhat differently from replaceable designs. The pad conforms to the foot with double bevels providing arch conformity. This does not provide antipronatory therapy.

The lateral border then follows a straight edge in metatarsal space 2–3, bevelled so as not to make shoe fit too bulky. All edges are top-bevelled in order to achieve maximum conformation (Fig. 11.12).

Hallux valgus oval (HVO). If cushioning is the aim, Tubifoams or Silipads make the best replaceable dressings. The adhesive dressing is again temporary, as its main function lies in protecting open wounds, sinuses and ulcers.

Classically, the felt or foam HVO pad is ovoid (egg) in shape but tailored to contour the individual foot; this pad is cavitied if redistribution of pressure from the prominent medial aspect of the first MTPJ is required (Fig. 11.13). The main indication for this modality is to protect a lesion over the medial first MTP joint. The exact position of the bony prominence dictates the precise position of the pad, but the following points should be observed: dorsally it should not extend over the tendon of extensor hallucis longus (EHL) and thus interfere with tendon sheath function; distally it should not extend as far as the IPJ; the full thickness of the pad should not extend plantarly under the foot, although it is acceptable if the bevelled area does so for a short distance. If footwear accommodation does prove a problem, a viable alternative is the hallux valgus crescent. This has the same shape as the oval, except that the anterior portion is crescented to the bony prominence. As with the oval, all edges are singly top-bevelled, except for the crescent which is back-bevelled or left unbevelled.

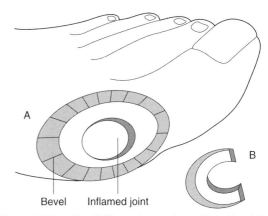

Figure 11.13   The HVO can be used on either side of the foot and can be shaped appropriately to conform to footwear and provide protection from cutaneous irritation. A cavity (A) or crescent (B) is provided, the latter being most suitable where the distal end is too bulky.

A *'Tailor's bunion' oval* has the same specifications as the HVO but is used on the lateral side of the fifth MTPJ.

Tendon or saddle pad. This pad is used for dorsal protection of the EHL tendon. Roughly oval in shape and top-bevelled, it has a central channel of adhesive removed for the EHL tendon and may have a deeper cavity cut within the channel to accommodate a lesion. The pad is placed on the dorsal surface of the first MTPJ, with the lateral edge lying over the first intermetatarsal space and the medial edge lying on the line of the dorsomedial aspect of the first MTPJ.

Discussion

Adhesive padding should only be employed for short periods of time. Success is based upon a number of factors, such as patient acceptability and occupational requirements, i.e. shoe types may not allow sufficient room for the pads. The obstacle presented by padding to good hygiene, the detrimental effect on the skin with long-term use, and the short life of the materials used dictate the need for eventual progression to a replaceable or alternative form of orthosis or footwear adaptations.

LIMITING FOOT AND ANKLE MOVEMENT

Adhesive tape may be used to limit function and provide rest to an injured part in an acute condition, or periodically to give support to repetitive strain injuries, for instance in sports enthusiasts. Movement can also be limited by casting the area in question.

Neither adhesive taping nor casting is a long-term solution to relieving foot pain, but they both inhibit movement without taking up too much room in footwear.

Recently introduced products provide splinting by pumping air into plastic air sacs, e.g. Aircast. While rather expensive, these devices are easily removed and replaced by patients with little technical instruction.

Taping

This technique can be used successfully for short periods on the ankle, as low- and high-dye taping, on the arch structure of the foot, and on the first MTP joint. Some patients can replace the taping at home to continue the effect, and this is commonplace with sports people. You should note the following points when applying taping to the skin:

- tension should be applied without skin wrinkling
- taping should not encircle parts likely to be vascularly compromised
- taping should be contoured to ensure that it does not ruck up and peel back from socks or shoewear
- a skin tactifier such as tincture of benzoin can be helpful
- hair should be shaved first to avoid damage
- taping should never be used directly on known sensitive skin, infection, or bullous or oedematous tissues
- taping is best overlapped evenly

- the joint position should be corrected before applying the tape.

First metatarsophalangeal joint support

In the case of an acutely painful first MTPJ, strapping can provide rest by limiting dorsiflexion and abduction (Fig. 11.14).

The patient is laid supine with the foot over the edge of the treatment table. If required, the relevant skin area may be prepared with a tincture of benzoin (BPC) or Opsite (Smith & Nephew) to assist skin adherence. The tape used is non-stretchable and 2.5 cm in width. With the hallux placed in the desired position, which is neither dorsiflexed nor plantarflexed, the first strip of tape is placed longitudinally on the superior lateral aspect of the hallux, starting at the mid-portion of the distal phalanx and extending proximally to the base of the first metatarsal. Additional strips are placed to slightly overlap each previous strip in a medial direction, continuing downwards and onto the plantar aspect of the toe and foot. When applying these strips, no traction should be applied in case it dorsiflexes the hallux, but the tape must never be allowed to remain slack because this will result in a decreased effect.

Anchoring strips are then applied to secure the longitudinal strips. In order to avoid any risk of compromising circulation, the anchoring strips around the toe should never completely encircle it, but should terminate at the margins of the interdigital space. In order to avoid tightness, anchoring strips around the longitudinal arches should terminate at either end on the dorsum of the foot.

Low-dye taping

This is a form of taping which can be used for symptoms of plantar fasciitis and which has also been found to have an antipronatory effect (McCloskey 1992; Fig. 11.15). McCloskey found a positive effect using low-dye (LD) taping with Kistler force plate analysis ($P < 0.05$) for 75% of patients studied ($n = 16$). Again, the same width of tape is employed and the patient lies supine with the foot extending over the table edge and at right angles to the leg. The first of three strips is applied, starting proximal to the fifth MTPJ. After the tape is secured on the outside of the foot, the end is grasped in one hand and wrapped around the heel while simultaneously inverting the heel slightly. The end of the tape is then attached to the medial side of the foot, terminating just proximal to the first MTPJ.

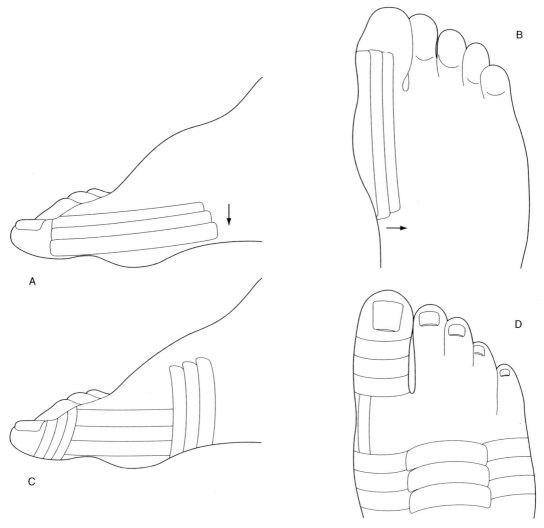

Figure 11.14 Fan strapping is a useful method for painful joints associated with transient synovitis, hallux limitus and acute trauma to the first MTP joint. A–D: 1.25 cm wide strips, usually zinc oxide (ZO) tapes, are placed around the first toe joint, overlapping each other. The proximal ends are left loose until all the ends can be pulled into tension and secured at the base as well as at the distal end around the great toe.

This is repeated twice, each subsequent tape overlapping the previous by two-thirds. Finally, transverse strips of 5 cm width should be placed without dragging the skin and causing discomfort. They are placed across the foot from dorsolateral to dorsomedial and should extend from the base of the fifth metatarsal to just proximal to the first and fifth MTP joints.

False fascia taping (for fasciitis)

Tapes applied from the toe sulci to the posterior heel support the three bands of fascia when discomfort has been clearly identified. Figure 11.16 illustrates rigid zinc oxide taping supported with Mefix to ensure good skin attachment. Elasticated plaster rolls provide additional support and are ideal for limiting tensile stresses. Smaller feet will require two tapes of 5 cm width, whereas large feet will require three.

Ankle support

Support for the ankle (Fig. 11.17) may be necessary in the following cases:

- following inversion sprains, where taping is

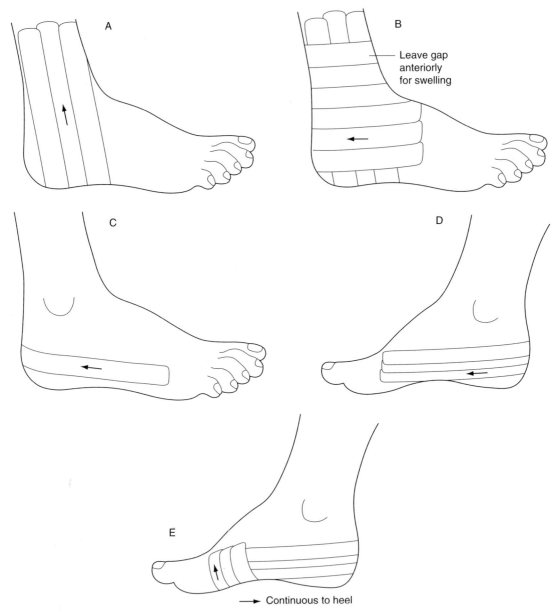

Figure 11.15 The high-dye (HD) strapping (A, B) and low-dye (LD) strapping (C–E) act as a basic orthosis for controlling the ankle and subtalar joint (HD) and the subtalar joint (LD), respectively. Taping in an inverted position takes the stress off the fascia and may be applied in a neutral STJ position.

needed to support the lateral ligament of the ankle without unduly restricting joint motion

• following eversion sprains
• as a general support for the structures of the ankle in an attempt to prevent sprains.

In the first two cases, two types of tape are needed—a 3.75 cm wide non-stretchable and a 5 cm wide elastic adhesive bandage. Two gauze 'diamonds' are positioned, one on the anterior of the ankle to prevent undue constriction from the tape upon ankle dorsiflexion, and one posteriorly to protect the Achilles tendon and prevent undue skin shear. An assistant may be needed to maintain these in place initially.

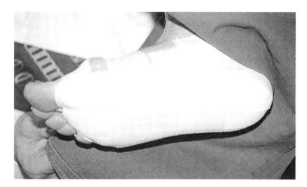

Figure 11.16 False plantar fascia. An alternative system illustrates rigid taping used in longitudinal strips to support the fascia. Elasticated taping is preferred but the principal direction of application is the same and follows the main bands of fascia. Transverse 5 cm taping with Mefix (a hypoallergic tape) supports the zinc oxide-based false plantar fascia tape.

Strips of non-stretch tape are used at first. With the lower leg extended over the edge of the table, the first strip is placed on the medial side of the lower leg and is taken vertically downwards under the heel and up onto the lateral side of the foot and lower leg as a 'stirrup'. Further strips are added, each slightly overlapping the previous one, until the final strip finishes well in front of the malleolus.

Using the same type of tape, horizontal strips are now applied. The first starts on the lateral side of the foot and passes behind the heel and along the medial aspect of the foot. Further strips are added in overlap fashion until the malleolus is covered. To complete the ankle support, the elastic adhesive bandage is used to form a 'figure of 8'. This begins with placement on the lateral aspect of the leg above the malleolus and passes downwards and medially across the instep, under the foot, up and over the lateral aspect of the foot, and finally upwards and medially to pass above and behind the medial malleolus and terminate at its origin.

In eversion sprains the directions are reversed; the vertical strips are applied from lateral to medial, and the figure-of-8 is applied in the opposite direction.

In order to prevent sprains, a 5 cm crepe bandage is better than a tape. The limb is positioned as before. The end of the bandage is placed on the medial side of the lower leg, and encircles it before passing down and over the instep to the lateral side of the foot. The strap is then taken under the foot, up and over the instep, and then under the foot once more. On emerging at the medial side, the bandage forms a heel lock by passing obliquely backwards and around the heel to the front of the leg. It then encircles the leg, passes over the instep in a medial direction and under the heel to form a heel lock on the opposite side. Finally it is secured with a short piece of tape horizontally around the leg.

In some cases it may be advantageous to incorporate an adhesive pad, such as a valgus pad, to assist with a medial foot influence, stabilising the midtarsus.

Cautions

There are some disadvantages associated with taping. Plaster allergy dictates that tape cannot be adhered to the skin; it is sometimes possible to overcome this by covering most of the foot/lower leg with tubular bandage which is adhered at either end with hypoallergenic tape. The taping is then placed on the tubular bandage rather than directly onto the skin. However, the intimacy of contact is lost and the effect is likely to be less than adequate. Occupational constraints allied to limitations of hygiene may make taping therapy inappropriate, but these constraints need to be balanced against the severity of the condition under treatment.

Discussion

Taping for the acute condition is but one stage in a comprehensive treatment plan. Once the acute phase has passed, the practitioner must consider the next or adjunctive stage in the plan. This may take the form of physical therapy, such as contrast foot baths, infrared irradiation, ultrasound, injection, imaging for further diagnosis above X-rays and oral/local medication. Rehabilitation may involve passive stretching or exercises. The success of the taping regime may suggest that a form of orthosis is indicated; this is particularly the case with low-dye taping. To be effective, taping should only be used for short periods. If there is an obvious benefit, patients can be taught to apply their own tapes.

Casting

Casting is a very useful method for enforcing rest. The following four systems are briefly described, with notes on how to apply the casts safely:

- foot cast
- back slab
- full below knee cast
- pre-moulded plastic walker.

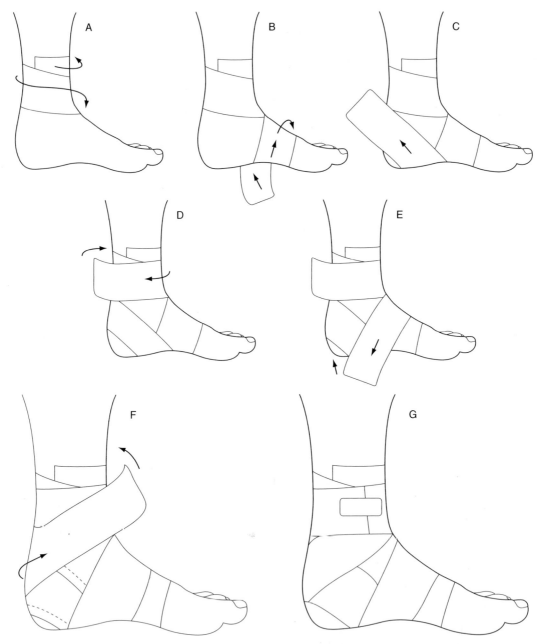

Figure 11.17 A–G: The application of ankle supportive taping in order to lock the talocrural and subtalar joints. The material used should be of a heavy-duty nature, 2.5–5 cm wide, and ideally should have a longitudinal stretch. Indications include ankle pain without gross swelling and lateral/medial ankle sprains, especially where bone and joint pathology has been ruled out by X-ray first.

General indications

Foot pain without a clearly defined source can be assisted once the practitioner is satisfied that there is no specific underlying pathology. Apart from use in fractures, casting techniques can provide a valuable tool in managing acute pain.

Cautions. In each of the cases described, the technique offers rest and alignment of the joints of the foot—the ankle is completely limited if splinting is raised above the malleoli. Once a joint is immobilised, it will stiffen as a result of disuse and will thus need rehabilitating afterwards. Bone and muscle will atrophy, as the tissues are not normally exercised. Deterioration of bone during lengthy periods of casting can be limited by bone growth stimulators, which are incorporated within casts to reduce the rate of osteopaenia.

Casts applied without sufficient care to protect bony prominences may cause ulcers and erosions of normal skin, blisters and nerve compression. Peroneal compression around the head of the fibula can produce foot drop. Additional padding is required at the heel, digits, lateral joints and malleoli. Patients must be advised to return to the clinic should any unexplained pain result or numbness occur. Digits are best left exposed so that their colour can always be inspected. An emergency contact number should be available for use outside clinic hours, or arrangement should be made with accident and emergency departments in advance. It is good practice to give patients a note advising any other practitioners of the reason for treatment. This is particularly helpful if someone else has to remove the cast.

Weight-bearing is highly desirable to avoid deep vein or pulmonary thromboses following injuries. Patients should be advised that some limb exercise is necessary by contracting calf muscles and moving the knee joint where the foot and ankle are restricted.

Inappropriate casting can also leading to cast disease (wasting and pain due to swelling), and sympathetic and ischaemic dystrophy.

All casts are applied similarly—a tubular bandage is used as the first layer and this is followed by wool (Velband or similar) to protect the skin. The wool is wrapped around the limb, overlapping at each turn. Additional padding is applied over the prominences highlighted. Finally, synthetic casting material is taken (7.5 or 10 cm) from a sealed packet and firmly unravelled following the route taken by the wool. All casting techniques *must be demonstrated* by experienced practitioners and practice undertaken with supervision.

Foot cast

The application of a slipper cast below the ankle has the advantage of allowing ankle motion and exercise. In some cases, mobility may be undertaken without crutches (Fig. 11.18A) while still protecting the foot. Because the technique used requires a light plastic material, a cast cutter is essential for trimming in front of the ankle, to allow normal dorsiflexion and to remove any potential pressure against the skin likely to cause necrosis or nerve compression (Fig 11.18B). Sometimes patients find that the roof of the cast presses, and sometimes swelling is expected; in both cases the cast can be bivalved (cut in half). This

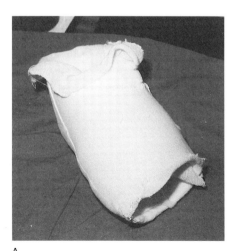
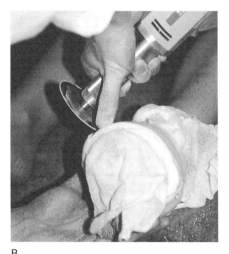

A   B

Figure 11.18   A: The foot cast shown should provide support under the toes, and not impinge the lateral digits or prevent the ankle from dorsiflexing. The heel should be sufficiently thick to allow weight-bearing without premature cracking. B: Removal of the synthetic cast requires an oscillating saw held at right angles to the material. The patient should be warned of vibration and occasionally heat. Soft cast wadding should prevent skin damage. These cast cutters should only be used with appropriate training.

adaption allows the roof of the cast to be replaced with additional orthopaedic wool and 7.5 cm bandage such as crepe to prevent the cast slipping or rubbing.

Where a foot cast would not provide sufficient rest and limitation of function, a below-the-knee design might be more appropriate. In both cases, the foot must be over-dorsiflexed to allow normal walking, otherwise the patient will be liable to fall over and hurt themselves. Crutches may be used optionally where patients are less steady; however, a walking cast shoe is preferred over the old rubber walkers bound to the bottom of the cast.

Backslab

This technique allows complete rest around and about the ankle, with the potential for removal should any pressure points develop with swelling. This is useful where the patient would be unlikely to seek help early or is going away, or if the practitioner does not have a cast cutter. The practitioner can design this cast for use as a night splint, forming a clinical ankle foot orthosis (AFO). Two forms of cast exist: a plaster model (Jones cast) and a synthetic plastic cast. Plaster can be applied in lengths from below the knee to the toes, over padding as described above. Synthetic models are harder wearing but have to be trimmed to remove the anterior portion of the cast following bivalving (Fig. 11.19).

Below-knee cast

This technique is similar to the backslab, except that the cast is not bivalved (Fig. 11.20). Again, plaster or synthetic cast materials can be used over padding. Plaster takes 24 hours to dry thoroughly and is very heavy, causing limb atrophy when left on for long periods. The lighter cast made from polyester, while more expensive, is more popular and much stronger but is not waterproof.

Casts should not be immersed in water and patients should be advised not to use hair dryers to deal with waterlogged casts. There are a number of products now available that are suitable for limited immersion during showers and baths. Seal-Tight (Brown Medical) can be used to cover below-knee casts adequately (Tollafield 1995). The Seal-Tight forms a gasket below the knee to make the bag water-resistant; it is not, however, designed for swimming. XeroSox (George Medical) provides a heavy duty latex bag which conforms to the leg so well that its US distributor advertises its use in a swimming pool. Air is expelled by sucking via a plastic tube. The advantage lies in

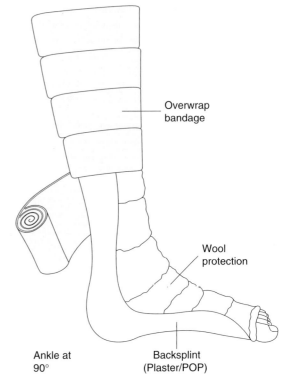

Overwrap bandage

Wool protection

Ankle at 90°

Backsplint (Plaster/POP)

Figure 11.19 A backsplint. This can be made of Plaster of Paris (POP) or synthetic material once the anterior part of the cylinder has been cut away. Replacement is not easy at home and only patients who can follow clear instructions should be offered this type of cast. The illustration depicts a backsplint alone, although the Jones splint (POP only) includes a stirrup which supports the lateral sides of the ankle. Plenty of protective wadding is required, which also absorbs water from the POP. An alternative system is the pneumatic walker (Aircast UK Ltd; see Fig. 11.21).

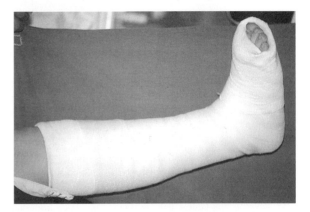

Figure 11.20 A below-knee (BK) synthetic cast must be placed on the foot and leg in the correct position. Compression of nerves and soft tissues warrants special caution.

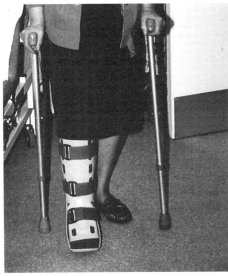 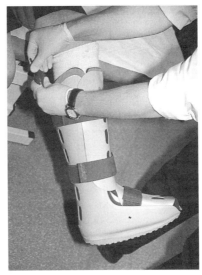

A   B

Figure 11.21   A: The prefabricated (Aircast UK Ltd) cast shown is available in three sizes—small, medium and large—and is easily removable. B: A small bulb pump similar to a stethoscope is used to introduce air at four different sites.

its ability to seal without the need for a gasket. Such modalities can assist the practitioner greatly. The inability to bathe remains a major disadvantage of long-term dressings and casts.

Pneumatic walkers

There are a variety of splinting methods that use air in their design. These light splints, which include a walking cast (Aircast UK) as shown in Fig. 11.21, provide a replaceable, light but strong design. These systems are indicated where repeated casting is likely and regular bathing is desirable. Once inflated, the cylinder is easily positioned and requires no additional skills.

Discussion

Casting offers a valuable tool for dealing with foot pain, provided that infection, tumours and open fractures have been managed appropriately first. The foot cast allows unimpeded ankle motion and walking in a light cast system; above-ankle casts result in a greater level of immobility. For the reasons given above, patients should not use casts, or be immobilised, for indefinite periods.

REPLACEABLE ORTHOSES

Where previously pads as 'chairside appliances'

were designed to have a longer effect than adhesive padded dressings, many off-the-shelf materials or stock orthoses are gaining in popularity. The advent of pre-manufactured orthoses has reduced the need to spend valuable time in producing chairside appliances during consulting sessions.

Traditionally, replaceable padding has been made from clinical felt and foam. Handcrafted materials were bevelled using nail drills, and adhesives were on hand during the clinical consultation to manufacture latex or elastic toe and tarsal loops and covers for insoles.

The other form of orthosis commonly made in the clinic was based on an insole design. Wedged insoles with dense felt, and those with plantar pads, are still used, although pre-manufactured pads are available which offer a variety of different functions. Replaceable pads and insoles will be considered separately.

Replaceable padding

If an adhesive dressing has been selected, the next stage of the foot care programme is progression to a replaceable facsimile.

While proving as effective as the adhesive form, replaceable padding has certain additional advantages:

- It is far more hygienic and easy removal allows for unhindered bathing.
- The non-occlusive effect creates a healthier local

environment, avoiding the effects of excessive moisture from heavy perspiration; the pad may be removed at will and allowed to dry. Replaceable padding has a longer life than adhesive dressings.

• Allergies are far less likely to occur (although it is true that the modern hypoallergenic backing has reduced this problem with adhesives).

Patients generally prefer replaceable padding because it allows them to bathe normally. Those who have used adhesive dressings for years tend to become dependent on them. In these cases, patients should be encouraged to convert to replaceable padding in order to improve hygiene as well as to decrease the frequency of clinical visits required.

There are, however, some disadvantages of replaceable padding:

• Where dressings are necessary for longer periods, for example in the case of ulcers, adhesive dressings provide better protection than replaceable padding as less movement will arise on adherence to the skin.
• Replaceable padding does not conform to the foot as well as adhesive dressing. There is a potential for reduced accuracy with replaceable forms because of slight movements of the pad.
• The practical problems of removal and replacement by a physically compromised patient negate some of the potential benefits. (Even so, an alternative to adhesive padding for long-term use must still be sought if detrimental effects to the skin are to be avoided.)

Replaceable padding may be made from clinical materials such as felt and foams or from more durable materials. The advent of new products on the market,

such as Silopad, is likely to reduce the popularity of chairside manufacture.

The way is open, then, for a staged progression in the foot care programme; just as replaceable padding follows as the next logical step from adhesive, so the results of replaceable padding will indicate the desirability of advancement to more durable orthoses. Most of the adhesive pads described earlier may be converted into a replaceable form. While the range available is very wide, only a few examples are discussed.

Digital

Protective function. A number of off-the-peg padded 'sleeves' or 'tubes' can be utilised for digital protection; examples of these include Tubular foams, sizes A–D (Table 11.1), and Silipos (Silopad) digital pads comprising a thin wafer of gel (Shanks 1991; Fig. 11.22). The advantage of the gel products lie in their ease of application, their clear effectiveness as they release an emollient oil softening the keratotic lesion, and good shoe fit acceptance. Silipos may obviate the need to manufacture IDW, apical and dorsal dressings, although ulcers should first be resolved and any infection cleared.

Semi-corrective function. Darco and Berkemann have produced a range of soft and hard day and night splints for a variety of digital deformities. Originally designed for the hallux, lesser digits can be splinted during the day with Velcro loops. There now seems to be a place for such modalities, although marked deformity is unlikely to be corrected permanently without surgical intervention first (Fig. 10.4).

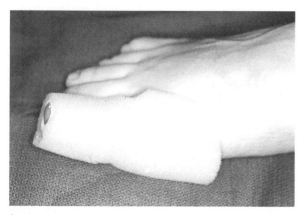
A

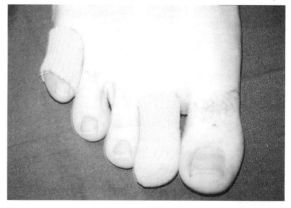
B

Figure 11.22 Protective digital devices. A: Tubifoam for hallux. B: Silopad for the second and fifth digits.

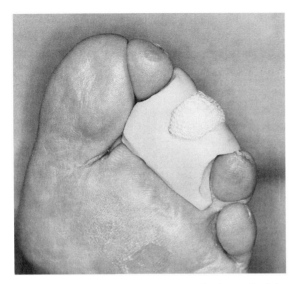

Figure 11.23 A silicone device in seen in situ on the left foot. Toes 2–4 cradle the third toe which has a tubular bandage dressing underneath.

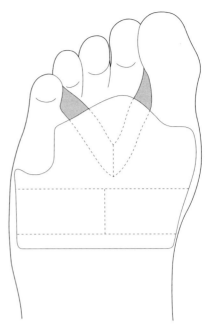

Figure 11.24 Replaceable single-winged plantar cover manufactured in the clinic.

Digital props can also be made from silicone gum (Fig. 11.23) or from pre-prepared leather-covered foam props. Care must be taken with single toe loops, especially where toes swell or circulation is less than satisfactory.

Forefoot

All the forefoot pads previously described may be constructed as replaceable pads. Tubipad offers a method of protection as an elasticated bandage and can be trimmed from a roll. This is essentially a 'Tubigrip' (Seton) with a polyurethane open-cell foamed uncovered lining. This is a temporary cushioning material and is amenable to adhesive padding additionally attached to its foam surface.

Leather-covered stock pads are available in many shapes as arch fillers, metatarsal pads or domes. Toe and tarsal loops are used to keep the pad securely attached to the foot. Many of these systems have been unpopular amongst practitioners because of their lack of specificity. Foam and felt replaceable pads made in the clinic still have a place (Fig. 11.24). The figure illustrates one of many designs that can be covered by thin leather. Temporary forms may use Tubegauz for toe loops instead of elastic.

Silipos materials are also available as covered and uncovered gels. The benefit is the same as stated previously, except that the thin dimensions and potential for compensating for loss of adipose tissue across

the metatarsal heads make it highly desirable for a wide range of patients.

A cheap range of forefoot pads is available in the form of a latex foam pad from Scholl. Frequently, these pads are inadequate for the medically compromised foot problem. The attachment relies on a single toe loop and therefore is less likely to stay in position. The material used has a limited life and is easily abraded by the shoe. Tight toe loops are a distinct disadvantage and should not be used in patients with poor pedal circulation.

Valgus pads. Valgus pads as arch fillers have been found to be valuable for fascial strain, as previously mentioned. Where the practitioner wants to use an arch filler for a functional purpose, these are best designed on an insole base. Arch fillers are available with single tarsal loops, although many traditional practitioners still design their own where appropriate facilities exist.

Heel padding

Traditionally the practitioner would adhere foam to an insole template for the treatment of plantar heel pain. Padding designed for the heel may come in the form of a flat or a cupped pad. Figure 11.25 illustrates some of the stock designs available. The heel may need plantar or retrocalcaneal protection, and appro-

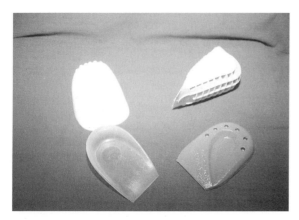

Figure 11.25 Forms of heel pad: Viscolas, stippled heel cup (Comed), Tuli heel and Wonderzorb (Silipos) with variable density centre.

priate selection must be based on its individual quality. Simple foam inserts exist for the heel and can be found at most large stores, often from the Scholl counter.

Viscolas (Orthopaedic Systems) can be used for central heel pain in ambulant patients, as the centre is designed to be removed. Elasticated Tubipad and Silipos can be used in patients who are sedentary. The pad is incorporated around the heel and held in place as an elasticated dressing. Silipos around the heel is not recommended for walking but does offer some retrocalcaneal protection. There is a wide and interesting range of heel cup products and they vary from a simple pre-formed polyethylene cup to the Tuli pad which has a waffle network that collapses on pressure. The waffle was designed by a podiatrist in the USA to mimic the fat pad structure.

Complex and much more expensive forms of heel pad are available and these often incorporate Achilles tendon pads, as well as protecting the malleoli (Bauerfeind). Bauerfeind and Silopad (soft silicone as Wonderzorb) offer cup-type pads with centres of variable density. Viscolas fairs less well despite its popularity amongst orthopaedic departments—the reason for this is that it is recommended to be used only with a single pair of shoes because of its highly tacky undersurface. The side that comes into contact with the foot has a fabric covering to prevent adhesion.

Insoles

The insole starts life as a simple cardboard template taken from the insock outline of a shoe. The advantage of an insole, with a pad adhered under a cover, is

that its position is maintained by the shoe, thus avoiding the need for foot straps. The disadvantage of insoles, however, arises from the need to ensure that placement in the shoe is correctly aligned with the foot and the difficulty in ensuring patient compliance. Patients who have more than one pair of shoes need more than one insole.

Template making

The outline of the insock area of the shoe is carefully trimmed in cardboard until it fits accurately. Using a felt-tipped pen, relevant bony landmarks and lesions are highlighted on the plantar surface of the foot (see Figs 12.6B and C, p. 224); the complete shape of the pad-to-be may be drawn in this way, if required. The insole is then sprayed with a liquid, such as a spirit-based pre-operative skin cleanser. The foot, or feet (if two are being replicated), is then placed in the shoe(s) and the patient is requested to walk a dozen or so steps. The shoes are removed and the felt-tipped pen markings are observed, having been transferred to the insole. The spirit-based liquid dries quickly and the forefoot pad can now be drawn accurately onto the cardboard template and sent away to a laboratory (as a prescription), or, alternatively, a pad can be adhered directly to the template which now becomes the insole base. To complete the insole, the pad is covered with non-stretch strapping, e.g. Mefix, which can then be lightly dusted with talcum powder. The foot can now slide into the shoe with the covered padding offering less resistance.

A more accurate method of obtaining a clearly marked base for the insole involves a more dynamic impression. Any base material may be used but 3 mm Plastazote is particularly suitable as it compresses well. This is inserted into the shoe unaltered, and when the patient returns after a period of use, a clear imprint is formed in the soft material, thus indicating precisely the required position of the padding.

Another method of chairside insole construction is described by Kippen (1982b). An impression on a base material is obtained as previously described. A pad is then adhered to this impression using double-sided tape. This method allows the use of those more durable padding materials traditionally associated with the construction of long-term orthoses. Double-sided tape is again used to adhere a covering material such as Yampi. This is a longer-term form of device which is constructed easily and quickly in a chairside form.

The heel pad adhered to a card base still has a useful place in the clinic, as does the Cobra pad. The latter is illustrated in Fig. 15.9 (p. 311) and serves as a useful short-term antipronatory insole prior to selecting stock or prescription orthoses. High density (high

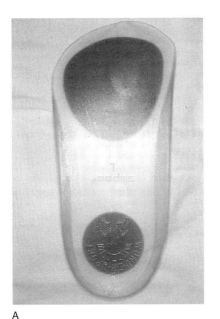

A

durometer) felt is used to form a wedge at the heel; this extends forward, incorporating a valgus-type filler. In busy practices, however, the use of the Frelon insole (Mediforce; Figs 11.26B and D) offers a cheap time- and cost-effective method providing similar assistance to the foot. This useful stock insole is well designed and is used frequently by many practitioners, since it lasts well, is easy to cut to shape (Fig. 11.26B) and is offered in six basic sizes. Unfortunately, no small sizes exist for children. Wedging, now purchased in sheets, can be obtained and tilted in varus, with a 2° and 4° canting (Fig. 11.26D). Once adhered to the Frelon or any similar base, the mechanical effect of wedging on the foot offers considerable orthotic control. Stock orthoses are worth trying as a first line attempt before turning to prescription orthoses.

Three designs of stock orthosis have recently become available in the UK. The Alphathotic (UK distributors, Nova Instruments) is a dense polyurethane orthosis (Fig. 11.26C) and comes as a basic shell to which EVA can be adhered. Sizes are available for children.

The AOL orthosis (Fig. 11.27; UK distributors, CPL) is an Australian-designed EVA-type orthosis which can be suitably wedged/posted using pre-formed

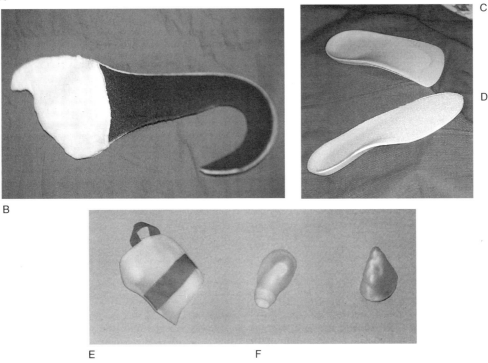

B

C

D

E   F

Figure 11.26 A: Wonderzorb (Silipos). B: Frelon trimmed to fit shoe, with felt extension added. C: Alphathotic. D: Stock premoulded orthosis. E: Plastazote clinically constructed plantar cover. F: Digital Plastazote cover with padding sandwiched between Plastazote.

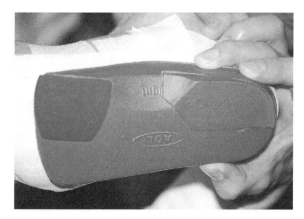

Figure 11.27 AOL. A stock orthosis with an in-built 4° varus heel to which forefoot and rearfoot wedging can be added by heat-moulding or adhesive backing. Three densities are available, red, green and blue, red being the most dense and blue the least dense.

wedges, but these need to be adhered again. The basic shell is canted to 4° initially. Three colour coded densities assist practitioner selection.

The MBS or Multi-Balance System (Langer Biomechanics Group) is formed in hard plastic and has clip-on wedges which fit pre-drilled holes for a snap-on fit. Valgus and varus wedges are created by reversing the direction of the wedge, making this system very flexible. No adhesive is required and wedges (posts) can be altered between 2° and 4°. Each MBS pack comes complete with eight wedge/post variations, whereas the AOL device wedges have to be purchased separately.

The Alphathotic and AOL orthoses have a heel cup of moderate height and will not fit all shoes, but they are available in a range of sizes, including children's sizes. The MBS comes in a wide range of sizes above size 3. The manufacturers claim that these off-the-peg orthoses can be customised.

Because of the flexibility of these and other stock systems, which are part of an ever-growing market of competitors for prescription-casted orthoses, cost is likely to be a key factor in their favour.

Stock and modular insoles

This section would not be complete without indicating some of the newer orthoses and insoles available. These differ from the previous orthoses in that they have no moulded heel cup and a minimal arch (valgus) filler.

Wonderzorb soft silicone (Silipos) orthoses, Tuli insoles (Mercury's Shadows) and Viscoped (Bauerfeind)

have all been developed as an extension of their heel pad and cup designs.

Few studies have been undertaken to evaluate the effectiveness of insoles, although the Frelon-type systems are becoming the standard against which comparisons are made. Many gimmicks have been marketed in newspapers, such as the water-filled insole, which displaces with each footstep to reduce forefoot load. Another innovation is an orthosis which is injected with fast-setting resinous compound material. The advantage of this product is its instant adjustability for clinical use.

A small number of modular manufacture systems exist which can be costly to set up initially and time-consuming to use in a busy department, unless an orthotist is available to support this kind of activity. Nonetheless, these systems have a particular role to

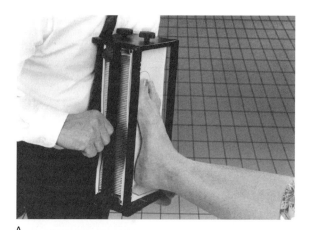

A

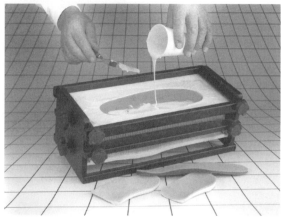

B

Figure 11.28 The Irving Insole Device in use. A: Taking the impression. B: Filling with liquid resin. (Reproduced with permission from Taylor Therapy.)

play, as they can be formed to each patient's specific foot shape; one of these, the Irving Insole Device (Taylor's therapy), is illustrated in Figure 11.28.

Discussion

Where time and resources are available, the practitioner can still offer the patient a chairside appliance. Companies such as Footman make a wide selection of pre-moulded pads which can be adhered to a base of the practitioner's choosing. Leather insoles are still available, with valgus fillers and ready-placed metatarsal pads. Experience is the only real basis on which to make a sensible selection.

SILICONES AND MOULDED THERMOPLASTIC ORTHOSES

Silicone moulds

This group of thermoset orthoses gained popularity at the end of the 1970s and they are still a very popular method in the UK for managing digital lesions. Thermosetting plastics, once formed, cannot be reheated. Silicones (polysiloxanes) may also be used for HVO shields and for orthoses for the heel, and have even been advocated for forefoot padding on a non-cast insole (Garrow 1979). While silicone can be used to make up full foot orthoses, the greatest disadvantage lies in its weight. As seen in the previous chapter, silicones have rubber-like properties. In effect, this means that they compress without losing their original form, although they are often heavy and bulky in shoes. Silicones are a group of compounds whose properties are a blend of the silicates and paraffins, both of which are characterised by a considerable degree of chemical inertness (Ch. 10). They can be used on the skin without fear of allergic response.

Early products were adapted from dental denture liners and impression materials, e.g. the Verones coloured green and red, in which a catalyst was added to make the product set. Shrinkage following curing was less than 0.8%. While all modern silicones still require an additive, the modern generation of mouldable silicones are lighter and have greater tensile strength. The first silicones to be used in podiatry were fluid in composition and were mixed with a liquid catalyst. Once a hardener paste or catalyst has been added, the silicone forms a cross-linking thermoset material as the polysiloxane polymer undergoes cross-linking. Silicone devices are usually ready to use immediately, although some practitioners like to wait an hour to ensure adequate curing.

Indications

When adhesive dressings are undesirable because of irritation or because of inability to wash the affected part, a silicone digital device should be considered. The treatment may be curative with some callus and corn-type lesions, where the underlying pathology has not created chronic inflammatory change. The lesion should not be open or have any discharge. Open lesions should be dressed appropriately.

Silicone devices can be used as prostheses following digital amputation. The prosthesis can take the form of a simple toe wedge or a moulded toe(s) copied from the patient's contralateral foot (Ch. 12).

Orthodigita. Correction in younger patients can be applied to flexible deformities, especially those affecting the 2–5 toes. Black & Coates (1981) suggested that in young children deformities were conducive to manipulation, but this will depend upon the age that treatment commences. Soft tissues can be stretched by applying Davis's law. This states that as long as a tensile force is applied to the tight structure, some elongation will take effect (Ch. 15).

Protection. This is achieved by building the silicone around the area of maximum pressure and stress (Fig. 11.23). Continual use can provide impressive results and the treatment is quick and cost-effective despite the lack of good scientific research to support these observations. Protective silicones can be used as interdigital spacers, apical, dorsal and medial/lateral MTP joint protectives. Tight extensor tendons can be protected and holes fashioned to help distribute stress away from the traumatised area. Debridement of callus and corns should be undertaken after the mould is applied. The lesion is deemed to be better protected in this way because a natural depression is created.

Clinical application

Silicone elastomers can be applied either (1) during the phase transition, i.e. as the silicone changes from its free flowing malleable state to an elastic solid, or (2) before the phase transition begins. Whether using (1) or (2), the site of application must be clean and free from debris and the skin unbroken. The amount of paste or putty to be used should be measured. Putties (Otoform, Dreve) are more convenient to handle than products packaged in a free flowing viscous form, such as KE20. The amount required for the device prior to mixing is easier to gauge when it is in putty form. This is not possible with paste and the ability to assess amounts without wastage comes with experience. Generally it is better to begin with too much material and later discard the excess than to begin with too little. Some silicones, such as Verone 'RS' and 'G', will accept additional material following an initial set, while others, such as Otoform, will not. When using pastes, a measured amount is placed on a mixing board. It is usual to add a plasticiser at this stage. Baby oil or paraffin liquid is commonly used and the amount applied should not exceed more than about one-third of the paste. The oil acts as a plasticiser, making the silicone more malleable as it penetrates between the polymer chains and forces the molecules further apart. The strength may, however, decrease if an excessive amount is used. The catalyst is added following the plasticiser. Each brand of silicone carries its own instructions regarding the ratio of catalyst/putty (or paste) to be used. Catalyst is added until a uniform colour is produced; this normally takes about 30 seconds, although it may vary between brands. The mix is then applied to the foot and manipulated to the size and shape required.

When the paste is used, it is quickly spatulated together with the plasticiser and catalyst again for about 30 seconds. When the mix reaches a sticky consistency, it may be handled and placed in position on the foot and manipulated.

Setting times will be affected by the amount of catalyst used and the room temperature—the higher the room temperature, the quicker the set. Hot water can accelerate the setting process. Individual manufacturer's instructions should be followed to achieve the optimum strength of cure by accurately mixing the catalyst. Once set, minor alterations may be made using a power burr.

The manufacture of HVO shields and heel cups require a larger surface area of silicone material. The mix used needs to be more liquid than solid, and this can be achieved before the phase transition begins. The application is easier at this point as the silicone flows more readily than during the phase transition. Application to the foot is made with a spatula in a direction where the bulk of the device is needed.

Discussion

While cost-effective, silicones will not help every patient. Silicones are not designed to correct hallux deformities, and bulky designs are often rejected by patients, while thin designs tear easily. Catalysts and their additives contain colouring; this can be a source of sensitivity in some patients. The practitioner should attempt to use a thin construction, protecting the lesion at the point of maximum stress by increasing the thickness. Correction of long standing, e.g. contracted toes such as digiti adductovarus, is less satisfactory. Silicone material offers poor tensile stretch to tissues but excellent resilience to compression. Often bulk is used to achieve adequate strength. This product has a shelf life and careless storage can have an adverse effect.

Thermoplastics

Thermoplastics are materials which can be remoulded and shaped. This group of plastics offers a number of advantages for the production of orthoses, with the potential for clinical adjustment as needed; heat guns are useful when making adjustments.

Low-temperature thermoplastics are particularly valuable in that they do not require expensive ovens. Perhaps the best-known of these plastics are Hexcelite and Aquaplast, which were among the first of this type of material to be given a podiatric application.

Hexcelite is made up of a cotton mesh impregnated with a thermoplastic resin. Initially marketed as a splint material, it can be regarded as a semi-rigid plastic (Smedley 1982) and has been used as heel cups to protect pressure sores (Woods 1982), as functional devices for biomechanical disorders (Smedley 1982), in the management of hallux rigidus (Monaghan 1984), and as resting splints for foot drop (Hicks & McFetridge 1993).

Hexcelite is a light, durable easy-to-use material in the clinic. Although thermally stable up to at least 200°C, it only needs to be heated to 72°C to become pliable. As it is not associated with an exothermic reaction, it can be moulded directly to the foot. The desensitised foot may need to be protected with a tubular bandage. The working time is about 3 minutes, by which time it will have regained its semi-rigid qualities. Modifications are easily carried out by re-warming. Upon heating it is self-bonding, so that thickness can be increased as required. The mesh construction ensures good ventilation, negating any potential perspiration problems. The only heat source required is a container of hot water. The manufacturer claims that the product has an indefinite shelf life.

Disadvantages associated with Hexcelite include cost. It is made expensive by the fact that construction time is increased with the need to line the device to avoid skin irritation and damage to hosiery.

Aquaplast has similar qualities to Hexcelite. It is solid rather than having a mesh form, and is off-white in colour, becoming translucent, and workable, when heated. It softens at a lower temperature than Hexcelite, about 60°C, and takes slightly longer to become rigid, the amount of time varying with the thickness of Aquaplast used. Aquaplast has been compared with rigid high-temperature thermoplastics and was found to be superior in terms of its convenience of construction (Kippen 1982a).

Foamed thermoplastics

Materials in common use include Plastazote and Evazote. Plastazote is a closed-cell, cross-linked expanded polyethylene. Evazote is ethyl vinyl acetate, a closed-cell cross-linked copolymer foam, and is marginally softer than Plastazote.

When preheated to a temperature of 140°C, those materials are readily moulded to contours of the foot. Although they may be directly moulded to the skin, it is wise, initially, to cover the desensitised foot with a tubular bandage. On rapid cooling, the moulded shape is retained. Rapid cooling necessitates a high level of dexterity and swift action in moulding if reheating is to be avoided. The rate of heat loss is dependent on the thickness of the material and the room temperature. Reheating does allow the materials to return to their original shape.

Auto-adhesion. At 140°C these thermoplastics are auto-adhesive upon compression, but below this temperature this quality is lost and an adhesive such as Neoprene is required. High-temperature, non-rigid foamed thermoplastics also have a part to play, although only high-density forms last. Two pieces of Plastazote of different densities can be combined by auto-adhesion, as shown in Figure 12.21 (p. 236). In this way, properties of both low- and high-density foams combine to offer a soft contour with stiff infrastructure to prevent collapse. This type of modification produces an orthosis that lasts longer than one of softer low-density material alone.

Plastazote is chemically inert and may be applied to the foot without fear of skin irritation. As insulators, polyethylene foams are extremely effective in preventing heat loss from the foot. Plastazote material is often prescribed as an accommodative orthosis which serves to protect against chilblains. On the other hand, this is a disadvantage in the case of patients with hyperhidrosis, necessitating the creation of ventilation holes if an alternative material is not considered.

Orthoses made in the clinic from Plastazote or Evazote are quick to produce and can often be made as chairside appliances; such devices are inexpensive, but resilience is comparatively low and re-fabrication is often necessary. Both types of material may be used for lining devices constructed from other materials such as Hexcelite. The versatility of Plastazote is demonstrated by the fact that it is used in the construction of orthoses for all areas of the foot. Plastazote may be used to mould arch fillers on simple insoles or to produce orthoses from casts with heel cups. Plastazote has been used for toe props and protection of hallux valgus in the past, and can be quickly moulded to shape (Figs 11.26E and F). Additional material can also be sandwiched between the Plastazote to offer greater protective or functionally corrective properties.

SUMMARY

This chapter has considered the management of foot problems with dressings, pads and a range of available stock orthoses which offer accommodation, rest, redistribution, stabilisation, immobilisation and compensation.

The whole area of clinical padding has received scant research and has been relegated to small clinical studies without controls. However, many materials and products have now been made available for easier dispensing, affording greater efficiency in the clinic. Further investigation is warranted if the practitioner is to remain vigilant, as the ever-increasing range of new products requires constant changes in practice.

REFERENCES

Black J A, Coates I S 1981 Silicones: their uses and development in chiropodial orthotic and prosthetic management. The Chiropodist 36: 237–251
Garrow A 1979 The silicone insole: a chairside appliance. The Chiropodist 34: 137–138
Hicks S, McFetridge L 1993 Foot drop resting splint. Orthopaedic Systems promotional literature
Kippen C 1982a Low temperature thermoplastics – application in chairside foot orthotics. The Chiropodist 37: 36–41

Kippen C 1982b The simple insole? The Chiropodist 37: 410–414
McCloskey P J 1992 A study of the effect of low dye taping on the foot. British Journal of Podiatric Medicine & Surgery 4(3): 6–9
Monaghan M M 1984 The use of Hexcellite in the management of hallux rigidus. The Chiropodist 39: 435–438
Shanks J 1991 Silopad – a clinical trial. The Chiropodist 46(10): 193–196

Smedley R 1982 The fabrication of a semi-rigid orthosis in Hecellite material. The Chiropodist 37: 338–340

Woods P 1982 The use of Hexcellite splinting material in the prevention and treatment of pressure sores occurrng on the feet. The Chiropodist 37: 333–335

FURTHER READING

Coates I S 1979 Silicone orthodigita: principles, aims and prognosis. The Chiropodist 34: 137–138

Kippen C 1989 Insoling materials in foot orthosis manufacture – a review. The Chiropodist 44: 83–87

12

Prescription orthoses

D. R. Tollafield
D. J. Pratt
K. Rome

INTRODUCTION

This chapter provides a broad insight into the principles underpinning prescription orthoses. The practitioner who prescribes orthoses needs to have a fundamental knowledge of mechanics and also of the properties of the materials that are used in their manufacture. In the absence of these, practioners will have difficulty in providing adequate solutions to the problems they meet.

A practitioner will justify the choice of a particular orthosis in terms of the benefit that is likely to be gained from it. A prescription can be determined once the clinician understands:

- normal lower extremity function (as a basic prerequisite)
- the origin of the biomechanical dysfunction
- the influence of the proximal limb on the foot
- the ideal material properties required of the orthosis
- the role of footwear in relation to the intended orthosis
- the psychological requirements of the patient.

The use of orthoses as part of mechanical therapy in the clinic can complement any programme of treatment. A prescription orthosis is produced from an impression, usually on an individual basis. Usually, they are required because there is no equivalent device available as a stock item or because the problem to be treated does not lend itself to stock materials, as their physical properties cannot achieve the desired effect.

Functional orthoses have already been described in Chapter 10. In this chapter, we will discuss the ways in which the forces applied to the foot are incorporated into their design (Lundeen 1988).

Orthoses described in this chapter fall into three main categories—*digital, foot* and *ankle foot orthoses*

(AFO)—and may bear some similarity to those described in Chapter 11. In the case of AFOs, there are few stock orthoses available that offer satisfactory functional control. The majority of the principles and designs described in this chapter fall into the 'rigid' category, which refers to the firm plastic shells or orthotic plates that form the basis of control and allow additional material to be incorporated into their design.

The term *prescription* is used to describe the situation where a mould of the foot or of the foot and leg is referred to a laboratory with a written prescription attached from the practitioner or orthotist, and the orthosis is dispensed at a later consultation. No attempt will be made to describe manufacture, partly because this is not the aim of this chapter and partly because the manufacturing process requires a clear manual of instruction which can best be found in other texts, such as Bowker et al (1993), Wu (1990), Philps (1990), Spencer (1978) and Sgarlato (1971).

The hindfoot or midtarsal components of a functional orthosis are easily modified. The necessary changes may be achieved simply by altering a plaster cast. The incorporation of extensions and posts (the latter are used to pitch an orthosis in an everted or inverted direction) may be best achieved by combining a number of different materials, e.g. acrylic (PMMA), EVA and foamed polyurethane, such that their individual properties are used to greatest effect.

Prostheses are introduced in this chapter because they have a clear prescriptive function as well as a contribution to make in controlling unstable feet with poor prognoses. Prostheses can be used to make up for a deficit in foot function, often associated with amputation, as well as to provide a better foot outline for fitting a standard shoe, thus avoiding the need for bespoke footwear (Figs 12.1A and B). Of course, many bespoke shoes are made in order to accommodate complicated prostheses, but these fall outside the scope of this book.

DIGITAL ORTHOSES

The number of digital problems that rely upon prescription management are becoming fewer, because of the clinical modalities that are available, as already described in Chapter 11. Tollafield (1985) discusses the manufacture of latex digita, but these devices are no longer popular because they often cause more

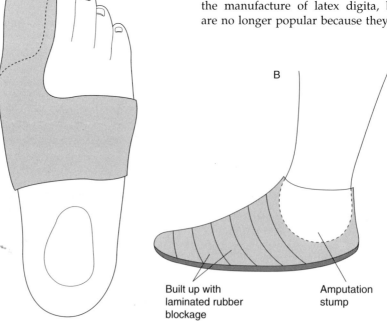

A

B

Built up with
laminated rubber
blockage

Amputation
stump

Figure 12.1 Prostheses. A: Prosthesis for amputation in a case where the foot was involved in a railway accident affecting the whole first ray. B: Prosthesis for post-Syme's amputation after reconstructive surgery following Buerger's disease of the whole foot.

problems than they alleviate, due to the fact that the interaction between latex and skin is less satisfactory than that between skin and other materials.

There are two types of prescription orthosis worthy of particular mention: the digital prosthetic and the hallux orthosis. Both can be combined with other orthotic designs depending upon their desired function.

Indications

Once the structural integrity and functional efficiency of the forefoot becomes impaired because of digital dysfunction, a variety of pathologies can result which would benefit from orthotic management.

Lesions. Dorsal lesions over the IP joints or apices may develop as a result of hammer toes. Patients may benefit from orthodigita. Redistribution and accommodation are essential to prevent tissue damage over a joint prominence.

Prosthetic function. Toes that have been amputated will subsequently allow adjacent toes to deform into the remaining gap. A replacement digital prosthesis can be made for either single or multiple toes, or, if necessary, a whole forefoot cover can be made. Toes are often associated with massive dislocation at the metatarsophalangeal joints (MTPJs) in severe arthritides, and they lose their spring in gait. A prosthesis offers not only a better 'toe-off' action, but also improves shoe fit. Metatarsal head areas may require cushioning and the plantar material may be extended back under the foot to improve shock attenuation.

Prophylactic protection. The hallux may require a prescription orthosis to prevent recurrence of ulcers in diabetics. A hallux shield can be extended to protect the medial eminence and to deflect shear forces from the plantar interphalangeal joint (IPJ), often associated with a spur or accessory ossicle.

Dysfunction from a hallux rigidus can create pressure over IPJ and MTPJ areas. If footwear cannot be adapted to rock over the great toe joint, a hallux orthosis may provide better propulsion and protection at the same time.

Replication technique

Material

The orthotic laboratory requires sufficient detail to avoid guesswork. The favoured materials include alginate moulding (DeTrey—Dentsply, Zantalgin), as alginate offers greater skin detail as well as making the mould easy to remove because of the material's plasticity (Ch. 10). Plaster of Paris bandage may be used for large areas that need to be captured.

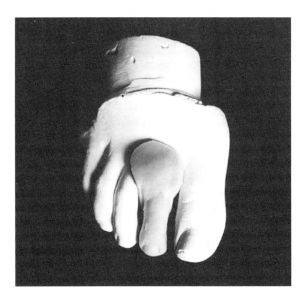

Figure 12.2 A prosthetic toe has been created using a normal toe encased in alginate for detail. The forefoot has been casted separately in alginate and plaster.

Plaster of Paris (POP) bandage is used with alginate to achieve adequate detail around the toes and to support the alginate impression material. A gap must be left for the finished prosthetic toe (Fig. 12.2). The opposite foot provides an accurate impression of the missing toe. If this is deformed or also missing, another patient may consent to being casted.

The alginate is mixed according to the instructions provided; some products may vary but each includes graduated scoop spoons and tumblers. Alginate dries quickly and then shrinks, rendering the technique useless if this is not prevented with moisture. A small hole can be made at the end of the toe to allow any air to be forced out upon filling with plaster of Paris; in this way the end of the digit is not distorted by an air bubble.

Plaster can be used alone but does not offer the same detail as alginate. When it is used alone, greater preparation in the laboratory may be necessary.

This combined casting technique using both POP and alginate can be adopted for any part of the forefoot, including the great toe. The practitioner must bear in mind that it is important to have sufficient proximal detail to form a good base for the prosthetic toe. The cast must therefore be extended back as far as is reasonable. In the case of replacement toes, silicones are used to obtain greater detail. A mixture of KE.20 and Verone RS is used to allow a liquid fill, the Verone RS providing the flesh coloration. When the toe is worn under stockings or tights, it is often indistinguishable from the unaffected foot. This is a device which is expensive but ideal for patients who wear sandals frequently.

Single toes

Replicating digits is achieved by using a 'dummy' silicone toe which has been casted from a suitable 'donor', usually the opposite foot.

Multiple toe prosthesis

Figures 12.3A and B illustrate the use of a leather moccasin prosthesis to compensate for the congenital loss of toes (phocomelia). Although the toes are shorter than in normal feet, foam digital prostheses allow the toe box to fill out adequately. The benefit, as previously stated, is that this creates a snug fit for the foot in the shoe, as well as preventing slippage. The laboratory will make these prostheses as leather or half-latex devices. A latex outerskin provides an element of washability. The prescription should state the material preferred and whether the device is to have ventilation perforations.

Hallux and first MTPJ

Paraffin wax sheets for taking bite impressions can be used to make a bunion shield. This thin material only needs to be immersed in water at 40°C before it can be comfortably moulded around the first metatarsophalangeal joint, with no need to protect the skin from heat. The open edges are pinched around the toe and the whole cast is removed, retaining its shape. It is then instantly ready to be filled with plaster powder mix. Bunion shields from thermoplastics, leather and latex can be manufactured after preparing a plaster model.

Foot prosthesis

A whole foot can be made into a moccasin prosthesis (Fig. 12.1B). This device will provide a block of foam rubber which often obviates the need for orthopaedic footwear as stock shoes can be worn. A full foot cast must be taken—the description given here can be applied generally for a number of foot impressions.

The impression is taken using either alginate, for easy removal, or plaster, bivalved or spirally casted (see 'Ankle foot orthoses', p. 244). The bivalve technique is very useful where the practitioner wishes to avoid a knife or cast cutter. Two-four ply plaster bandage is applied with the patient lying supine on the couch.

The posterior leg bandage is applied first and an obvious ledge is made as shown in Figures 12.4A and B. This hardens and the ledge is smeared with a simple emollient to allow separation. The anterior section is placed over the first, marrying the second ledge to the posterior section. Once set, the cast can be split easily along the seam. The seams are then sealed

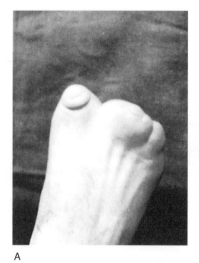 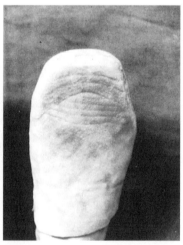

A   B

Figure 12.3 Multiple toe prosthesis. A: The foot has abnormally shortened toes as a result of developmental failure. B: The finished leather moccasin prosthesis which has a latex foam infill for the toes.

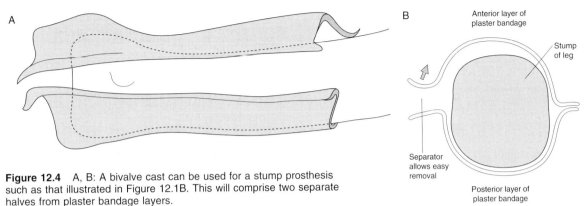

Figure 12.4 A, B: A bivalve cast can be used for a stump prosthesis such as that illustrated in Figure 12.1B. This will comprise two separate halves from plaster bandage layers.

with more bandage, the cast is labelled with the patient's name, date of casting and the practitioner's name, and it is dried naturally. If alginate is selected, it must be stored wet and supported with plaster bandage encased in bubble wrapper.

The cast cannot be sent off to the laboratory until a replica of the insock has been cut out of cardboard or regenerated leatherboard. This will provide the laboratory with the width. The girth can either be supplied as toe box, height and girth measurements across the metatarsals and midfoot, or a cast can be taken of the inside of the shoe.

Casting the shoe. This is undertaken with plaster fill, mixing powder with water and placing the mix into a strong plastic bag. The shoe is replicated and the laboratory staff thus have an accurate model to follow.

Prescription

In addition to taking personal details from the patient and noting specific points required to provide foot dimensions, the practitioner should decide on the materials and request any additions on the same form. Using an experienced orthopaedic or podiatric orthotist can make a great difference as far as avoiding problems associated with poor fit.

Prostheses must be made from material which avoids friction at graft sites and scars or areas that have poor circulation. Where loss of muscle has arisen due to injury, the lack of bulk tissue overlying stumps will have to be supplemented with additional hydrogel protection such as second skin (Spenco) or Silipos covers, which are made to fit the lower limb. All materials selected should be light but durable.

After the positive cast preparation, the cast is covered with chamois. Where seams are employed, it is important to ensure that they do not come into contact with amputation scars, as this can cause irri-

tation to the suture line. The seams will be reinforced by the laboratory for added strength.

Diagrams and written itemised details are helpful, especially where small variations in design are anticipated.

Discussion

Ulceration and gangrenous changes may be averted in digits by considering a digital prosthesis. Replacements should be ordered before any previous prescription deteriorates. Patients will become dependent on their prostheses and they will be unhappy if relieved of them, albeit temporarily, in order to make a copy. Keep all casts and details as necessary unless footwear changes are anticipated. Patients are advised to use similar styles of footwear, wherever possible, to avoid incurring additional costs.

FOOT ORTHOSES

The field of foot orthoses forms a very large part of the foot specialist's work. The available prescriptions are divided into *insoles* and *functional orthoses*. Insoles play a less important role than functional orthoses and as such they will be illustrated but not described in any detail. Nonetheless, insoles do have a role to play, and circumstances may dictate the need to offer patients a range of orthotic designs based on an insole system which uses manufactured pads shaped to the practitioner's requirements.

INSOLES

The greatest advantage of insoles lies in their low cost. Thin 1.5 mm polypropylene sheets have been used for insole bases, with wedges of EVA to reduce base deterioration by decomposition—a common problem associate with insoles. Unfortunately, even these functional designs will fill the toe box of many styles of shoe. Casted orthoses finish behind the metatarsals instead of running the full length, and therefore fit into more than one pair of shoes more easily.

Designs of insole

Ten insole variations are illustrated in Figure 12.5. Each design comprises a stiff or soft insole base. Materials include a firm neoprene (Spenco), latex foam rubber or polyurethane foam pad (Poron, Cleron).

Composite materials

The use of different materials combined offers a variety of properties in a single insole. Firm polyurethane foams can be mixed with foam latex rubber buttons to produce cushioning and compensation, with redistribution or accommodation around rigid deformities on the sole. The use of wedged EVA will provide an element of realignment.

Many of the designs suggested have been described in Chapter 11 and will not be described again.

Replication technique

Templates for insoles have already been described for chairside appliances. One problem with taking templates is the poor correlation that is afforded when marking lesion sites. Ink paper Shu-Track and mats such as Harris-Beath mats offer alternative dynamic systems of acquiring information for use in bespoke manufacture (Fig. 12.6A).

The Shu-Track system comes in the form of a sandwich consisting of a top sheet to walk on, a transfer sheet to provide the ink, and a bottom sheet on which the image is formed. There may be an additional transparent sheet which is used to cover the resulting image to prevent smudging and to allow incorporation in the case notes. The individual sheets come in the form of a roll which can be laid on the floor so that the subject being studied can walk on a number of them to obtain a realistic representation of their angle and base of gait. The footprint shows a composite picture of the plantar pressure history but does not indicate where in the gait cycle the pressures peaked. However, this image, together with an examination of the subject, will often be sufficient for a foot orthosis to be made. The drawback of this system

is that it is quite expensive, although it is quick and clean. Cheaper variants are now available under different trade names.

Prescribing

Specific information should be recorded, as shown in Figures 12.6B and C:

- date, patient's name, practitioner and clinic
- metatarsal head positions
- limits for padded additions, such as styloid process, toe sulci, navicular and central heel point
- lesions (areas of callus, IPK, verrucae, cysts)
- materials required, thickness, density, pad, insole base and stiffener
- position of materials, drawn onto template
- relevant shoe information.

Discussion

Insoles are formed on a soft or hard base and may have a short life of 6–9 months. Three-quarter length (to metatarsal head) orthoses taken from plaster casts appear to have a greater success rate due to improved shoe fit. As previously mentioned in Chapter 11, many new stock items have made insole therapy redundant. While some research work has been carried out into the scientific value of this type of orthosis, the greater part of study has involved the shock attenuation properties, as these are more easily measured. Insoles with redistribution pads rarely remove the long-standing plantar lesion, but they do minimise the load over specific points, thereby reducing symptoms.

CASTED ORTHOSES

The step from the insole to the casted orthosis is largely emphasised by the need to increase foot control, particularly pronation. The cost increases because of the need to take an impression (casting to produce negative plates), and because there are clinical costs and laboratory charges (manufacture). Many types of orthosis exist; two main categories are considered—the functional orthosis and the accommodative orthosis. The most common orthotic designs are described below, under general headings: standard foot orthosis, high/low profile orthoses, heel orthoses and, the latest addition, talar control orthoses.

The functional orthosis

The use of the term 'functional' implies that an orthosis will restore the time sequence associated with

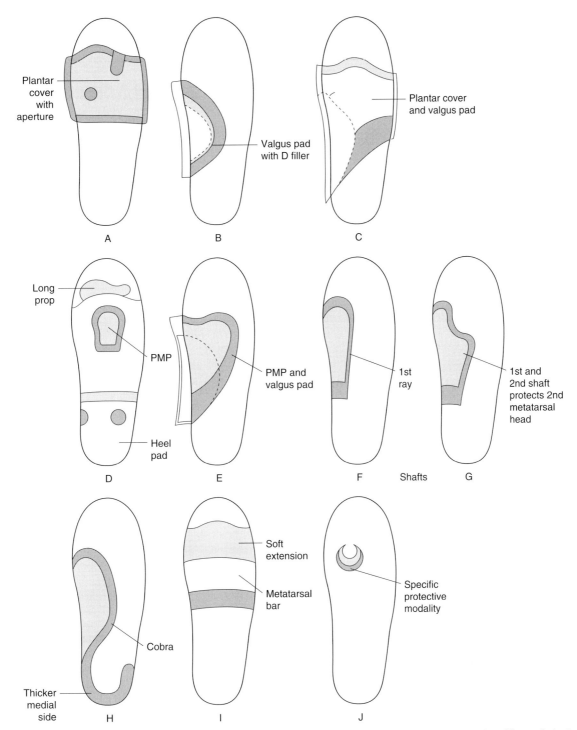

Figure 12.5 Insole designs suitable for manufacture. A, plantar cover; B, valgus filler; C, combined valgus filler and plantar cover; D, long prop and PMP combined with a heel pad with two point cut-outs for pressure distribution; E, PMP combined with valgus filler; F, first ray shaft; G, shaft extended as L pad; H, the successful Cobra pad comprising heel meniscus and valgus filler; I, metatarsal bar with soft extension to toe sulci combining cushioning with redistribution; J, insole showing simple crescentic redistribution pad; any shaped design can be used alternatively as in (J).

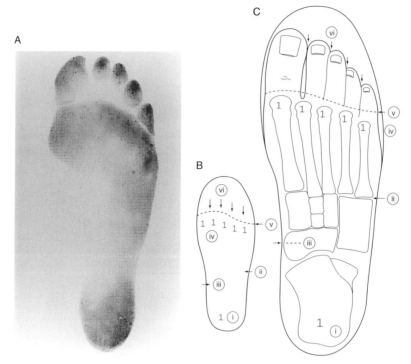

Figure 12.6 A: Insole template used to manufacture a bespoke orthosis from a patterned and inked rubber mat. B: Information is transferred from the foot onto a cardboard base cut around the inside of the shoe, recording: (i) heel centre, (ii) base of fifth metatarsal, (iii) level with navicular, (iv) metatarsal head centres, (v) toe sulci, (vi) interdigital spacing. C: Points (i)–(iv) recorded onto the cardboard template for laboratory manufacture.

ground contact by reducing abnormal compensation as a result of foot pathology.

The purpose behind the functional orthosis has been described by many authors, too numerous to cite; suffice to say that this is not a new innovation. The orthosis is produced from a cast or impression of the foot in order to reproduce the contour of the foot in a neutral position. The reason for adopting a neutral position around the subtalar joint (STJ) is associated with the belief that the foot creates an ideal functional platform during *midstance*. Some authors believe that this theory is flawed and that a position of inversion might be more appropriate during casting. Many different views are held and as long as the laboratory receives adequate instructions, then any orthosis should be able to satisfy the practitioner's prescription requirements.

However, one advantage to be gained by taking the impression in STJ neutral is that a useful comparison can then be drawn between the clinical measurement (foot) and the cast alignment after replication, namely the extent of varus and valgus deformity.

Unless there is an obvious valgus or varus, the heel contour will not pick up the minor deformity. The neutral negative plate provides information about forefoot relationship only. Naturally, no rearfoot-to-leg relationship exists once the cast has been removed from the foot. Supinatus, a triplane forefoot deformity similar to forefoot varus, cannot be detected either.

Accommodative orthosis

Accommodative orthoses occupy a position between clinical therapies (Ch. 11) and prescription therapies. The terms so described need clarification: 'clinical' means that the orthosis can be wholly dispensed as part of the patient's treatment at the time of consultation, while 'prescription' implies that the orthosis will be sent away to be fitted on a further consultation.

The Irving Insole Device (Taylor Therapy) is an example of an orthosis that can be dispensed within a single clinical visit.

Accommodative prescriptive orthoses are made

from casted plaster models, as are functional orthoses, although the practitioner may select a wider variety of techniques than the neutral technique. This type of orthosis usually has a softer design and is made to cushion and protect areas where considerable pressure builds up.

Orthotic designs and specifications

As the selection is very wide, only a few designs will be described to illustrate the varying specifications. Modifications to these orthoses will be elaborated upon later in the chapter.

Standard foot orthoses

The most common types of orthosis are Root and Shafer. The Shafer orthosis predated the Root orthosis in the UK. The plate was trimmed to provide a heel cup with sufficient depth to assist rearfoot control, and therefore flared medially with a moderate arch height, although one that was lower than the UCBL device. The application of a lateral modification or addition prevented any sharp edges sticking into the foot (see under 'Prescriptions', p. 233). The Shafer system used extrinsic posts (Fig. 12.7A).

The Root orthosis (Fig. 12.7B) adopted a number of modifications called 'additions' in order to provide a good shoe fit, as well as selecting an intrinsic forefoot post system. Originally, the Root heel cup was lower than its predecessor.

High profile orthoses

The UCBL orthosis, designed at the University of California Biomechanics Laboratory, from which its name is derived, has a very deep heel cup, and the lateral and medial sides of the orthosis extend equally up either side of the foot (Figs 12.8A–C; Mereday et al 1972). No medial or lateral additions are used and the device offers the ultimate foot orthotic control for marked pronation. Posts can be applied to the polypropylene plate, although success will depend heavily upon shoe designs accepting this type of orthosis.

The standard orthotic productions follow Root and Shafer designs (Fig. 12.7). These consist of a plate which is shaped to conform to most Oxford shoe designs, although it may need to be made narrower for Court shoe designs.

Low profile orthoses

Langer Laboratories has, without doubt, had the greatest influence on the world market and has single-handedly innovated many design changes to assist shoe fit. Their Halfthotic™ has an interesting trim based on the Cobra insole (Fig. 12.9). The lateral portion of plastic is removed, leaving a well-trusted shape proximally, similar to the Rose-Schwartz meniscus. The orthosis is strengthened with EVA and offers an effective design without losing key components for high-heeled shoes and for shoes in which it is difficult to fit the full orthotic plate.

Talar control foot orthoses

Pratt et al (1993a) described an innovative orthosis from the US. The resulting shape, illustrated in Figure 12.10, is known as a talar control foot orthosis (TCFO; Brown et al 1987). The difference between this and other orthoses stems from the fact that the arch is not contoured. The orthosis has been designed from the viewpoint that control is better with a total dorsal contact foot orthosis. The cast technique for the TCFO is different from those described earlier. A spiral cast system is preferred, as for ankle foot orthoses (AFOs) which are described on page 244.

Heel orthoses

The heel cup has been described in Chapter 11 as being available as a stock item. Where a prescription orthosis is required, mainly to improve heel contour and rearfoot stability, fabrication will be made from

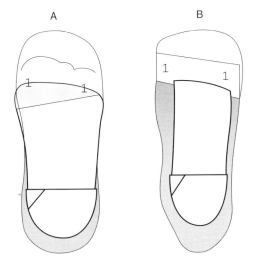

Figure 12.7 A: Root plate trim. B: Shafer plate trim shown on casts (adapted from Anthony 1992).

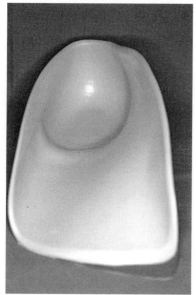

A

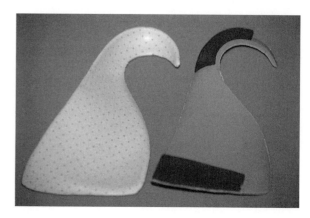

Figure 12.9 Low profile orthosis to allow for fitting in narrow, high-heeled shoes showing posting on one side.

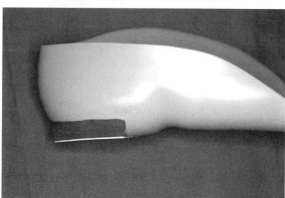

B

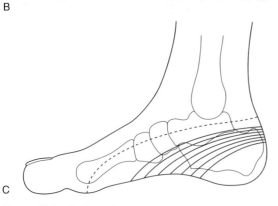

C

Figure 12.8 A: The UCBL. A small modification made over the cuboid attempts to prevent the calcaneocuboid joint subluxing. B: UCBL outline with rearpost. C: Trim lines conforming around the heel with a high specification to capture and control the sustentaculum tali. (Adapted from Pratt et al 1993b.)

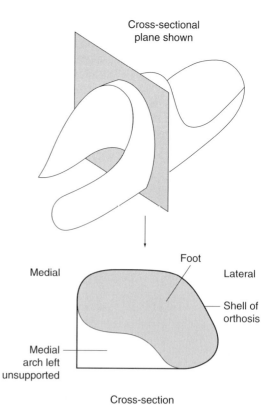

Cross-sectional plane shown

Foot

Medial   Lateral

Shell of orthosis

Medial arch left unsupported

Cross-section

Figure 12.10 The talar control foot orthosis (TCFO) is designed without direct arch contact. It must be taken using a spiral cast technique rather than a slipper-shaped cast. (Adapted from Pratt et al 1993b.)

a whole foot cast as previously described. The heel orthosis is valuable in children, where the practitioner does not wish to influence the developing forefoot. In adults, it can be used to enhance foot control without compromising the amount of space in the shoe.

Laboratories take the positive cast and can remove the anterior part of the orthosis once the material has been vacuum-formed.

One design involves the use of an extended medial arch, which can extend to either the first ray or the talonavicular joint. As many practitioners have different preferences, no detail is offered here regarding heel cup designs. As with the TCFO, casts can be adapted by having small areas of plaster removed, which in effect creates greater pressure against the foot. This resisting force can help to create further stability, especially around the sustentaculum tali.

Research

Despite the use of many modern materials in the production of foot orthoses, much of the research has been devolved to material sciences rather than looking at specific physical effects upon foot pathology. Tollafield & Pratt (1990a,b) looked at the effects of the Shafer and Root designs of functional orthosis on a normal foot, using pedobarographs, video filming and Kistler force plates (without synchronomy). Acrylic posts were used to angle the pressed plastic plate made from polymethylmethacrylate (PMMA). Little difference between the Shafer and Root plates was noted, except that the Root design offered greater shoe comfort. The trace taken from the Kistler force plate altered between the various angles of tilt, and the sensitivity between $0°$, $4°$ and $8°$ was difficult to interpret with any real significance. The fact that pressure was distributed differently was shown more clearly by the pedobarograph. The rearpost showed some off-loading of the forefoot, presumably due to its larger surface area.

Indications

The influence of the foot on the proximal skeletal structures is now slowly being accepted. It is clear from previous evidence that the subtalar joint has a profound relationship with the leg and that disruptions in its action do lead to proximal disorders (Inman 1969). The proportional knock-on effect of subtalar frontal plane motion on transverse plane motion within the leg and knee, and vice versa, emphasises that walking is more than just putting one foot in front of another. Any surface that can change the

ground contact relationship will influence rotational movement. These rotations are greater at the top of the leg, reducing movement in a distal direction. However, there are still considerable rotations at the ankle level. If, for example, the subtalar joint is immobile, for whatever reason, these rotations of the leg have to be accommodated elsewhere in the kinetic chain of the leg and trunk. If the ankle cannot cope with the extra rotation, the knee joint is affected next, with a change in the Q angle, causing patella tracking problems (D'Amico & Rabin 1986).

Orthoses function predominantly by reducing the effect of prolonged pronation. The aim of control is to restore the time sequence, i.e. to an acceptable pronation of about 25% of the stance phase when it reaches its optimum pronated position. During midstance, the leg can be influenced by an inlay appropriately balanced to ensure that the subtalar joint is supinated and continues supinating, with consequential external rotation of the leg until final propulsion.

Compensatory pronation at the subtalar joint everts the rearfoot and supination inverts the rearfoot. As the rearfoot moves, the forefoot will also move to remain in contact with the ground. The ability of the forefoot to fully compensate depends on there being sufficient joint motion, requiring inversion during subtalar pronation and eversion during subtalar supination. This midtarsal joint motion takes place largely about the longitudinal axis but is limited by its small range (Root et al 1977).

The effects of foot pathology do not stop at the knee; the hip is able to accommodate some of the rotation but will not then provide the motion needed for normal gait. Thus, gait changes follow an exaggerated transverse plane body rotation and create the need for shorter stride lengths. Conversely, if there are symptomatic problems in the proximal structures associated with excessive rotations, they may be addressed by controlling subtalar pronation or supination. This is more common in sporting activities, where every possible deficit is examined and treated in an attempt to improve performance.

A sagittal plane relationship exists between the foot and the proximal body structures. Principally, this is reflected in an equinus position of the foot and the ankle joint. If this position is fixed then the knee and hip must flex sufficiently to allow walking to take place, usually with the toe as the initial contact point between the foot and the ground. This requires an increase in muscle activity in the knee and hip extensors to stabilise the limb, which can tire rapidly. Additionally, discomfort can be experienced at the knee, particularly due to the much increased joint loading from the flexed position. This foot position can also lead to hip hiking (lifting up) and circumduction of the leg to obtain ground clearance if knee and hip flexion is not possible. All of these processes consume more energy than normal gait and can lead to arthritic changes later in life. Orthotic contribution can smooth out some of these determinants.

The subtalar joint (STJ) is the anatomical structure that is responsible for accommodating transverse rotations and it thus enables the leg to rotate on a fixed foot. By tilting the supporting orthotic platform, both midtarsal and proximal joint motions are influenced.

Flexible feet are characteristically easier to control than rigid feet. Nonetheless, the additional effects of abnormal axes within flexible feet can make orthotic control difficult. The foot can easily slip off the inlay despite careful manufacture, because a flexible foot with a high midtarsal joint oblique axis can move over the inlay within the shoe.

Marked rigidity is associated with limited joint movement and may be typified by a forefoot equinus, pes cavus or congenital talipes foot with triplane deformity. A rigid foot with fixed deformities may need to be accommodated with thin foam materials incorporating good shock-absorbing properties and forefoot extensions to reduce contact pressure. As with any orthotic design, good shoe fit is essential and, as part of good prescribing, both shoe and foot pathology must be considered.

Replication technique

Casts can be taken using POP in a variety of ways. Most common methods use non-weight-bearing techniques, with the foot in subtalar joint neutral (the neutral position cast) (Tollafield 1985, Anthony 1991); other techniques have the subtalar joint pronated or weight-bearing in a neutral position:

- *Non-weight-bearing techniques*
  —suspension technique, patient supine
  —modified suspension technique, patient prone
  —direct pressure technique, patient prone or supine
  —semi-pronated technique, patient prone or supine
  —fully pronated technique, patient prone or supine
  —vacuum casting in neutral (in the shoe)
- *Weight-bearing techniques*
  —semi-weight-bearing on a foam pad
  —foam impression (Birkenstock).

Suspension technique

This is the traditional way in which neutral foot casts

are taken. The patient is positioned in a supine (sitting or lying) relaxed position.

The practitioner's forearm, wrist and fingers are held in a straight line and placed over the dorsum of the foot, with the thumb in the sulcus of the fourth and fifth toes (Fig. 12.11). The advantage of the finger position lies in the fact that the cast contour is not deformed by thumb pressure. The foot is extended in order that some weight-bearing lengthening is created.

While holding the foot firmly, it is moved through its full range of subtalar pronation and supination, at the same time palpating the head of the talus (Fig. 12.12). When the medial and lateral prominences of the talar head are felt to be equal, the subtalar joint

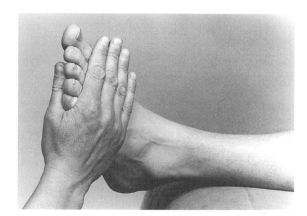

Figure 12.11 The foot is shown being held in subtalar joint neutral with the midtarsal joint maximally pronated and the ankle dorsiflexed. The leg is suspended over the couch. This is the initial position for holding the forefoot for the suspension technique with the patient supine.

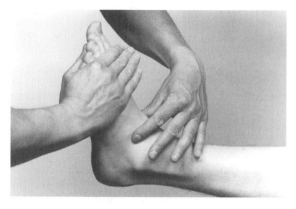

Figure 12.12 The head of the talus can be easily palpated in the supine position.

is thought to be in neutral. This can be confirmed quickly by checking that the superior and inferior curves of the lateral malleolus are symmetrical (Root et al 1971).

With the foot held in this neutral position, it is lifted slightly from the couch and a small force is applied to pronate the midtarsal joint and to dorsiflex the ankle joint to resistance (note—this will not necessarily bring the foot to 90° to the leg). During the above procedure, the rest of the leg should be observed to maintain the correct relationship with the foot. In order to avoid dorsiflexion of the fourth and fifth toes, the wrist needs to be rotated to bring them back into alignment with the other toes, as shown in Figure 12.12.

Double or twin ply plaster bandage is usually used: 20 cm wide for adults and 10 cm/15 cm for smaller feet. The process of applying the plaster bandage is the same for all of the techniques and so will be explained in detail here.

Applying plaster bandage. The first length is taken and about 15 mm of one long edge is folded over to form the reinforced top edge. This strip is then immersed in slightly warmed water and the excess water squeezed out. This length is applied around the back of the heel (Fig. 12.13) and brought forward to its correct position distal to the first and fifth metatarsal heads, with the reinforced top edge aligned with the first and fifth metatarsal shafts, respectively. In addition, the top edge must also extend at least to the lower limit of the malleoli. This will allow correct cast evaluation later and provide a deep enough positive model of the foot.

The plaster is smoothed onto the sides of the foot and then across the plantar surface, with the two parts of the strip overlapping. The fold at the heel produced by this overlap can be pushed to the back of the calcaneus. It is important to obtain a good impression of the plantar surface, and so all the air must be expelled from under the bandages before proceeding to the next step.

After preparing and soaking the second plaster strip as was done for the first, it is wrapped around the toes to overlap with the sides of the first piece (Fig. 12.14), leaving space at the end of the toes to prevent pressure on them during positioning of the foot; this forms an apron. This second piece is folded over the plantar surface in the same way as the first, with the excess plaster being pushed into the sulcus. The foot is now positioned as required and is held until the plaster sets, which usually takes just a few minutes. A piece of absorbent paper will help to prevent the fingers slipping.

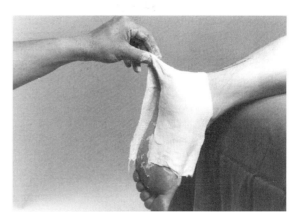

Figure 12.13 The first strip of plaster applied to the rearfoot and being smoothed over the plantar surface.

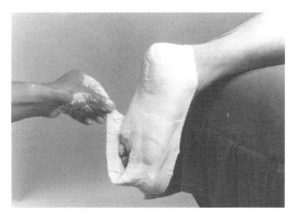

Figure 12.14 The second strip of plaster applied to the forefoot, overlapping the first and being smoothed over the plantar surface.

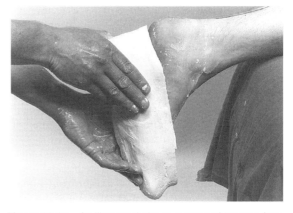

Figure 12.15 As illustrated, the cast removal process has just begun, with the cast clear of the heel and ready to push down along the plantar surface.

To remove the cast (Fig. 12.15), the skin along the top edge is carefully eased away from it and then the foot is shaken firmly, holding it just above the ankle. The fingers of both hands are then placed along the posterior reinforced top edge of the cast and pulled plantarly with a constant force until the cast is eased from the heel. Patients should not assist in this, nor should they move their toes. Once free from the heel, the cast is pulled along the plantar surface and then inverted to clear the forefoot. The cast is now complete and ready for evaluation.

Clinical comment. This technique produces a good plantar impression without distortion. The supine position allows ready visualisation of the extensor tendons to ensure that they remain inactive during casting. The talus is accessible to palpation, which makes detection of the subtalar neutral position simpler. The main drawback of this technique is that it is probably the hardest one to master. Most errors using this approach are a result of the grip used to take the impression; the alignment of the hand and the fingers may be incorrect, so that the resulting cast is easily supinated and the toes can be dorsiflexed.

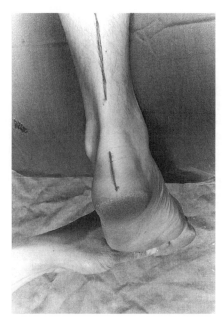

Figure 12.16 The prone suspension technique showing the correct hold.

Modified suspension technique

This is a very similar technique to that described above except that the subject is prone. The same arm, wrist and finger positions are used as above and the subtalar joint is positioned in neutral much as before. To pronate the midtarsal joint, the leg is not lifted from the couch but pulled downwards and a dorsiflexion force is applied to the ankle joint much as before (Fig. 12.16). Again, the wrist position is checked to ensure alignment of the fourth and fifth toes, and the whole procedure is repeated as necessary as a dry run to become familiar with the position required without the plaster. Plaster is prepared and applied exactly as described above and the foot is repositioned and held until set. Removal is the same as for the supine casting.

Clinical comment. This technique allows better visualisation of the forefoot to rearfoot relationship than does the supine position, and the curves above and below the lateral malleolus are easily seen, making confirmation of subtalar neutral simple. The extensor tendons are not visible and so cannot be checked to ensure inactivity, and there is thus greater potential for some distortion of the cast without the practitioner's knowledge. There may also be some discomfort of the anterior leg at the ankle level as it is pulled into the couch during casting. This could result in the subject repositioning themselves and causing unwanted movement; this discomfort can be prevented by using a softer edge on the couch.

Direct pressure technique

This can be carried out with the patient prone or supine and is probably the most universally used and preferred technique.

The hand position is slightly different from that adopted for the suspension technique; the thumb is placed on the plantar surface of the fourth and fifth metatarsal heads in line with the sulcus of the toes (Fig. 12.17). The foot is moved through its full range of subtalar pronation and supination while the other hand is used to palpate the talar head and identify subtalar neutral. With the subtalar joint in neutral, pressure is applied to the fourth and fifth metatarsal heads to fully pronate the midtarsal joint about both axes and to dorsiflex the foot at the ankle joint to initial resistance.

The plaster is applied as described above. Having a piece of paper or gauze under the thumb during this stage sometimes helps to prevent the thumb slipping on the wet plaster. Removal of the cast is as has already been described.

Clinical comment. While this is the most common casting technique, it is not without its problems. The forefoot can be forced laterally if the pressure applied

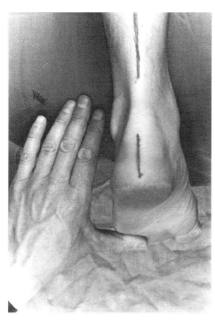

Figure 12.17 The position of the thumb during the direct pressure technique.

to the metatarsal heads is not applied directly in line with the long axis of the leg. Direct pressure can also distort the true position of an unstable fifth ray. A depression created in the cast has to be filled later on unless pushed out at the time of cast removal. In either case, this will introduce some inaccuracy into the forefoot impression which, for some purposes, may be unacceptable.

Vacuum casting in 'neutral'

The vacuum cast was popular in the USA in the 1980s. A cast is applied as previously described, with a plastic bag wrapped over the foot and a flexible tube placed inside the bag so that the whole foot slips into the shoe easily while the plaster is still wet. The tube connected to a vacuum pump produces compression around the foot, ensuring a very accurate in-shoe impression. Neutral position is selected by talar head palpation and dorsiflexion under the lateral sole of the shoe.

Clinical comment. This technique, again developed in the USA, means that sensitive feet, especially following surgery, can be casted in the corrected position without painful manipulation. The vacuum builds up sufficient compression to provide an adequate mould without causing discomfort. Furthermore, patients with court shoes do well with this technique due

to a better orthotic fit, although no studies confirm these advantages.

Semi-pronated technique

Where a neutral subtalar joint position is not indicated, a semi-pronated cast may be more appropriate. The prone position is preferred as it improves visualisation of the forefoot to rearfoot relationship. This is important in eliminating an inverted forefoot by pronating the subtalar joint. The forefoot is held and the whole foot is moved into a sufficiently pronated position at both the subtalar and midtarsal joints. The forefoot should be aligned at 90° to a bisection of the calcaneus and held until the plaster is set.

Clinical comment. Different practitioners use different variations on this technique. For example, forefoot supinatus may be reduced by vertical pressure at the base of the first ray or this amount of soft tissue deformity may be left in the cast. The advantages and disadvantages of the technique are similar to those already described.

Fully pronated technique

If the subtalar joint motion is restricted, the foot may have to be maximally pronated during casting. Joint bridging from bony bars, painful sinus tarsi and arthritides are best managed with a pronated cast. The orthosis plays an inhibitive rather than a functional role. The procedure outlined above is still used. In some cases, there may be insufficient motion at the subtalar and midtarsal joints to reduce fully the forefoot supinatus.

Weight-bearing casting techniques

Casts for producing accommodative orthoses can be taken while the foot is bearing weight or by using impression blocks (Fig. 12.18). This technique is clearly unsuitable for any foot which requires significant positioning during casting.

The cast is taken with the foot on a foam pad (covered in plastic), maintaining a neutral position (if required) by rotating the leg to obtain talar congruency. In all other respects, the technique is the same as before.

Impression systems. Where an accommodative type of inlay does not require a high corrective specification, all that is required is an outline impression of the foot. If the foot is essentially rigid but needs some protection from internal stresses, then it is clearly inappropriate to attempt to position the foot in any particular orientation. It is far better to capture the true position of the weight-bearing foot including the spread of soft tissues. This can be done by getting the subject to stand in putty (Pratt et al 1984), but it is often a messy procedure and the putty needs to be stored in specific conditions so that it remains usable for a reasonable time. A better and cheaper way is to use foam impression blocks, which consist of a box, each half containing foam. This foam has no rebound, and when an object is pressed into it, it permanently deforms to take up the plantar shape, in a similar manner to 'oasis' used by flower arrangers. By pressing the foot into the foam, a good impression of the plantar surface is obtained quickly and with little mess (Fig. 12.18), to make a plaster positive of the foot.

The Irving (impression) system has been described in Chapter 11 (Fig. 11.19) and offers the practitioner a weight-bearing orthosis which can be produced immediately from an accurate replication technique.

Clinical comment. Weight-bearing cast techniques have the disadvantage of creating a broader positive cast, which can create footwear fitting problems. For this reason, the non-weight-bearing cast technique seems, on the whole, to offer a better shoe fit.

Discussion. There are some doubts about the non-weight-bearing casting procedure. It has been suggested that it does not represent the true forefoot to rearfoot relationship and that it often produces a false inversion of the forefoot (Kidd 1991); this belief arises from the fact that the cast contours the soft tissue rather than the bony structure.

There has been limited research into the effects of neutral foot casting. No controlled studies have been conducted to establish whether variations introduced into casting are significant enough to influence the technique selected.

Measured inverted or everted forefoot deformity can be diagnosed. Large variations of deformity are more visible than small changes. Metatarsal sagittal plane deformities cannot be differentiated from frontal forefoot deformities unless the metatarsal can be visibly identified. If an inverted deformity exists, the rearpart of the plate tilts the same number of degrees in an everted direction. Conversely, an everted deformity will cause the plate to tilt in an inverted direction. Some allowance for error, perhaps ±3°, should be made when transposing the values from the measured tilt of the rearpart of the cast.

General cast critique

The practitioner should determine the accuracy and quality of the negative impression before sending the plate to the laboratory.

A clean cast should be produced without lumps or bulges that do not conform to the foot; the plate should appear smooth inside. The more lumpy a cast, the more work a laboratory has to carry out and the more likely it is that there will be inaccuracies in the finished product. Such casts should be rejected at the clinical stage. A 12 point checklist can be used to evaluate the quality of a neutral cast taken in the clinic:

1. Does the cast appear to replicate the same deformity as in the neutrally held foot?

2. Using the plantar surface as a reference, draw an imaginary line through the heel. A line projected distally should end up between the second and third metatarsals, unless of course there is a transverse plane deformity. If the deformity was soft tissue, this should have been corrected in the cast first.

3. A 'C' shape along the lateral border indicates either a true metatarsus adductus or the fact that

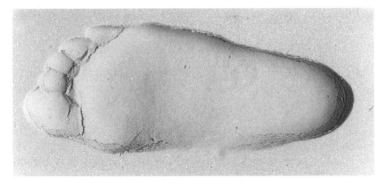

Figure 12.18 A foam impression of a foot, commonly used for accommodative orthoses.

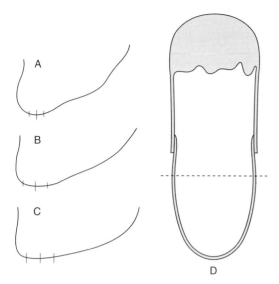

Figure 12.19 The plaster negative shell has been sectioned as shown. A: Supinated. B: Correct alignment. C: Pronated. D: The position of the cast cross-sectioned. Note the varying widths of the shoulder associated with the fifth ray.

the practitioner has adducted the foot with supination of the oblique midtarsal joint axis.

4. The inside contour over the calcaneocuboid joint is normally flattened across the lateral furrow. This needs to be seen in transverse perspective (Fig. 12.19). Semi-weight-bearing casts tend to have a flattened area (Tollafield 1985).

5. When using the suspension technique, the toes should be in alignment, and in particular the lateral fourth and fifth toes should not be dorsiflexed. This type of error would ultimately plantarflex the metatarsals.

6. The direct pressure technique thumbprint should only cover those lateral metatarsals. It is not unusual to find the plantar surface of the cast rucked up from aggressive and careless casting. In the suspension technique, the lateral side of the cast should not be pinched excessively.

7. Viewing the lateral arch from inside the cast, one should see a gentle curve in the sagittal plane. A high arch may suggest that the cuboid has been plantarflexed.

8. The rearpart of the cast should reflect a high lateral and medial side to a point just below the malleolus. A low rear heel part will make filling very difficult and will make a shallow cast for the purpose of vacuum-forming.

9. Excessive pronation, a likely result of using the direct pressure technique, will cause the heel to widen

medially. If when looking inside, the talonavicular area is flattened in a 'normal' shaped foot, or a lateral crease is observed under the fibula, then it is likely that pronation has occurred and a new cast should be taken.

10. The first metatarsal head should leave a clear imprint with skin striae demonstrable. A faint or poor impression suggests that the longitudinal axis has been supinated.

11. The surrounding rim of the cast should be strong to prevent deformity of the rear section when it is removed. If the rim has been deformed, this means that the cast has been removed carelessly.

12. The two pieces making up the plate on the inside should have no join. If care is taken, the orthotist is likely to have greater confidence in the practitioner.

PRESCRIBING CASTED ORTHOSES

All practitioners should routinely undertake a joint and soft tissue evaluation, whether or not orthoses are intended. A more in-depth examination will be necessary to assist with the prescription, particularly in the case of a functional orthosis.

Many claims, particularly emanating from the USA, have been made in support of a variety of prescribing theories. Without doubt, more research is required to assist prescribing decisions. However, in recent years, much interest in the UK has focused on the accuracy of measurements used in prescription fabrication.

Measurement techniques used for prescriptions

Clearly, the techniques required to cast and complete an examination rely on two basic skills:

1. the ability to bisect a limb segment accurately
2. the ability to determine reliably the subtalar joint neutral position.

There are a number of problems associated with these as they are both prone to error. Such errors may be greater than the accuracy with which the measurements are required for any clinical value. Studies have been carried out to examine the ability of practitioners to perform these fundamental tasks.

It is well known that the skin of the body moves as the limbs move. The accuracy of the measurements of skin, determined from lines drawn over joints, limits the accuracy of measurements of motion derived from this activity. Various studies have been highlighted below to illustrate this point.

Subtalar joint (STJ) assessment

The proportion and range of excursion of the STJ seem to vary widely. Kidd (1991) questioned the accuracy of measurements and bisectors and the validity of the (1/3):(2/3) ratio (Root et al 1971) as a viable technique.

Bailey et al (1984), using radiographic tomography, found a number of subjects with a ratio of 3:1 (3/4:1/4), as did Tollafield & Pratt (1990a,b) using a hand-held tractograph. The wide ranges of subtalar joint movement measured by various clinical authors are well-documented, illustrating the variability among the different methods employed. Bailey et al (1984) found a mean of 30° total motion for 20- to 30-year-olds, Tollafield & Pratt (1990a) found a mean of 37° in a group aged 19–51, Inman (1976) found a mean range of 40° ± 7° with a spherical goniometer, and McMaster (1976) found a total range of 30° with a calcaneal pointer.

Griffith (1988) set out to examine the reliability of measurements. In a large study, using nine examiners, he examined the inter- and intra-observer errors associated with the measurements of ankle joint dorsiflexion, subtalar joint motion (in three ways) and the angle of the hallux. The findings of this study revealed the following accuracies:

1. calculated neutral position—an average of 2.63° varus with a standard deviation (SD) of 4.31°
2. measured neutral position—an average of 6.02° varus with an SD of 3.06°
3. stance neutral position—an average of 4.04° varus with an SD of 2.59 degrees.

When compared with a radiographically determined neutral position, work on the neutral position of the subtalar joint shows that all techniques produced a varus position, with the 'calculated' approach being the most accurate, while the 'measured' technique showed the least variability. Further reference to calculated and measured neutral positions forms part of patient assessment and data can be found in other sources (e.g. Tollafield & Merriman 1995).

There are many reasons for this inaccuracy which are not due to observer error. For example, the positioning and lining-up of goniometers with the limb are critical if measurements are to be accurate and repeatable. Add to this the fact that the subtalar joint is triplanar in action, and positioning of the single axis goniometer with respect to the joint is bound to produce some discrepancies in measurement. Ball & Johnson (1993) found errors similar to that found by Griffith (1988) when using a flexible goniometer. In fact, when all of these matters are taken into account, it is surprising that the accuracy is as high as it appears to be.

Phillips et al (1985) used goniometers to measure the calcaneus and lower third of the leg, followed by rigorous mathematical analysis. No allowance was made for the possibility that the measurements used in the equations produced were themselves open to the kinds of error detailed above.

An unreported study carried out in the Orthotics and Disability Research Centre at Derbyshire Royal Infirmary, UK (D. J. Pratt, unpublished work) showed that the most experienced practitioners could not bisect by eye the lower third of the lower leg to an accuracy of better than about 3°. The less able practitioners were even less accurate than this. It was possible to increase the accuracy to about 1.5° if the width of the limb was accurately measured with callipers. However, this took far too long to perform so that many of the practitioners said it would not be suitable for use in the clinic.

If the lines drawn on skin are unreliable, then the measurements taken from them will likewise be suspect, and it is these derived angles that have been more often recorded and used to determine the accuracy of the whole approach. Despite concerns about reliability, recent evidence suggests that assessment by eye can produce adequate repeatability and accuracy. A study by Cook et al (1988) examined 138 subjects and measured the neutral position of the subtalar joint in three ways: by palpation of the talus; by equalising the proximal and distal curves of the lateral malleolus; and by observation of the skin over the sinus tarsi. They found a 95% correlation between the three methods but had assumed that a ±2° error was clinically acceptable.

The triplanar motion of the subtalar joint complicates the essentially two-dimensional assessment techniques usually used. This matter was addressed by Engsberg et al (1988) in an in vitro study on nine cadaveric lower legs and feet. They found that the monitoring of the inversion/eversion and abduction/adduction orientations of the talocalcaneal/talocrural complex is more valuable in predicting pronation and supination positions than using inversion/eversion alone.

Components of prescribing

The laboratory requires information that will allow technicians to convert a negative plate into a moulded inlay that conforms to the practitioner's requirements. Any omission of information will lead to further error. The primary aim of the orthosis is that:

- patient symptoms will be relieved
- the foot will feel more stable
- less abnormal shoe wear will be observed
- the patient can use the orthosis in a number of shoes.

The heel shape and skin contours will be affected by different positions adopted when casting the foot. A non-weight-bearing cast should require less plaster work but frequently will need adaptations to allow a weight-bearing simulation, most notably the medial and lateral expansions. Weight-bearing casts may need some surface reduction to improve their shoe fit.

Medial additions

When the flexible foot contacts the ground, the medial long arch descends about the long axis of the MTJ. If the cast is taken while the foot is non-weight-bearing, the arch will appear higher than it would functionally when on the ground. In this case, an addition should be ordered to prevent the plastic from gouging the foot. It was Tollafield & Pratt's (1990a) belief, when comparing the Shafer plate (without medial addition) with the Root plate (with medial addition), that including an addition does not alter the efficacy of an orthosis. The fascial band of the plantar aponeurosis may be prominent and easily irritated. Early concerns with functional orthoses creating fibromatosis have been reported in American podiatric literature. A medial addition, or even an additional channel, to avoid arch irritation may be ordered by asking the laboratory to add plaster to the positive cast. This adaptation will deflect the plastic material when moulded away from any areas of sensitivity. The negative cast must be marked accordingly.

Lateral expansions

An additional ledge of plaster to the cast will prevent the skin becoming pinched. In deciding whether to utilise an expansion, the practitioner will consider the ultimate height of the heel cup first. A high heel cup set at 20 mm (adult foot) is less likely to require a lateral addition than would a low 10–12 mm cup. In the case of the lower specification, an addition is useful and will prevent pinching from the orthotic plate. In other words, when high heel cups are ordered, little additional value is gained from expanding the cast edge, as shoe fit, as well as some hindfoot control, will be compromised. Medial and lateral additions are shown in Figure 12.20.

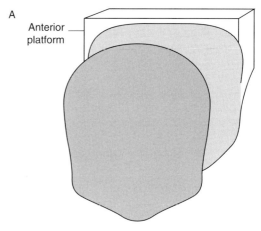

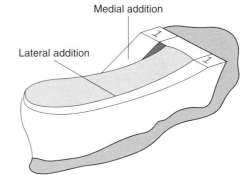

Figure 12.20   A: The intrinsic post is fabricated on the positive plaster cast. B: Medial and lateral additions blend in as shown. (Adapted from Anthony 1992.)

Materials

Choosing materials can be problematic because the current array of plastics have very different mechanical properties yet they all look alike (Rome 1990). The acrylics and polythenes are perhaps the most popular, although soft materials for accommodative orthoses vary, from Birkenstock or woodflour (sawdust with latex) to EVA sheets, which are ground by hand to provide a firm but yielding inlay. Leather laminates have fallen from popularity but can be made into acceptable orthoses if the skin type precludes the use of plastics. Top covers can be used to cover surface defects but may lead to the need for early replacement. Top covers are optional and usually depend on the desired cosmetic finish.

Polycarbonates, carbon fibre and fibreglass orthoses are less popular. Early PVC materials were found to fracture initially (Ch. 10).

Two further matters need to be considered: first, the type of orthosis to be used for the problem; and second, the required thickness and durability of the material selected for any occupational and additional activities. Orthoses should not break as a result of normal walking cadence stresses. Sporting activities naturally impose forces of greater magnitude in all orthogonal planes. An acrylic device will need to be around 4 mm thick to cope with this stress in the case of an adult, while a polypropylene or high density polyethylene of 3 mm thickness will be more satisfactory, with less likelihood of fracture, for the same individual.

The patient's weight is a determining factor. Materials can be made thicker, although selecting a material above 4 mm does provide additional shoe fit problems. Arch strengthening can be ordered with foam infills, which are popular additions provided by some orthotic laboratories, particularly those dealing with podiatrists. Lightness has become a serious factor for runners and other athletes. Trainers have become lighter over the years and orthoses have become heavier with the use of elaborate additions and fillers. Ballet shoes often do better with a high density moulded Plastazote orthosis (Fig. 12.21). The practitioner should study the range of materials on offer to suit the different needs.

Three other factors need to be discussed to fulfil the prescription: elevators, trim lines and addition specifications.

Posting

Posting is the method used for controlling an orthosis by tilting the contoured plate against the foot. Two types of posting are currently in vogue: extrinsic and intrinsic. Initially, as with shoes, wedging was applied to the outer surface (extrinsic post). In the 1980s, an intrinsic method was introduced by a number of practitioners in the UK. Little scientific follow-up has been conducted comparing the merits of intrinsic and extrinisic methods.

Intrinsic. An intrinsic post or step is one that is created within the plastic. The forefoot is usually intrinsically posted by adding plaster platforms to the cast (Fig. 12.20). The plaster additions effectively alter the lie of the positive cast, correcting its valgus or varus position. The anterior platform will create a flat edge to the pressed orthosis. It is usual to order intrinsic posts with medial additions to allow a smoother contour to the finished orthosis. The medial and lateral additions blend better with the anterior platform.

Plastic material will be vacuum-formed over the anterior platforms. Once a cast is angled intrinsically by more than a few degrees of varus, the control relies proximally on the plate of the orthosis across the position of the metatarsal shafts.

In fact, greater posting angles provide little additional benefit and can cause the patient to slide off the orthosis. The exception to this is that an intrinsic valgus wedge appears to offer more useful control and stability than higher values of varus wedging. Because the fifth metatarsal has minimal contour alterations, any such prescriptive requirement keeps the orthotic plate closer to the surface of the skin.

Selection of the intrinsic post, often associated with the Root orthosis, is particularly beneficial for patients whose shoes cannot accommodate forefoot extrinsic posts. Added to narrow trim lines, the acceptance rate has been found to be much higher. Intrinsic posts can be ground into some plastics more easily than others, particularly under the heel. The laboratory will advise on the most suitable material and technique if doubt exists.

Triaxial. Lundeen (1988) suggested that conventional systems can be used to produce a plaster positive, which can be adjusted by following a series of alterations. By sectioning through the cast at three predetermined points, corrections can be made that influence the position of the foot. A screw introduced through the heel along the length of the cast, and another screw across the foot, is loosened for adjustments. The cast is influenced predominantly through the midtarsal joint and first ray in three planes as necessary. Plaster is smoothed over the adjusted cast to create an orthotic plate. At present this system has not been received favourably in the UK.

Extrinsic. An extrinsic post offers more intimate

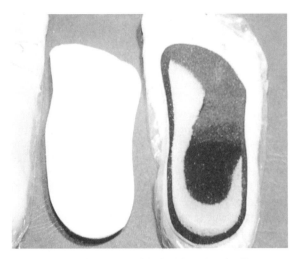

Figure 12.21 Combined high and low density Plastazote orthosis indicated for dancers. (Courtesy of Dr Tom Novella.)

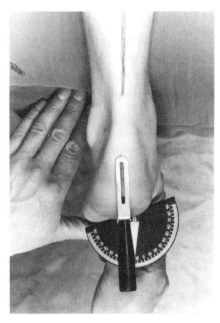

Figure 12.22 The measurement of the forefoot to rearfoot with a special goniometer designed to rest on the plantar forefoot and hindfoot.

control against the patient's foot than an intrinsic post. The wedge of plastic PMMA or EVA must be ground to blend in with the anterior edge of the orthosis, offering support to the foot without taking up additional room in the shoe. The proximal part of the orthosis is also blended to sit inside the heel counter and ground down to allow for the heel height. The main prescriptive consideration lies in how much of an angle to order.

The post cannot be balanced to the same number of degrees of deformity established from clinical examination (Fig. 12.22) because it would take up too much room in the shoe. Over-posted (balanced) orthoses are uncomfortable and affect the independent first and fifth rays adversely.

Two problems might arise as a result of extrinsic forefoot post design. Firstly, if the deformity in the adult has been present for a long time, the foot will have compensated to some extent, possibly without symptoms. Secondly, if any material is placed under an independent metatarsal, that ray will become elevated and cause impairment of movement at the MTP joint. If the metatarsal head appears elevated then some adjustment is necessary.

While practitioners will develop their own preference for either intrinsic or extrinsic posting, both types of system have advantages and disadvantages.

A less common practice of mixing intrinsic and extrinsic posts has been used in the US. In this prescription, the intrinsic work is carried out first and any additional extrinsic is added after the plate has been trimmed.

Position of the post. Each orthosis will have either a rearpost or a forefoot post, or both. Convention dictates, perhaps erroneously, that the rearpost should always have a varus/inverted cant. However, patients who have been provided with valgus/everted rearposts have not always suffered detrimentally. The simple rule-of-thumb that a valgus forefoot deformity be prescribed with a lateral wedge and a varus forefoot deformity with a medial wedge provides a useful place to start. Nonetheless, the absence of problems with everted rearposts does not mean that there should be a sudden change in prescribing fashion— the wary practitioner should use soft valgus wedges first, before converting to a permanent prescription format.

A varus rearpost is used with values of 0°–8° as a rule-of-thumb. Posts applied to the anterior and posterior ends of the orthosis appear to offer better control than a single post at one end only (Fig. 12.23).

Varus forefoot posts of values greater than 4°–6° create the types of problems alluded to above. Valgus posts can be tolerated until the fourth and fifth toes become irritated; this tends to restrict higher values above 5°.

There are only a few studies which consider the scientific basis of posting. Tollafield & Pratt (1990a) reviewed the dearth of literature supporting the use of both forefoot and rearfoot posts.

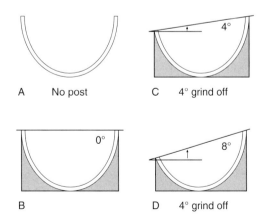

Figure 12.23 Rearposting and heel relationships. A: No post. B: Zero post for no motion. C: 4° degree varus post with 4° grind-off (common angle selected initially). D: 8° varus post. If motion is too great, an additional forefoot post is applied, i.e. 3° forefoot varus will limit motion to 5°.

Heel cup heights have been discussed above (p. 235). The height must be selected for the shoe first, and the type of pathology and intended control are considered next. As the post tilts laterally, the heel height on that side may need to be higher than for a lower post angle. This feature is the same for both distal and proximal posts.

Elevators. Ross & Gurnik (1982) pointed out that the stability offered by posts would be affected by variable shoe height. In fact, a point arises where an orthosis offers little benefit to a patient if the heel height is so great that both anterior and posterior posts rock uncontrollably. The adverse mechanical effects from this could cause more harm than assistance. The reasons for such adverse problems relate to the production of unwarranted sagittal or frontal plane rock, reducing the intended stability offered by the orthosis.

An elevator is a piece of plastic of known thickness (4–12 mm) used to account for heel pitch. Given that a shoe has a heel height, an elevator is used to ensure that the orthosis is appropriately balanced such that no adverse movement arises at the back of the shoe. Ross & Gurnick's (1982) main precept considered three bands of heel height: 0.5 inch (1.25 cm), requiring a 4 mm elevator; 1 inch (2.5 cm), requiring an 8 mm elevator; and 1.5 inches (3.75 cm), requiring a 12 mm elevator (see Fig. 12.24). Thus, the soft acrylic material or EVA post should be pressed or ground down, respectively, using an elevator to comply with the heel height determined above.

Trim lines. The orthosis, made from a plate vacuformed from thermoplastic, needs to be trimmed. The use of specific terms will assist the laboratory, although no doubt there is much diversity in the terms used internationally. The practitioner can dis-

cuss this with the laboratory, describe the trim lines in detail or specify a certain type of orthosis, such as a Root orthosis.

Trim lines also include specifications such as heel height, medial and lateral side heights, and additional flares, as in the Robert-Whitman orthosis, where the lateral cup has a flange extending up the calcaneus to grip the heel.

Additions to the orthosis. This part of the prescription is concerned with variations which, when added, have additional benefit upon foot function. In the main, such additions fall into two categories: extensions and adaptations.

Extensions are added to a functional orthosis to enhance further the redistributive, accommodative, stability, compensatory and rest qualities of general therapeutic objectives.

Polyurethane foam of thickness 1–3 mm is sometimes added under a vinyl or leather cover (Fig. 12.25). The extension may be full-length, in which case this will be trimmed to the shape of the shoe by the practitioner, or it may be trimmed to the toe sulcus. The latter is favoured, as the toe depth is compromised to a lesser degree. Padded materials in latex foam, neoprene, PU foam, PE foam and PVC foams can all offer redistribution and rest to part of the forefoot, as well as compensating for loss of adipose tissue.

Adaptations are considered to increase surface control. A flared post can be beneficial medially and laterally, to increase pronatory resistance and reduce lateral heel sprain, respectively, by altering moments of force about heel contact. When ordering a flared post, the extent of the flare should be stated, e.g. 1–6 mm, as well as which side (or perhaps both) is to be flared. A Thomas heel, which extends from the medial side anteriorly to fill in part of the long

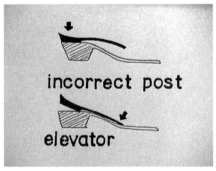
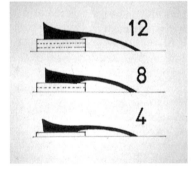

A   B

Figure 12.24   A: Incorrect elevator selection will produce instability where a rearpost should be stable. B: Correct elevator selection is measured in mm (see text).

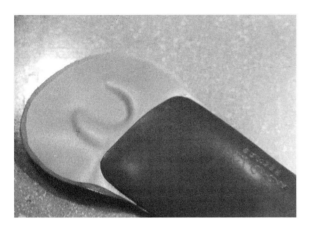

Figure 12.25 An extension placed on a standard orthotic plate offers protection over the forefoot at a specific site of high shear pressure.

arch, has been used in much the same way as a medial flare.

Some anterior posts will need to be trimmed to minimise the vertical forces applied over the independent first and fifth rays.

Many patients, when first issued with rearposts, complain of being lifted out of their shoes. Posts in EVA are capped with thin plastic to prevent material compression, but the capping may need to be removed if the lifting effect is too great. On the whole, an orthosis will bed into the insock and settle after a few weeks.

Tollafield & Pratt (1990a) noted that the function of the rearpost provided a large surface area to stabilise the STJ and ankle joint. The varus angle allowed motion to function around a specific STJ axis (low, normal or high).

Posts may be omitted altogether. In this case, the rounded heel cup allows considerable rolling movement at contact. A zero post is a flat post (Fig. 12.23) which will confine the heel (calcaneus) and allow less STJ movement. A zero post may have greater value in cases where patients suffer from arthritic pain in the hindfoot and require limitation of joint movement. If the prescription is likely to work, a higher than normal heel cup should be requested, otherwise the heel will force its way out of the cup with foot rotation. The ability of a foot orthosis to exert this type of control is limited and, if failure is suspected, the practitioner should consider an ankle foot orthosis (AFO) or a supramalleolar orthosis (SMO), which increases heel/ankle control.

The usual initial request for a varus is 4°. The use of a varus tilt of 8° can be equally helpful, creating

a greater antipronatory force, and is often made more effective with concomitant forefoot posts.

Weed et al (1978) found that the use of a post without grinding off to allow some pronation resulted in back pain. It is probably for this reason that all hard posts made from acrylic have some element of grind-off. EVA posts, being less dense, do not suffer from the same problem. Tollafield & Pratt (1987) found no evidence to support the practice of varying orthotic post prescriptions by single degrees; increments of 0°, 4° and 8° are commonly used and work satisfactorily.

Forefoot posts should always be added first and rearposts afterwards; this is because the anterior edge is always used as a reference for rearpost positioning. Rearposts contribute less to the measured values of deformity and predominantly affect heel placement. Any adjustments are best undertaken by a laboratory, as considerable experience is required when working with plastics—furthermore, any warranty that exists may become invalid if this is not done.

The prescription should always indicate how much motion ground into the medial rearpost is required. A summary of the prescription components is included in Box 12.1.

Dispensing a functional device

When fitting a functional orthosis, consideration must be given to the accuracy of plate dimensions, adequate foot-to-orthosis contact and comfort. An optimum fit is essential if the device is to be well tolerated. The orthotic plate and post should conform to the previously examined deformity (Fig. 12.26). The orthosis should be checked during both non-weight-bearing and weight-bearing. The alignment of the lower extremity is checked while standing on the orthosis both with and without shoes. Any adjustments for fit, comfort or biomechanical alignment are made at the initial consultation or after a period of acclimatisation.

Compliance and expectations

Another important consideration is the fitting of the orthosis in footwear; many problems arise simply from a failure to prescribe orthoses appropriate to the patient's footwear. The patient should be told in advance what shoes the orthosis is designed for and ideally should be shown a sample. Confusion over these simple issues can lead to poor patient satisfaction. The side of the shoes should be as high as possible to aid orthotic accommodation and should have a deep heel counter to prevent slippage. Elevators must

Box 12.1 Prescribing a functional orthosis. The orthotic prescription comprises many component factors which need to be taken into consideration

- *Patient details*
  —problem, aim, define pathology
  —morphology: weight
  —occupation/sports activity

- *Cast (shell) enclosed*
  —state method used
  —pour plaster to perpendicular/inverted/everted
  —cast marked: metatarsal heads, lesions, points of pressure

- *Intrinsic post*
  —balance to perpendicular
  —degrees forefoot varus/valgus

- *Additions on the positive*
  —lateral expansion
  —medial addition
  —fascia

- *Material*
  —acrylic, polypropylene, ortholen (HD polyethylene), PVC, foamed HD polyethylene (Plastazote), carbon fibre, polycarbonate
  —thickness: 2–5mm (stock-dependent)
  —*accommodative orthoses*—leather laminate, Levy mould (rubber latex/wood flour), EVA (HD/LD)

- *Orthotic plate/trim lines*
  —Shafer, Root, UCBL, Robert-Whitman, TCFO
  —modification, width, ray cut-outs, heel cups
  —heel cup height (after rearpost applied); state lateral/medial/both symmetrical in mm
  —anterior edge cut-outs, 'clips' (medial/lateral ray)
  —lateral flare (very high lateral edge)

- *Posting*
  —forefoot varus or valgus 2°–6°
  —rearfoot varus 0°, 4°, 8°, with 4° grind-off (acrylic), no grind-off (EVA)
  —elevator 4, 8, 12 mm (for shoes)
  —flare medially/laterally 1–6 mm

- *Finish (additions)*
  —vinyl/leather cover/foam cover/perforated
  —full PU 3 mm extension
  —extension to toe sulcus, PU 3 mm
  —PU 6 mm pad as on diagram

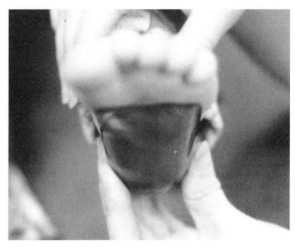

A

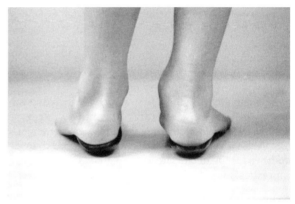

B

Figure 12.26 The orthotic plate is held against the foot while in a STJ neutral position. The forefoot and rearfoot relationships should conform to the prescribed posting. B: Poor fit shown here only on weight-bearing. Insufficient width and poor design have lead to an orthosis which has little control over the calcaneus.

correspond to the heel height. The patient should be warned about selecting heel heights for the best orthotic function. The patient should be examined while walking to ensure that the device is comfortable and that it controls any abnormal compensations for which it has been prescribed.

All patients should be warned, before they have committed themselves to an orthotic treatment programme, of the damage that orthoses can inflict

upon shoes. Post indentation at the heel and forefoot insock can cut any delicate material. Because of their width, most trimmed orthoses may protrude medially against the upper, sufficiently to crease and deform this permanently.

In cases where there has been a large degree of correction, the prescription change mentioned may be too great. Patients may complain of aching knees, hips, thighs and back after 3–4 consecutive hours of wear. Pain or discomfort may also be felt on the plantar surface of the foot. Muscle and ligament adaptation particularly affects the leg, while the foot has to cope with the new sensation of an object interfacing between the foot and shoe.

A compromise must be sought to allow a comfortable wearing-in period. When dealing with children and handicapped persons, it is essential that a responsible parent or guardian is informed of the 'wearing-in' process. In these situations, the acclimatisation period may need to be longer.

Acclimatisation period. A suggested regimen for wearing an orthosis, where one has not been worn before, includes use for 1 hour only on the first day of issue. This is then increased by 1 hour each day until the devices are comfortable all day long. The patients are usually asked to return to the clinic 2–4 weeks after dispensing the orthosis in order that any problems can be dealt with. If, after 6–8 weeks, the orthosis persists in causing discomfort, the patient should be re-examined, with a view to making adjustments or re-making the foot device.

Production changes

In the last decade, the development of orthoses from computerised analysis has become more sophisticated. In future, orthotic laboratories will make use of computer-aided design (CAD) and computer-aided manufacture (CAM) of orthotic devices to eliminate human error from the fabrication process (Stats & Kriechbrum 1989, Michael 1989). Computer hardware has been developed to scan a foot and digitise the information to generate a computerised cast model.

Prescriptions can be developed on a table-top computer and then sent, via floppy disk, to a computer-controlled manufacture process. While plaster positives can still be used to access dimensional data on foot shape, orthoses are manufactured from the digital information by a computer-controlled milling machine. This system can bypass the process of pressing plastics by sculpturing directly from solid plastics. At present, this type of orthotic manufacture is only available in the USA, and UK practitioners have to send negative casts by airmail. The Ammon and Orthocam CAD/CAM production systems can evaluate computer-generated casts as well as generate positive casts for the fabrication of other functional orthoses. Figure 12.27 illustrates a positive cast made from wood resin.

Discussion

The functional prescription orthosis differs from the insole or arch support in two respects. Firstly, the orthosis is commonly taken from a neutral cast. Secondly, the orthosis is balanced so as to reduce the need for foot compensation via intrinsic or extrinsic

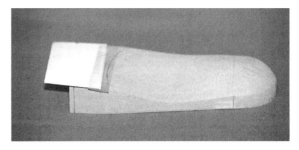

Figure 12.27 Positive cast from wood resin. (Reproduced with permission from Fifth Avenue Hospital, Seattle.)

posts. The intention behind treatment is therefore to improve the ground–foot interface with the shoe and to improve the timing of foot contact so that the foot supinates and pronates in the correct sequence.

The prescription must define the required orthotic design and include, where helpful, a diagram labelling any variations clearly. The practitioner must convey to the patient that the bespoke orthosis is not an arch support and does not function by supporting the arch. All such devices attempt to control abnormal foot function by restoring some of the time sequence to re-establish useful contact and propulsive phases.

Depending upon the design, orthoses will:

- reduce unwanted foot motion at the MTJ and STJ
- create a stable platform
- use materials to apply forces against the sustentaculum tali, calcaneus and lateral border, as well as over the talonavicular complex
- create specific foot influences using hand-made cast adaptations.

The medial long arch has not been shown to influence pronation significantly. The concept of creating a painful supinatory reflex offers poor justification for a high arch prescription, although feet with high arches do benefit from contoured infills. The concepts above are still broadly misunderstood. While the stock orthosis works, few cheap designs can create any of the biomechanical properties inherently incorporated by those prescription orthoses described.

ANKLE FOOT ORTHOSES

The ankle foot orthosis (AFO) is one of the most commonly prescribed lower limb orthoses. Despite its apparent simplicity, it has proved disproportionately effective in restoring function when compared to modalities such as 'callipers'.

Indications

The influence of AFOs can extend beyond the joints of the foot and ankle encompassed by the device to proximal joints; often it is this indirect effect which is being sought. Thus, AFOs may be used to reduce swing phase problems and to influence stance phase characteristics.

The nature of the pathological conditions producing the locomotor functional disorder can be usefully arranged into three groups:

- conditions which result in weakness of the muscles controlling the ankle–foot complex
- upper motor neurone lesions which result in hypertonicity or spasticity of the muscles
- conditions which result in pain or instability due to loss of structural integrity of the lower limb and/or foot–ankle complex.

In the first of these categories, weak or absent dorsiflexors, plantarflexors, supinators and/or pronators are included. In the first case, the foot tends to adopt a plantarflexed attitude and the AFO helps to maintain a more dorsiflexed foot to reduce compensatory mechanisms such as excessive knee flexion during swing, circumduction of the leg and hip hiking. It may also prevent the toe from being caught, resulting in trips or falls, and would reduce the energy required to walk. With weak or absent plantarflexors, the swing phase is not affected, but during late stance, excessive dorsiflexion occurs at heel-off, accompanied by a total lack of push-off. Here an AFO has to prevent the excessive dorsiflexion and actively assist plantarflexion, usually via an ankle hinge. However, other techniques, such as the anterior ground reaction AFO (Glancy & Lindseth 1972), can be used.

Subtalar joint instability, resulting in excessive pronation or supination, can be controlled with an AFO in which a stabilising three-point force system (Ch. 10) is used, with the forces applied on the upper calf, proximal to the ankle and on the border of the foot. Whether these forces are applied medially or laterally depends upon the instability being controlled.

Weak knee extensors, usually unilateral, cause the person to walk with an anteriorly flexed posture of the trunk to induce a knee-stabilising moment via the anteriorly positioned ground reaction force. In cases of moderate weakness in lighter subjects, an AFO may be able to provide the knee stability without the need for the subject to adopt the ungainly and potentially injurious posture.

In upper motor neurone lesions, such as cerebral palsy, head injury, multiple sclerosis and CVA, abnormal muscle tone is produced. This may be static or variable and introduces high intrinsic forces and joint moments which the AFO has to control in addition to those due to weight-bearing. In addition, if the AFO is not fitted correctly or causes discomfort, it may stimulate reflex activity, resulting in higher tone throughout the body. A well-fitting AFO, on the other hand, can reduce whole-body tone (Meadows et al 1980). The function of the AFOs for this category of patient is similar to that mentioned above, although the reason for the prescription will differ, i.e. to resist overactive plantarflexors as opposed to assisting weak or absent dorsiflexors.

Impaired structural integrity takes many forms which can result from trauma or, more commonly, from an arthritic condition. Whatever the underlying pathology, the functional consequence of this impaired integrity is pain during essentially normal ranges of joint motions and loading levels. If joint motion causes the discomfort, then restriction of the painful motion is the aim of the AFO. Often the pain due to joint motion is only part of the problem, which includes discomfort on weight-bearing or heel strike. Footwear adaptions can be used to provide shock absorption, as can inserts in the heel (Pratt 1990), but in some cases the foot needs to be off-loaded. This can be achieved using a patella-tendon-bearing AFO (McIllmurray & Greenbaum 1958), which uses the same concept as employed in prosthetics to transfer some limb load to the AFO via the patella tendon, thus bypassing the foot. Only a proportion of the limb load can be redirected, an absolute maximum of 50% having been demonstrated (Lehmann & Warren 1973).

Wapner & Sharkey (1991) reported on the results of the use of moulded AFO night splints for the treatment of plantar fasciitis in 14 patients. All patients had symptoms for greater than 1 year and had previously undergone treatment with non-steroidal agents, cortisone injections, shoe modifications and physical therapy without resolution. All patients were provided with a custom-moulded polypropylene AFO in 5° of dorsiflexion, to be used as a night splint. In combination with non-steroidal anti-inflammatory drugs, heel cups, shock-absorbing insoles and general stretching exercises, successful resolution occurred in 11 patients in less than 4 months. This suggests that the use of night splints provides a useful adjunct to current therapeutic regimens of plantar fasciitis.

AFO designs

There are two main forms of AFO, the older con-

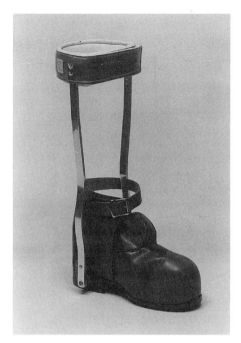

Figure 12.28 An ankle calliper with bespoke shoe is necessary to prevent deterioration of the heel counter. A leather calf band is shown.

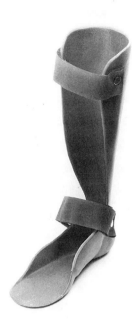

Figure 12.29 An ankle foot orthosis made from thermoplastic material has two points of fastening. In the illustration, Velcro is shown as the most popular system of orthosis/leg retention.

ventional metal and leather 'callipers' and the newer thermoplastic types.

Rigid bracing

The metal and leather AFOs (Fig. 12.28) employ a calf band connected to one or two metal side bars attached to the shoe, usually at the heel. Variations on the style can include the metal bar connecting posteriorly to the shoe, the inclusion of motion at the heel insert or addition of hinges at the ankle level. These AFOs are made by shaping the metal components to a full-sized outline of the limb, drawn by an orthotist, together with details of limb girth. Leather straps are often added to induce or control medio-lateral motion, and are called T or Y straps because of their outline shape. Recent changes to metal alloys and metal production techniques have resulted in the weight of these AFOs being reduced while still maintaining their performance. However, in many instances they have been superseded by the thermo-plastic design of the AFO.

Semi-rigid bracing

The thermoplastic design is more complicated to pro-

duce than the metal and leather AFO, as a cast of the leg is required (Fig. 12.29). This is taken with the foot–ankle complex held in its corrected position relative to the leg, and from this negative a positive model is made. The positive is modified in line with the orthotist's directions and then a thermoplastic sheet is heated and vacuum-formed to the model. Once cooled, the sheet is cut off, producing a plastic shell which is cleaned, and straps are now added to produce the AFO. The most commonly used plastic for these is polypropylene (homopolymer or copoly-mer), but polyethylene is also used in some cases (such as night splinting), as are more mechanically weak materials such as Orthoplast.

Thermoplastic AFOs, being a total contact design, are more difficult to fit than the conventional type but offer many advantages such as improved cosmesis, lighter weight, more precise control and less restricted choice of footwear. However, they are of no value if large diurnal limb volume changes take place or if the patient has anaesthetic skin or peripheral blood flow problems. They are also less successful in treating heavy patients and cost more than the conventional orthosis. In many cases, the advantages of their use outweigh the disadvantages, and improved treatment of lower limb functional impairments has resulted from their development. As development continues, newer techniques are being found to control the foot–ankle complex, and the role of the thermoplastic AFO continues to strengthen (Brown et al 1987).

Replication

A spiral cast is used for the AFO as well as for UCBL and TCFO devices. The POP bandage is wrapped circumferentially around the foot and leg and allowed to set. The negative cast should capture the contours of the foot and ankle sufficiently for these orthoses to be made. Unlike the types of cast discussed under 'Foot orthoses', the foot needs protecting before casting to prevent the plaster sticking to hairs on the dorsum of the foot and the lower part of the leg. This protection can be either a cream which is washed off later or, more commonly, a thin tubular bandage (e.g. Tubifast), extending from the toes to above the height of the finished cast.

As these casts cannot be pulled off like a plantar cast, a strong plastic tube is inserted under the sock, running from one end of the sock to the other and protruding well beyond both ends. Plaster bandage is wrapped around the foot, extending as far proximally as required, usually to above the malleoli for UCBL orthoses or higher in the case of AFOs. A total of about five to six layers of plaster is required, at which point the foot is positioned as required. This may be in subtalar neutral and, if so, the foot will need to have been positioned using one of the techniques described earlier in the chapter. Often this is not indicated and the basic requirement is to obtain a specific forefoot to rearfoot relationship after a full assessment of the subject. The best position for taking such casts is with the subject seated with their foot at a comfortable height for the practitioner.

Once the plaster has set, it is cut along the tube with a sharp knife and the cast is opened out to remove the foot (Fig. 12.30). The plaster is sufficiently flexibile to allow this process and still enable the cast to be closed up afterwards to re-create accurately the full shape of the foot. This is the technique used to cast for ankle foot orthoses where the upper level of the cast would end just below the knee.

A useful variation of this technique is to use one of the newer quick-setting plaster alternatives, such as Scotchcast, to take the cast. This will set fast enough that the subject can walk in the cast and thus an assessment of the foot position and likely functional result of the orthosis can be readily obtained. Such

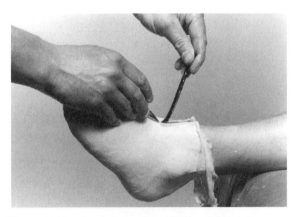

Figure 12.30 A spiral cast for a UCBL orthosis being removed by cutting with a knife onto a dorsal tube. This system of casting can be extended proximally to replicate feet/legs for AFOs or TCFOs.

Box 12.2 The key points considered when taking an impression and prescribing an AFO

- *Patient details*
  —biomechanical problem, orthotic aim, define pathology
  —morphology: weight
  —occupation
- *Cast taken*
  —taken weight-bearing or non-weight-bearing
  —mark malleoli, navicular, metatarsal heads, lesions and any points of pressure
- *Cast rectification*
  —before filling, check angles
  —after filling, set up for additions to be made
- *Cast additions/modifications*
  To include some, but not all of the following:
  —forefoot intrinsic posting
  —rearfoot intrinsic posting
  —Carlson modification (Carlson & Berglund 1979)
    (i) three point pressure
    (ii) calcaneal grip
    (iii) hinging alterations
- *Material*
  —polypropylene 3, 4.5 or 6 mm
  —polyethylene for night splinting
  —foam for padding (often PU foams)
- *Trim lines*
  —forward or behind malleoli
  —behind or on metatarsal heads or full foot
  —include (or not) first or fifth metatarsal heads
  —three-point presure trim
- *Posting*
  —rigid or flexible
  —forefoot or rearfoot

casts are more difficult to remove, usually requiring the use of an oscillating plaster saw as it is too hard for a knife. In addition, this does add to the cost of the process but may save an inappropriate orthosis being made.

Prescribing

Many of the principles described under foot orthoses can be applied to AFOs. Box 12.2 summarises the steps to be followed when considering taking an impression and prescribing an AFO.

Discussion

By the very nature of their design, ankle foot orthoses do not allow normal foot function, as the ankle cannot plantarflex and torque conversion is affected. They are used to provide a larger scale control over the foot and leg in order to influence such factors as spastic toe walking, knee hyperextension and excess pronation. As such, the re-establishment of normal foot contact timing sequences is not on the agenda, but the control of potentially damaging abnormal positions of the foot, leg and spine is required.

What is fundamental to the success of AFOs, apart from accuracy of the casting and manufacture, is the correct biomechanical description of the requirements of the AFO. Without this, there is little chance that the optimum orthotic performance will be realised. This takes considerable training and understanding of the practical aspects of the interrelationship between the human being and a plastic orthosis. It should always be remembered that the orthosis should satisfy the three 'S's—straight, stable and symmetrical.

SUMMARY

The process of treating patients has been described on the basis that the practitioner has a clear idea of the products available and their physical and chemical properties (Ch. 10). Mechanical therapy is provided in a variety of ways. In this chapter, the focus has been prescription orthoses as opposed to clinical padded adhesive orthoses or stock devices.

Occasions arise where clinical materials are unsatisfactory. Prescription orthoses may offer materials with better physical properties, made-to-measure designs which should fit shoes more effectively, and prescriptions that can offer a better foot–ground interface for the biomechanical requirements of foot function.

The practitioner is faced with an ever-increasing range of methods to help patients; at present, research has not provided sufficient understanding as to how they work. McCourt et al (1994) undertook a realistic sample size survey and found that all types of orthosis—bespoke, clinical insole and stock designs—showed >80% effectiveness in each case.

The scientific practitioner must strive to consolidate any process that can offer the most consistent rewards within a cost-effective framework. The aim of treatment is to remove pain, reduce dependency on medication, increase mobility, restore normal function and moderate abnormal footwear patterns.

Too many subdivisions exist to be able to describe all the orthotic designs possible within the limited space available in a text such as this. Readers are therefore directed to Bowker et al (1993) for further references to foot orthoses and AFOs. The examples provided in this chapter should assist the new practitioner in selecting orthoses using the basic principles described.

REFERENCES

Anthony R J 1991 The manufacture and use of the functional foot orthosis. Karger, Basel

Bailey D S, Perillo J T, Forman M 1984 Subtalar joint neutral: a study using tomography. Journal of the American Podiatric Association 74(2): 59–64

Ball P, Johnson G R 1993 Reliability of hindfoot goniometry when using a flexible electrogoniometer. Clinical Biomechanics 8: 13–19

Bowker P, Condie D N, Bader D L, Pratt D J Wallace W A (eds) 1993 The biomechanical basis of orthotic management. Butterworth Heinmann, Oxford

Brown R N, Byers-Hinkley K, Logan L 1987 The talar control ankle foot orthosis. Orthotics and Prosthetics 41: 22–31

Cook A, Gorman I, Morris J 1988 Evaluation of the neutral position of the subtalar joint. Journal of the American Podiatric Medical Association 78: 449–451

D'Amico J C, Rabin M 1986 The influence of foot orthoses on the quadriceps angle. Journal of the American Podiatric Medical Association 76(6): 337–340

Engsberg J R, Grimston S K, Wackwitz J H 1988 Predicting talocalcaneal joint orientations from talocalcaneal/talocrural joint orientations. Journal of Orthopaedic Research 6: 749–757

Glancy J, Lindseth R E 1972 The polypropylene solid-ankle orthosis. Orthotics and Prosthetics 26: 14–26

Griffith C J 1988 An investigation of the repeatability, reliability and validity of clinical biomechanical measurements in the region of the foot and ankle. BSc thesis, Polytechnic of Central London

Inman V T 1969 The influence of the foot–ankle complex on the proximal skeletal structures. Artificial Limbs 13: 59–65

Inman V T 1976 The joints of the ankle. Williams & Wilkins, Baltimore, p 45–66

Kidd R 1991 An examination of the validity of some of the more questionable cornerstones of modern chiropodial diagnosis. Journal of British Podiatric Medicine 9: 172–173

Lehmann J F, Warren C G 1973 Ischial and patella-tendon weight-bearing braces: function, design, adjustment and training. Bulletin of Prosthetics Research 10: 6–19

Lundeen R O 1988 Polysectional triaxial posting. Journal of the American Podiatric Medical Association 78(2): 55–59

McCourt F J, Bevans J, Cluskey L 1994 Report of a survey on in-shoe orthoses provision. Journal of British Podiatric Medicine 49(5): 73–76

McIllmurray W J, Greenbaum W 1958 A below-knee weight-bearing brace. Orthotics and Prosthetics Journal 12: 81–82

McMaster M 1976 Disability of the hindfoot after fracture of the tibial shaft. Journal of Bone & Joint Surgery 58B: 90

Meadows C B, Anderson D M, Duncan L M et al 1980 The use of polypropylene ankle foot orthoses in the management of the cerebral palsied child. A guide based on clinical experience in Dundee. Tayside Rehabilitation Engineering Services, Dundee

Mereday C, Dolan M E, Lusskin R 1972 Evaluation of the University of California Biomechanics Laboratory shoe insert in "Flexible pes planus". Clinical Orthopaedics and Related Research 82: 45–58

Michael J W 1989 Reflections on CAD/CAM in prosthetics and orthotics. Journal of Prosthetics and Orthotics 1: 116–121

Phillips R D, Christeck R, Phillips R L 1985 Clinical measurement of the axis of the subtalar joint. Journal of the American Podiatric Medical Association 75: 119–131

Philps J W 1990 The functional foot orthosis. Churchill Livingstone, Edinburgh

Pratt D J 1990 Long term comparison of some shock attenuating insoles. Prosthetics and Orthotics International 14: 51–57

Pratt D J, Rees P H, Butterworth R H 1984 RTV silicone insoles. Prosthetics and Orthotics International 8: 54–55

Pratt D J, Iliff P M, Ward J B 1993a Talus control foot orthoses. The Foot 4: 31–33

Pratt D J, Tollafield D R, Johnson G R, Peacock C 1993b Foot orthosis. In: Bowker P M, Pratt D J (eds) Biomechanical basis for orthoses. Butterworths, London, p 72–98

Rome K 1990 Behaviour of orthotic materials in chiropody. Journal of the American Podiatric Medical Association 80(9): 471–478

Root M L, Orien W P, Weed J H, Hughes R J 1971 Biomechanical examination of the foot. Clinical Biomechanics Corporation, Los Angeles, vol 1

Root M L, Orien W P, Weed J H 1977 Normal and abnormal function of the foot. Clinical Biomechanics Corporation, Los Angeles, vol 2

Ross A S, Gurnik K L 1982 Elevator selection in rearfoot posted orthoses. Journal of the American Podiatric Association 72: 621–624

Sgarlato T E 1971 A compendium of podiatric biomechanics. California College of Podiatric Medicine, San Francisco

Spencer A M 1978 Practical podiatric orthopaedic procedures. Practical podiatric monograph series. Ohio College of Podiatric Medicine, Cleveland

Stats T B, Kriechbrum M P 1989 Computer-aided design and computer-aided manufacturing of a foot orthoses. Journal of Prosthetics and Orthotics 1: 182–186.

Tollafield D R 1985 Mechanical therapeutic coursework laboratory I & II. First year Chiropody. Nene College, p 193–202, 210–212, 242–256

Tollafield D R, Merriman L M 1995 Assessment of the locomotor system. In: Merriman L M, Tollafield D R (eds) Assessment of the lower limb. Churchill Livingstone, Edinburgh, p 170–173

Tollafield D R, Pratt D J 1987 An analysis of the effects of posting on casted functional orthoses. In Pratt D J and Johnson G R (Eds) The Biomechanics and Orthotic Management of the Foot. Orthotics and Disability Research Centre, Derby, UK

Tollafield D R, Pratt D J 1990a The control of known triplanar forces on the foot by forefoot orthotic posting. British Journal of Podiatric Medicine & Surgery 2: 3–5

Tollafield D R, Pratt D J 1990b The effects of variable rear posting of orthoses on a normal foot. Chiropodist 45(8): 154–160

Wapner K L, Sharkey P F 1991 The use of night splints for treatment of recalcitrant plantar fasciitis. Foot and Ankle 12, 3: 135–137.

Weed J H, Ratliff F D, Ross B A 1978 A biplanar grind for rearposts on functional orthoses. Journal of the American Podiatric Association 68: 35–39

Wu K K 1990 Foot orthoses: principles and clinical applications. Williams and Wilkins, Baltimore

FURTHER READING

Anthony R J 1992 The fabrication protocol for the manufacture of a functional foot orthosis. Journal of British Podiatric Medicine 47(5): 91–98

Bates E H, Chung W K 1988 Congenital talipes equinovarus. In: Helal B, Wilson D (eds) The foot. Churchill Livingstone, Edinburgh, ch 14

Birke J A 1991 Rehabilitation of the diabetic patient. In: Frykberg (ed) The high-risk foot in diabetes mellitus. Churchill Livingstone, New York, p 497–512

Blake R L, Ferguson H 1991 Foot orthosis for the severe flatfoot in sports. 81(10): 549–555

Blake R L, Ferguson H 1992 Extrinsic rearfoot posts. Journal of the American Podiatriatric Medical Association 82(4): 202–206

Brodke D S, Skinner S R, Lameroux L W, Johanson M E, Moran S A, Ashley R K 1989 The effects of ankle foot orthosis on the gait of children. Journal of Pediatrics and Orthopaedics 9: 702–708

Carlson J M, Berglund G 1979 An effective orthotic design for controlling the unstable sub-talar joint. Orthotics and Prosthetics 33: 39–49

Condie D N, Meadows C B 1993 Ankle foot orthoses. In: Bowker P, Condie D N, Bader D L, Pratt D J, Wallace W A (eds) The biomechanical basis of orthotic management. Butterworth Heinmann, Oxford, ch 7, p 99–123

Diamond J E, Sinacore D R, Mueller M J 1987 Molded double-rocker plaster shoe for healing a diabetic ulcer. Physical Therapy 67: 1551–1552

Edwards J, Rome K 1992 A study of the shock attenuating properties of materials used in chiropody. The Foot 2(2): 99–107

Eggold J 1981 orthotics in the prevention of runner's overuse injuries. Physical Sports Medicine 9: 125–128

Elveru R A, Rothstein J M, Lamb R L, Riddle D L 1988 Methods for taking subtalar joint measurements: a clinical report. Physical Therapy 68: 678–682

Freeman A C 1990 A study of inter-observer and intra-observer reliability in the measurement of resting calcaneal stance position and neutral calcaneal stance position. Journal of Podiatric Medicine and Surgery 2: 6–8

Geary N P J, Klenerman L 1987 The rocker sole shoe: a method to reduce peak forefoot pressure in the management of diabetic foot ulceration. In: Pratt D J, Johnson G R (eds) The biomechanics and orthotic management of the foot. Orthotics and Disability Research Centre, Derby, ch 17

Gibbard L C 1968 Charlesworth's chiropodial orthopaedics. Balliere, Tindall and Cassell, London

Hice G A 1984 Orthotic treatment of feet having a high oblique midtarsal joint axis. Journal of the American Podiatric Association 74(11): 577–582

Hice G A, Solomon W, Fashada P 1983 The plaster-synthetic cast. Journal of the American Podiatric Association 73: 427–431

Holmes G B, Timmerman L 1990 A quantitative assessment of the effect of metatarsal pads on plantar pressures. Foot and Ankle 11(3): 141–145

Isman R E, Inman V T 1969 Anthropometric studies of the human foot and ankle. Bulletin of Prosthetics Research, Spring: 97–127

Johnson G R 1990 Measurement of shock acceleration during running and walking using the Shock Meter. Clinical Biomechanics 5: 47–50

Lange L R 1990 The Lange silicone partial foot prosthesis. Journal of Prosthetics and Orthotics 4(1): 56–61

McCourt FJ 1990 To cast or not to cast? The comparative effectiveness of casted and non casted orthoses. Journal of British Podiatric Medicine 45(12): 239–243

Mann R A 1986 Biomechanics of the foot and ankle. In: Mann R A (ed) Surgery of the foot. Mosby, St Louis, ch 1

Manter J T 1941 Movements of the subtalar and transverse tarsal joints. Anatomical Record 80: 397–409

Milgram C, Giladi M, Kashtan H 1985 A prospective study of the effect of a shock-absorbing orthotic device on the incidence of stress fractures in military recruits. Foot and Ankle 6: 101–105

Novick A, Birke J A, Hoard A S, Brasseaux D M, Broussard J B, Hawkins E S 1992 Rigid orthoses for the insensitive foot. Journal of Prosthetics and Orthotics 4(1): 31–40

Odom R D, Gaskwirth B 1987 San splint orthoses. Journal of the American Podiatric Association 72(3): 98–101

Root M L, Orien W P, Weed J H 1978 Neutral position casting technique. Clinical Biomechanics Corporation, Los Angeles

Rose G K 1986 Orthotics: principles and practice. William Heinemann Medical Books, London.

Ross F D 1986 The relationship of abnormal foot pronation to hallux abductovalgus: a pilot study. Prosthetics and Orthotics International 10: 72–78

Schaff P S, Cavanagh P R 1990 Shoes for the insensitive foot: the effect of a "rocker bottom" shoe modification on plantar pressure distribution. Foot and Ankle 11(30): 129–140

Schuster R O 1974 A history of orthopaedics in podiatry. Journal of the American Podiatric Association 64(4): 332–336

Sinacore D R, Mueller M J, Diamond J E et al 1987 Diabetic plantar ulcers treated by total contact casting. Physical Therapy 67: 1543–1549

Sutton R 1989 The thermoplastic elastomer foot orthoses and the thermoplastic eloastomer biomechanical foot orthoses. Journal of Prosthetics and Orthotics 2: 164–172

Taillon D M, McCormick D 1992 Tone reducing orthoses; myth or reality? Proceedings of the International Society of Prosthetics and Orthotics 7th World Congress, Chicago, p 446

Tollafield D R 1986 A foundation in podiatric orthopaedics. Nene College, p165–166

Tooms R E, Griffin J W, Griffin T P 1987 Effect of viscoelastic insoles on pain in nursing students. Orthopaedics 10: 1143–1147

Volshin A S, Wosk J 1985 Low back pain conservative treatment with artificial shock absorbers. Archives of Physical Medicine and Rehabilitation 66(4): 145–148

Weatherwax R J 1980 The plaster slipper cast. Clinical Orthopaedics and Related Research 154: 327–328

13

Footwear therapy

M. Lord
D. J. Pratt

INTRODUCTION

Footwear influences the treatment of many foot problems. For example, no matter how effective an orthosis may be, it will have no therapeutic effect if it cannot be accommodated in the patient's footwear. Conversely, the most effective treatment plan will not achieve its desired results if the patient continues to wear shoes which exacerbate the problem. The use of footwear as a therapeutic tool may involve:

- advice on the purchase of footwear
- prescription of bespoke footwear
- modifications to footwear.

Most patients will benefit from advice about the purchase of suitable footwear. The majority should be able to purchase appropriate footwear from general or specialised retail outlets. For a minority, the only way they can obtain good-fitting footwear is to have it specially made for them (bespoke footwear). Sometimes it is possible to improve foot function by modifying the patient's existing footwear. These three aspects of footwear therapy will be considered in detail in this chapter.

ADVICE ON THE PURCHASE OF FOOTWEAR

Footwear protects the foot from extremes of temperature, moisture, hard surfaces, knocks and scratches. However, for many people its cosmetic value is more important than its functional purpose. The choice of footwear is affected by appearance and current fashion trends as much as, if not more than, by functional purposes. For those with foot problems, however, the choice of footwear may be influenced by supplementary requirements, e.g. to reduce excessive pressures on sensitive structures, to improve walking ability or to accommodate an orthosis or prosthesis.

This section will discuss the following issues related to the purchase of footwear:

- types of footwear
- where to purchase footwear
- advice to patients on the purchase of footwear.

It is important that the practitioner is familiar with the range of footwear types. The practitioner should also be conversant with the availability of footwear locally, as well as that of specialist footwear which may only be obtainable from farther afield. Advising patients that they need 'better footwear' is a futile exercise if it is not backed up with specific advice as to what is needed and where to get it from.

TYPES OF FOOTWEAR

Footwear can be classified in a number of ways. For the purposes of this chapter, the following classification will be used:

- mass versus specialist production
- general versus specific purpose footwear.

Mass versus specialist production

Most footwear is mass-produced from a statistically determined set of lasts (Fig. 13.1A). The shoe last is not the same shape as the foot which will fit the shoe; indeed, making a shoe directly over a plaster cast of a foot would produce ill-fitting shoes. The last is generally deeper in the midfoot region, has a sharp 'feather edge' where the upper surface meets the sole, is clipped in along the topline (around the ankle) and is faired over and extended in the toe region. This provides a shape which applies appropriate tension when the shoe distorts to contain the loaded foot.

It is interesting to note that for female fashion footwear, the tread width across the joint is usually less than the foot outline width by up to 10 mm, and the joint girth may be 10 mm or so less than the foot joint girth. This often results in the sole of the foot spreading outside the shoe insole, and the fifth metatarsal being hammocked on the overhanging upper.

Mass-produced footwear can be produced in *single size/width* or *half size/multiwidth fittings*. Most mass-produced adult footwear is produced in single size and width fittings, whereas children's footwear is more likely to be produced in half size and multiwidth fittings. Inevitably, the cost of producing half sizes

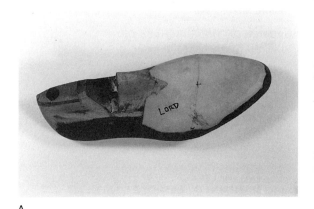

A

Figure 13.1 A: A shoe last. B: Components of a shoe.

and multiwidths is far greater and the additional cost may deter many people. However, as feet come in various shapes and sizes, the use of a range of length and width fittings is more likely to lead to well-fitting footwear.

For those who cannot find well-fitting mass-produced footwear, even when made in half size and multi-width fittings, there are a number of alternatives:

- stock footwear
- modular footwear
- bespoke footwear.

Stock footwear. There is now a wide range of footwear targeted at the orthopaedic market which is variously described as stock, off-the-shelf or ready-made. As well as providing depth for a removable cushioning insert, these shoes often have a wider fit than normal, particularly in the forefoot. They may be offered in a range of overall widths, from normal to extra wide, with a variety of styles and fastenings.

Most companies supplying stock orthopaedic shoes use a limited range of last styles, perhaps up to five different fundamental shapes, which are then produced in a range of sizes. Some companies give details of the lasts and associate these with the styles in their catalogues, which is helpful in making a good choice for an individual patient. Shoes can be bought with confidence if the last shape is known to suit. Lasts can be designed with particular orthopaedic features in mind. For example, the normal straight-edged last can be substituted by a last with the forepart angled with respect to the backpart to provide for supination or pronation (Fig. 13.2). Other lasts are specifically designed to give extra deep toe boxes to accommodate claw toes, or have toe plan shaping to suit hallux valgus.

The use of stock shoes has risen dramatically over the past few years in the UK, spurred on by the increased choice and rapid availability. They cost more than mass-produced shoes but are around a fifth to a quarter of the price of bespoke shoes.

Modular footwear. This type of footwear is fabricated using stock lasts to which minor adaptations are made. The orthotist can conduct a trial fit using the standard stock shoe, and then specify a number of fixed modifications to be made. This enables the special shoes to be delivered at the second visit. The John Locke system is one of the well-known implementations of this technique.

Bespoke footwear. This is footwear which is custom-made for an individual, and involves the production of a last specific to that individual's foot. Bespoke footwear can be obtained either privately or via the NHS. Because of the production and fitting costs, this type of footwear is considerably more expensive than that purchased in the high street.

General or specific purposes

Ideally, footwear should be purchased with a view to its intended use. Unfortunately this is often not the case—consider, for example, the habitual wearing of trainers by teenagers in all weathers and for all purposes. Those who wear open-toed, sling-back shoes in the depth of winter are inviting problems with chilblains. Wellingtons, walking boots, safety boots, trainers designed for specific sports, golf shoes and boots are all examples of footwear designed for specific purposes and usually with the intention of pro-

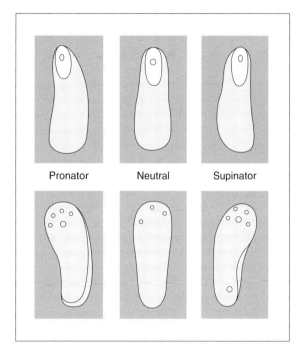

Figure 13.2 Plan views of lasts designed to encourage pronation or supination.

tecting the foot in adverse situations. Patients should be encouraged to buy shoes to meet specific purposes.

Where to purchase footwear

Footwear can be purchased from:

- general high street shops
- specialised high street shops
- mail order
- specialist retail outfits.

Additionally, stock, modular and bespoke footwear may be obtained free via the *National Health Service*.

General high street shops. The majority of people purchase mass-produced footwear from general high street shops. Such footwear is designed to meet most general-purpose needs, but is often only available in single size and width fittings. Much of the footwear is imported and, because of the restriction in sizes, it is usually the most inexpensive type of footwear to purchase.

Specialised high street shops. In most towns and cities it is common to find at least one shop which stocks multiwidth as well as half size fittings. These shops primarily sell children's footwear although they often have adult departments where some of the footwear is in multiwidth fittings. There are also shops which specialise in the adult half size/multiwidth market. The cost of this footwear can be up to two or three times more than that purchased in general high street shops.

Mail order. Mass-produced as well as specialised footwear can be purchased via mail order. Usually companies produce catalogues illustrating their range. Unfortunately there is no opportunity to check the fit prior to purchase, although most firms operate a return service. Most of the popular sizes and styles of these shoes are made in bulk and held in stock at the manufacturers, and are thus available by return of post. Shoes made-to-order from stock patterns and lasts may have a delivery period of a few weeks.

Specialist retail outlets. These cater for specific markets, e.g. those with very long feet. A wide range of specialist footwear is now available and patients can be guided to those most suited to their needs. Suppliers are listed in the *Disabled Living Foundation service handbook*. This encompasses the whole spectrum of special needs—from suppliers of standard shoes in extra small/large or extra narrow/wide ranges, odd and single shoes, and rehabilitation and temporary shoes, through to suppliers of orthopaedic footwear. Bespoke footwear can be provided by some specialist footwear retailers.

NHS footwear. NHS footwear is usually supplied via a prescription from a hospital consultant. The proposal of direct access for general practitioners is gaining favour. Under this scheme, patients could be referred directly to a footwear clinic rather than through a consultant.

Stock, modular or bespoke footwear may be provided. Stock footwear in the UK must meet standards of construction laid down by the NHS in order to be supplied to NHS patients. Some company orthotists carry their own stock of a few styles, enabling them potentially to fit and supply at the first visit. However, there is a compromise between choice and speed of supply, since holding a stock of more than a few styles would be prohibitive for the normal turnover at most foot clinics.

Bespoke footwear is made via a prescription which is expanded into a full specification either by an orthotist employed by a NHS Trust or by one who works for a private company. Whereas 5 years ago the vast majority of shoes were supplied by contractor's orthotists, it is now more common for hospitals to employ their own orthotist. Other members of the clinical team may be involved in designing the prescription, e.g. a podiatrist or physiotherapist. Bespoke footwear is usually produced off-site by a contractor for subsequent delivery at a later clinic. The NHS contract normally requires that such footwear is available for fitting 6 weeks after the measurements are taken. Adaptations and shoe inserts may be made on-site by NHS staff or by the contractor.

ADVICE TO PATIENTS ON THE PURCHASE OF FOOTWEAR

Whether patients are purchasing mass-produced, stock orthopaedic or modular footwear, the need to take into account the following:

- fit
- comfort
- cosmesis.

Fit

The concept of a well-fitting shoe involves many factors, which relate as much to characteristics of an individual's foot as to the construction of the shoe. The fit of the shoe should allow for a snug approximation around some areas of the foot, while in other areas a clearance over the skin is required. Excessive tightness and excessive clearance could both constitute poor fit, although these are difficult to determine in any quantitative sense. Additionally, the shoe needs to change shape in concert with the foot during weight-bearing and walking.

Because fit is an individual characteristic, a trial fit of footwear is essential when it is supplied for the first time. The assessment of shoe fit is made both subjectively and objectively. For normally sensate feet, the subjective impression is valuable for reporting tightness and discomfort, but where sensory deficits are present this is less so, and the burden of ensuring fit falls to the fitter.

Subjective perception of fit depends on the wearer's preference for tightness and habituation to foot deformation in the name of fashion. It may be necessary to educate some patients to accept a looser fit in the forefoot than that to which they are accustomed. If purchasing from a shoe shop, the patient should be encouraged to walk around to test the fit of the shoe.

Objective assessment by observation and touch is always important in a trial fit. The first requirements for any shoe are those of normal good sense. The shoe should not compress the joints of the forefoot, should be a good fit and capable of secure fastening to prevent slipping, and should be of an appropriate heel height for optimum foot functioning. The following points should be routinely checked (Fig. 13.3):

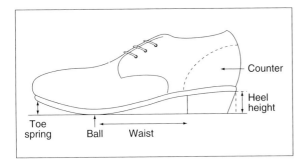

Figure 13.3 Features of a shoe which should be taken into consideration when fitting.

- location of the metatarsophalangeal joints at the widest part of the shoe
- adequate width across the joint of the foot
- clearance in the toe region
- adequate length for extension of the foot during walking (10 mm)
- snug fit in the midfoot, noting particularly whether the lace panel, when fastened, is too spread out or overlapping
- snug fit at the rear of the heel—excessive space is indicative of a shoe size too large or too great a depth or width across the throat, allowing the foot to slip forward; or an excessive length of the rearpart of the shoe
- gaping at the topline of the shoe, which can be caused by inappropriate shaping, incorrect heel height for the shoe or clearance under the malleoli at the topline
- localised tight spots over bunions or other protuberances
- back seam height not excessive so as to cause irritation over the Achilles tendon

Table 13.1 Changes in foot dimension due to weight-bearing for 26 women in the age range 18–60 years, of average foot size and with normal feet.

	Average dimension non-weight-bearing	Change in dimension to weight-bearing	
	(mm)	(mm)	(%)
Foot length	242	6.8	2.8
Joint* girth	231	5.4	2.3
Joint width	89	5.0	5.6
Waist* girth	226	5.4	2.4
Instep* girth	229	3.4	1.5
Heel width	59	3.0	5.1

*The joint is the widest part of the forefoot, the waist is the narrowest part of the midfoot, and the instep is around the highest point of the longitudinal arch.

- rearfoot fit in depth and clip adequate to prevent heel slip during walking.

Heel height is important for correct foot function, particularly if it is too high. A steep heel to forefoot angle will tend to cause the foot to slip forward and impact against the end of the shoe. Heel heights are generally age-related, with up to 18 mm for children, 37 mm for adolescents and women, and 21–25 mm for men.

Differences in foot dimensions between weight-bearing and non-weight-bearing vary between individuals, depending on the flexibility and mechanics of the foot (Table 13.1). During walking, the foot flexes primarily at the metatarsal break, i.e. approximately along the line of the metatarsal heads (Fig. 13.4). Shoes are also designed to flex in this region. The match of the location of the break, and the degree of flexibility are important for correct shoe fit (Chen 1993).

When selecting shoes, the manufacturer's marked

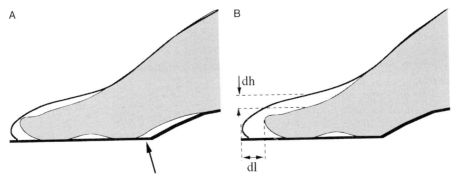

Figure 13.4 Correct fitting of the forepart of the shoe. A: Ill-fitting shoe with ball incorrectly located. B: Well-fitting shoe with the ball correctly located and adequate toe clearance in both length, dl, and height, dh.

size should be treated only as a guide (Rossi 1983). There can be no fixed definitions of shoe sizing because this depends on the shape of the shoe as well as the overall length. The sizing system is graded in length, historically in steps of 8.4 mm per full size in the UK and USA systems, and in steps of 6.5 mm in the European sizing system. The increments in the UK and USA system are the same, but the sizing systems do not share the same starting point. European sizes cannot be converted exactly into equivalent UK or USA sizes because of the different grading increment.

Because the difference between sizes in the UK and USA systems is quite large, interim half sizes are sometimes used to improve the fitting range. This, however, incurs extra costs in the manufacture and in maintaining stock levels in shops. Cheaper shoe ranges and many of the special orthopaedic shoe ranges are only stocked in full sizes.

Width is usually measured from the forefoot girth, with the increase in one width fitting equivalent to 5 mm for whole sizes up to children's size 13, and 6.5 mm for whole sizes above this. It may also be expressed in terms of the linear width of the shoe across its forefoot.

Special fitting considerations

For certain purposes, problem feet can usefully be categorised into the *hypersensitive* (*painful*) or the *insensate* (*anaesthetic*) foot. In the case of the former, the pressures exerted on the foot by the shoe must be minimised; this can be achieved by underfoot cushioning, light-weight construction of upper and soles, seamless construction of the upper, use of shock-absorbing heels and sole materials, and perhaps by providing a rigid shoe sole or a boot to immobilise the joints.

Controlling the pressures exerted on the foot is also imperative in the case of the insensate foot. Even though the tolerance of this type of foot to pressure may be normal, excessive pressure from foreign bodies or simply from overuse will not result in the usual pain-avoidance responses. Furthermore, abnormally high plantar pressures are often present in the forefoot with conditions such as diabetic neuropathy (Boulton et al 1983), and these correlate with the location of ulcers. Provision of cushioning and moulded inserts to effect pressure redistribution can be effec-tive in managing the condition (Cavanagh et al 1987). A study by Chantelau & Haage (1994) showed that the recurrence rate of neuropathic ulcers was considerably reduced in diabetic patients who wore cushioned protective footwear for more than 60% of each day.

The second categorisation which can be useful is that of the *hypermobile* versus the *rigid* foot. A hypermobile foot may require a degree of support or correction to maintain the joint orientations. This can be achieved by insole contouring, internal or external wedging and supportive shoe upper design. In extreme cases, the foot may need to be immobilised by the use of a rigid sole, which will require a rockered design to enable roll-off. The rigid foot, by contrast, cannot be corrected, and therefore must be supported in its fixed position and accommodated. Wedge soles can be used which result in there being no definite heel breast (Fig. 13.1A). Such a sole will impart intrinsic stability to the waist which may benefit some foot conditions. It is essential that, of these two, i.e. correction versus accommodation, the correct strategy is chosen.

Extra deep footwear may be required to accommodate orthoses or clinical padding. Ideally, if orthoses are being prescribed, the patient should be encouraged to purchase new shoes. The function of an orthosis may be adversely affected if the patient is wearing well-worn shoes which have noticeable wear marks on the heel and sole. Worn shoes may adversely affect the patient's gait and reduce the therapeutic value of the orthoses.

Comfort

In order to be classed as comfortable, footwear should:

- be as light-weight as possible
- have adequate thermal conductivity
- be permeable to moisture
- not produce excessive pressure or friction
- prevent excessive movement of the foot in the shoe.

Clearly some of these may be mutually exclusive, so it is important to identify which features are most important to assure the patient's foot comfort. Thermal conductivity, permeability to moisture and excessive pressure and friction are considered in detail below.

Thermal conductivity

The temperature inside shoes affects foot comfort. Foot temperature is largely determined by blood flow, as about 10% of the total blood volume exists within 2 mm of the skin surface. When the average foot temperature drops to below about 18°C, most people complain of cold feet. Below about 10°C feet often

Table 13.2 Thermal conductivity (Boulanger et al 1976). All measurements in W/m² °C × 10². PU = polyurethane, rh = relative humidity

Material	28% rh	65% rh	77% rh	100% rh
Microporous PU	7.7	8.0	7.9	8.2
PU-coated non-woven fabric 1	7.7	7.9	8.1	8.1
PU-coated non-woven fabric 2	8.8	9.1	9.6	10.0
Corrected grain leather	9.4	11.2	12.0	14.0
PVC-coated full-grain leather	9.9	11.0	11.2	14.6
PU-coated woven fabric	12.5	13.4	14.1	16.1
PVC-coated woven fabric	17.8	18.1	18.0	18.8

become painful. This is significant because the foot is generally insensitive to cold—the number of cold receptors on the foot is small (3–$6/cm^2$) when compared with the rest of the body (9–$13/cm^2$).

The thermal conductivity of footwear materials varies considerably (see Table 13.2). Patients suffering from vasospastic disorders and poor arterial blood supply need to be mindful of which materials provide the best insulation from external temperatures. The insulation properties of footwear can be improved by the use of fleece linings or thermal insoles. A simple Plastazote insole may be beneficial for some patients.

The feeling of discomfort due to heat is often confused with that due to sweatiness, which suggests that the rate of heat dissipation is more relevant to discomfort than the temperature per se. Studies have found that temperatures of about 32–35°C are the upper limit for general comfort, and that a temperature of about 45°C is painful (Bunten 1983).

Many people complain of a burning sensation as a source of discomfort. This is a difficult sensation to characterise as excessive shoe tightness and perspiration do not in themselves produce this feeling. It is thought to be due to type C pain fibres (Rothman 1954). A study by Murray & Peet (1966) suggested a link between temperature and this sensation, but Burry (1956) suggests a number of other possible causes:

- chemical irritation due to excess acidity in the insole or allergy to substances from the hosiery or shoes
- poor shoe fit causing creasing of skin and friction between the foot, sock and shoe
- overheating of the foot due to vapour-impermeable materials in the shoe, overly warm clothing or excessive physical activity
- pathological conditions such as Morton's neuroma or fungal infections.

Permeability to moisture

Perspiration within footwear is principally produced by the eccrine glands and is slightly acidic (pH 3.8–5.7). However, as it cannot evaporate quickly within footwear it decomposes and becomes alkaline. The foot typically perspires about 4 mg cm^{-2} h^{-1} of water via insensitive perspiration (water loss without noticeable skin surface moisture). Sensitive perspiration of sweat is dependent upon environmental conditions and the health of the person, and varies from about 2.5 mg cm^{-2} h^{-1} to as high as 35 mg cm^{-2} h^{-1}. The water vapour permeability of footwear materials is an important factor to take into consideration (Table 13.3). This property varies considerably in materials used in the manufacture of footwear.

It is doubtful if wetness of the skin due to perspiration is itself uncomfortable, but the indirect effects can be very marked. Wet skin, however produced, tends to reduce the cooling effect of the evaporation of perspiration and may stop it completely. Hence, the foot will tend to feel uncomfortably hot. Other indirect effects may arise from the higher heat conductivity of the epidermis if soaked in water such as the softening of the skin, which could make it more susceptible to damage from friction or pressure. Moisture also encourages fungal growths which can be irritatingly itchy.

Pressure and friction

Plantar pressure within shoes has been measured by a number of people over the years (Lord 1981, Lord et al 1986, Alexander et al 1990) and now interest is also being shown in the measurement of shear forces (Pollard et al 1983, Warren-Forward et al 1992, Lord et al 1992). There is an established link between excessive pressure and shear, and the development of skin damage, particularly in feet considered to be 'at risk' (Bennett et al 1979).

Table 13.3   Water vapour permeability (rh = relative humidity)

Material		Environmental conditions		
	(Inside) (Outside)	21°C, 50% rh 21°C, 0% rh	21°C, 100% rh 21°C, 50% rh	39°C, 100% rh 21°C, 50% rh
Sheepskin		1.39	1.25	1.16
Belly leather		0.63	0.80	1.16
Kip leather		0.31	0.23	0.22
Patent leather		0.02	0.01	0.01
PVC on fabric		0.01	0.01	0.02
PVC on polyester		0.08	0.08	0.08
Perforated PVC on fabric		0.05	0.04	0.04

The dorsum of the foot is more sensitive to pressure than the plantar surface. Excess pressure is the most common source of foot discomfort. The extent of foot pathology, e.g. rigid plantarflexed first ray, will dictate the level at which discomfort is felt. In some cases where the disease process may result in insensate feet, such as diabetes and Hansen's disease, patients do not feel discomfort. Damaging pressures may have been acting for a long period of time and may have led to significant damage.

Continued static pressure between the foot and shoe is more likely to cause general discomfort than the high transient pressure associated with walking or running. This is probably due to the static occlusion of blood flow, a subsequent reduction in sweating and an increased perception of discomfort because the foot feels hotter without the cooling effect of the perspiration (Bunten 1983). Hence, a foot will feel hotter when subjected to pressure in a hot environment. The converse happens in a cool climate as the reduction in blood flow caused by the pressure cools the foot, as it is relying on blood circulation to keep it warm. In addition, the soft tissues are compressed by the pressure and suffer anoxic damage which accumulates unless the pressure is removed for sufficient time to allow recovery. A good description of the interface problem is to be found in Bader & Chase (1993).

Repetitive transient pressure which may occur during walking can cause localised tissue damage via a more direct mechanism than blood flow occlusion. This involves mechanical injury to tissue and/or formation of callus, leading to skin lesions which can themselves become the source of discomfort and pain.

Pressure exerted by the shoe upper may be exacerbated by swelling of the foot. Footwear must accommodate the change in foot shape during weight-bearing in addition to daytime volume changes associated with orthostatic pressure of the blood and the dynamics of the venous and lymphatic systems. Normal daily changes in foot volume are of the order of 3% (range 1.5–5.3%), with a further increase of between 1 and 3% due to increasing foot temperature (Bunten 1983). In cases of venous insufficiency and lymphoedema, these increases will be much larger, and the choice of materials and design of footwear become much harder. The ability of footwear materials to respond to changes in foot shape which occur during the day is an important consideration when selecting appropriate shoes. In particular, the tensile properties of the material will influence the feeling of comfort (Table 13.4).

To reduce friction, all parts of the shoe which contact the foot should be smoothly lined. The vamp should be reinforced by the toe box or toe puff as this helps to protect the toes from knocks and stubbing, and helps to preserve the contour of the vamp.

Cosmesis

The fit of a shoe and its appearance are linked. It is impossible to achieve a satisfactory fit for 'at risk' feet with high-heeled shoes with pointed toes. However, it is often possible to maximise the cosmetic appeal within the constraints of what is required functionally. The old adage 'beauty is in the eye of the beholder'

Table 13.4   Tensile properties at two extensions in N/cm

Material	2% extension	10% extension
Calf	1.8	4.6
Suede calf	1.3	3.2
Veal suede	4.5	8.2
Grained side	1.6	2.9
Clothing leather	0.15	–
Softee leather	2.0	3.5
Clarino 1 (synthetic)	3.1	2.7
Ortix 1 (synthetic)	2.1	1.9

certainly applies to shoes. What one person accepts as pleasing may be totally abhorrent to another, so an element of individual choice is always necessary. Cultural influences and social patterns can also dictate preferences. Whereas the recent UK fashion for Doc Martens and trainers has provided a welcome temporary remission from the more damaging aspects of some fashions, this will probably not continue.

The psychological effects of the appearance of footwear must not be dismissed lightly. For many, shoes are the item of dress which first mark the person out from their peer group as different. Many a pair of orthopaedic shoes lies unworn in the wardrobe. Conversely, compliant patients often restrict their lifestyles solely because of the appearance of the footwear. Costigan et al (1989) reviewed 82 patients given shoes 2–3 years previously at the General Hospital in Nottingham, of whom 59 were women and 23 were men. Of the 82 original patients, 66 continued wearing the footwear, but 'even patients who still wore their surgical shoes were often dissatisfied, the reasons being the inability to fasten the shoes themselves... and the appearance of the shoes'. Fisher & McLellan (1989) similarly reported that some patients found their shoes too heavy or clumsy, or of poor appearance.

The balancing of functional needs with aesthetic acceptability is a matter of judgement of the clinical staff. Patient education is advisable.

PRESCRIPTION OF BESPOKE FOOTWEAR

Bespoke footwear is made to fit an individual patient's foot measurements. The process from measurement to delivery usually takes around 2 months in the UK. As already highlighted bespoke footwear may be purchased privately or obtained free or at reduced costs via the NHS for those referred by a consultant.

Initial assessment

It is essential that a thorough assessment is undertaken, which includes an examination of foot mobility and alignment, presence of sensory neuropathy, skin lesions, prominences and deformities, oedema, alignment and gait. It is also important that the patient's lifestyle requirements and perceived problems and needs are taken into consideration. Additional consideration should be given to educational needs and compliance.

The patient should be shown a catalogue of styles and offered a wide choice of colours, perhaps from swatches of leather. Often the most basic style of shoe can be made more attractive by good colour selection and attention to details such as punch hole patterns on the front part, or contrasting topline padding, careful placement of ornamentation and balanced designs (Fig. 13.5).

There are two main shoe styles used in bespoke footwear, the Derby or Gibson and the Oxford (Fig. 13.6). With the Derby shoe, the manner in which the quarters and vamp are cut and attached enables the shoe to be fitted more easily, because the tongue can be reflected completely back and the shoe can be opened wider than with the Oxford style. T-bar styles can be used for certain categories of patients. More recently, trainer styles have been added to the range of many companies, in response to fashion demands, although these usually have a traditional sole construction rather than the moulded soles of the volume shoe. In addition to shoes, boots are also available which extend more proximally, to help keep them on in the case of forefoot amputation, or to impart extra support around the ankle.

Measurement (BS 5943)

Foot measurement can be taken with a pencil of 7 mm diameter, paper and a 6.25 mm wide tape measure. The following procedure should be adopted:

- The outline of the foot with the patient standing should be recorded. The pen should be held vertically but angled in under the longitudinal arch.
- The height over prominent toes or bony features should be indicated.
- Sites of skin lesions should be marked.
- The girth of the foot should be measured while the patient is standing. The tape measure should be slipped under the foot and wrapped over the prominences of the first and fifth metatarsal heads: the tape should be pulled tight then released slightly so as not to compress the tissues. The position of the girth is marked on the outline by dropping the tape flat onto the ground and scoring either side of it (Fig. 13.7).
- Similarly, the girth at the waist (narrowest dimension) and instep (over the navicular prominence) are recorded and the positions marked.
- Long and short heel (minimum) measures should be taken. The long heel measure is taken to the same point (navicular prominence) as is used for the instep measure.

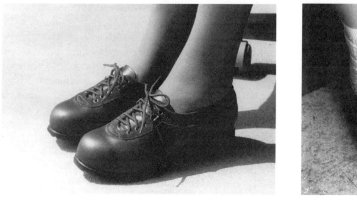

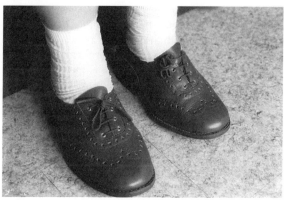

A

B

Figure 13.5 Well-designed shoes have a traditional shape detailing sufficient toe depth, good quarter fit below the malleoli, facings and tongue with a small gap not giving rise to pressure over the dorsal midfoot bones. A: Adult. B: Child.

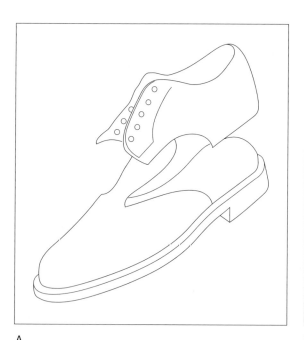

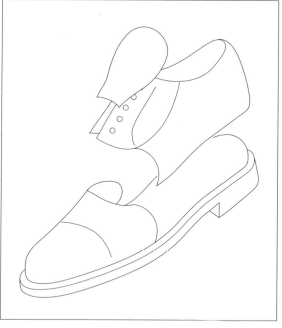

A

B

Figure 13.6 A: Derby or Gibson style shoe. B: Oxford style shoe.

• Foot length should be measured along the medial border with a size stick, with the foot weight-bearing or semi-weight-bearing.

For more severe cases, a plaster cast of the foot may be taken to represent the overall contours. This is usually done with the foot in its non-weight-bearing neutral position as described by Root et al (1971), although some practitioners prefer weight-bearing casts.

An impression of the foot bed is required for moulded inserts. This can be taken with a slipper cast, or by pressing the foot into a special-purpose box of foam, or by the use of vacuum bag casting which is

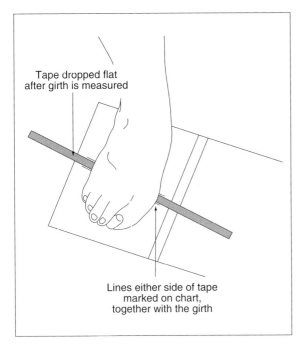

Figure 13.7 The position at which girth measurements are taken should be noted on the outline, so that the measurements can be matched at the same location on the last.

Table 13.5 Suggested average last allowances for orthopaedic shoes

Dimension	Last allowance (mm) (last measurement minus foot measurement)
Length	10
Joint girth	10
Long heel	−5
Joint width	0
Heel width	0

favoured in continental Europe. Other direct methods of making insoles are now available; for example, a device may be used where the foot shape is captured by impressing the sole into a bed of closely packed rods from which a silicone insert can be directly fabricated. A high technology approach can also be adopted—for example, the measurement can be taken with the patient standing on a bed of round-ended tubes which are forced up through pre-shaping templates by a constant, adjustable pressure. The resulting shape is captured on an adjacent computer, where shape compensations can be made before the insert is milled from a preform in a computer controlled machine alongside.

Bespoke lasts

These are made either by modification of the contours of a stock last by the addition or reduction of material to suit the individual's measurements, or by producing a custom last. The dimensions of the custom last do not correspond to those of the foot. The differences in key dimensions are known as the last allowances. There are no hard and fast rules for these, although generally the lastmaker works to a notional standard when making the first attempt at the last. As a general guidance, the values in Table 13.5 are used, although these can be changed in accordance with last shaping and the fit required. For example, it is reported that curvature of the bottom surface of the last can affect the girth allowance and an extra 2 mm of depth above normal is equivalent to an increase in joint girth of 3.5 mm (Browne 1993). Individual allowances may also depend on the foot conditions, e.g. increased joint allowances for sensitive forefoot and reduced instep girth for supportive footwear.

The allowances do not provide space for inserts, which require further allowances on the forefoot girths of twice the insert thickness (or less if compressible)—preferably, the lasts are made to the normal allowance and an equivalent thickness of the insert is blocked onto the bottom of the last before the shoe is constructed.

Construction

Although there are many ways of constructing a shoe, the recommended method for bespoke shoes is by welt construction. This method produces a shoe which is smooth inside, facilitates internal modifications, is simple to repair and retains its shape well.

In a well-constructed bespoke shoe, there are two soles, inner and outer. The outer sole, in contact with the floor, is often leather but is increasingly being made from a synthetic material. The inner sole of leather lies under the foot, and between these two soles is a compressible filler.

Patients have complained about the weight of bespoke footwear. This was in the past determined by the standards of leather, and heavy leather soles and construction dictated by the NHS guidelines. More enlightened interpretation of the guidelines now permits the use of different materials, such as Microlite soles. This allows the possibility of a lighter shoe for patients with occasional or indoor use.

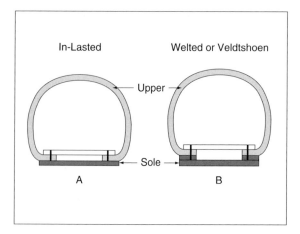

Figure 13.8 Diagram of an in-lasted (A) and a welted (B) shoe construction.

Generally, heel heights for bespoke shoes should not exceed 42 mm and heels should be straight-sided and have a low pitch. The heel is nailed to the outsole and the whole shoe is polished ready for delivery.

There is an alternative method for making bespoke shoes called the in-lasted method, in which the upper material is wrapped around and under the last and the sole is attached to the bottom (Fig. 13.8). This produces a close fit but is more difficult to alter and repair, as is so often required for users of special footwear.

Trial fitting

Bespoke shoes provided at the rough finishing stage should have a temporary heel of the correct height attached. It is important to ensure that the final versions of any removable inlays are provided with the shoes. These should first be removed from the shoes, and a check made with the patient standing barefoot on the inlay. If satisfactory, the inlays are put back into the shoes. In all cases, the patient should then put on the shoes while wearing the customary hosiery, paying attention to any problems of entry or fastening. With the fastening firmly done up, the patient should be asked to stand. The check list outlined in the section above on fit should be used.

For minor modifications to bespoke shoes or for minor adaptations to the uppers of a stock shoe, positions of local alterations may be marked onto the upper with an erasable pencil. Other fitting observations must be recorded. If the fit requires major modifications, a remeasure should be undertaken, and a further trial fit will be required.

One variant on this process, practised in continental Europe, is the use of shell shoes. At the stage when the last is first made, a plastic shell is fabricated by vacuum-moulding over the last and inset (Fig. 13.9). With the addition of a temporary heel of the correct height, this shell is then sent for trial fitting, as opposed to a rough-finished shoe. The advantage of this method is that the shell can very quickly be ready for trial fitting, cutting perhaps 2 weeks off the supply time. More adventurous pattern designs can be undertaken once the last is closer to its final shape.

Delivery

Delivery should be at a clinic where a final fit assessment can be made. Some problems with fit may not come to light until the shoes have been worn. These include creases in the vamp, excessive pressure on the dorsum of the foot, pain due to mismatch of foot

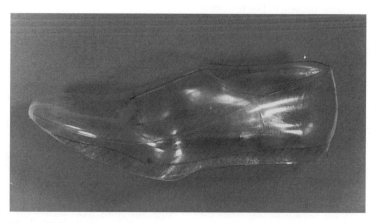

Figure 13.9 A clear shell shoe.

and shoe function, and rubbing due to prominent seams. It is important, therefore, to check the shoes a few weeks after delivery. The lack of any signs of wear on the sole or upper can be quite revealing about usage.

Changes in UK practice

It is hoped that the introduction of computer-aided design techniques will improve the production of bespoke footwear without incurring excessive overheads. It may even allow for the possibility of link-ups with volume manufacturers for subsets of their current ranges (Lord et al 1991). The use of shell shoes to expedite fitting is being introduced into the UK by several contractors. The contractors are also introducing computer-aided design and manufacture for bespoke shoes, which may improve the speed of delivery and quality of the product.

FOOTWEAR ADAPTATIONS

Many adaptations can be made to a patient's footwear. The purpose of such adaptations is to achieve one or more of the following:

- accommodate fixed deformities
- improve the stability of the foot
- relieve discomfort.

Adaptations may be fitted to the exterior or the interior of the footwear, although most are fitted to the exterior. External adaptations do not usually result in the shoe-fitting problems which often occur with internal footwear adaptations, e.g. insoles and orthoses,

nor should they distort the shoe. Any adaptation should be as light-weight as possible so as not to adversely affect what might already be a poor quality, high energy consuming gait.

Before an adaptation is fitted, it is essential to ensure that the footwear is a good fit. To achieve this, the footwear, usually a shoe, needs to:

- extend proximally on the foot to grip the rearfoot and help control the subtalar joint
- be effectively fastened to the foot by means of laces or straps (elasticated straps or inserts should be avoided)
- have a firm heel counter to help control the calcaneus
- have a broad heel for overall stability.

Malalignment of the foot joints, plus involvement of the more proximal joints in conditions such as arthritis, may lead to severe pain up through the ankle, knee, hip and spine. It is therefore important to consider the whole body alignment when assessing for footwear adaptations. The design of the footwear also needs to take into account the gait. In the typical rheumatoid gait, for example, the foot is placed flat onto the ground and lifted in the same way, without the usual heel strike and roll-over pattern of normal gait. The provision of rockered soles can assist in establishing a more normal gait both by pain relief and by reduction of the effort needed from weakened calf muscles (Dimonte & Light 1982).

Any changes aimed at achieving realignment via changes in heel height or wedging must be carefully managed and gradually introduced in order not to induce stresses in more proximal joints.

A range of adaptations can be made to footwear. These are listed in Table 13.6 and discussed below.

Table 13.6 Footwear adaptations for specific conditions as alternative methods to other systems of management

Condition	Objectives	Possible adaptations
Arthritis (traumatic or rheumatoid)	Limit motion Accomodate valgus/varus Pressure relief	Rocker sole, use of boot, ankle stiffener, heel flare, Thomas heel Sach heel, cushioning inserts
Ankle or subtalar arthrodesis	Improve gait pattern Accommodate short leg and equinus	Rocker sole Heel/sole raise
Ankle and subtalar instability	Support unstable joints	Heel flare, boot with ankle stiffener, orthosis with frontal plane control
Diabetic neuropathy	Plantar pressure redistribution and relief	Soft uppers (digits) Shock attenuation, moulded inlay or rocker sole
Pes valgus and similar variations	Limit eversion at hindfoot Control forefoot	Use of boot with broad heel, use of long medial stiffened counter, orthotic inlay for forefoot varus/valgus wedge or on outer sole (less control)

Table 13.6 (contd)

Condition	Objectives	Possible adaptations
	Limit midtarsal compensation	Additional heel adaptations, Thomas heel, extend heel breast, medial flare on orthosis and shoes
	Contour long arch	Longitudinal arch fillers
Pes equinus	Assist foot in plantarflexed position (rigid)	Heel raise internal/external to shoe
	Decrease equinus (flexible)	Remove heel or elevate sole
	Hold foot in shoe	Use boots, add collar to shoe
Pes cavus	Plantar forefoot redistribution	Increase heel height
	Foot contour problem	Deeper shoes, use of boot, deep toe puff, soft tongue pad. Inlay to balance heel with forefoot
	Varus heel/valgus forefoot	Heel and sole wedges on shoe
	Metatarsalgia	Insole contoured for arch and metatarsal pressure areas and to cushion shock
Talipes equinovarus	Accommodate deformity	Use of boots for improved control, high heel counters extended forward, breast extended anteriorly, lateral heel extended, lateral heel and sole wedges/flares, shank filler
	Flexible deformity, attempt to assist stretch out deformity	Lower/remove heel, use Bebax design (Ch. 15), use modified (outflared last)
Calcaneal pain	Shock attenuation	Cushion heel material, strong heel counter, Sach heel
	Pressure relief	Insoles/heel pads, heel elevation, remove heel counter
Metatarsalgia and metatarsal depressed transverse arch	Pain relief	Ensure sufficient shoe length for spread forefoot, lower heel height, excavate insole
	Redistribution	External metatarsal bar, add Denver bar, internal metatarsal pads, lower heel to off-load forefoot
Flexion toe deformities	Relief from IPJ pressure	Deep toe box, balloon patch, soft or Norwegian vamp
	Stabilise metatarsals and hindfoot problems	Attention to valgus/varus as above
Hallux valgus and exostosis	Provide adequate room	Broad last with long vamp, add balloon patch. Build adequate depth into shoe design, hindfoot may be narrow (see splay foot). Go for snug fit across vamp to prevent movement
	Prevent deformity	Width compression reduced as above. Allow room for orthoses
Splay foot	Narrow heel problem	Stiffen and narrow heel counter
	Accommodate Tailor's bunion	Balloon patch over fifth metatarsal or stretch shoe
	Stabilise foot	Use various orthotic modalities or modify heel, elevate heel, use boot and ankle stiffener
Hallux rigidus	Prevent motion and reduce pressure if enlarged	Toe box depth, add rocker sole across metatarsal heads or long rocker sole. Steel sole plate
Foot shortening	Fill room in forefoot	Extra insole, tongue pad, split shoe sizes, filler in toe part with steel sole plate. Extreme cases—bespoke shoes
Leg length discrepancy	Achieve symmetrical posture *Additional objectives:* Improve gait determinants Keep heel in shoe	Internal heel elevation to 12 mm maximum. Use collar or boot if fit problems. Go for external raise on heel and sole. Metal skate for large discrepancies. More conspicuous extension boot with foot placed in equinus

The sole and heel of the shoe

Heel flares. These can be applied to either side of the heel to provide a correctional moment of force at the heel during heel strike (Fig. 13.10A). They do this by moving the point of initial foot contact medially or laterally such that the moment created by the ground reaction force opposes the deforming moment. They can be used to help stabilise the subtalar joint in arthritic or unstable foot conditions, which often lead to recurrent ankle sprain. Flares do not alter the resting position of the foot, they only help to correct the foot motion at foot contact. Wedges are used to alter the resting foot position.

Wedges. These can be applied to either side of the heel, over the whole length of the sole, a localised area of the sole (e.g. fifth metatarsal head area) or any combination of these, to achieve a tilting of the inside of the shoe relative to the ground (Fig. 13.10B). It is unusual to have a wedge of more than 6 mm, with 4 mm being typical, as higher values than these tend to cause the foot to slide down the incline created without providing any additional benefit. It must be remembered that for wedges to work satisfactorily, there must be the appropriate joint motion in the foot. Wedges can be of value in managing mild cases of pes planovalgus (medial heel wedge) and pes cavus (lateral heel and sole wedges), either on their own or in conjunction with other orthoses, their principal action being to promote inversion or eversion of the foot, particularly via the calcaneus.

Metatarsal bars. These are added to the sole of the shoe, proximal to the metatarsal heads, in an attempt to relieve pain and decrease pressure from the metatarsal heads (Fig. 13.10C). Their effectiveness depends upon the sole material and thickness, with better results found with thinner soles. They are generally less successful than metatarsal pads placed within the shoe.

Sole plates. These are used to stiffen the sole by the insertion of a spring steel shank. They are useful in the treatment of pain associated with hallux limitus, by preventing or limiting flexion at the metatarsophalangeal joints. Rocker soles are used for established cases of hallux rigidus.

Thomas heel. This is an anteromedial extension of the heel which can be used to provide additional support to the medial longitudinal arch of the foot (Fig. 13.10D). Thomas heels may be used in conjunction with a medial heel flare or wedge in managing pes planovalgus or to increase the effectiveness of insoles or foot orthoses in the heavier patient. The use of shoes with a wedge sole has a similar effect.

Heel and sole raises. There are a variety of reasons why raises may be used. Leg length discrepancy is a common factor. Care should be taken when adding raises to footwear, as flexibility of the sole is important for walking. If this cannot be maintained, an additional rocker sole should be considered. Any increase in heel height requires an increase in the amount of dorsiflexion at the metatarsophalangeal joints, i.e. about 1° for each 5 mm of additional heel height. An increase in heel height can also lead to an increase in forefoot loading (Gastwirth et al 1991). Common practice suggests that up to 12 mm may be added to the heel before it is necessary to raise the sole; this could be split by adding 6 mm inside the shoe (providing it has sufficient depth at the heel) and reducing the contralateral shoe outside by 6 mm. The actual prescription must be decided on an individual basis as it is not always advisable to include heel raises in cases of neurological damage such as cerebral palsy. It is also necessary to monitor the person with the raise regularly, as not all patients respond in the same way.

Sole rockers. These are used to alter the forward progression of the ground reaction force so that loads can be taken off susceptible metatarsal heads. This is particularly relevant in the management of diabetic foot ulceration (Geary & Klenerman 1987; Fig. 13.10E). The reduction in toe dorsiflexion that rocker soles induce often helps to relieve metatarsal discomfort. Rocker soles can also be used as described above to augment other shoe adaptations and orthotic devices, and to replace motion required for gait which has been lost elsewhere in the foot, e.g. through an arthrodesis of the ankle joint.

Cushioned heel. These can be used to help relieve the discomfort associated with the shock of heel contact during walking. A compressible material is inserted into the posterior heel as a wedge which compresses during heel strike and cushions the foot— this is sometimes called a Sach heel (Fig. 13.10F). Heel pain may be due to a calcaneal spur, and cushioning alone may not be sufficient to relieve symptoms. In these cases an excavation in the heel of the shoe can be used to off-load the tender area.

Torque heel. This is a rubber device which can be attached to the heel of a shoe. As the heel is loaded, the rubber wings of the insert are forced over, causing the shoe to twist, usually outwards. This can be used to assist children who walk with their feet internally (or externally) rotated, provided there is no significant spasticity present (Fig. 13.10G).

Calliper. The portion of the sole between the ball and the anterior border of the heel is called the waist.

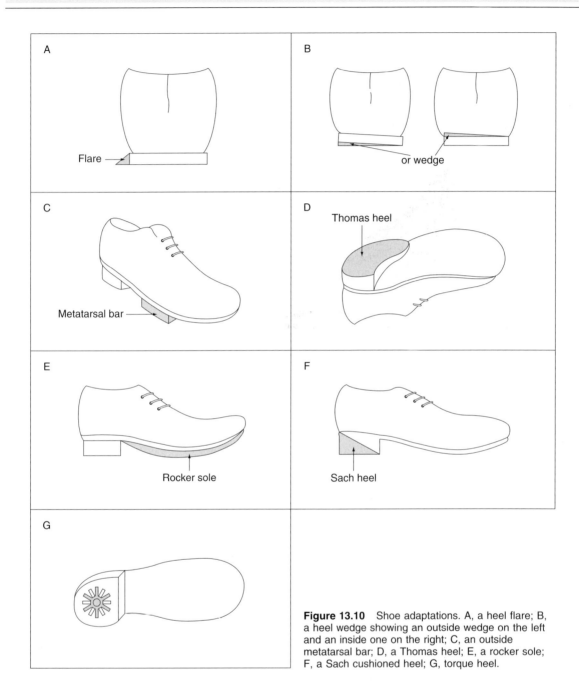

Figure 13.10 Shoe adaptations. A, a heel flare; B, a heel wedge showing an outside wedge on the left and an inside one on the right; C, an outside metatarsal bar; D, a Thomas heel; E, a rocker sole; F, a Sach cushioned heel; G, torque heel.

This area is usually reinforced with a metal insert called the shank piece, which must be sufficient to prevent unwanted flexion of this area. This is particularly important if a calliper is to be attached to the shoe, as without this reinforcement there will be too much flexion in the waist and the calliper will not function correctly.

The shoe upper

Stretching and balloon patching. Shoe uppers can be modified to relieve dorsal pressure on, for example, claw toes or bunions. If selective stretching of the shoe does not relieve the discomfort then a balloon patch may be added. This is a patch of leather, often softer than that of the shoe itself, which is glued over a hole cut in the upper to provide pressure relief. Care has to be exercised to match this to the shoe colour and texture as closely as possible.

Stiffeners. Often shoes can be made more supportive and effective if they are stiffened, particularly around the heel. A more rigid leather or other material is inserted between the layers of the shoe counter, providing more stiffness and enhanced stability to the foot.

Tongue fillers. If the girth of the shoe is too large, a pad of material can be adhered to the underside of the tongue (in a lace-up shoe). This has the effect of taking up some of the excess room and also serves as a cushion.

Fastening. The means of closure of the footwear can be altered to take account of the clinical need and the ability of the wearer. As well as the usual laces, which may extend down to the toes for easier fitting, there are elastic laces and elastic gussets to accommodate swelling, zips and Velcro for quick easy adjustment, and buckles for extra grip on the foot.

There are ways of tying laces one-handed which enable those with only one functional hand to still get the benefits of stable footwear (Hughes 1982).

Toe caps. With some medical conditions, such as hemiplegia, the patient may have a tendency to rub the toe end of the shoe due to an inability to dorsiflex the foot. Reinforced toe caps can be added to slow down the shoe wear in such circumstances and prevent irreversible damage to the structure of the shoe.

SUMMARY

It is important that footwear therapy is not overlooked when producing a management plan. This chapter has demonstrated that footwear plays an essential role in the treatment of foot problems. Footwear therapy encompasses a range of activities, from advice to a patient buying a pair of shoes to footwear adaptations aimed at reducing discomfort and improving gait. Appropriate footwear therapy should always result in a reduction of symptoms and may sometimes cure the foot problem.

REFERENCES

Alexander I J, Chao E Y S, Johnson K A 1990 The assessment of dynamic foot-to-ground contact forces and plantar pressure distribution: a review of the evolution of current techniques and clinical applications. Foot & Ankle 11: 152–167

Bader D, Chase A 1993 The patient orthosis interface. In: Bowker P, Bader D, Condie D N, Pratt D J, Wallace W A (eds) The biomechanical basis of orthotic management. Butterworth-Heinneman, Oxford, ch 5, p 68–69

Bennett I, Kavner D, Lee B K, Trainor F A 1979 Shear versus pressure as causative factors in skin blood flow occlusion. Archives of Physical Medicine and Rehabilitation 60: 309–314

Boulton A J M, Hardisty C A, Betts R P, Franks C I, Worth R C, Ward J D, Duckworth, T 1983 Dynamic foot pressure and other studies as diagnostic and management aids in diabetic neuropathy. Diabetes Care 6: 26–33

BS5943 British Standards Institution 1980 A method for measuring and casting for orthopaedic footwear. HMSO, London

Browne R 1993 Better lasts, better fit. Shoe and Allied Trades Research Association Bulletin, April: 57–58

Bunten J 1983 Foot comfort. Shoe and Allied Trades Research Association Report SR 44

Burry H S 1956 Some objective data on a case of burning sensation of the feet. Shoe and Allied Trades Research Association Memorandum TM 1192

Cavanagh P R, Sanders L J, Sims D S, Jr 1987 The role of pressure distribution measurement in diabetic foot care. Rehabilitation Research & Development Progress Reports 54

Chantelau E, Haage P 1994 An audit of cushioned diabetic footwear: relation to patient compliance. Diabetic Medicine 11(1): 114–116

Chen C 1993 An investigation into shoe last design in relation to foot measurement and shoe fitting for orthopaedic footwear. PhD thesis. London University

Costigan P S, Miller G, Elliott C, Wallace W A 1989 Are surgical shoes providing value for money? British Medical Journal 299: 950

Dimonte P, Light H 1982 Pathomechanics, gait deviations, and treatment of the rheumatoid foot. Physical Therapy 8: 1148–1156

Disabled living foundation service handbook. *Obtainable from DLF, 280–384 Harrow Road, London W9 2HU*

Fisher L R, McLellan D L 1989 Questionnaire assessment of patient satisfaction with lower limb orthoses from a district hospital. Prosthetics and Orthotics International 13: 29–35

Gastwirth B W, O'Brien T D, Nelson R M, Manger D C, Kindig S A 1991 An electrodynographic study of foot function in shoes of varying heel heights. Journal of the American Podiatric Medical Association 81: 463–472

Geary N P J, Klenerman L 1987 The rocker sole shoe: a method to reduce peak forefoot pressure in the management of diabetic foot ulceration. In: Pratt D J, Johnson G R (eds) The biomechanics and orthotic management of the foot. Orthotics and Disability Research Centre, Derby, ch 17

Hughes J (ed) 1982 Footwear and footcare for disabled children. Disabled Living Foundation, London

Lord M 1981 Foot pressure measurement: a review of methodology. Journal of Biomedical Engineering 3: 91–99

Lord M, Reynolds D P, Hughes J R 1986 Foot pressure measurement: A review of clinical findings. Journal of Biomedical Engineering 8: 283–294

Lord M, Foulston J, Smith P J 1991 Technical evaluation of a CAD system for orthopaedic shoe-upper design. Engineering in Medicine, Proceedings of Institution of Mechanical Engineers 205: 109–115

Lord M, Hosein R, Williams R B 1992 Method for in-shoe shear stress measurement. Journal of Biomedical Engineering 14: 181–186

Murray D L, Peet M J 1966 Summary of work on burning sensation. SATRA Internal Report 219

Pollard J P, Le Quesne L P, Tappin J W 1983 Forces under the foot. Journal of Biomedical Engineering 5: 37–40

Root M L, Orien W P, Weed J H, Hughes R J 1971 Biomechanical examination of the foot. Clinical Biomechanics Corporation, Los Angeles, vol 1

Rossi W 1983 Footwear and the podiatrist: the enigma of shoe sizes. Journal of American Podiatry Association 73: 272–274

Rothman S 1954 Physiology and biochemistry of the skin. University of Chicago Press, Chicago

Warren-Forward M J, Goodall R M, Pratt D J 1992 A three dimensional force and displacement transducer. Institute of Electrical Engineers – Proceedings A 139: 21–29

FURTHER READING

Shereff M J, DiGiovanni L, Bejjani F J, Hersh A, Kummer F J 1990 A comparison of non weight-bearing and weight-bearing radiographs of the foot. Foot & Ankle 10: 306–311

Snow R E, Williams K R, Holmes G B 1992 The effects of wearing high heeled shoes on pedal pressures in women. Foot & Ankle 13: 85–92

Tappin J W, Robertson K P 1991 Study of the relative timing of shear forces on the forefoot during walking. Journal of Biomedical Engineering 13, 39–42

Managing specific client groups

14

The adult foot

D. R. Tollafield
T. E. Kilmartin
T. D. Prior

INTRODUCTION

Describing the management of every manifestation likely to arise in the adult foot is notoriously difficult. One of the greatest difficulties in outlining any chapter on treatment is that it relies on a certain amount of common agreement between professionals that certain strategies are effective. The fact that many treatment strategies have unclear outcomes is evident from a paucity of effective audit. Journals dedicated to the scientific study of feet are reluctant to print unsubstantiated work. We have therefore been left with the problem of dovetailing historical treatment methods with scientific fact.

This chapter sets out to achieve three aims: firstly, to provide a summary of common conditions affecting the foot that can be treated by conservative and surgical means; secondly, to integrate treatment philosophy highlighted in previous chapters with conditions typically seen in the adult patient group; and finally, it is hoped to describe common approaches to treatment for foot problems related to articular/bone conditions, deformity, corns and callus, soft tissue pain and some miscellaneous conditions not covered elsewhere in the book.

TREATING THE ADULT PATIENT

Effective management of foot problems will only succeed if the following factors are taken into consideration:

- correct diagnosis
- patient compliance
- avoidance of secondary complications
- patient mobility or disability
- financial status.

The planned strategy of care will need to be recorded. The type of care selected will depend upon the available resources and the factors listed above. A broad discussion on general treatment planning has already been presented in Chapter 1. The following points will therefore have to be considered before treatment commences.

Correct diagnosis. Quite often, foot disorders are misdiagnosed or dismissed because there are insufficient clinical signs to suggest the likely trend in pathology. In the United States, financial and legal pressures have created a need for expensive diagnostic centres. Fortunately in the majority of foot complaints, diagnosis is relatively straightforward, and extensive investigations are unnecessary. Where a condition fails to improve, the practitioner is duty bound to expand the network of investigation, adjust the management plan within moderation, or refer to another specialist.

Patient compliance. No matter how dedicated a practitioner might be, an unresponsive patient will make management of a problem more difficult. A lack of compliance may relate to one or more of the following:

- limited finance
- misunderstanding
- inability to understand English
- inability to travel to the centre
- poor personal attitude.

In all cases, except the last, supportive help can be given; in the case of language difficulties, translators should be engaged as part of good *Patient Charter* practice.

Secondary complications. This creates two problems. Firstly, an associated condition may be exacerbated by treatment for a primary complaint; for example, pre-existing metatarsalgia is known to be greatly aggravated by excisional arthroplasty for a painful metatarsophalangeal joint (MTPJ). Secondly, an underlying disease or concurrent medication or treatment may complicate management or delay treatment response. Cardiovascular disease, diabetes mellitus, medication such as steroids and anticoagulants, malnutrition, alcoholism, drug abuse and pre-existing joint replacements or implants will all have significant implications for the success of any treatment. Some of these implications have been described in other chapters.

Patient mobility. Disability or immobility affects both young and elderly patients. Treatment is sometimes limited to strategies which are less than ideal. Injudicious management may contribute to a patient's existing disability. The practitioner must select the appropriate treatment, which is sometimes very different from the ideal treatment.

Financial status. While it is insensitive to ask someone how much they earn, a very different question will reveal their status. Do they work? Can they afford time away from work? Many foot problems may be alleviated by changing footwear, but this will usually mean that the patient has to buy new shoes. The practitioner should consider any financial limitations before suggesting that the patient contributes financially to their treatment.

ARTICULAR AND BONE CONDITIONS

This section is subdivided into three areas associated with joint and bone conditions:

- arthritis
- stress fractures
- neoplasia.

ARTHRITIS

Degenerative joint disease may lead to pain, swelling and deformity. In severe cases it will restrict mobility. All joints can be affected and treatment must differentiate between crystal arthritis, rheumatoid arthritis, the seronegative arthritides and degenerative (osteo-) arthritis.

Crystal arthritis

Crystal arthritis can affect the first MTPJ as well as the lesser toes and ankle. The pathogenesis is very different from degenerative arthritis, but there are similarities between the signs and symptoms. Gout and pseudogout (pyrophosphate arthropathy) are the two main members of this group (Klenerman 1991)—other variants exist and must be identified.

Principles of management

It is necessary to identify the active process causing inflammation, which should be reversed by systemic medication. Control of the metabolic pathway is usually preferred to using anti-inflammatory drugs alone. Secondary changes associated with the loss of articular surface, soft tissue calcinosis and tophi, synovitis and reduced movement should be managed on the basis of radiographic changes and clinical symptoms. Diagnosis is principally provided by blood assay and joint aspiration.

Gout. Hyperuricaemia diagnosed by raised uric acid

serum levels does not always provide a positive confirmation of gout, as it may not always precipitate an acute gouty attack. It can, however, lead to kidney stone formation or even cardiomyopathy. X-rays may be normal initially. Chronic deposition of sodium urate crystals may cause tophaceous gout, where hard nodules or tophi may become apparent subcutaneously and bone erosions are seen on plain X-ray. In cases of gout which appear as an isolated swollen toe, psoriatic arthritis should be considered.

Pseudogout. There will be crystal deposition within the cartilage (chondrocalcinosis) in older patients, and calcium pyrophosphate dihydrate will be present. The latter condition may be associated with a systemic manifestation such as hyperparathyroidism or haemochromatosis.

Hydroxyapatite arthropathy. These crystals will cause inflammatory changes in joints, although the pathogenesis of this form of arthritis is controversial (Rees & Trounce 1988). Large quantities of collagenase and neutral proteinase may be identified within the synovial fluid. Deposit over the first MTPJ tendons can mimic gout (Klenerman 1991).

Conservative management

Medical care. The use of diuretics causes gout; cessation of their use must be considered appropriate to the condition being treated. NSAIDs, particularly indomethacin, naproxen, ibuprofen and piroxicam, are valuable as an alternative to colchicine for acute attacks. Corticosteroid injection will abort an acute attack.

Where attacks are frequent, hypouricaemic drugs such as allopurinol will block the last stage of the metabolic pathway in urate crystal production. The daily dose is 300 mg, but this will need to be adjusted according to the serum level of urate. Allopurinol is generally cited as the drug of choice and is beneficial where renal disease or stones complicate the picture. Dietary care will have to be considered, moderating excesses of alcohol and offal meats high in purine.

Orthoses and footwear. Soft shoe uppers and firm thick soles will reduce the pressure over tender enlarged joints and limit first MTPJ movement. Bunion shields made from latex or foam, or over-the-counter products may offer some skin protection. These latter products are not tolerated in the acute phase of disease. Tophi can cause ulcerations and the skin will need to be protected by soft redistributive dressings. Low density, heat-moulded polyethylene (Plastazote) foam may also be used over the joint. Larger shoes will have to be prescribed where the midtarsal area is

affected. Soft orthoses may be used to protect the medial foot against the shoe, as well as to stabilise the foot where pathology has weakened the foot architecture.

Skin care. The skin should be protected at all times and non-viable areas should be prevented from ulcerating. Tophaceous gout can cause considerable shoe wear pressure problems.

Surgical management

Surgery can be used to remove tophi, in order to limit tissue degeneration and inflammation (see case history in Box 14.1). Arthrodesis has been used successfully in psoriatic arthritis, and arthritis caused by tuberculosis and gout (Yu 1992) to limit the extent of movement and secondary changes. Small joints of the toes should be excised and arthrodesed to prevent ulceration. Surgery should be performed between periods of active disease. The gouty patient may have a postoperative gouty attack due to local trauma or dehydration, particularly after general anaesthetics.

Degenerative osteoarthritis (OA)

This form of arthritis is not very likely to arise in the young adult unless injury or disease has damaged the joint cartilage. Often the patient complains of toothache-type pain in the joint(s) which is made

---

Box 14.1   Case history: unusual presentation of gout

An 18-year-old wrestler presented with pain in his right first MTP joint. There was no previous history of injury. Symptoms included 'throbbing', which was made worse by weight-bearing. An examination revealed no swelling. The presence of mild erythema over the plantar aspect of the first MTP joint was noted. There was tenderness over the medial sesamoid, and dorsiflexion elicited moderate pain. Orthoses initially provided some relief from symptoms. Radiographs taken at 10 weeks revealed cystic changes in both the proximal and distal segments of the partitioned sesamoid. An exploratory incision revealed an inflamed capsule and chalky white material which contained monosodium urate crystals; this was later reported to be consistent with gout upon haematoxylin and eosin staining together with Gomori's methenamine-silver stain. The latter stain, when combined with Gomori's stain, shows positive for tophaceous gout. The serum uric acid level was 7.8 mg/dl (normal levels 3.5–8.0 mg/dl). History was determined in the family on the paternal side. There was no history of renal disease, nor a use of diuretics or alcohol. This unusual case was reported by Mair et al (1995).

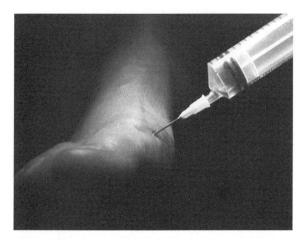

Figure 14.1 Joint aspiration of first MTP joint to rule out gout, infection and presence of blood.

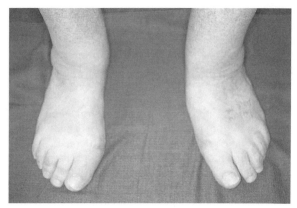

Figure 14.2 Distorted foot shape associated with progressive midfoot arthritis. Note that the left foot looks pronated, but that the STJ is not affected.

worse by activity. Frequently, patients will also confirm that the condition is exacerbated by cold or damp weather. When in the advanced stages, crepitus may be noted on examination of the joint. In many joints, synovitis rather than cartilage destruction causes the primary symptoms. Provided that localised heat of an acute inflammation, general pyrexia, sinus tracking and effusive swelling are not present, septic arthritis may be excluded clinically. Aspiration of the joint should be performed under sterile conditions in combination with plain X-rays beforehand (Fig. 14.1).

The midtarsal and first metatarsophalangeal joints are perhaps the most common foot joints that present with degenerative osteoarthritis. The first metatarsophalangeal joint may be damaged due to repetitive jamming of the joint secondary to a long or dorsiflexed first metatarsal. Excessive pronation of the foot may malalign the tarsal joints and the subsequent incongruity will predispose the joint surfaces to degeneration. The midfoot may show signs of palpable osteophytes, tenderness and distortion. The misalignment gives the forefoot an abducted, pronated appearance (Fig. 14.2). Osteophytes may rub against soft tissue, causing localised discomfort on specific foot movement. A number of ossicles can become incorporated at joint lines, mimicking osteophytes.

A clinical history may provide evidence of trauma, or the patient may complain of difficult footwear fit without any knowledge of how and when the problem started. X-rays may provide some evidence of degeneration but they often lack the clarity afforded by CT or MRI scans. Patients admitted to casualty with injury may be dismissed as having simple bruising. Midfoot trauma without obvious X-ray changes can easily mislead the inexperienced casualty doctor. Early discharge may result in lack of a correct diagnosis. This type of problem may well develop active degenerative change several years later.

Principles of management

Once degenerative arthritis has been identified from clinical and radiographic examinations, footwear and general activity may need to be modified. Supportive footwear, particularly above-ankle lace-ups, will reduce pain by controlling joint movement. It is unlikely that footwear alone will resolve the problem without some modification to lifestyle and physical activity.

Analgesics. Paracetamol is a useful analgesic which has few side-effects and may be recommended to be taken as necessary. If paracetamol does not help, NSAIDs such as ibuprofen or diclofenac sodium may be used, although gastric irritation arises with long-term use.

Strapping to limit joint movement can be initiated as a short-term measure, but this is only a temporary measure as long-term use will almost certainly cause skin irritation.

Orthoses may be applied to increase support and further reduce joint mobility, particularly in the subtalar, midtarsal and tarsal joints. The beneficial effect is likely to be reduced where these joints are already subluxed.

Physical therapy in the form of heat is beneficial in acute and subacute stages of the disorder. Infrared and interferential forms of physical therapy should be considered in order to suppress inflammation.

Corticosteroid injection is valuable in the joints of the foot but should not be repeated too frequently. The action of the drug is directed at the synovium rather than the cartilage. Corticosteroid given in small quantities will reduce inflammation and relieve spasm and reduce effusion. Reliance on this powerful agent is discouraged and the benefit can be reduced if injections are overused. Certain corticosteroids, such as methyl prednisolone (Depo-Medrone) and triamcinolone (Kenalog), may cause a localised flare-up of symptoms in the immediate post-injection phase. Betamethasone (Betnesol) may have a lower propensity to post-injection flare-up as it is water-soluble but appears to act for a shorter period of time.

Surgery is indicated where the arthritic condition does not improve with conservative care or medication. Arthritic joints can be approached in the following manner:

- *excisional arthroplasty*—replacement of joint surfaces
- *interpositional arthroplasty*—involves placing soft tissue, usually joint capsule, between the resected bone surfaces
- *osteotomy*—decompresses and realigns the joint surfaces in the earlier stages of arthritis
- *joint replacement*—used for irreversibly damaged joints
- *arthrodesis*—immobilises the joint permanently, thus preventing further pain. The joint is destroyed by fusion. Restricted footwear height becomes a problem.

While all these measures can be very effective, the foot is a complex structure with interconnecting joints that need to function in equilibrium. There is a high risk that surgery at one joint will have potentially damaging implications for other previously normal or asymptomatic joints. The effects of both conservative care and surgery on the following individual joints are considered below:

- interphalangeal joints
- metatarsophalangeal joints
- midtarsus
- ankle.

Interphalangeal joints

The interphalangeal joints (IPJs) are not commonly affected by degenerative arthritis but may develop a fibrous union, limiting movement. The fibrous change creates a fixed flexion deformity due to contraction. Upon dissection, few of these joints show the erosion or damage typical of larger joints. However, the main complaints associated with acquired digital problems are corns and callus caused by footwear irritation. Common sites include the dorsal aspect of the IPJ and, because of weight-bearing, the apex of the digit. Joint pain associated with arthritic degeneration is less common.

Conservative management. In many cases, the primary cause of lesser digit problems is hallux valgus, which causes crowding of the lesser toes. Definitive treatment involves correcting the hallux valgus in order to achieve an effective prognosis. In the case of lesser digital deformities unrelated to hallux valgus, it is possible to treat individual toes. Protection of pressurised skin areas over the joints will be discussed in greater detail under corns and callus, and surgical correction will be discussed under deformities.

Lesser digit problems may be conservatively treated using silicone props or crescents (Figs 11.3–11.6 and 11.23).

While excisional arthroplasty or arthrodesis (Fig. 7.23) has been the traditional surgical approach to painful toe joints in the adult foot, small joint implants have recently become available. These silastic prostheses usually have two stems with a small disk spacer in-between. While these devices prevent bone to bone apposition following joint arthroplasty, they are unlikely to resist deforming forces from muscles or adjacent toes.

First metatarsophalangeal joint

Trauma. The effects of acute injury to this joint will reduce with immobilisation and ice therapy in the first 2–24 hours. Pain can be managed with analgesics, elevation and ice applied over the affected part every few hours for 10–20 minutes. Forced rest can be assisted with elbow crutches (see Appendix 3 on crutch use). The toe joint may need to be splinted with *fan strapping* for 2 weeks (Fig. 11.14). The patient can be shown how to replace this every 2–3 days. A foot or below-knee leg cast should be used if pain does not subside, or if the patient cannot rest the foot adequately (Fig. 11.20). Long-term follow-up may establish the early development of osteoarthrosis.

Hallux limitus is a common condition whereby extension/dorsiflexion of the great toe (MTPJ) is limited either by a mechanical jamming of the joint or by a large osteophytic projection over both the head of the first metatarsal and dorsal proximal phalanx. A compensatory ring of fibrocartilage can develop, limiting the first MTPJ further. The exuberant osteophytes will erode the synovial lining and cause the capsule to thin. X-rays will show diminished joint

Box 14.2   Case history: epiphyseal trauma

A 14-year-old male sustained an epiphyseal injury to the base of his first proximal phalanx following a judo kick. Upon X-ray, the epiphysis showed early closure on the lateral side. While Salter–Harris classification was difficult to determine, a linear split was probably created across the phalangeal epiphysis with some distraction away from the main body of bone. Failure of early treatment led to degenerative changes across cartilage of the first metatarsal head. The hallux was limited at the MTP joint, with pain on movement. The joint was exposed and the metatarsal was shown to have tram line tracks depressed into the soft cartilage. The metatarsal was decompressed to open up the joint line, stabilised with a 2.7 mm screw and the patient was allowed to mobilise at 7 days with crutches.

Conclusion. Epiphyseal injury may settle without treatment but early recognition of such trauma should be followed up. The effects of degenerative arthritis may be reversed and symptoms ameliorated if conservative surgery can be offered as soon as possible. The patient in this case remained pain-free at 12 months, but requires routine monitoring. Joint motion has been improved, establishing normal lubrication (Fig. 14.3).

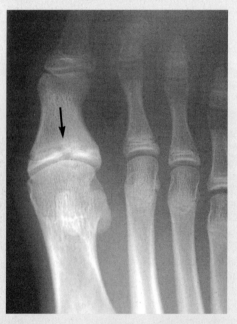

Figure 14.3   Epiphyseal trauma associated with joint changes following a judo kick. Note the irregular proximal (hallux) epiphysis typical of a Salter–Harris fracture.

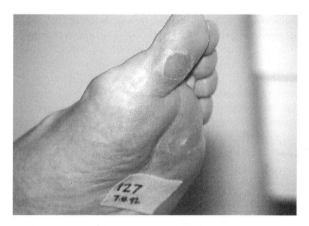

Figure 14.4   The first MTP joint is affected by dorsal lipping with an elevated first metatarsal and will affect normal first MTP joint function. Lateral X-ray view.

space and sclerosis (increased density) underlying the cartilage. The presence of lucent (dark areas) suggests synovial/lipid-filled cysts, which occur when bone to bone contact forces synovial fluid into the subchondral bone.

Hallux flexus. The hallux may flex to gain purchase in the presence of an elevated first metatarsal (metatarsus primus elevatus). In this condition, plantar callus under the IPJ will cause discomfort (Fig. 14.4). Proximal postural symptoms may arise as the patient attempts to compensate by supinating the foot.

Hallux rigidus presents as a stiff first MTP joint. Because there is no movement within the joint, there is usually no pain other than footwear irritation associated with joint thickening.

Hallux valgus is commonly associated with hallux rigidus. Degenerative joint disease arises from this condition because it creates incongruity at the first MTP joint. Incongruity affects joint loading. Shear and compressive forces will be abnormally directed over the lateral joint surface. The medial surface becomes atrophied, with thinning of cartilage due to ineffective joint lubrication and reduced pressure to stimulate normal cellular strength. Where the hallux valgus is associated with an elevated first metatarsal, normal rotation of the hallux over the dorsal articular surface of the first metatarsal head will be impeded. With damage to the articular surface, the joint will become stiff, and new bone and fibrocartilaginous tissue deposited around the joint margin will limit normal motion.

Conservative management. In the early stages of osteoarthrosis affecting the first MTP joint, the patient will complain of intermittent toothache-type pain from within the joint. Symptoms are exacerbated by activity, high-heeled footwear and cold, damp weather. On clinical examination there is slight thickening of the joint and pain on plantarflexion of the hallux; dorsiflexion may be restricted but is rarely painful. X-rays will indicate a loss of joint space and possibly the presence of osteophytes on the lateral side of the first metatarsal head (Figs 14.5 and 14.6). At this stage, in-shoe orthoses may be extremely effective in alleviating the joint pain. Any orthotic that extends under the first metatarsal will restrict first metatarsal plantarflexion which will reduce mobility of the hallux and thus relieve pain.

In more advanced cases of osteoarthrosis, the joint is enlarged. Pain will arise from damaged articular cartilage interposing against bone or from bone against bone. Footwear may compress the dorsal and medial metatarsal head osteophytes against soft tissue, causing deep tissue shear, inflammation and soft tissue bursae

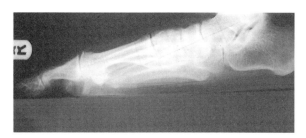

Figure 14.5 An elevated first metatarsal is frequently associated with callus under the hallux

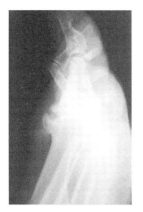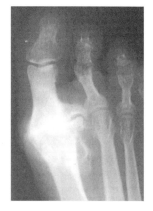

Figure 14.6 Complete loss of joint space and metatarsal lipping form extensive degenerative radiographic changes associated with osteoarthrosis. Two views are required to determine the extent of pathology. Note the parrot's beak effect on the lateral side of the first MTP joint (hallux rigidus).

(Fig. 14.7). X-rays will show an almost complete loss of joint space and prolific osteophytes all around the metatarsal head. In the most advanced cases, osteophytes may also be seen on the base of the proximal phalanx (Fig. 14.8). Joint movement will often be limited to 20° dorsiflexion or less. Orthoses will do little to relieve joint pain at this stage and indeed they may cause further footwear irritation as they fill up the shoe.

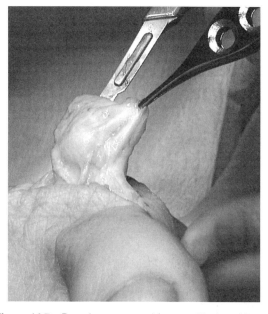

Figure 14.7 Bursal sac removed from an 80-year-old female after aspiration failed to resolve her bunion pain.

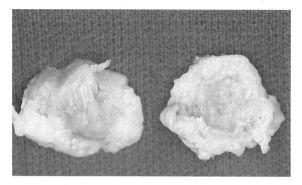

Figure 14.8 Excised joint surfaces of the first metatarsal (left) and the base of the proximal phalanx (right). Pathology shows loss of cartilage, hypertrophic deepening of the base of the phalanx with exuberant osteophytic lipping. The diagnosis is hallux rigidus with gross OA changes.

Footwear adaptation. Shoe accommodation with balloon patches receives little favour these days, but would be valuable in patients unsuited or unwilling to undergo surgery. Alternatively, latex or foam covers can be applied over the first MTP joint to reduce skin irritation. Stiff-soled shoes will restrict movement of the first MTPJ and may relieve joint pain. The application of a rocker bar assists the propulsive phase of gait by allowing the foot to roll over the forefoot. The need to extend the first MTP joint will be reduced.

Injection. Synovitis is a feature of degenerative joint disease which often responds to intra-articular corticosteroid injection. A single injection of 0.1–0.3 ml of dexamethasone has been found to be beneficial. A Mayo or metatarsal ring block of local anaesthetic using 1% xylocaine for short duration will remove any spasm from the flexor hallucis brevis. Not only does this allow painless joint injection with corticosteroid medication, but the technique also offers a differential diagnosis in the presence of spasm associated with traumatic change versus true rigidus where clinical signs are unclear. Loose bodies and marked articular inflammation will cause spasm; some of these symptoms may be reduced by heat therapy. Manipulation of a stiff joint under local anaesthetic will help to break up adhesions after corticosteroid injection. The joint should be physically distracted and circumducted (rotary movements). This exercise can be continued at home or in combination with foot spa baths or hydrotherapy pools. If this technique fails, the practitioner must suspect that advanced stages of pathology have developed.

Surgical management. The surgical management of the adult with first MTPJ pain involves a number of different techniques, depending upon the physiological age of the joint and the extent of pathology. The objective of surgery should be the restoration of a normal (45°–65°) pain-free range of movement and the removal of dorsal and medial osteophytes. The surgical procedure should be based on the degree of cartilage loss, severity of osteophyte formation, first metatarsal length and sagittal plane position. The patient's age and activity level should also be considered. Where there is still adequate joint space on X-ray, and only moderate loss of articular cartilage when the joint surfaces are viewed intra-operatively, an osteotomy can be performed to decompress the joint and restore pain-free movement. The osteotomy illustrated in Figure 14.9 shortens the metatarsal length as well as correcting other problems such as hallux valgus.

Gross changes associated with complete cartilage

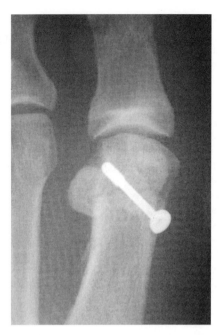

Figure 14.9 An osteotomy performed to decompress the joint, alleviating synovitis and improving joint congruency.

loss and severe osteophytosis can be managed with either a Keller's excisional arthroplasty (Fig. 7.4) or joint replacement (Fig. 7.5). In both cases, pain relief should be experienced within the first week following surgery, with reasonable mobility. Casts are seldom required. Joint replacements come in many varieties and opinion varies as to which is most suitable. Hinged silastic implants are probably the most popular (Ch. 7). Research indicates an average life expectancy for an implant of 8 years. This suggests that they should be avoided in patients much younger than 65 (Kilmartin & Wallace 1992). The joint implant may well have to be replaced earlier in very active patients.

Arthroplasty without joint replacement does lead to shortening of the toe and is known to cause metatarsalgia. This problem can be limited if the extent of proximal phalanx resection is not very aggressive. No more than 33% of the bone length should be removed, in order to avoid marked disturbance of the great toe plantarflexors.

The use of arthrodesis for joint pain depends upon surgical preference. Fusion of the joint has met with success where movement is very painful. A fused first MTPJ can also be very awkward for the patient to tolerate, especially as it limits the range of shoe heel height. In some cases, fusion fails to occur because

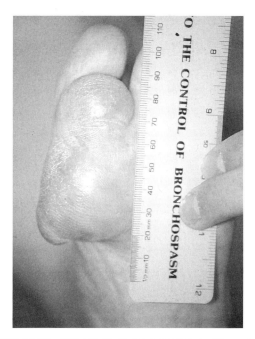

Figure 14.10 The effects on the deep tissues 30 years after a poorly positioned arthrodesis (see Fig. 14.28).

of inadequate bony compression. An overextended hallux brought about by an arthrodesis can disturb the plantar soft tissue, as illustrated in Figure 14.10.

Lesser metatarsophalangeal joints

Overloading of the lesser MTP joints may occur in hallux valgus or following hallux valgus surgery. If the first metatarsal is dorsiflexed, as it will be in the advanced stages of hallux valgus, or if the first MTP joint has undergone an excisional arthroplasty, the load borne by the first metatarsal will transfer laterally and the second metatarsal will be subject to overloading. This will manifest clinically as tenderness under the metatarsal head, which can be aggravated by direct palpation of the metatarsal head.

Abnormal metatarsal length may also cause painful tenderness on weight-bearing. It is usual to find that the second ray has the longest metatarsal in the foot. The first metatarsal is the same length as the third, and the fourth is longer than the fifth. A long second metatarsal or a short first or third is a particularly common finding in cases of plantar tenderness associated with the second metatarsal head. Soft tissue bursae are discussed later under skin/subcutaneous tissues.

Freiberg's disease, rheumatoid or psoriatic synovitis, painful accessory ossicles, traumatic capsulitis and stress fractures may also cause pain in the lesser metatarsal joints. Any symptoms in this area must always be differentially diagnosed from intermetatarsal neuroma.

Principles of treatment. Immobilisation of the lesser MTP joints can only be accomplished with below-knee or slipper casting of the foot. It is possible, however, to redistribute some weight-bearing pressure away from the metatarsal heads by using insoles or orthoses.

Corticosteroid injections will have a dramatic effect on synovitis, and often a single injection will bring sustained relief. Repeated injections into the lesser MTP joints can lead to degeneration of the articular cartilage, collateral ligaments of the joint, as well as atrophy of the volar (plantar) plate. Subluxation of the joint is an undesirable side effect of such overuse.

Degenerative arthritic change, often associated with old Freiberg's disease, will only temporarily respond to corticosteroid injections. Excision of the base of the proximal phalanx will, however, eliminate the bone to bone contact that causes the pain. Joint replacement may also be considered but tends to act only as a joint spacer. Loss of the load-bearing function of one metatarsal head may cause transfer metatarsalgia of the adjacent metatarsals.

In psoriasis, quite severe erosive changes may destroy the normal metatarsal head. Excision of all the metatarsal heads will reduce joint pain and metatarsalgia but will shorten the foot and destabilise the digits. As with most active forms of arthritis, the disease should be in remission before surgery is considered.

Midfoot arthritis

Trauma to the midfoot foot is an important cause of long-term disability (see case history in Box 14.3). Any significant trauma, especially from road traffic accidents, should be carefully investigated. Further sequential X-rays should be taken if pain persists. CT and bone scans may be necessary to determine any intra-articular damage.

First metatarsal cuneiform exostosis

Osteophytic thickening at the first metatarsocuneiform joint may present clinically as footwear irritation over the midfoot area (Fig. 14.11). The condition is associated with a hypermobile plantarflexed first metatarsal and develops as a consequence of low grade but repetitive impaction of the base of the first metatarsal against the medial cuneiform. The

Box 14.3 Case history: midfoot arthritis

A 46-year-old overweight male caught his foot on a conveyor belt while at work. Initial (plain) X-rays showed no abnormal changes, despite extensive bruising recorded in the medical records. A backsplint cast was applied to the leg and foot, but the period of non-weight-bearing was complicated by a deep venous thrombosis which had to be treated as a medical emergency.

X-rays taken at 1 year revealed arthritic changes around the second to third metatarsocuneiform joint. Two years following the injury, the patient was still considerably disabled.

Treatment for this form of arthritis initially limited daily pain. Casted orthoses used to splint the midtarsus reduced the effects of movement between the damaged joints. While rest limited symptoms, the patient gained weight. NSAIDs were helpful but the patient preferred to use them only occasionally. In the long term, arthrodeses of the affected joints may be necessary if symptoms persist.

Conclusion. The prognosis is somewhat unpredictable. Early diagnosis might have used other imaging techniques, such as bone scans and CT, to provide a clearer picture of the damage. A combination of orthoses and NSAIDs will alleviate the symptoms of joint degeneration.

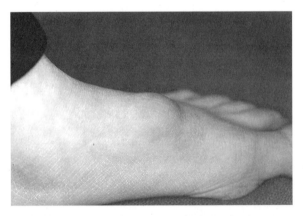

Figure 14.11 Enlarged metatarsocuneiform exostosis and bursa can make shoes difficult to wear. The bursa shown was too established to aspirate and therefore underlying bone was flattened by open surgery.

osteophytic thickening is best visualised on a lateral weight-bearing X-ray but often looks worse clinically because of the presence of an overlying cartilage cap. In severe cases where there has been considerable footwear irritation, a soft tissue bursa may form dorsomedial to the joint.

Principles of management. Footwear advice should be given initially. Certain footwear designs will avoid the area; trainers with a soft upper and well-designed lacing system will prevent further irritation of the soft tissues overlying the exostosis.

Protective felt padding can be used to deflect pressure from the area, although the use of felt rings may cause further extrusion of soft tissues. While functional orthoses restrict motion at the first MTP joint (Kilmartin et al 1991), it may be that they could also restrict motion at the first metatarsocuneiform joint and thus prevent further impaction and damage to the joint. To date, however, the role of functional orthoses in this condition remains uncertain. Surgical removal of the exostosis is reserved for recalcitrant problems. Sensitive scarring over the area can be a source of further irritation, especially if the scar becomes thickened postoperatively. Cheilectomy may deal with the prominence, but may not deal with the primary mechanical cause. Recurrence does occur.

Ankle joint

Osteoarthrosis of the ankle occurs much less frequently than degenerative joint disease of the knee or hip. Unlike the hip and knee, when the ankle does become arthritic there is usually a history of trauma, i.e. repeated low grade injuries, such as recurrent inversion sprains, or a more severe high impact injury causing fracture of the component bones and derangement of the articular surfaces. In the case of the subtalar joint, intra-articular fracture has a poor prognosis.

Chronic osteoarthrosis of the ankle may be seen on plain X-ray. Acute injuries are better evaluated by CT to account for subtalar involvement and damage to the central mortice of the talus.

The practitioner must exclude tendon inflammation and repetitive strain during examination, as confusion between articular and soft tissue problems may arise.

Principles of management. Having excluded a history of trauma, the ankle and subtalar joints should be assessed for motor power, range of motion and specific pain points, which are sought in an attempt to locate the pain over specific anatomical structures, such as the lateral ligaments, sinus tarsi, trochlear surface of the talus and posterior talar process.

Acute pain will be managed as in the case of any joint. Ankle splints can be made or below-knee casts applied. The dorsal (top) part of the cast over the foot and leg can be removed as a night splint. Forced rest and elevation are essential in the early stages to allow repair, assisted by NSAIDs, ice therapy (Fig. 7.25) and the use of crutches. X-rays may fail to show any early changes and will have to be repeated after 2–6 weeks.

Posterior ankle pain. Pain arising behind the ankle is often associated with repetitive plantarflexion of the ankle in soccer or ballet. The posterior process of the talus and the overlying synovial capsule of the ankle become impinged between the posterior lip of the tibia and the calcaneus. The condition occurs more commonly when there is an enlarged posterior or Steida process present, or when the accessory ossicle os trigonum is present.

Pain can be elicited by forced plantarflexion of the foot and sometimes by firm palpation of the area. Inversion/eversion of the subtalar joint and dorsiflexion of the ankle prove asymptomatic. Plain X-ray is essential to rule out fracture of the posterior process or separation of the os trigonum from the main body of the talus. Rest and corticosteroid injection into the posterior capsule of the ankle prove to be effective.

Anterior ankle pain. Painful limitation of dorsiflexion of the ankle may result from an exostosis on the dorsal neck of the talus. This will impinge on the anterior aspect of the tibia and will present clinically as a painful stiff ankle. The dorsiflexion range of the ankle should be examined with the knee flexed to reduce any soft tissue restriction caused by a tight Achilles tendon/gastrocnemius soleus muscle. Movement will be limited and the range of motion will come to an abrupt bony end. Lateral weight-bearing views of the ankle and a stress view with the ankle dorsiflexed will confirm the presence of a bony block, which can be removed arthroscopically.

Tenderness along the plafond of the talus may indicate degenerative pathology, cartilage defects and synovitis. Unilateral, non-pitting oedema is suggestive of any chronic degenerative change, unless an acute injury or disease process can be excluded. Treatment for each of these conditions will depend upon the extent of symptoms and the patient's age, mobility and occupation. The most severe, disabling pain requires subtalar arthrodesis. However, patients find ankle orthoses to be of value, especially where footwear enables higher ankle-conforming orthoses to limit hindfoot motion. The heel seat should have a 0° or flat post, or should be manufactured to have a flat heel seat. Both modifications will limit subtalar joint movement. The use of ankle splints or braces, along the lines of the inflatable Aircast (Fig. 14.12), offers a useful off-the-shelf semi-immobilisation system for the ankle and subtalar joints.

Lateral ankle sprains. Ankle sprains are not exclusive to sportspersons, but the principles are similar. The principle approach is rest, elevation, ice, anal-

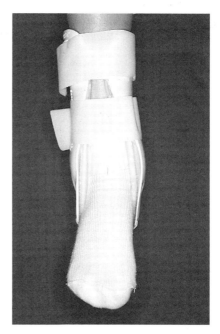

Figure 14.12 Aircast ankle brace can be fitted around the ankle using easy to adjust Velcro straps. The sides can be inflated to improve the fit.

gesia, support, gentle rehabilitation and restoration of activity. Because subtalar damage can arise, patients should be followed up carefully for 3 months to ensure that X-rays can be repeated and CT imaging used early. Chapter 16 covers ankle injury recovery in greater detail.

FRACTURES

Stress fractures associated with the foot will most commonly affect the metatarsals (Ch. 16). The patient will present with pain following a history of direct injury or a recent episode of vigorous athletic activity. March fractures were so named because of the high incidence of fractures in military recruits, forced to march while undergoing basic training.

Fractures which extend through the epiphyses are particularly significant because they will disrupt bone growth and, in a long bone, premature fusion due to closure of one side of the growth plate. As in the case history in Box 14.2, joints may become extensively involved and require fusion.

Conservative management

The principal method of managing any fracture is to

limit movement; this will in turn reduce pain and swelling. Stress fractures do not present with any marked deformity, so reduction of the fracture is not necessary. Movement should be reduced initially by crutches or a stiff walking shoe, and simple analgesics should be used for pain.

Direct application of felt dressings and taping is valuable for central metatarsals. Toes can be taped together but must not be bound tightly, so as not to restrict circulatory flow. This treatment should be continued for 3–6 weeks with a review at that point if progress is satisfactory. A below-knee walking cast or foot cast (below-ankle) should be applied where pain is unremitting, where other soft splinting techniques fail, or where analgesia is ineffective. The patient should be counselled to avoid excessive movement and to rest the foot for up to 6 weeks. Bone growth stimulators have been popular in some centres, using a form of piezo-electric field to attract osteogenic activity within the hydroxyapatite salts.

Retention of movement is important for healthy repair of bone but, in rare and unfortunate cases where patients are restricted by long periods of rest, a deep venous thrombosis or reflex sympathetic dystrophy syndrome can arise, both with disastrous effects.

Surgical management

Fortunately, surgery is rarely necessary in stress fractures. Toes may be better pinned with Kirschner wires as a closed technique under fluoroscopy. The Jones fracture associated with the base of the fifth metatarsal is the exception to the rule. Due to poor blood supply, this fracture may take many months to settle and will cause pain and swelling. Avulsion fracture of the fifth metatarsal must be excluded and not confused with a Jones fracture which is usually more distally sited. Physiotherapy exercise and manipulation are not indicated and can make the condition worse. A screw to compress the site of the fracture by open reduction provides the most expedient method for young active patients. Casts may assist in the older patient but can cause an element of demineralisation.

Displacement and fragmentation should be managed by open reduction, especially where anatomical structures such as nerve pathways and blood vessels are damaged. Joints should be decompressed and deformity corrected as soon as possible. The presence of infection may complicate management and external fixators may be applied. Bone grafts may also be necessary to replace lost bone, either at the time of injury or as a secondary phase of management.

NEOPLASIA OF BONE

Few bone tumours resolve without surgical intervention. Conservative management relies on monitoring the progress of any swelling and diagnosing the tissue type through X-rays, bone scans and magnetic resonance imaging. Aspiration of tumours is generally considered unwise.

Two main considerations must be observed when dealing with tumours after diagnosis has been made. First, the whole lesion should ideally be excised. Secondly, because removal of bone will leave a weakened structure, surgical planning must include the possibility of bone graft requirements. In bones affected by malignant disease, prosthetic implants are commonly used together with adjuvant chemotherapy.

Treatment must be managed by multidisciplinary cooperation. The principles of management include the following approaches:

- accurate diagnosis
- surgical planning
- surgical biopsy to plan further management/diagnosis
- complete excision
- replacement prosthesis/bone graft/skin grafting
- chemotherapy/radiotherapy
- postoperative prosthesis
- bespoke footwear after resection surgery.

Subungual exostoses

Subungual exostoses cause pain under the nail and, in more severe forms, footwear fitting difficulties (Fig. 6.8). Surgical excision provides the most acceptable long-term solution. In order to expose the exostosis, it is usually necessary to remove the nail plate. The tissues overlying the exostosis will be thin and dystrophic, and difficult to reflect. Moreover, once the underlying exostosis has been removed, these tissues are often difficult to close because they are so friable. The area is also somewhat prone to infection because of the presence of a variety of bacterial and fungal elements under the nail. Once a toenail has been removed, it is likely that it will re-grow somewhat thickened because of damage to the nail matrix which occurs on avulsion of the nail.

An apical approach has been developed in order to avoid nail removal. This is useful for smaller exostoses, but the technique may lead to temporary skin necrosis at this site. Subungual exostosis excision may cause considerable postoperative pain and tenderness, and a combination of NSAIDs and paracetamol/codeine compounds is advised.

DEFORMITY

The most common deformities seen in the forefoot are conditions associated with hallux valgus and hammer toes. The most common whole-foot deformity is pes planus; this condition shares similarities with pes cavus in that it may be mild, moderate or severe. Classification of digital deformity has been considered in greater detail elsewhere (Merriman & Tollafield 1995).

LESSER TOES

Conservative care

Footwear should be evaluated to establish adequate fit and design. Patients are more likely to follow advice if they understand the reason for the problem, realise the limited approaches to treatment and appreciate the long-term effects of unsuitable footwear. This part of management may not be easy if the patient only wishes to have palliative care. Shoe adaptations, as previously mentioned, seldom appeal to patients. Skin and nail management can be provided on a re-petitive level and are preferable for elderly patients or patients where surgery would be inappropriate.

Toe deformities respond well to surgery and this form of treatment should certainly be considered, the alternative for many patients being years of palliative care.

Surgical management

A fixed toe deformity can exist at the interphalangeal joint (IPJ) or at both the IPJ and the MTPJ. The goal of digital surgery is to return the proximal phalanx to a neutral position (i.e. neither dorsiflexed nor plantar-flexed) relative to the metatarsal head. Once this has been achieved, equilibrium will be restored to the digital muscles whilst simultaneously neutralising the deforming forces. If the proximal phalanx is left dorsiflexed, the flexor muscles will be kept under tension and the distal and intermediate phalanges will be pulled into plantarflexion. As the intermediate phalanx plantarflexes, a retrograde force will be exerted on the proximal phalanx, forcing it into further dorsi-flexion. When the proximal phalanx is in neutral, however, the flexor and extensor muscles are in equilibrium and the digit remains straight.

Hammer toe. The single toe with a fixed sagittal plane deformity can be corrected by excising the head of the proximal phalanx. This will relax the passive stretch on the flexor muscles caused by the dorsiflexed position of the proximal phalanx and will also reduce the bony prominence causing corn formation.

In younger patients, where there is a chance of long-term recurrence, flexor tendon transfer and arthro-desis of the proximal IPJ may be considered. This procedure will ensure that the flexor tendons, which are transferred into the extensor apparatus, actively contribute to holding the proximal phalanx in a neutral position. Furthermore, a good position of the digit should be retained relative to the relevant meta-tarsal head and other toes. Moreover, while most digital surgery will heal within a fortnight, swelling can sometimes persist for many months.

Retracted toe. A toe deformed at more than the IPJ will need to be managed in stages. The toe deformity is corrected by eliminating each deforming factor. The IPJ is dealt with first, then the tendon, then the capsule of the MTP joint, and finally the flexor surface of the metatarsal. Even using all these stages, the deformity may not be eradicated if the metatarsal is badly plantarflexed. Metatarsal surgery is then required.

Mallet toes. The excisional arthroplasty is also popu-lar for single toe deformities. Excision of the head of the intermediate phalanx is performed through a double ellipse. Insufficient removal of bone may result in only partial correction. Sometimes it is necessary to remove the entire intermediate phalanx. The wound is closed using the double ellipse to draw the distal toe into extension.

Multiple toe deformities. The second, third and fourth digits should be arthrodesed simultaneously. Correc-tion of an isolated deformity, where more than one toe problem exists, can be a mistake. This is because the altered vector of forces pulling equally from the shared extensor tendons causes inequality if only a single tendon is transected; furthermore, isolated toe surgery will leave asymmetrical shortening, or uncor-rected adjacent digits will continue to underride and deform the remodelled toe. Abnormal digital parabola caused by surgery can lead to buckling of long toes and necessitate further surgery. Excessive shortening of single digits may cause plantar metatarsalgia.

Dislocation at the MTPJ. Deformity of a toe that has an associated dislocation should be easy to diagnose. The range of motion is unrestricted and the toe sits in an abnormal position above or, less commonly, below other adjacent toes. A second toe deforms either as a result of injury or, alternatively, as a result of pres-sure from an adjacent hallux valgus pushing the digit dorsally and laterally. Disease processes such as rheumatoid arthritis and psoriatic arthritis can cause multiple digital disturbance at the MTP or IP joints. If a congenitally retracted fifth digit sits too high, rubbing against the shoe can arise. Options available include amputation (Fig. 7.19), arthrodesis or soft tissue correction. The choice of treatment is influenced by age, occupation, adjacent toe position and likely success.

Amputation may be considered in a patient who has toe pain associated with shoe-fitting difficulties. An adjacent hallux valgus deformity that is asymptomatic in an older patient may be left uncorrected, instead carrying out a whole or partial toe amputation. The decision must, however, depend upon the patient's preference. If the patient fears losing a toe, then the hallux must be corrected and the second toe brought into alignment with the other toes by arthrodesis. In this case, a pin (Kirschner wire) is passed through the MTP joint and antegraded (or moved forward) 3 weeks later to avert a stiff toe. An alternative procedure may preserve the toe by excising the base of the proximal phalanx. Care must be taken not to remove too much of the base, and the capsule must be correctly repaired. Failure in either of these methods will lead to a floppy and unsightly toe which is very much foreshortened between the hallux and second digits.

Adductovarus of the fifth toe. The fifth toe may adopt various positions of deformity. Adductovarus rotation and overriding (clinodactyly) can be corrected together using a V-Y plasty incision (Fig. 6.19A), with or without an arthroplasty to the IPJ. The tendon is initially transected to see how much the toe will drop into alignment with the other toes. The capsule is incised (capsulotomy), which again removes tension from a retracted deformity. As a rule, fifth toes are never arthrodesed because they will cause pressure between the skin and the shoe due to their rigidity. Incisions made around the MTP joint are very important, as lengthening of the contracted skin is required by V or Z incison. In resistant cases, an ellipse of tissue may be removed from the plantar aspect of the toe in the area of the proximal skin crease; this will resist further recurrence.

HALLUX DEFORMITY

Hallux valgus

The deformity of hallux valgus includes a large medial eminence, broadening of the forefoot, and dislocation and rotation of the great toe. The condition is often complicated by lesser toe deformity, arthritic changes, a splay forefoot or metatarsus adductus. Unfortunately, once developed, little conservative care can be offered; the main choices of care are accommodation and surgical correction.

Conservative management

Bunion. The medial eminence frequently produces a bursa overlying fibrous cartilage and bone. The medial eminence is in fact the medial metatarsal head made prominent due to subluxation of the first MTP joint. *Footwear* may be adapted with balloon patches, or a bespoke shoe made to accommodate the broad foot. The accommodation of the additional width of the foot is important to limit tissue breakdown and sinus tract formation. A case for prescription footwear is greatest for those high risk patients suffering from vascular ischaemia, neuropathy or gross arthritic degeneration.

Aspiration. Enlarged bursae are fluctuant sacs which can become infected. Aspiration can be performed using up to 0.5 ml of plain anaesthetic, 0.5–1% xylocaine, and drawing off fluid with a 19G needle and a syringe (20–60 ml) using an aseptic technique. The pressure required is considerable and the fluid should not be allowed to return. The colour of the aspirate can be checked for blood, pus and crystals. In chronic cases, bursae contents are viscous and gelatinous, have a translucent colour and are flecked with blood. If the aspirate is too viscous, it may be difficult to draw off. The effect of aspiration may only last for 6 weeks. The bursa that is too thick for a needle to enter it may prove impossible to aspirate and will need to be resolved by surgery (Fig. 14.7).

Sinus tracts. At one time it was fashionable to apply phenol or silver nitrate to destroy the organised bursa. However, this is ill-advised because it may lead to tissue breakdown or increased sensitivity. Drainage should be established and swabbed for infection.

Orthoses. The aim of orthotic treatment in hallux valgus must be to:

- prevent further progression of the deformity
- prevent the development of secondary problems, such as lesser digit deformity and related nail and skin pathology
- alleviate pain within the first MTP joint or metatarsalgia of the lesser MTP joints.

A bunion shield can be made from latex dip casts, Plastazote moulded around the enlarged joint or replaceable foam ovals (Fig. 14.13). Protective adhesive dressings offer local protection from potential ulceration, but are limited to short-term use only (Ch. 11). Animal wool dressings are useful for chilled skin

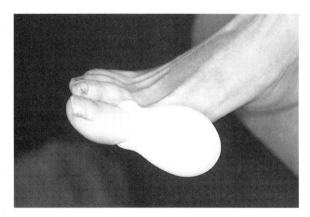

Figure 14.13 Foam to protect a bunion from pressure—available as a stock item.

but should not be wrapped around the toe, in order to avoid constriction. The wool nests use fibres running longitudinally. If care is not taken and the wool is haphazardly wrapped 'around' the toes, when wet the fibres will contract, endangering tissue viability.

Hallux deviation

Orthoses. Attempts to wedge material between the hallux and adjacent second toe may alleviate inter-digital corns. Prevention of further deviation is limited because the second toe is easily pushed over by the bulky insert. Moreover, the work of Hardy & Clapham (1951) indicated that when the hallux abuts the second toe it forms a retrograde force at the MTP joint which pushes the first metatarsal into further varus.

In a study of 25 Argentinian children, Groiso (1992) found that hallux valgus night spl...
metatarsus primus varus static w...
hallux valgus by on average 3°. Th...
used for an average period of 2 y...
valgus showed no sign of furthe...
years follow-up. The night splin...
be expected at least to prevent fu...
of hallux valgus in the child. It i...
ment that requires considerable p...
because if the device is not worn...
cannot be guaranteed.

While Groiso's work on juvenile...
promise (Groiso 1992), little evid...
support the use of night splints i...
in advanced hallux valgus. It sl...
considered as a possible conservati...
The success of night splints can...
6–12 months with a digital gon...
bearing dorsoplantar X-rays wl...
alignment of the first MTP joint.

While casted orthoses have often been recommended for hallux valgus to limit excessive pronation of the foot, longitudinal studies have shown that in children, functional orthoses will not prevent the progression of the deformity (Kilmartin et al 1994).

Antipronation orthoses may, however, be used to reduce the first MTP joint pain associated with loss of joint congruity. One reason for this effect is that orthoses have been shown to restrict first MTP joint movement; this relative immobilisation reduces irritation within the joint (Kilmartin et al 1991). It is important that the patient is advised that the functional orthosis will not prevent progression of hallux valgus and night splints should therefore be used in conjunction with orthoses.

Surgical management

Where night splints have failed to prevent progression of the deformity, or orthoses have failed to relieve joint pain, surgery should be considered as the next appropriate option.

Another important criterion for surgical intervention is the stage when the hallux begins to abut the second toe. At this point, the deformity is likely to progress rapidly (Hardy & Clapham 1951). The condition is no longer just affecting the first MTP joint but is also beginning to deform the lesser digits as well.

Over 150 operations have been described for hallux valgus, but many are simply modifications of original ideas. Essentially, seven approaches exist, a number of which have been illustrated in Chapter 7 (see Table 14.1)

... deal with the following

... rsal angle

... the transverse and

... cal management of hallux

	Example of procedure
	McBride
	Keller
	Silver
	Austin
	Akin
	Various
	Trethowan

Failure to achieve long-term correction of the deformity may be due to inadequate correction of any one of these components of hallux valgus.

Bunion. The medial eminence, or bunion, was thought by Haines & McDougall (1954) to be a traction apophysitis caused by movement of the medial sesamoid, and consequently traction on the medial sesamoid ligament's insertion in the metatarsal head. The medial eminence can be safely reduced provided that good capsular repair is achieved. No more than the enlarged fibrocartilaginous bone should be removed, to prevent narrowing of the articular surface ('staking') and the creation of a hallux varus (adductus) (Fig. 14.14). Bursae can be removed at the same time and redundant tissue plicated at both capsular and skin levels. This procedure does not, however, correct the position of the hallux, sesamoids or first–second intermetatarsal angle.

Mild hallux valgus. Capital osteotomies are valuable where the toe has not created any pressure against the second digit but the toe (hallux valgus angle) is deviated by greater than 15°. The type of osteotomy selected will depend upon whether the joint needs to be decompressed. In achieving decompression, first metatarsal shortening may arise. Wherever possible, therefore, the first metatarsal length should always

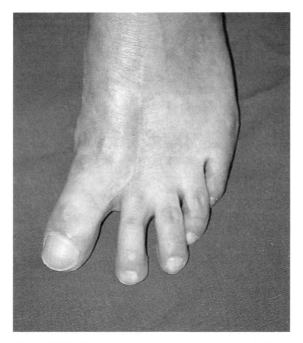

Figure 14.14 Iatrogenic hallux varus from overcorrection of hallux valgus. The metatarsals were splinted together with an internal wire.

be retained relative to the second metatarsal. The act of shortening a metatarsal will slacken tight tissues to assist hallux correction, but the transfer of load to a second or third metatarsal is undesirable. Elevatory osteotomies must be used with caution, whether using a capital or proximally placed osteotomy. A number of factors should therefore be considered in deciding the appropriate capital osteotomy:

- articular set angle (Fig. 7.8)
- intermetatarsal angle between the first and second metatarsals is around 10°–13°
- soft tissue contracture
- extent of dorsiflexed position.

Severe hallux valgus. Where the characteristic angles that are associated with a large hallux and intermetatarsal position arise, the general approach is to select a proximal osteotomy. Faults lying at the first metatarsocuneiform joint may even require an arthrodesis. In some cases a capital osteotomy may have to be used to correct the proximal articular set angle (PASA) at the same time. The association of distal articular set angles (DASA) within the phalanges may require an osteotomy within the phalanx but should never be used alone to correct this deformity to avoid failure. The concept of joint congruency is an important diagnostic feature that must be corrected within the surgical procedure.

Hallux abductovalgus. The presence of a single transverse plane deformity is less complicated to manage than a deformity which has a rotatory twist. Rotation arises when the joint attempts to define a new axis and, consequently, soft tissues shorten. The frontal plane rotation is best corrected by performing a closing wedge osteotomy or Akins operation on the hallux. Double osteotomies may have to be used, and in cases of degeneration, a Keller's excisional arthroplasty can be used with a capital osteotomy.

Degenerative hallux valgus. As with hallux rigidus, the options may vary depending upon patient requirements: arthrodesis will correct a moderate angle; Keller's excisional arthroplasty will shorten the hallux and reduce the retrograde force, which drives the first metatarsal into varus. A replacement joint cannot be used unless the intermetatarsal angle (IMA) is small, as too much stress will be placed on the implant.

Postoperative care. Early ambulation is the goal of all foot surgery. First of all, this lowers the risk of deep venous thrombosis, and secondly, weight-bearing will stimulate osteogenesis around an osteotomy site. Early joint motion reduces stiffness as it divides adhesions associated with postoperative haematoma formation. However, swelling arises from too much motion in the early postoperative stages. Patients should be asked to rest with their foot elevated as much as possible during the first 2 weeks postoperatively, to allow for normal wound healing.

In older patients with impaired venous return, postoperative swelling can be very long-standing. Less complicated surgery is suggested, in order to minimise tissue dissection and to avoid problems associated with bony union failure in cases where poor mineralisation is present.

Trigger hallux

The trigger hallux, or retracted great toe, is associated with pes cavus, where plantarflexion of the first metatarsal arises with tightening of the extensor hallucis longus tendon. The patient may complain of footwear irritation on the dorsal aspect of the IP joint and sesamoiditis associated with the plantarflexed position of the first metatarsal. Treatment can, however, be provided to manage the trigger toe in isolation in some cases.

Conservative management

In the early stages of deformity, an insole with a shaft pad extended under the first metatarsal can be used. This is made from a firm foam material such as polyurethane or neoprene rubber. The objective is to dorsiflex and extend the first MTPJ, lessening the dorsal contraction of the capsule and extensor tendons. Conservative management is in most cases aimed at preventing soft tissue damage from footwear over the IPJ and cushioning the plantar surface of the first metatarsal head and sesamoids. Silicone or Otoform putty can be moulded to redirect pressure from the IPJ. Silopos digital sleeves and Cica care gel (Smith & Nephew) can also be used.

As the deformity progresses, the shoe toe box will need to be deepened to accommodate the deformed toe. More substantial plantar cushioning will also be required. A flat 6 mm Spenco insole is most suitable if it can be accommodated within the shoe. However, difficulties do arise when added plantar cushioning fills the shoe and causes further dorsal irritation.

Surgical management

Arthrodesis of the IPJ with a single screw or two wires (sited percutaneously), will prevent the toe from flexing. The joint must be in good condition. The extensor tendon is transferred through a hole made in the metatarsal head in order to elevate the ray. This proce-

dure should not be used in the presence of the following three factors:

- If the metatarsal is rigid in plantarflexion, the tendon cannot be relied upon to provide normal hallux ground purchase.
- If the forefoot is everted badly, as in the case of pes cavus, multiple surgery may be needed, affecting the other metatarsals or tarsus.
- Poorly mineralised bone and marked joint degeneration are unlikely to form a satisfactory union. In this case, an excisional arthroplasty can be performed as a salvage procedure in the event of deep ulceration.

Hallux varus

This condition is associated with metatarsus adductus in the younger patient, but also commonly arises from overcorrection of the hallux valgus deformity or by staking the head due to overzealous bone resection (Fig. 14.14). Abductor hallucis release, and division and resection of the lateral capsule may be used; alternatively a reverse closing wedge osteotomy of the proximal phalanx may be performed.

FOREFOOT DEFORMITY

Metatarsus adductus is rarely noted in adult feet, as compared with children. This may be a consequence of spontaneous improvement or secondary compensations; both concepts are discussed further in Chapter 15. In the adult, significant forefoot deformities include splay foot and plantarflexed metatarsals.

Splay foot

In the normal foot, the angle between the first and second metatarsal is between 7° and 9° (Kilmartin et al 1991). The angle between the fourth and fifth metatarsals is between 4° and 5°. A pathological increase in the angles between the first and second, and fourth and fifth, metatarsals is known as splay foot and manifests clinically as a widened forefoot with hallux valgus and Tailor's bunion.

Conservative treatment

Footwear fitting is the primary problem in splay foot. Soft wide shoes or trainers are most appropriate, although bespoke footwear is worthy of consideration. Another primary complaint is irritation of the dorsomedial aspect of the first MTPJ and lateral aspect of the fifth. Latex rubber and foam shields may be used to palliate this complaint (Fig. 14.13).

Surgical management

The objective of management is to reduce the width of the foot. Osteotomies which reposition the distal end of the first and fifth metatarsals toward the midline of the foot are indicated. Whether such osteotomies are performed at the proximal or distal end of the metatarsal is determined by the degree of deformity. Higher intermetatarsal angles (i.e. greater than 16° between the first and second metatarsals, or greater than 10° between the fourth and fifth metatarsals) require proximal metatarsal osteotomy.

Metatarsal plantarflexion

Normally, load should be distributed evenly across the lesser metatarsal heads. When load becomes focused on one metatarsal head, tenderness, callus or even bursae arise.

Unequal load distribution may cause plantarflexion of a single metatarsal. Shortening of a single metatarsal or dorsal displacement of a metatarsal will also cause overloading of an adjacent normal metatarsal. This situation is particularly common in hallux valgus where the first metatarsal, which has a independent axis of motion is dorsiflexed by the force of ground reaction, leading to overloading of the adjacent second metatarsal.

In the cavoid foot, overpull of peroneus longus will plantarflex the first metatarsal and significantly increase loading of the metatarsal head. Painful callus of the fifth metatarsal head is also commonly seen in pes cavus. This is due to the tendency for rapid supination of the foot after forefoot loading when the plantarflexed first metatarsal makes ground contact first. Forefoot load then rapidly moves laterally. This is, of course, the reverse of the normal situation where the lateral border of the foot and the fifth metatarsal usually make ground contact first.

Conservative management

Metatarsalgia due to plantar pain should initially be managed with shock-attenuating orthoses. Alternatively, depressed metatarsals may be accommodated inside the shoe with an insole. A cut-out using a cavity or build-up around the metatarsal will achieve the same effect. The load placed over the metatarsal will be distributed across the remaining metatarsals. Symptomatic relief is very successful and will depend

on good shoe design to accommodate the extra material. Plastazote material makes a useful temporary substitute for loss of adipose tissue, as well as forming a natural depression. For long-term use, this is not appropriate. The best resutlt often comes from trial and error (Pratt et al 1993).

More complex prescriptions can be considered with off-the-shelf orthoses such as AOLs, Alphathotics and MBS (Multi Balance System), which are mentioned in more detail in Chapter 12, or by taking a neutral cast to balance the effect of the metatarsals. Contemporary philisophy emphasises the need to control the hindfoot to influence the forefoot about the midtarsal joint. The converse philosophy may be true as well.

Forefoot varus. In the case of forefoot varus, a medial forefoot wedge will prevent the hindfoot from compensating by leaning in medially. The medial long arch is improved by placing a rearfoot wedge or post on the orthosis so that both wedges act to create a reactionary force during forefoot loading (Tollafield & Pratt 1990). Talar and cuneiform alignment are improved while the orthotic is worn. This type of orthotic modification will reduce the strain created in the tibialis posterior and anterior tendons by actively supinating the hindfoot about the midtarsal joint to counter pronation. The use of posting above the deformity value will have deleterious effects on the first ray. Tollafield & Pratt (1990) found that two-thirds of the deformity could be accommodated without elevating the first metatarsal excessively.

Rearfoot posting often commences with a 4° post. Footwear fit and patient tolerance often dictate alterations necessary. The MBS off-the-shelf system (Langer Biomechanics Group) provides an interchangeable posted orthosis without the need for glue or heat guns. This aptly named (Multi Balance System) product allows practitioners to move between 2° and 4° posts by using a press stud fit, for both varus and valgus wedges (Fig. 14.15).

Forefoot valgus. This deformity arises when all the metatarsals are everted in the same plane. A high arch foot may be apparent, but the typical plantarflexed first and fifth metatarsals seen in pes cavus are not present. A lateral wedge or post is provided on the orthosis to prevent the foot supinating around its midtarsal and subtalar joint axes. Unfortunately, if toes are already retracted on the lateral side of the foot, they can easily rub against the shoe upper, making tolerance less practical. An intrinsically posted orthosis may fare better.

First ray involvement. The first ray may be dorsiflexed (metatarsus primus elevatus, MPE). MPE is quite common and has already been described as part

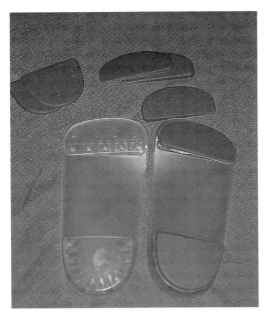

Figure 14.15 MBS orthosis (Langer Biomechanics Group UK Ltd). The wedging (posting system) clips on, making this easy to adjust and dispense.

of the contributing aetiology in hallux rigidus and hallux limitus.

The first ray may be plantarflexed in three different positions (plantarflexed first ray, PFFR): rigid, semi-rigid or flexible. Each has a slightly different management when prescribing orthoses:

- *Flexible.* Cast the first ray out as much as possible by pushing the first metatarsal dorsally while the negative cast is being taken. Pain at the first MTP joint associated with use of the orthosis may indicate that the first metatarsal has been dorsiflexed too much and that the joint has begun to jam because the hallux can no longer rotate around the metatarsal head.
- *Semi-rigid.* The first ray should be dorsiflexed to reduce any marked plantarflexion in the cast. An extrinsic or intrinsic forefoot post is used along the lateral anterior edge. The aim is to limit compensation through the long axis of the midtarsal joint and subtalar joint, and to prevent abnormal dorsiflexion of the first ray.
- *Rigid.* The first ray is casted as it is assessed in a plantarflexed position. A cut-out in the orthosis can be used at the anterior-medial first ray edge and a bar can be used from the second to the fifth metatarsal to bring the forefoot surface to a level position. Alternatively, a lateral anterior wedge (full or tip post) is prescribed on a firm casted orthosis. Another variation

involves the use of softer orthoses with a depression to allow the first ray to find its own level.

Many of these orthotic concepts were developed by Root and his co-workers in the USA during the 1960s. Experienced practitioners find that they prefer their own variations and frequently develop new concepts in casting and orthotic prescription on the basis of experience.

Surgical management

Plantarflexed metatarsals can cause significant pain from bruising, bursae, sesamoiditis, nerve entrapment or keratomata. Osteotomy or excision of the metatarsal head has a part to play in relieving symptoms. There are a number of operations for managing this problem; essentially, the principle involves elevating the metatarsal. This can be done at the base or head of the metatarsal by an osteotomy. The incidence of pain following operations for metatarsal elevation is commonly associated with non-union of bone and with skin transfer lesions and is high (Grace 1993). Where the deformity is rigid, the plantar pressure is greater. In the presence of microangiopathy or neuropathy, ulceration can arise. The views held by foot surgeons vary, but many believe that all three central metatarsals should be operated on simultaneously, as they tend to act mechanically as one unit. This might be less true for an obvious isolated plantarflexed metatarsal.

Rheumatoid patients have the additional problems of forefoot ulcers and large bursae with nodules on the plantar surface. The multiple excision metatarsal was originally described in 1912 by Hoffman. The approach to removing the metatarsal heads may utilise the plantar surface or the dorsum. The plantar approach allows repositioning of the distal fat pad proximally and allows easier removal of the metatarsal head. This type of surgery has had good results, according to Grace (1993).

Removal of the metatarsal heads is, however, a very drastic operation with immense implications for forefoot mechanics. Excision tends to be used for sedentary patients, those with extreme forefoot pain and those with digital deformities unresistant to other forms of surgery. Where some digital function can be retained, excision is less approriate.

A lesser metatarsal osteotomy through the cartilaginous head may appear to be inappropriately placed, but has been recorded as being highly effective for a wide range of patient groups, including those with rheumatoid deformity. The metatarsal head is

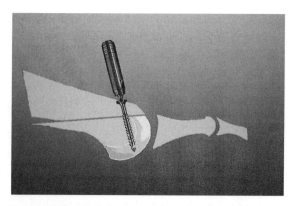

Figure 14.16 Osteotomy associated with Barouk/Weil. Because internal fixation (screw in situ) is used, failed bone union has not been reported in the literature at present. The osteotomy allows decompression of the lesser MTP joints and lateral displacement if required. This technique has distinct advantages over freely displaced osteotomies.

elevated by the thickness of the power saw blade. The metatarsal can be shortened and displaced transversely. This type of osteotomy has become very popular with podiatrists and orthopaedic surgeons in France because it is more predictable; non-union is unrecorded and the movement is controlled. The success also lies in the fact that unlike many elevatory lesser metatarsal osteotomies, this type of procedure is fixed with a wire or screw (Fig. 14.16). When used for plantar corns, many of the common complications associated with osteotomy do not appear to arise (Barouk 1994).

HINDFOOT DEFORMITY

Serious deformity is rare, but when it does present, as in the case of congenital talipes equinovarus (CTEV), treatment is highly specialised. The adult foot is less amenable to correction because of completed growth and serious contracture. Specialised footwear plays a very large part in accommodating problems. Plantar pressure points can be reduced by orthoses.

Haglund or retrocalcaneal bump

A prominent calcaneal bone may cause significant problems at the posterior dorsallateral edge of the heel. Radiographically the picture is unclear unless the lateral contour is affected, causing a spur to form (not to be confused with the plantar spur).

Conservative management

The heel bump can be protected by felt and foam dressings in the early stages of the problem. Gel pads such as Silopos of Cica Care (Smith and Nephew) will protect the skin overlying the bone.

The heel counter should be soft, but during flare-ups patients should use open-heeled shoes. High heels should be avoided, especially those with a deep heel counter which have the effect of cutting into the skin. Soft heel lifts placed in the shoe will elevate the calcaneus above the heel counter. Socks should always be worn to minimise direct pressure and friction against the skin. High ankle training shoes will also help to redirect pressure from the posterior lateral corner of the calcaneus.

The rearfoot condition is often associated with a rigid plantarflexed first ray or partially compensated rearfoot varus. The movement created by these foot problems is thought to act in causing shearing stresses over the skin and periosteum as the heel moves from inversion through to eversion. An orthosis that uses a rearfoot varus wedged post can limit this movement and provides an acceptable treatment regimen. Posted orthotic therapy is often started at a varus cant of 4°. The heel cup should fit the shoe and, if prescribed, should be moderately deep (15–18 mm).

Surgical management

Heel bump surgery should not be entered into lightly. Recurrence, sensitive scarring, damage to the sural nerve, weakening/rupture of the tendo Achilles and prolonged swelling are all possible complications (Fig. 14.17). The procedure may only require the bone to be levelled; unfortunately, because of the bone contour and the poor pre-operative value of X-rays, the surgeon can easily continue to resect bone until the area around the calcaneus has been weakened. This can lead to tendo Achilles rupture. Because surgery is often performed close to the tendinous insertion of the tendo Achilles, pain related to movement is not uncommon afterwards. A below-knee cast is required for 6–8 weeks.

Retrocalcaneal exostectomy may require a period of rehabilitation of up to 3–6 months. The position of the incision line is very critical to limiting nerve damage of the sural and calcaneal branches of the tibial nerve. An alternative procedure is used for dorsal spurs. A V-osteotomy is performed in the sagittal plane to move the proximal superior edge closer to the main body of the bone; this is known as the Keck and Kelly procedure.

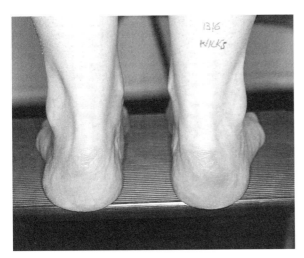

Figure 14.17 Sensitive scar lines affecting both heels following transverse incision. Both scar lines are flat and soft, but the hyperaesthesia leaves the patient with few solutions other than soft shoe counters and heel pads. Incisions placed lateral to the heel may avoid this problem.

DEFORMITIES ASSOCIATED WITH ARCH SHAPE

Pes planovalgus, pes cavus and congenital talipes equinovarus are rare and are helped considerably by footwear modifications and orthoses in adults. These deformities are often associated with hindfoot pathology but may be complicated by forefoot pathology. There is further discussion on this subject in Chapter 15.

Conservative management

Soft tissue problems arise because of hypermobility affecting a less mobile structure or because the foot is rigid. The hindfoot may be structurally abnormal but it is often the midtarsus that takes the brunt of the pathology through compensation.

Pes planus. The talus, navicular and medial cuneiform may all become involved with compensation (Fig. 14.18). The hindfoot should be stabilised early by varus posted casted orthoses. The medial side of the heel cup may be made high to limit the effects of the talus declining and adducting by influencing the sustentaculum tali. The cast should be marked appropriately so that the laboratory technician knows where to increase the heel cup effect.

A University of California orthosis (UCBL) should be considered for ultimate control for the flexible flat foot, providing that no neuromuscular disease

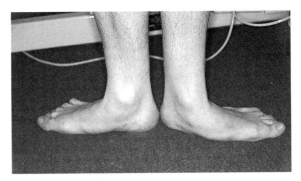

Figure 14.18 This male patient had six pairs of simple insoles which failed to maintain foot comfort for his pes planus. Because the foot is flexible, UCBL or SMO may be considered more appropriate.

is present (Fig. 12.8). Proximal weakness is likely to require an ankle foot orthosis (AFO) to stabilise the ankle and the subtalar joint. Supramalleolar orthoses (SMOs) occupy a position midway between AFOs and foot orthoses (Fig. 14.19). Control is offered around the ankle, providing ultimate stability to a foot with postural strain. Assessment of the flat foot deformity may require simple forefoot and rearfoot posting to bring the ground up to the foot, as mentioned earlier with forefoot varus. The more significant modifica-

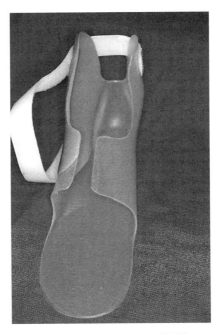

Figure 14.19 Supramalleolar orthosis (SMO). (Reproduced with permission from David Pratt, Derbyshire Royal Infirmary.)

tions, such as UCBLs and SMOs, will make acquisition of shoes more difficult, a point that should be discussed with the patient before casting.

Simple orthoses based on insoles, such as the Cobra design, have a place in flexible and rigid flat feet. A trial in compressed felt is worthwhile, or pre-moulded foamed orthoses such as Frelon, AOL, Alphathotics and MBS, to name but a few, can be selected as economical orthoses (Ch. 11). Stretching exercises should be used in all but the very contracted cases of ankle equinus to ensure that the patient does not lift out of the shoe.

Shoe stiffeners, heel cups and Thomas wedges designed to reduce pronation have found favour in the past. The practitioner will find that an orthotic prescription for inside the shoe is more economical and easier than adapting footwear.

Cavus type feet. The conservative approach to problems associated with this foot type will depend upon the rigidity of the foot. Shock attentuation will relieve major pressure areas under the first/fifth metatarsal. Flexible cavus feet are treated similarly to those feet with forefoot valgus or plantarflexed first ray. In some feet, Haglund's deformity will have to be protected or operated on, depending upon the symptoms. Retracted digits are difficult to deal with, although some patients find plantar metatarsal pads (PMPs) incorporated into insoles to be of some value. Rigid and semi-rigid toe deformities can easily become forced into shoes if insoles are made too bulky. The secondary, iatrogenic corns which develop are not an uncommon problem.

Rigid foot problems. Conservative management has been considered for flexible feet. Rigid feet should be treated differently, in that no orthosis will correct an established deformity, and this is particularly the case if the deformity is not corrected in childhood. Shoes may have to be soft along the medial border and patients must be warned that early replacement is expected because of the marked pronatory forces. Heel wear will cause a problem; repair is easier in bespoke footwear than in off-the-shelf shoes because of the construction design. However, some UK manufacturers, such as Clarks, will replace the polyurethane soling unit. This is worthwhile where the uppers are still in good condition. Soft foamed orthoses will protect skin and offer some relief from foot strain and will hopefully limit proximal stress problems in the leg and knee.

Surgical management

Mixed deformities affecting different parts of the foot

may be better dealt with in stages. The reason for this is to allow one part to settle and return to adequate function before another part is dealt with. The best example of mixed deformity is club foot (CTEV), but problems such as pes valgus and pes cavus tend to be more common.

The club foot has a tight tendo Achilles. This needs to be lengthened by a tendon lengthening procedure. Surgery on the other tendons is designed to restore equilibrium to the evertors and invertors of the foot as well as the dorsiflexors and plantarflexors. Surgery can be quite major in older established deformities or where they have recurred over time, but is less so in a younger child where soft tissue that has contracted can be released before degeneration is reversible.

Pes valgus will only require surgery if there is pain which cannot be controlled with conservative measures and evidence of progressive deformity and joint degeneration. Again, a combination of tendon balancing and osseous correction is indicated. With regard to osseous correction, an important component of pes valgus is abduction of the forefoot. This may be reduced by lengthening the lateral column of the foot by placing a bone graft in the lateral border of the calcaneus (Fig. 7.9). The low medial longitudinal arch with subluxation of the talonavicular and naviculocuneiform joints can be corrected by taking a triangular wedge from the medial cuneiform, the apex of the triangle being placed dorsally. Closure of the wedge will plantarflex the forefoot and raise the medial longitudinal arch. If the forefoot is abnormally adducted and the tarsus is not severely affected, the metatarsals will be divided by closing wedge osteotomies.

Where the flat foot deformity cannot be resolved with less radical surgery, correction by ankle arthrodesis may be required. This form of fusion immobilises the ankle at one to three joints (Fig. 7.6). Pain and disability often provide the main deciding factors for a procedure which is preferred as the last resort.

Pes cavus is characterised by a high arch. Fascial release and calcaneal osteotomy may be used to lower the arch height (Fig. 7.10). The tarsus is frequently 'humped', causing an excessive declination of the metatarsals which cannot be managed without midtarsus osteotomy. Digital deformity may have to be managed by tendon balancing and osteotomies, as described under the section on forefoot deformity.

Pes cavus and CTEV have similarities in that the foot is rigid and experiences pressure points. Treatment of these complex deformities is managed with a mixture of soft tissue and bone techniques. Details of these procedures fall outside the scope of this text.

CORNS AND CALLUS

The types of problem encountered at the skin and subcutaneous levels must be considered carefully as some overlap in management may be required, as the underlying deformity and deeper tissue pathology may be influenced by different forms of therapy. Callus is usually a response to mechanical pressure associated with shear and friction. Remove the physical irritation and the condition will reverse, leaving the skin soft and pliable again.

Underlying deformity, such as exostoses, should be protected with orthoses or removed by surgery. However, while not exclusive to the plantar metatarsal area and IP joints of toes, callus causes fewer symptoms elsewhere. Penetrating injuries associated with foreign bodies such as glass can cause an irritant effect on deep tissues, leading to thick scarring. Neuroma involvement and synovial cysts have been identified in patients with otherwise typical intractable plantar keratoma (IPK).

Conservative management

The use of debridement skills (Ch. 6) is valuable in reducing the irritant effect of thicker layers of epidermis on sensitive nerve endings. Emollient products can be applied when the skin is thin enough to allow effective penetration. Areas of the foot experiencing localised pressure will develop characteristic concentric centres or corns (clavus). Enucleation will temporarily reduce pain sensation, particularly in younger patients. Recalcitrant lesions will manifest, creating subepidermal thickening, bursa formation and even sinus tracking over joints. The most painful form of corn is associated with fibrous infiltration around sweat glands and nerve endings, often involving blood vessels.

Continuous debridement may cause repetitive trauma, and over long periods offers proportionally less relief and may require more frequent attention. Callus and corns overlying bone areas are therefore more obdurate to treat. Surgery of the underlying cause may be necessary. Nonetheless, non-osseous-related lesions, as cited in the case history in Box 6.2, illustrate some of the problems which can be encountered when no direct irritant factor can be identified.

Orthotic management. The use of distributive felt padded dressings with apertures and cavities has proved effective in reducing symptoms. A successful outcome might be measured by reducing the need for frequent debridement. Silicone orthodigital splints are valuable in that they are replaceable and easy to mould to toes. Other ready-made devices include digital Tubifoam and Silipos sleeves and a wide variety of insole bases to which felt may be added. The simple insole used for plantar redistribution invariably reduces symptoms, but does not eradicate the build-up of callus completely.

Medication. Injectable medication such as vitamin B_{12}, sclerosing agents such as alcohol and even steroids have been used to break down the fibrous tissue with some success. Balkin (1972) advocated implants of fluid silicone injection under lesions. This has been shown both to reduce keratoses and to improve ulcers.

Local application of emollients under plastic occlusion in hard vehicles such as firm pastes has been recommended to hydrate lesions. *Keratolytics* such as salicylic acid preparations can be used in solution, collodion or paste. The availability of similar products in corn plasters causes much controversy. Patients often fail to apply these over-the-counter treatments with appropriate caution. Injudicious application can result in tissue breakdown and infection. Professional treatment is always advocated and Lang et al (1994) concluded that the length of treatment relied upon clinical judgement and patient tolerance. Keratolytics can provide a valuable approach to desquamation. The optimum period of application of corn plasters as 40% salicylic acid was studied over 3 weeks in 240 patients. Some adverse reactions were shown, even in controlled conditions (1.3%). Maceration around the area of application increased with duration of application; only patients with healthy tissue should be selected.

Silver nitrate in varying strengths has been advocated to astringe (dry up and cause contraction) corns. Lack of scientific evidence and audit has meant that the long-term benefits of these products has not been proven, although pyrogallic acid (50%) does appear to be beneficial in reducing the size of lesions when applied and debrided over 4–8 weeks. The telltale brown stain should lead the practitioner to suspect that either silver nitrate or pyrogallol has been used previously.

A combination of topical medicament and redistributive insoles has been valuable. It would appear from empirical experience that success with all the above treatment strategies relies on early management before chronic subdermal tissue changes occur. Silicone sheeting and Silopos products have provided an alternative philosophy in the hydration of lesions. These products still have to be adhered to skin or applied as a replaceable appliance, which may affect the integrity of skin contact. Orthoses to correct underlying pronation should be considered as an adjunct to the above therapy rather than as a cure for the corn or callus; symptom improvement, however, has only been noted empirically.

Seed corns. These small plugs of keratin form in the creases of the epidermal surface of the foot. Research has shown little proof of a different aetiology from those lesions found over weight-bearing surfaces. Emollient applications temporarily improve skin elasticity. Orthoses that can improve pressure distribution serve as a useful adjunct to emollient application. E45 and urea preparations are popular, although any lubricant will provide similar properties. With the exception of excision, little has been written on the subject of surgery for this condition. Regular enucleation, while highly beneficial, still risks further damage to the local skin structure.

Surgical management

Surgical management of corns provides an attractive solution and falls into four categories: skin excision, correction of fixed deformity, elevation of metatarsal head and correction of forefoot/hindfoot alignment. Callus can be helped by the latter three surgical methods.

Skin excision. Excision should only be considered where an underlying dermal problem such as bursa, inclusion cyst, fibroma or foreign body has arisen (see case history in Box 14.4). Furthermore, the lesion should ideally be over a non-weight-loading area such as the metatarsal head area. Removal of such plantar lesions should be followed by a period of assisted weight-bearing (e.g. with a cast) or non-weight-bearing (with crutches). Early forefoot pressure will strain the incision site.

Correction of fixed deformity. Digital deformity contributes considerably to skin lesions. If conservative treatment fails to relieve the problem within 6 months, surgical excision of the head of the phalanx will

---

Box 14.4 Case history: excision of a corn

A 63-year-old male presented with a corn under his right foot which had previously been removed by his GP. The appearance (Fig. 14.20) showed the lesion to be a long-standing IPK with a well-defined border but with minimal callosity beyond the periphery. The lesion measured 1.5 cm and was excised. A large cyst was identified underlying the hyperkeratosis (Fig. 14.21) and was reported by histopathology as having an epithelial lining of cuboidal cells. A blunt seeker shows a central punctum through the dermis. The depth was recorded as 1.5 cm taken from an ellipse measuring 3.5 cm × 0.8 cm. A small drain was inserted into the wound before closure and removed 2 days later.

Conclusion. The following criteria: intense pain, traumatic origin, length of duration of symptoms, lack of biomechanical abnormality, may lead the practitioner to have doubts about a simple corn arising. In the case of IPKs presenting with these findings, surgical care may have to be considered. Because the lesion in this case was not directly over a metatarsal, and a definitive subdermal cause could be found, the wound healed uneventfully.

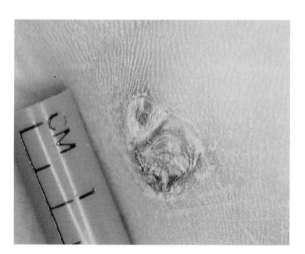

Figure 14.20 Corn overlying synovial cyst. The appearance is atypical of a corn as this had already been excised once 3 years previously.

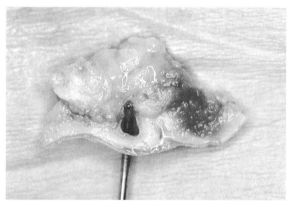

Figure 14.21 Cyst removed from tissue (shown in Fig. 14.20). The central punctum communicates with a cavity in the dermis. Histology shows acanthosis and hyperkeratosis. The cyst was lined with cuboid epithelium surrounded by fibrosis. The diagnosis is a synovial cyst.

improve the lesion dramatically in those patients suited to surgery. The dermal changes have often been found to be seriously altered upon excision with small bursae/cysts present. Without ameliorating the cause, patients are often destined to retain persistent corns in perpetuity.

Apical and interdigital lesions respond equally well to arthroplasty or arthrodesis. Hallux valgus correction and exostectomy should be appropriately selected for medial or phalangeal problems associated with the great toe.

Elevation of metatarsals. The metatarsal head that lies below the other four adjacent metatarsals will become overloaded with pressure. Bursa development (see under bursitis) or callus arises as a response of the soft tissues to mechanical stress. Single elevation osteotomies can be undertaken. Some controversy exists concerning the view that, once divided, the bone should be fixed, since a single non-union can have devastating effects and, on the whole, fixation stabilisation is safer (Fig. 14.12). Over-elevation will create two problems. Firstly, the adjacent metatarsals may become overloaded with new callosity forming within a few months, if not weeks; and secondly, the MTP joint may become stiff, as an elevatus will reduce joint range excursion.

Where very severe lesions exist, metatarsal head excision may be preferred because symptom relief is immediate. However, transfer lesions may still arise and should be anticipated using an insole to protect the other metatarsals. Excision is usually a last resort associated with multiple toe deformities and digital retraction and forms a salvage type of operation.

Forefoot/hindfoot alignment. The splayed forefoot, pes cavus and club foot will all give rise to metatarsal callosity. Surgical correction may need to be staged, but these tend to involve both forefoot and hindfoot deformities. Some of these surgeries have already been discussed earlier.

SOFT TISSUE PAIN

Many inflammatory soft tissue problems relate to stress and strain episodes and are associated with repetitive injuries following sporting activities. The adult patient frequently presents with such problems with no recollection of injury. Conservative management is called for in the majority of cases where soft tissue injuries present.

Complete rupture of tendons may require surgical repair rather than immobilisation in a soft splint or cast. Chapter 16 considers tendon injuries in greater detail.

HEEL PAIN SYNDROMES

Heel pain is responsible for a high proportion of podiatric referrals. Pain on the plantar aspect of the heel is a common problem which has a number of aetiological factors (Sunberg & Johnson 1991). Most heel pain relates to soft tissue.

Accurate history taking should rule out less common conditions such as gout, Reiter's disease and ankylosing spondylitis. Back pain and referred S1 nerve pain can be excluded by careful examination of the hip and lower back. Haglund's has already been described under deformity. Tendo Achilles pain and problems associated with calcaneal and Achilles bursitis/tendinitis are usually located at specific points—these conditions are dealt with in Chapter 16.

Calcaneal tumours are rare, but X-rays are required to rule out unicameral bone cysts, osteoid osteomas, fractures, and radio-opaque foreign bodies and metastatic tumours. X-rays should be taken only when no other history fits the symptoms. Nocturnal, non-weight-bearing pain that does not resolve with aspirin or paracetamol may in rare cases suggest a malignant tumour.

Although nerve entrapment is dealt with as a separate subject, recent evidence suggests that the practitioner should be aware of variations in the branches of the tibial nerve which might contribute to heel pain (Campbell & Lawton 1994, Davis & Schon 1995). Nerve entrapment, as with tarsal tunnel syndrome, can be associated with a frequently found anomalous nerve branch supplying the abductor digiti minimi. If the branch divides proximally and close to the medial calcaneal tuberosity, compression can easily arise.

Plantar heel pad pain

Heel pain most commonly affects the plantar surface. Generally, the pain may present as sharp burning or an intense ache which is reproducible on direct pressure. Pain is increased on walking and standing, and eased by rest. Pain is worse on activity, after a rest period, or when first getting out of bed. There are several factors associated with the cause of plantar heel pain; each needs to be considered and rectified where possible within the treatment plan. Common causes include increased activity, inappropriate footwear design (Fig. 14.22), sudden increased weight, as in pregnancy, and abnormal foot function.

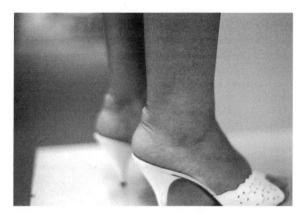

Figure 14.22 Fatty heel bumps in a patient with highly unsuitable shoes. Note that the soft calcaneal tissue is allowed to hang over the edge of the sling back shoes, leading to further problems—fissuring and hard skin.

While a calcaneal spur may be diagnosed, asymptomatic spurs may be found on the contralateral heel. Unilateral heel oedema suggests chronic heel pad strain, although this can be confused with a bursa. Plantar fasciitis and heel pain syndrome must be distinguished from S1 referred pain, infection and osteoid osteoma.

Conservative treatment

Heel pain, especially on the medial aspect, is often related to excessive pronation although a supinated foot type may influence symptoms due to inadequate shock absorption. Care should be taken to control the rearfoot and forefoot with appropriate orthoses to allow first ray plantarflexion, particularly if there is a tight medial band of the fascia. Rigid orthoses should have a groove or indent to accommodate tight fascial bands. There is a range of heel orthoses available, and no one product has been shown to be superior. Foot or even below-knee leg casts have been used to limit strain or as night splints designed to rest the foot.

Muscle stretching should be included in the management plan and may typically include the calf and hamstring muscle groups. Flexibility exercises for the former will stretch both the muscle and the plantar structures. If a fracture is suspected or ultrasound over the site causes pain on treatment, an X-ray is indicated. Physical therapy has a part to play in rehabilitating the patient with heel pain. Heat, ultrasound, laser and TNS units all have a role.

Chronic heel strain does not resolve with analgesics and NSAIDs as successfully as acute strain. Many patients attend the clinic once the chronic stage has developed, some 7–18 months after symptoms were first recognised. Footwear, insoles and heel cup advice can afford much improvement with occasional analgesic use.

Specific sites of pain with swelling and balottement point to the diagnosis of a plantar *bursa*, which some call policeman's heel. The bursa can be infiltrated with 0.25–0.5 ml corticosteroid such as methylprednisolone or triamcinolone hexacetonide. Cut-outs within heel pads and insoles can provide some relief, as can injection therapy. Flare-up is not uncommon in patients, accounting for 1–2% of cases (Tollafield & Williams 1996). Patients should be warned about this side-effect which usually lasts for no more than 2 days.

Elasticated support stockings or compressive heel pads are valuable if worn before placing the foot on the floor first thing in the morning (Fig. 14.23). The elasticated support compresses the heel and improves the venous return to alleviate congested tissues. Where orthoses and all the other conservative measures fail, the patient may require walking casts or Aircasts to retain mobility while ensuring that rest continues. Crutches are not recommended, as the patient should maintain weight-bearing wherever possible (see Appendix 3). If rest therapy fails, surgery to release the fascia may have to be undertaken.

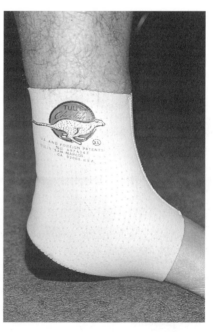

Figure 14.23 Stock heel cushion with elasticated ankle sock (bright green; Tuli pad design).

Heel pain will generally respond well to conservative management. However, no single isolated treatment must be relied upon. It is often a combination of therapies that is most effective. Heel pain may resolve unaided, often after a prolonged period of 2 years.

Fasciitis and plantar spurs

Tenderness along the medial and central bands of the fascia can be located at the insertion point of the calcaneus (associated with an enthesis or projection), although spurs are generally deeper to the insertion (Powell & Gilchrist 1996). Current literature is divided over the origin of the spur; some take the view that spur resection is the only answer. The tenderness produced by dorsiflexing the toes, dorsiflexing the ankle and palpation will reveal one or more specific areas of pain. While obesity is not the only factor involved, weight loss is to be encouraged, although exercise may not be possible because of the fasciitis; the cycle of events must be broken.

Rupture of the fascia should be ruled out if clinical examination identifies a gap in the fascia or if the patient reports a history of a sudden snap along the band. Injudicious use of steroid injections has been known to cause weakness.

Conservative management

Physical therapy, fascia strapping and single injection therapy with a corticosteroid medication offer an approach to reversing inflammation, resting the fascia and limiting swelling and pain (Fig. 14.24). Relief is

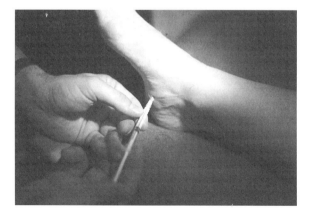

Figure 14.24   Corticosteroid (methyl prednisolone) in heel given from the medial side with a 3.75 cm 27G needle (Sterican, Braun). Patients should be warned to rest and told that 'flare-up' can occur.

usually very rapid, with patients reporting up to 70% relief within 2 weeks. If the pain does not resolve quickly, the practitioner should seek further diagnostic investigation or supplement treatment with varus canted heel cups, heel pads and orthoses, much as for heel pad strain. Repeated steroid injections should be used cautiously; lack of improvement implies that steroid treatment is unhelpful and provocative of further pain. NSAID analgesics have an unpredictable effect and rarely ameliorate a long-standing problem. Ibuprofen or diclofenac sodium may offer valuable supportive therapy in assisting reduction of swelling and inflammation, but complications as a result of long-term use are well recognised (Ch. 8).

Fasciitis may involve the heel fat pad and can complicate the clinical picture. Patients should monitor the association of symptoms at work or at home, to rule out exacerbating factors. Heel lifts in felt and foam can reduce tendo Achilles tension. As mentioned earlier, stretching is an important strategy in resolving fasciitis.

Orthotic management of pronation is essential in order to prevent recurrence of the condition. Pes cavus feet require shock attenuation because the taut band is easily traumatised. Plantar fasciitis associated with pes planus requires antipronation (orthoses/strapping) to prevent the fascia lengthening and causing strain.

Surgical management

A small percentage of patients with heel pain will require surgery; most will respond to conservative measures. Surgical intervention is determined by the diagnosis:

- plantar fasciitis is dealt with by division of the plantar fascia from its insertion into the calcaneus (Barrett & Day 1993)
- heel neuroma is dealt with by releasing and decompressing the medial calcaneal nerve as it passes under the abductor hallucis muscle belly. Surgery to release nerves and their associated branches has been cited by Campbell & Lawton (1994) to have provided good relief
- plantar bursitis requires excision, although this is very rare (in our practice).

In all cases the surgical approach should avoid areas of stress. The medial side of the calcaneus is often chosen where the plantar and dorsal skin meet. Avoidance of scarring must remain the key objective when selecting incision lines, while still allowing access to tissues involved.

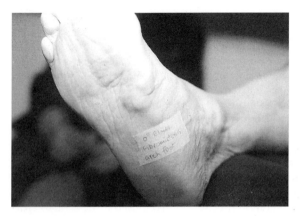

Figure 14.25 Fascia nodules form in plantar fibromatosis as in Dupuytren's contracture. Fibromatosis does not have to be symptomatic.

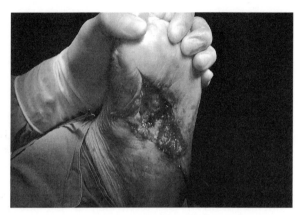

Figure 14.26 Surgery must be aggressive when dealing with fibromatosis. The illustration shows fascial resection following previous surgery. The fascia is stripped away from the underlying muscle. A drain (not shown) is used in situ to prevent haematoma formation.

Plantar fibromatosis

The soft tissue lumps appearing in the medial arch can arise with nodular lesions associated with subcutaneous tissue. This condition can develop as a proliferative fasciitis in young and old patients. The fibroma forms in the fascia and in the long plantar ligament (Fig. 14.25). In many cases, the condition is an inconvenience. Orthoses must avoid compressing the nodular structure and thus causing irritation. Casted orthoses must take account of the nodular area by marking the negative shell so that the laboratory can add plaster to the positive cast.

Where the digits are affected by marked clawing, or where pain arises, radicle resection is necessary, using Z-skin incisions or curved incisions to avoid inciting further scarring. The fascia and nodules are removed, exposing underlying muscle. Drains inserted into the wound reduce the possibility of haematoma becoming organised into further scar tissue (Fig. 14.26).

TENDINITIS AND BURSITIS

Tendinitis most commonly affects the Achilles tendon, although the posterior tibial tendon can be involved. Overuse can initiate the condition and therefore management is largely conservative in nature. Strapping and orthoses are highly effective, although in the early stages heel lifts can be used, providing that the heel cord is not encouraged to shorten and is monitored. Steroid injections are rarely recommended in the early stages of treatment. Stretching and strengthening are discussed in Chapter 16, but active maintenance of controlled tensile stress is essential to prevent contracture.

Bursitis around the Achilles tendon shows up as a collection of fluid which can be moved from side to side. A retrocalcaneal bursa may arise from direct irritation from hard or high heel counters; the shoe design should be changed. Aspiration can be attempted to collapse the wall; 20–60 ml syringes should be selected, with large guage needles, following infiltration of anaesthetic at the point of injection. The bursa is strapped down afterwards. Steroid injections have been found to be very useful in preventing further swelling. Underlying retrocalcaneal spurs or bumps may need resection.

Plantar metatarsal bursitis. This is another condition broadly classified as metatarsalgia. Inflammation of an adventitious bursa arises plantar to the MTP joint which is the result of shearing stress within the tissues. Located under one of the three central metatarsals when prominent, the condition may arise when the first metatarsal is dorsiflexed. An intense pain associated with burning, sharpness and throbbing is present on weight-bearing and will reduce on rest. Fluctuant swelling and tenderness provide some idea of the extent of pathology. Figure 14.27 illustrates the type of problem facing the practitioner if a bursa becomes chronically organised under a metatarsal head. Elevated first metatarsals causing plantar overload to second or third metatarsals may be balanced with a metatarsal shaft under the first ray. The disadvantage caused by this technique relates to limiting first MTP joint motion.

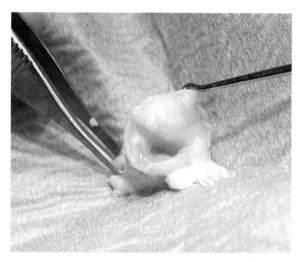

Figure 14.27 Adventitious bursa removed from under the second metatarsal head. The sac was well formed due to chronic organisation of tissue and failed to resolve with steroid injections. There were symptoms of metatarsalgia—burning pain. There was fluctuant presentation underlying skin.

Conservative management

Management for bursitis is similar to that for capsulitis. Although conservative measures using physical therapy may be beneficial, the plantar skin is difficult to penetrate. A felt pad for the sole of the foot, with a 'U' cut around the painful area reduces pressure. Corticosteroid infiltration will allow the bursa to shrink unless it becomes chronic.

Surgical management

Surgical excision must avoid the plantar weight-bearing surface. Incision lines must be made between the metatarsals. Displacement of metatarsals by vertical elevation and shortening may alter the weight-bearing balance effectively. The first metatarsal can in some cases be brought into greater plantarflexion.

NEOPLASIA

Skin tumours are far more common than bone tumours (described earlier). Diagnosis, to rule out infection, should be differentiated by biopsy and microbiological culture.

Principles of management

Conservative management may be appropriate for some lesions. Caustic sticks such as silver nitrate can limit epithelialisation. The use of any chemical agent around an undefined lesion may create malignant change; the practitioner should apply the following axiom: 'do not apply any agents to skin that might lead to damage or provoke an abnormal response'.

Lesions that discharge, show colour changes, have indistinct borders, show an insidious growth change or are irritant warrant appropriate specialist opinion. Corticosteroids have successfully been used for many inflammatory-based dermatological lesions, such as granuloma annulare (Rasanen et al 1993), but they are not indicated unless the diagnosis is distinct.

Hyfrecation and cryosurgery offer alternative destructive methods but destroy the quality of the lesion for the purposes of biopsy. Where the tumour is small, it is preferable to remove the lesion in one piece together with some of the healthy edge. This provides the histopathology laboratory with better material for analysis, and also improves the chances of complete removal. Care should be taken with excisional biopsy surgery to avoid interfering with skin involved with plastic surgery at a later stage. Inadvertent scarring may limit effectiveness of plastic surgery, therefore, careful planning of incision lines at biopsy is critical. Curettage is useful for skin warts (Ch. 15) and selection of this surgical technique will depend upon the likelihood of scarring and on the site. Keloid or hypertrophic scars (Fig. 7.27) are undesirable, especially on the plantar surface. Skin tags respond well to amputation by tying a fine thread around the base to cut off the local blood supply.

Surgical management will be determined by the site, depth and likely cause of the lesion. The object of surgery is to cause limited destruction, but primarily to allow correct identification. Amputation is used for cases with extensive invasive and malignant neoplasia. Plastic surgery by grafting is considered where a flap cannot be advanced over the defect left by the surgery (case history, Box 7.2; Fig. 7.18). A skin lesion may need to be traced through fascia and muscle to bone; drains may have to be used and the patient either admitted or appropriately discharged to home.

Ganglionic cysts remain common to the foot as a benign fluctuant swelling. Closely approximated to joint margins and tendon sheaths, aspiration will fail to achieve lengthy remission. Mucoid cysts over the distal IP joints have a similar appearance, although they are usually much smaller. Surgical excision is the best approach, allowing the foot to be correctly explored and part of the involved joint lining removed. Mucoid cysts affecting toes may require an excisional arthroplasty.

Tumours that cause no pain and remain the same size for years should be monitored. Monitoring consists of measuring the size in millimetres and drawing an outline using the adhesive side of clear tape to mark the lesion. The tape is then stuck securely in the records. An instamatic photograph on slide will provide visual evidence.

To treat or not to treat?

The reason for dealing with any growth falls into two categories: to identify the taxonomy of the lesion and to prevent space-occupying damage. Large cysts become organised with inflammatory material, cells and cholesterol deposits, and damage internal structures (Fig. 14.28) such as tendons, capsules, fascia and muscle. For the latter reason, the patient should have lesions removed which show a steady rate of expansion, even though they show no signs of discomfort, lymphadenopathy, lung, kidney or liver disease. Men should be questioned about prostate problems and women about breast examination and reproductive organ disorders. The patient should be referred to the appropriate specialist if doubt arises.

NEUROLOGICAL PAIN

Neurological pain is difficult to diagnose and may be the resultant effect of back and pelvic problems affecting the nerve pathways which descend into the foot. Pain located to a particular site within the foot may, however, result from local nerve entrapment.

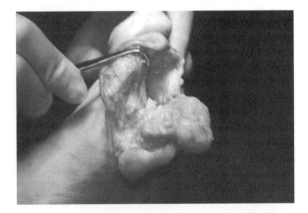

Figure 14.28 Space-occupying lesions may be painless but can cause marked destruction of underlying anatomy if left for years. Where lesions can migrate back in-between metatarsals, the appearance and size are deceptive (cf. Fig. 14.10). Both lesions come from the same site and patient.

Two common sites for nerve entrapment include the intermetatarsal spaces, particularly the 3–4 intermetatarsal space, and the tarsal tunnel which passes inferior to the medial malleolus; entrapment in the latter is a consequence of tibial nerve compression. Following a thorough examination of the locomotor system and failure of conservative treatment, these specific sites may require investigating and the tissue examined for pathology. The use of ultrasound in diagnosing nerve problems depends upon the available expertise of the radiologist, but as a test may not be wholly conclusive. While surgery should ideally be avoided, procedures are often undertaken as part of the diagnostic process.

Interdigital neuroma

This phenomenon is not a tumour but is associated with degeneration of the nerve due to stretching and compression. The symptoms associated with it include a sharp, shooting, pain radiating into the toes.

Conservative management

A recent study and review of steroid infiltration (Tollafield & Williams 1996) revealed that 30% improvement in neuroma pain was maintained in excess of 6 months' duration. Seventy per cent of patients may experience some immediate relief from injection therapy for 2–12 weeks. The use of corticosteroids for adventitious bursae is diagnostic as well as therapeutic, offering a sensible first line treatment. If the toes part (diastasis), an infiltrated bursa is suggested, as the fluid from the injection causes the separation.

In a report by Kilmartin & Wallace (1994), 50% of 21 patients studied found their neuroma symptoms relieved by an orthotic (Cobra) insole made from felt. Of the remainder, 30% required cortisone injections, while 20% required surgery. These recent studies allow us to focus on planned outcomes when advising patients.

Other forms of management include reflexology, osteopathy, plantar metatarsal pad (PMP) insoles and pads worn with toe loops. A PMP orthosis is believed to separate the metatarsals by extending the toe with an upward force on weight-bearing. Much of the success with conservative therapy is almost certainly related to early intervention and diagnosis.

Sclerosing agents such as alcohol and vitamin B_{12} (cyanocobalamin) have both been used for interdigital neuromata. Miller (1992) cites Dockery & Nilson (1986) who used 4% ethanol by mixing 2 ml of alcohol with 48 ml of anaesthetic. The injection is repeated every week for at least three visits.

Surgical management

Where the nerve has enlarged with fibrotic infiltration, excision is indicated. Pain may in fact result from an enlarged bursa. The literature reveals different approaches to removing a neuroma. A plantar approach is easier to undertake but can lead to problems from scarring and seed corn formation. The suture technique is of vital importance to prevent this; skin must be carefully apposed to prevent overlap. The plantar skin approach may vary between patients, but there may be resulting hyperkeratosis, wound dehiscence and scarring; these features are less common on the dorsum. The dorsal approach is technically more difficult, but postoperatively is more reliable. Although loss of sensation is a postoperative feature, this causes little symptomatic concern.

The dorsal- and web-splitting approach is useful if pain from an enlarged mass can be palpated in the intermetatarsal space. Interdigital healing may be slower in patients if the area becomes macerated with sweat; infection is not uncommon with interdigital incisions at 5–7 days.

Histology should always be used to confirm that a neuroma has been identified. It has been suggested that 75–95% of these neuromata can be resolved at operation (Mann 1978). Stumps of nerves can cause painful nodules where scarring has occurred. A repeat operation is often the only recourse, although patients can benefit from manipulative therapy where adhesions appear to respond by being broken up. Revision surgery is more certain to resolve the problem if a plantar approach is made.

Tarsal tunnel syndrome

Nerve entrapment causing pain in the arch and forefoot is attributed to tibial nerve compression. Pain, paraesthesia, dysaesthesia and hyperaesthesia around the ankle and along the distribution of the tibial nerve are common. A positive Tinel's sign, Valleix test (proximal pain along the nerve on pressure) and intrinsic muscle weakness are all suggestive of entrapment.

The use of a sphygmomanometer set at 100–150 mmHg is valuable in determining the extent of pathology. The toes and forefoot become sensitive and painful within 30 seconds of this test if positive. The sphygmomanometer pressure test allows reasonable judgement in referring patients on for nerve conduction and MRI, but is not in itself conclusive of tarsal tunnel syndrome.

The nerve conduction test may show altered sensory nerve conduction, i.e. slow or absent, decreased amplitude, increased duration of motor-evoked potential or increase latency of a distal motor nerve. Some patients find nerve conduction analysis quite painful.

Electromyography may show weakness in a muscle, as tarsal tunnel syndrome has been reported by Summarco & Conti (1994) to be caused by an anomalous hypertrophic or accessory abductor hallucis.

An MRI may be warranted to establish nerve and soft tissue entrapment, as in some cases the nerve has to be released at its distal as well as its proximal end. Enlarged or atrophic muscles will also be easier to identify. The patient should be thoroughly reviewed for other differential neurological conditions associated with peripheral sensory and motor disorders.

Conservative management

The foot mechanics should be stabilised with strapping or orthoses early into treatment, provided that temporary orthoses can be shown to resolve some symptoms. Pronatory problems are most likely to cause this condition.

Injection therapy has been used to good effect to reduce the intraneural and extraneural inflammation (Malay & McGlamry 1992). Casting for short periods to rest the inevitable traction along the nerve may reduce symptoms. NSAIDs and physical therapies may be tried to reduce fibrosis and improve movement around the nerve.

Surgical management

Intractable symptoms can lead to a disabling condition. The nerve in this case is not removed but released from scarring, causing tethering to adjacent tissues. Nerves must have the freedom to elongate with foot movement. The tibial nerve courses through the tarsal tunnel and is involved with the tibialis posterior tendon, flexor digitorum longus, neurovascular bundle and flexor hallucis longus. Surgery to expose these tissues should take care not to damage the vascular tissue or nerve (Fig. 14.29). The nerve is traced distally where it will divide into a medial and lateral portion. The medial portion is larger and runs between the abductor hallucis and flexor hallucis brevis, having passed through a fibrous opening between the abductor hallucis and spring ligament. Any fibrous constrictions are released, preserving nerve motility. Symptoms should be relieved once the tibial

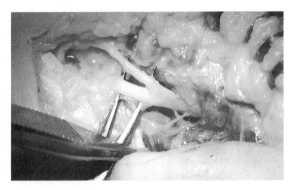

Figure 14.29 Nerve decompressed in the tarsal tunnel showing lateral and medial branches of the tibial nerve. (Reproduced with permission from Scott Hosler, Fifth Avenue Residency Programme.)

nerve is no longer compressed. Tarsal tunnel surgery may not always be successful as scarring can recur.

Cutaneous neurological pain

Any nerve close to the surface can be damaged, especially on the dorsal surface of the foot where it can become impinged by compression between shoe and bone. Pain from the superficial peroneal nerves may radiate onto the dorsum of the foot. The practitioner should initially exclude all medical causes, but surgery may provide assistance where all other forms of management fail and where diagnosis casts a high degree of suspicion on a neurological problem.

Surgery certainly cannot assist with nerve problems unless a physical cause can be shown to have caused the problem in the first place. Neuritic bunion pain has been described in the absence of fixed deformity (Rosen & Grady 1986). Symptoms were associated with shooting pain into the big toe. Diagnosis of medial dorsal cutaneous neuritis was established when at operation a fibrous band was shown to compress the nerve.

Miscellaneous nerve entrapment

While entrapment may arise above the ankle, tarsal tunnel is considered the most common form of foot entrapment after Morton's neuroma. In some cases, metatarsalgia may relate to a plantar nerve entrapped under the metatarsal head. The nerve becomes tethered to the metatarsal and is continuously traumatised. The case history in Box 14.5 emphasises the need to keep an open mind during examination.

Box 14.5 Case history: nerve entrapment

A 75-year-old female had been suffering for many years with pain under her first metatarsal. More recently, the symptoms had become more distressing. Examination of the foot provided a diagnosis of plantarflexed first ray causing sesamoiditis. Insoles and careful footwear selection had all been tried, but to no avail. Lateral X-rays were taken and a large medial sesamoid confirmed the suspicion that the first metatarsal pain was related to the ossicle. The surgical plan included planing of the sesamoid to trim it back, or removal if it was too large. Planing provided a less than satisfactory result. Once the sesamoid had been removed, the skin flattened sufficiently to diminish the accentuation of the first ray with its enlarged sesamoid. The interesting point about this case involved the identification of a thickened plantar nerve which had become invested within the tissues underlying the medial sesamoid (Fig. 14.30).

Conclusion. Trapped nerves must be excluded from foot pathology. Because the anatomical pathway of nerves varies, some of the symptoms associated with nerves may not be that obvious. Removal of the sesamoid was felt to be prudent because of significant pain, although in this case disruption of the flexor pull against the hallux must always remain a concern.

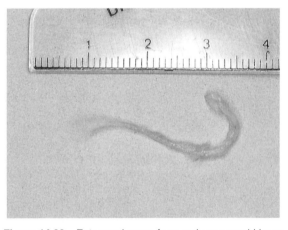

Figure 14.30 Entrapped nerve from under sesamoid bone (see case history in Box 14.5).

MISCELLANEOUS PAIN

Differentiating pain

Rarer forms of pain arising in the foot and lower limb include reflex sympathetic dystrophy (Ch. 7) and compartment syndrome (Ch. 16). Associated neurological pain with evidence of local swelling should be ruled out, and compartment syndrome, localised nerve compression from a tumour and localised damage to the nerve with fibrosis should be differentiated.

Acute vascular problems arise with disease processes such as diabetes and peripheral vascular disease, and these patients need to be urgently assessed and sent for appropriate investigations. Differentiation between vascular ischaemia and neuropathic ischaemia is important, and sensory, vibration and pressure testing can be performed in clinic.

Anatomical variation arises in the foot. Venous malformation can arise causing the same symptoms as tarsal tunnel syndrome (Julsrud 1995). More commonly, the types of structures likely to appear in some but not all patients are accessory ossicles. The pain produced by such structures varies, causing dysfunction, fracture, inflammatory change or contributing to arthritis.

PAIN FROM COMMON ACCESSORY OSSICLES

Accessory ossicles of the foot are often clinically insignificant as a radiological finding. While as many as 15 accessory ossicles have been documented within the foot (Romanowski & Barrington 1991), it is the ossicles affecting the tarsus that most commonly give rise to symptoms. The *os trigonum* is one of the largest and most frequently encountered of accessory ossicles; it lies posterior to the lateral tubercle of the talus and may be bipartite. Symptoms may arise from compression of the soft tissues between the talus and tibia when the foot is frequently plantarflexed in activities such as ballet dancing or soccer.

Diagnosis is made with lateral radiographs of the ankle, although bone scans may be helpful in confirming increased inflammatory activity.

The accessory navicular situated medial and posterior to the main body of the navicular is another commonly encountered ossicle. It can take several forms, the most common being the ossicle united to the navicular by a synchondrosis of 1–2 mm width. Symptoms are often related to the insertion of the tibialis posterior tendon. Contraction of the tendon causes displacement of the ossicle and stress on the synchondrosis. Eventually, the synchondrosis will fuse to form the corniculate navicular. Symptoms may subside at this point or the prominent navicular tuberosity will continue to be subject to footwear irritation.

Another form of accessory navicular is a sesamoid bone within the tibialis posterior tendon. This sesamoid is quite separate from the navicular and is best referred to as *os tibiale externum*. Apart from increasing the prominence of the navicular, which may cause footwear irritation, this form of accessory navicular is often asymptomatic.

Diagnosis of accessory navicular may be made clinically in the presence of an enlarged navicular tuberosity. Plain radiographs will allow a more accurate assessment. Excision of the ossicle is the definitive treatment for symptomatic cases. Careful planning is required in order that the mechanical advantage offered by the insertion of tibialis posterior is not affected as it inserts into the navicular tuberosity.

Os talonaviculare dorsale is worth mentioning as it can present an irregular appearance on a lateral X-ray, appearing as arthritis. Many different ossicles are apparent within the foot. Pain and dysfunction suggest that removal is required. Well-made conforming orthoses and sensible footwear selection play a primary part in managing problems associated with tarsal ossicles.

INFECTION

Infection has been described in Chapter 7 in relation to postoperative management. The principles of management do not differ when infection arises outside of surgery. Infection of the foot without an obvious cause may pose a different dilemma.

Surface infection may arise from fissures of the skin, paronychia, dermatomycosis, deep-seated abscess tracking to the surface, or focal infection from another part of the body. In children, haematogenous osteomyelitis can cause long bone pain. In adults, more often than not it is an injury that brings about osteomyelitis.

The principles of infection management remain straightforward: identify the signs, take a good history and rule out the less obvious causes of non-specific infection. Furthermore:

- establish drainage
- treat infection
- debride necrotic tissue
- protect with a dressing against further infection
- prescribe rest and elevation.

Conservative management

Drainage is not easy to establish unless access can be gained. Protein-breaking enzymes create a sinus. This can be assisted with a sterile scalpel. Low-strength antiseptic flush or 0.9% saline can be used to clean out the wound. Where the infection is localised, the wound is left to heal with the aid of a surface antiseptic and dressings. Antibiotics should not be used in this instance unless evidence of cellulitis, distressing pain or vascular damage is present. If the patient can cope with low grade analgesics, the wound should settle with rest. Rest may involve casts, crutches and short bed rest. Suitable absorbent dressings should be changed, depending upon the nature of discharge and whether the wound needs regular lavage.

Problems do, however, arise with wounds that do not establish drainage, particularly in patients who are compromised. Their health status must be checked to assess the best form of management, which will undoubtedly include antibiotics.

Surgical management

Once infection shows signs of tracking, bone destruction or surface necrosis takes place, surgery is indicated. Debridement and drainage will improve the chance of healthy granulation (see case history in Box 14.6). Surgical exposure will ensure that deep tissue is decompressed from swelling and pressure to avoid additional necrosis. The body's defence mechanisms are allowed to reach the site of infection. Antibiotics will be given intravenously to provide high tissue levels of antimicrobial activity at the time

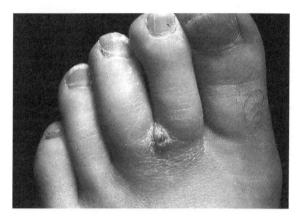

Figure 14.31 A granuloma is apparent between this man's left second and third toes. This is an example of a cutaneous infection that was maintained by antibiotics.

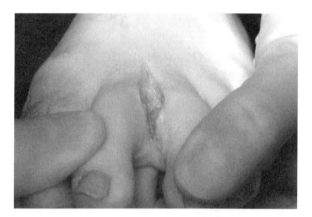

Figure 14.32 Infection being managed. The same lesion as in Figure 14.31 has been opened up and drained, resulting in a complete resolution (see text). The granuloma was removed and shown to be unremarkable. The organism was *S. Aureus.*

of surgery. The patient will be maintained on oral antibiotics specific to the organism. Heavily infected wounds are always left to drain. Closure may not be necessary, although further debridement may still be required. Clean open wounds may even be grafted over once the swelling has subsided and infection abated.

SKIN DISORDERS

While many texts on dermatology exist, the principles of management involve a multidisciplinary approach which includes the GP or dermatologist. Psoriasis, eczema and dermatitis are the commonest conditions.

Box 14.6 Case history: surgical drainage

A 46-year-old male factory worker developed an interdigital problem. Antibiotics were used by his GP, but the lesion did not clear (Fig. 14.31). The lesion presented as a granulomatous mass that had been present for 8 weeks. Access to the site was not possible and surgical drainage was required (a) to establish drainage; and (b) to identify the organism (Fig. 14.32). Deep tissue inflammation with a thin collection of pus was removed. Light sutures only were used with a vacuum drain. Flucloxacillin 250 mg q.d.s. was continued for a further 10 days. Postoperative resolution was immediate, within 7 days, with return to work at 3 weeks.

Conclusion. The diagnosis was an infection without an identifiable cause. The organism was *S. aureus.* The lesion was a granuloma and there was strong suspicion of a secondarily infected interdigital dermatomycosis associated with athlete's foot. Interdigital clefts pose problems from secondary bacterial infection. The cleft is moist, warm and able to sustain bacterial growth well. Once through the epithelial tissue, the spread of infection can travel between the metatatarsals quickly. In this case, the patient was fortunate enough to be healthy and maintained from cellulitic spread by his GP.

Other conditions that are treatable include disorders of keratinisation and nail disorders. The principles behind the treatment of nails are discussed in Chapter 6.

Inflammatory conditions associated with psoriasis are difficult to manage because of the underlying abnormality of keratinisation, which at best can be suppressed rather than treated. Blisters and fissures may complicate other skin problems, and concern for primary or secondary infection may arise. The patient usually becomes concerned when any skin problem on the foot becomes irritated by shoes. Interdigital spaces, paronychial tissue and the skin around the long arch, heel or ankle may cause pain, itching or simply ooze, as in the case of varicose eczema. In the latter case, ulcers may form around the ankle and medial side of the foot (Ch. 18).

Principles of management

• Keratin disorders may need debriding regularly. Caution should be taken with plaques because small bleeding points can be exposed. Reduction of tissue will maintain comfort.
• Inflammatory bases of hyperkeratosis should be dampened with corticosteroids when highly active.
• Keratolytics are valuable to soften areas, particularly around the heel and plantar metatarsal area in lieu of mechanical debridement.
• Creams and ointments can maintain suppleness and deliver various medications, e.g. allowing penetration of corticosteroids or assisting preparations such as urea, dithranol, antiseptics and antifungal agents.
• Cleansing agents—aluminium acetate 0.65% in water provides an effective astringent, or Permutabs (Bioglan) can be used for weeping ulcers.
• Antiperspirants such as aluminium chloride hexahydrate in an alcohol base reduce excessive sweating.
• Barrier creams such as dimethicone or zinc and castor oil will help to protect sensitive skin.

• Antipruritics will help to keep patients comfortable and prevent excoriation of skin from scratching. Calamine and crotamiton are equally effective.

Agents known to cause irritation should be removed. Footwear and socks/stockings/tights should be evaluated to ensure that component materials do not cause specific site dermatitis.

SUMMARY

The management of pain or deformity in the adult foot requires a quite different approach from that used in a child's foot. Deformities in a child are often flexible and liable to spontaneous improvement. Deformities in the adult, however, are usually rigid and often aggravated by footwear fitting or occupational demands.

Pain is a rare feature in the child, whereas in the adult pain may present in a variety of forms. Most patients are unable to recall specific injuries and so the practitioner must approach the problem systematically.

Where treatment is instigated, it should usually begin with conservative measures, because these methods generally carry fewer potential problems than surgery. A central tenet of conservative treatment is the use of foot orthoses. The high value placed on orthoses reflects the fact that most foot pain occurs on weight-bearing, and orthoses have the capacity to enhance the efficiency of weight-bearing. Drugs should only be used for short periods. They often work best in combination with other treatment regimens. Surgery should not be considered until all conservative options have been exhausted. When surgery is used, the foot surgeon needs to apply the most appropriate procedure to retain/restore the dynamic function of the foot. For every practitioner, the primary goal must be: *first do no harm*; it is only with an understanding of the unique requirements placed on the human foot that that intention can be realised.

REFERENCES

Balkin S W 1972 Plantar keratoses: treatment by injectable liquid silicone. Clinical Orthopaedics 87: 235–247
Barouk L S 1994 Weil lesser rays osteotomy. Med. Chir. Pied 1: 22–23
Barrett S L, Day S V 1993 Endoscopic plantar fasciotomy: two endoscopic surgical techniques – clinical results of 65 procedures. Journal of Foot and Ankle Surgery 32(3): 248–256
Campbell P, Lawton J O 1994 Heel pain: diagnosis and management. British Joural of Medicine 52(8): 380–385

Davis T J, Schon L C 1995 Branches of the tibial nerve: anatomic variations. Foot and Ankle International 16(1): 21–29
Dockery G L, Nilson R Z 1986 Intralesional injections. Clinics in Podiatric Medicine and Surgery 3(3): 473–485
Grace D L 1993 Surgery of the lesser rays. The Foot 3: 51–57
Groiso J A 1992 Juvenile hallux valgus. A conservative approach to treatment. Journal of Bone & Joint Surgery 74A: 1367–1374

Haines R W, McDougall A 1954 The anatomy of hallux valgus. Journal of Bone & Joint Surgery 36B: 272–293

Hardy R H, Clapham J C R 1951 Observations on hallux valgus based on a controlled series. Journal of Bone & Joint Surgery 33B: 376–391

Julsrud M E 1995 An unusual case of tarsal tunnel syndrome. Journal of Foot & Ankle Surgery 34(3): 289–293

Kilmartin T E, Barrington R L, Wallace W A 1994 A controlled prospective trial of a biomechanical orthosis in the treatment of juvenile hallux valgus. Journal of Bone & Joint Surgery 76B(2): 210–215

Kilmartin T E, Wallace W A 1992 Update on hallux valgus surgery. A review of results in the recent literature. The Foot 2: 123–134

Kilmartin T E, Wallace W A 1994 The effect of a pronation and supination orthosis on Morton's neuroma and lower limb function. Foot & Ankle International 15: 256–262

Kilmartin T E, Wallace W A, Hill T W 1991 Measurement of the functional orthotic effect on metatarsophalangeal joint extension. Journal of the American Podiatric Medical Association 81: 414–417

Klenerman L 1991 The foot and its disorders, 3rd edn. Blackwell Scientific Publications, Oxford, p 134–135

Lang L M G, West S G, Day S, Simmonite N 1994 Salicylic acid in the treatment of corns. The Foot 4(3): 145–150

Mair S D, Coogan A C, Speer K P, Hall R L 1995 Gout as a source of pain. Foot & Ankle International 16(10): 613–616

Malay D S, McGlamry E D 1992 Acquired neuropathies of the lower extremities, 2nd edn. In: McGlamry E D, Banks A S, Downey M S (eds) Comprehensive Textbook of Foot Surgery. Williams and Wilkins, Baltimore, p 1095–1123

Mann R A (ed) 1978 DuVries' surgery of the foot. Mosby, Missouri, p 466–468

Merriman L M, Tollafield D R (eds) 1995 Assessment of the lower limb. Churchill Livingstone, Edinburgh

Miller S J 1992 Intermetatarsal neuromas and associated nerve problems. In: Butterworth R, Dockery G L (eds) A colour atlas and text of forefoot surgery. Wolfe, London

Pratt D J, Tollafield D R, Johnson G R, Peacock C 1993 Foot orthoses. In: Bowker P et al (eds) Biomechanical basis of orthotic management. Butterworth-Heinemann, Oxford, p 86–87

Rasanen L, Hasan T 1993 Allergy to systemic and intralesional corticosteroid. British Journal of Dermatology 128: 407–411

Rees P J, Trounce J R 1988 New short textbook of medicine. Edward Arnold, London

Rosen J S, Grady J F 1986 Neuritic bunion syndrome. Journal of the American Podiatric Medical Association 76(11): 641–644

Rowanowski C A, Barrington N A 1991 The accessory ossicles of the foot. The Foot 2: 61–70

Salter R B, Harris W R 1963 Injuries involving the epiphyseal plate. Journal of Bone and Joint Surgery 45(A): 587

Summarco G J, Conti S F 1994 Tarsal tunnel syndrome caused by an anomalous muscle. Journal of Bone & Joint Surgery 76A(9): 1308–1314

Sunberg S B, Johnson K A 1991 Painful conditions of the heel. In: Jahss M H (ed) Disorders of the foot and ankle, medical and surgical management, 2nd edn. W B Saunders, Philadelphia, ch 47

Tollafield D R, Pratt D J 1990 The control of known triplanar forces on the foot by forefoot orthotic posting. British Journal of Podiatric Medicine & Surgery 2(2): 3–5

Tollafield D R, Williams H A 1996 The use of two injectable corticosteroid preparations used in the management of foot problems – a clinical audit report. British Journal of Podiatric Medicine, 51(12): 171–174

Yu G V 1992 First metatarsal phalangeal joint arthrodesis. In: McGlamry E D, Banks A S, Downey M S (eds) Comprehensive Textbook of Foot Surgery. Williams and Wilkins, Baltimore

FURTHER READING

Bayliss N C, Klenerman L 1989 Avascular necrosis of lesser metatarsal heads following forefoot surgery. Foot & Ankle 10(3): 124–128

Laing P 1995 The painful foot. In: Merriman L M, Tollafield D R (eds) Assessment of the lower limb. Churchill Livingstone, Edinburgh

Skalley T C, Schon L C, Hinton R Y, Myerson M S 1994 Clinical results following revision tibial nerve release. The Foot 15(7): 360–367

Spooner S K, Kilmartin T E, Merriman L M 1995 Pathologic anatomy of the first metatarsophalangeal joint in hallux valgus. British Journal of Podiatric Medicine & Surgery 7(2): 35–40

Turbutt I F 1995 Radiographic assessment. In: Merriman L M, Tollafield D R (eds) Assessment of the lower limb. Churchill Livingstone, Edinburgh

15

The child's foot

T. E. Kilmartin
D. R. Tollafield

INTRODUCTION

The treatment of children's foot problems should not be instigated without careful thought as to whether treatment is necessary in the first place. Many paediatric complaints are simply normal stages of development which in time resolve spontaneously without treatment; the possibility of 'normal abnormality' must be appreciated before treatment is commenced. The practitioner's first aim should always be to reassure the parents with a sound explanation of the presenting complaint and the likely prognosis. Because so many foot and leg complaints are developmental in nature, review and monitoring provide the basis of many treatment plans; objective measurements should be used wherever possible to facilitate this. Each case must be considered on the basis of the likely success of any treatment regime.

The following chapter will describe the range of short- and long-term treatments, supported by scientific evidence where it exists. Suffice it to say that not all treatment has a sound scientific basis. This chapter is therefore subdivided into the following areas:

- abnormalities and deformities (congenital and acquired)
- pain associated with the foot, knee or leg
- gait and foot position.

ABNORMALITIES AND DEFORMITIES

METATARSUS ADDUCTUS

Metatarsus adductus has an incidence of 1 in every 1000 live births. Four per cent of all cases are hereditary, although if one child is affected, the chances are 1 in 20 that the second sibling will be similarly affected (Wynne-Davies 1964). In the series of cases

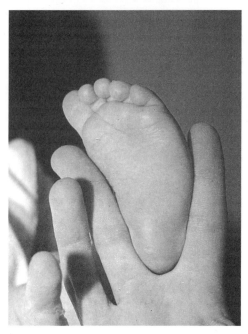

Figure 15.1 Metatarsus adductus. 'C'-shaped curvature of the lateral border of the foot is the key diagnostic feature.

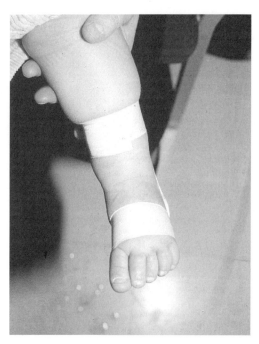

Figure 15.2 Strapping for metatarsus adductus. The strapping is wrapped around the forefoot, the forefoot is pulled into correction and the strapping is secured around the leg.

collected by Thomson (1960) and Rushforth (1978), the condition appeared to be slightly more common in females.

Treatment for metatarsus adductus is not necessary in every case. Spontaneous resolution is known to occur. Ponsetti & Becker (1966) found that only 12% of their patients required treatment, while Rushforth (1978), in an 11 year follow-up of 83 children, found that 4% retained severe deformity and another 10% displayed moderate deformity. The feet that are unlikely to resolve spontaneously can be identified on examination (Fig. 15.1). Rigidity within the foot makes manual correction difficult. A deep skin crease running along the medial plantar side of the first metatarsocuneiform joint generally indicates a more severely deformed foot.

Treatment

Strapping. This is a traditional treatment which can be demonstrated to the parents. The tape is wrapped around the forefoot, pulled proximally over the lateral malleolus and wrapped around the leg, as in Figure 15.2. Strapping used for any period of time may cause skin sensitivity. The practitioner will have to judge each parent's capability first before allowing participation in any treatment programme. Parents

may not be able to appreciate the complex anatomy of the foot, particularly as it is possible to create 'false correction' by abducting the forefoot, leading to pronation, without stabilising the subtalar joint first.

Reverse footwear. Wearing the right shoe on the left foot is another traditional treatment which carries a risk of false correction. It is poor practice to apply a significant corrective force to just one component of the foot, neglecting other parts that influence the foot deformity. Moreover, distortion of the shoe upper by the metatarsus adductus foot is very much a hallmark of the deformity. Reverse footwear may, therefore, be ineffective, the shoe simply taking on the shape of the foot; irritation of the skin is a common finding in this treatment.

Serial casting (see case history in Box 15.1). This technique was popularised by Kite (1950), who considered that using constant corrective force was preferable to 'corrective manipulation'.

A constant pressure could be better provided by a plaster of Paris cast placed above the ankle (see Box 15.2).

Not all cases of deformity are totally corrected by serial casting. It is, however, noteworthy that where feet have achieved only 60% correction of the

---

Box 15.1 Case history: metatarsus adductus treated with serial casting

A mother was concerned that her 13-month-old son was pigeon-toed. Shoe fitting was difficult due to the 'banana' shape curve of the child's foot.

On examination, a severe metatarsus adductus was noted with a pronounced medial first metatarsal-cuneiform skin crease. The adducted position of the forefoot could not be reduced with manipulation. On standing, the rearfoot was everted with notable dorsal humping of the midtarsal joint (Fig. 15.5). The complex variant of metatarsus adductus (skewfoot) was diagnosed on the basis of the rearfoot eversion in the presence of metatarsus adductus (Berg 1986).

Treatment consisted of serial casting. The child tolerated this well. After 7 weeks of casting, muscle atrophy of the leg was noted and the child had developed a painful pre-ulcerative lesion on the posterior surface of both heels. The adductus deformity of the foot had improved by some 60% but the heel remained in eversion on weight-bearing. Although far from corrected, the foot was much more flexible and could now be corrected by manipulation, which, according to Pentz & Weiner (1993), is an important prerequisite for spontaneous correction.

A suspension cast of the foot was then taken non-weight-bearing and a functional orthosis was made with a high medial flange and a deep heel seat to create a corrective abduction force on the forefoot while restricting excessive pronation of the rearfoot. Vitrathene clogs were also provided for night-time wear.

The child was reviewed every 2 months; improvement was noted at each follow-up, and by the time the child was 4 years old the metatarsus adductus had corrected. The foot, however, remained excessively pronated, with a low arch and medial bulging associated with the talonavicular joint. Orthotic management should be continued while the foot remains excessively pronated.

Clinical comment. Manipulation or casting under tension in an inappropriate manner can cause severe damage to the mesenchymal precursor to bone, and hence can lead to further deformity once the deformed cartilage has matured. Cartilage is easier to deform than tight ligaments or tendons and will yield without the inexperienced practitioner realising, causing such problems as rocker-bottom flat feet.

Box 15.2 Application of plaster of Paris casts— clinical comment

Plaster of Paris casts are applied using the following approach. A pre-cast tubular bandage (Tubifast, Seton) is slid over the foot and leg, ending above the knee. Orthopaedic wool (Velband, Johnson and Johnson) is used to wrap over the bandage in order to protect the bony prominences and overlying soft tissue. Two 7.5 cm rolls of wet plaster of Paris are applied from the subtalar joint to just below the patella. As the cast dries, the rearfoot is held very slightly supinated at the subtalar joint, with the ankle at 90°. By dealing with the anatomy in this systematic manner, the possibility of replacing one deformity with another, i.e. valgus rearfoot or ankle equinus, is limited. When the first section is dried, another roll of plaster of Paris is extended as far as the toes. The rearfoot is then cupped with the practitioner's dominant hand while the forefoot is pushed into correction using the soft thenar eminence of the other hand. The index finger is placed underneath the forefoot to ensure that the metatarsals do not overlap one another offering a false impression of correction. The ends of the tubular bandage should be rolled down, having first incorporated sufficient wool packing to prevent chafing of the skin or adverse circulatory compression.

The cast is kept in place for 7 days. The parents are then asked to remove it by soaking it off prior to the next visit. Three to six successive weeks of this treatment constitute the maximum period of time appropriate for this form of therapy. Longer than 6 weeks and it becomes almost inevitable that the leg muscles will atrophy and the skin will start to show rub marks or indeed frank ulceration. The most vulnerable site is the junction of the plantar and dorsal skin at the posterior heel. If ulceration occurs, casting can continue if necessary, although it is important to leave a window in the heel area of the cast.

Extension of the cast above the knee is required if the child has concomitant pathology such as medial genicular position or tibial torsion. Occasionally the infant will manage to repeatedly push the cast off. This can be overcome by extending the cast above the knee. Extension above the knee should be dealt with only when the foot and leg section is dry and applied in two sections.

---

deformity, they often correct spontaneously. Whether this is the result of greater flexibility created by corrective casting is uncertain. It is, however, noteworthy that manipulation of the foot by the parents prior to casting seems to shorten the length of treatment.

It is preferable to use serial casts before the child walks. Because of the child's activity level, weight, height and increasing musculoskeletal rigidity, serial casting is probably not appropriate after 20 months

of age. Follow-up treatment to prevent recurrence is often required. In some cases, however, children will not tolerate the plaster of Paris cast and alternative measures must be sought. Failure is often inevitable where casts are applied to children who are too old.

Adjustable shoes. Bebax boots are split into forefoot and rearfoot sections, connected by a ball-and-socket type hinge (Fig. 15.3). The multiaxial connector

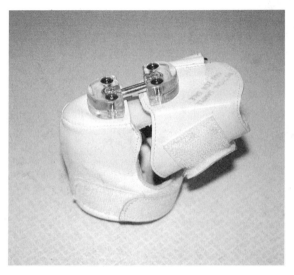

Figure 15.3 The Bebax boot. Triplane adjustment is possible—the ball-and-socket hinge allows the forefoot to be gently pushed into correction while the rearfoot is held in neutral.

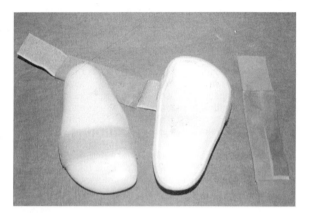

Figure 15.4 Vitrathene orthotic clogs for metatarsus adductus shown with separate velcro straps.

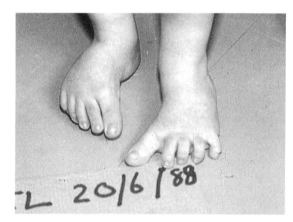

Figure 15.5 Skewfoot—where metatarsus adductus is complicated by rearfoot eversion.

allows the forefoot to be moved in any of the three body planes independently of the rearfoot position. Although expensive, the boots can be supplied in a number of different sizes and provide an excellent medium for correcting forefoot deformity; unfortunately, Bebax boots cannot be walked in without damaging the hinge mechanism.

Corrective orthoses. Vitrathene clogs made from polyethylene plastic form an inexpensive, custom-made orthosis which allows maintenance of corrective forces during walking. While the forefoot is held in a corrected position, a neutral suspension cast is taken. A high-sided Vitrathene clog is then vacuum-moulded around the positive cast. The inside is lined with low density polyethylene foam (Plastazote), and the finished orthosis is retained on the foot by Velcro straps as in Figure 15.4.

TALIPES EQUINOVARUS

While the incidence of metatarsus adductus appears to be increasing, the incidence of congenital talipes equinovarus (CTEV) appears to be falling (Kite 1950). More commonly known as club foot, this is a complex deformity which will restrict normal ankle dorsiflexion while at the same time holding the rearfoot in a supinated (inverted) position and the forefoot in adductus. By contrast, metatarsus adductus is relatively easy to manage compared to CTEV because the

deformity only affects the transverse plane. Treatment should begin as early as possible in the child with CTEV. The type of treatment is largely determined by the rigidity present and is assessed by manual manipulation of the ankle, subtalar and midtarsal joints. If each of these joints appears flexible, with adequate range of motion, the deformity may be corrected by the application of a plaster of Paris cast which extends above the knee.

Foot deformity is commonly associated with internal tibial torsion and this should also be dealt with during casting.

Corrective pressure should be applied to push the ankle up to 90°, the rearfoot into a vertical position and the forefoot straight. Casts should be changed weekly and the position of the three involved joints and their ranges of motion assessed. Failure to respond to casting should always be acted upon; surgical treatment should certainly be considered if serial casting fails to improve the deformity.

Surgery for CTEV is advocated within the first 6 weeks where there is an overt failure to improve the deformity by casting or manipulation alone. Surgical management consists of soft tissue division of tight tendons and ligaments, while bone and joint surgery is left until later in the first decade of life. Soft tissue surgery performed early gives encouraging results.

ARCH HEIGHT

The shape of the arch is a frequent concern for both parents and doctors. Parents are often advised to leave well alone, based on the possibility that the child will grow out of the problem. In many cases, arch supports are advocated. As the child grows out of a relatively flat foot, provided that normal foot development follows the expected pattern between 6 and 10 years of age, the indication for arch supports may well be questioned. Arch supports will not in themselves offer any lasting influence on the foot (Wenger et al 1989). The application of orthoses has been discussed in previous chapters. Further evidence expanding on the role of orthoses in assisting low arch feet will be covered later in this chapter.

As the height of the arch can vary so much, the question arises—should we treat it? Low medial longitudinal arches probably attract more concern than high arches. Afro-Caribbeans have a low calcaneal inclination angle, commonly resulting in a low arch profile without symptoms. Careful examination and family history must be undertaken, together with the judicious use of X-rays. X-rays should only be used to assess arch formation where the aetiology requires clarification and where a significant defect is suspected.

The algorithm outlining decisions to be made in treating flat feet (Fig. 15.6) emphasises the key points of concern that might require attention. To the existing criteria in Figure 15.6, we must add 'presence of symptoms'. As far as arch height is concerned, flat foot (pes planus) will be divided into flexible and rigid types (Tachdjian 1985). A high arch (*pes cavus*, which literally means 'hole' or hole through the foot) enables the practitioner to pass his or her fingers under the arch from medial to lateral. It is important not to forget the influence of neuromuscular conditions and systemic conditions such as juvenile rheumatoid arthritis which can have a marked effect upon the foot and its arch height; this will be considered later.

Flexible flat foot

In the pre-walking child or toddler, the medial longitudinal arch of the foot is poorly developed, largely because in the early years of life the calcaneus lies parallel to the ground (Wenger et al 1989). By 4 or 5 years of age, the calcaneus inclines to form an angle of 13°–18° with the ground. Low, or indeed absent, arches are therefore not a reliable sign of abnormal foot position or function. Medial bulging of the talon-avicular joint, Helbing's sign or heel valgus and forefoot abduction are more significant findings indicating excessive pronation of the foot (Fig. 15.7). In the newborn child where the foot cannot be assessed weight-bearing, these criteria may be difficult to appreciate. If the pre-walker's foot is pronated, and manipulation of the foot fails to correct this position, mild calcaneovalgus should be suspected and treatment should be considered (Fig. 15.8).

Treatment of calcaneovalgus in the newborn child aims to restore the foot to a neutral position and increase the range of plantarflexion available at the ankle joint. Flexibility of the foot is probably greatest in the younger child, so it is likely that the earlier treatment begins, the easier it will be to correct the condition. In very mild flexible cases, manipulation of the foot by the parents may be helpful. Manipulation involves placing the parent's hand on the dorsum of the child's foot and asking them to push the foot down into plantarflexion. Plantarflexion force will supinate the foot, bringing it into a neutral position while freeing up the ankle range of motion. The parent should hold the foot for several minutes at a time, regularly repeating the exercise. Such manipulation therapy should be closely supervised by the practitioner and if the foot fails to respond, with no obvious reduction of the pronated position, serial casting should be considered as the next line of treatment.

Applying plaster of Paris to the limb and then manipulating the foot into maximum plantarflexion is more effective than parental manipulation. The corrective effect is based upon *Davis's law*, where a continuous force creates soft tissue elongation along the line of tension; in the case of deformity along the parallel fibres of collagen.

The casting process is repeated for at least 3 weeks, even though, in the young child, correction may be achieved in 1 week. Recurrence of the deformity may be avoided by maintaining casting in this fashion. Once the episode of serial casting is complete, the parents should be encouraged to continue with manipulation of the foot in the pre-walker. In the toddler, an orthosis should be used to maintain the corrected position of

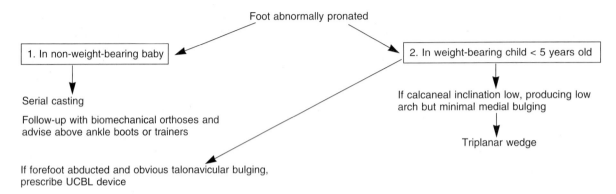

Foot abnormally pronated

1. In non-weight-bearing baby

Serial casting

Follow-up with biomechanical orthoses and advise above ankle boots or trainers

If forefoot abducted and obvious talonavicular bulging, prescribe UCBL device

2. In weight-bearing child < 5 years old

If calcaneal inclination low, producing low arch but minimal medial bulging

Triplanar wedge

Follow-up every 6 months, checking arch index and valgus index. Discharge when foot within normal values

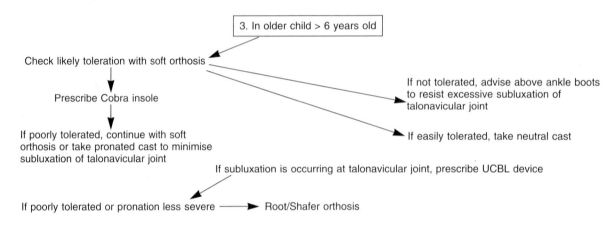

3. In older child > 6 years old

Check likely toleration with soft orthosis

Prescribe Cobra insole

If poorly tolerated, continue with soft orthosis or take pronated cast to minimise subluxation of talonavicular joint

If not tolerated, advise above ankle boots to resist excessive subluxation of talonavicular joint

If easily tolerated, take neutral cast

If subluxation is occurring at talonavicular joint, prescribe UCBL device

If poorly tolerated or pronation less severe ⟶ Root/Shafer orthosis

Review every 6 months, check for history of pain — if persistent, orthotic control inadequate. Also review shoe wear, Rose and Staheli index values

Figure 15.6 Flat foot algorithm.

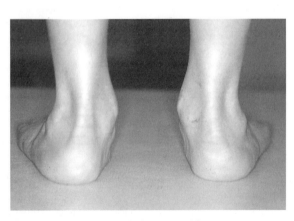

Figure 15.7 The excessively pronated foot.

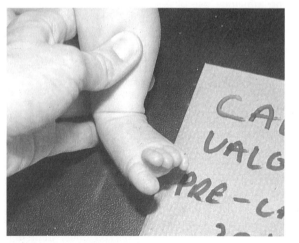

Figure 15.8 Mild calcaneovalgus in a 12-week-old infant.

the foot and prevent it from relapsing into pronation. An orthosis with a deep heel seat of 20–30 mm is vital to resist pronatory forces. The thermoplastic materials *Orthoplast* or *Hexcelite,* which can be rendered flexible by boiling water, can be used to fabricate such a device in the clinic. Continuous monitoring is advised until the child is at least 6 years of age.

Orthotic treatment applied to children under 6 years of age is a controversial issue. Theory based on the work of Elftman in the early part of the 20th century has led to the view that an orthosis can prevent normal ontogenetic valgus rotation of the talar head and neck creating a forefoot varus deformity. The neonate has a 'normal varus' which reduces by age 6 with talar head rotation. The theory regarding correction is poorly documented, remains inconclusive, and seems to arise from diverse US sources.

In a study which independently measured talar neck rotation and then the angle of forefoot varus in cadaver specimens, McPoil et al (1987) disputed whether there was any correlation between the two. No longitudinal study exists to support reducing the effect of forefoot varus with an orthosis to prevent a flat foot deformity occurring in later life, although empirically such treatment appears helpful.

All influence on the talar neck can be avoided before normal ontogeny, however, by prescribing a triplanar wedge, which may increase the calcaneal inclination angle (Fig. 15.9). Inclination of the calcaneus is vital

to the foot. If there is reduced calcaneal inclination, the plantar aponeurosis will lengthen. Lengthening of the plantar aponeurosis will impair the windlass effect. The windlass effect relates to raising the medial longitudinal arch as a consequence of dorsiflexion of the hallux at the propulsive phase of gait; this in turn tightens the plantar aponeurosis and pulls the rearfoot and forefoot together, elevating the arch of the foot. If the plantar aponeurosis is lengthened in association with a low calcaneal inclination angle, the foot will not easily achieve supination at the propulsive phase of gait.

Lengthening of the plantar aponeurosis arises when using prescription orthoses. It is suggested that orthoses act like a 'crutch' to 'jack up' the arch. In the long term, however, it is thought to weaken the foot, as the plantar aponeurosis has to stretch around the arch support.

Orthopaedic research has seriously questioned the value of the orthosis because a number of studies have found that the medial longitudinal arch is not raised after sustained wear (Mereday et al 1972, Penneau et al 1982, Wenger et al 1989). It must be emphasised, however, that the exponents of functional orthoses have never claimed that they would improve the arch. Orthoses are prescribed to prevent progressive subluxation of the midtarsal joint complex by reducing the need for compensatory motion.

Ironically, orthopaedic literature has also provided support for the prescription of orthoses in the treatment of flat feet. Rose developed a 'pronatormeter' which determined the effect of a Rose-Schwartz meniscus on the frontal position of the rearfoot by measuring external rotation of the tibia. The meniscus orthosis was found to produce much greater external rotation of the leg than the simple medial heel wedge (Rose 1958, 1962). This effect, noted by Rose, forms the precept of orthotic prescription by using antipronatory in-shoe devices to prevent progressive subluxation of the aforementioned midtarsal region through subtalar joint control.

Shafer and Root type orthoses assist rearfoot control by means of both forefoot and rearfoot posts (Tollafield & Pratt 1990). The arch area of the orthosis is important for no other reason than that it connects the rearfoot and forefoot posts. Indeed in the Root-type orthosis, the arch is deliberately lowered during fabrication of the device, in order to improve toleration of the device which is manufactured around a plaster of Paris impression of the non-weight-bearing foot.

The Cobra insole is a useful extension of the Rose-Schwartz meniscus incorporating a valgus filler

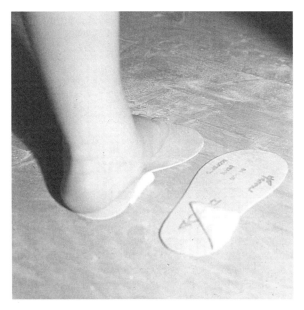

Figure 15.9 The triplanar wedge for limiting of excessive pronation of the under 5-year-old child's foot.

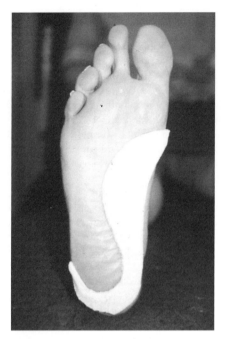

Figure 15.10 The Cobra pad is based on a valgus pad with a meniscus heel.

(Fig. 15.10). It can be fabricated in felt material as a temporary measure, during consultation, to determine the potential efficacy of prescription treatment. The control that such soft semi-functional orthoses can exert on an excessively pronated foot is likely to be less than a rigid functional orthotic device.

The child receiving orthotic treatment should be reviewed periodically. Details of any aches or pains should be documented. Orthotic fit should be reviewed as should signs of 'bottoming out' of the orthotic materials. Bottoming out is an expression used to indicate that a material has flattened sufficiently to provide no further functional use. Arch height and the degree of subtalar joint pronation should be evaluated with Staheli's arch index (Staheli et al 1987) and Rose's valgus index (Rose et al 1985). These evaluations are made from ink prints of the contact area of the foot using a Harris mat. The Staheli technique records the height of the medial longitudinal arch, while the Rose valgus index determines medial displacement of the medial malleolus which will occur as the rearfoot everts. Both techniques provide an objective means of recording the foot's abnormality which is useful when reporting the effect of treatment. The decision to discontinue treatment may be influenced by a significant improvement in the arch and valgus index values (see case history in Box 15.3).

Box 15.3 Case history: flexible flat foot

A 7-year-old boy complained of pain in the area of the tibialis anterior muscle belly and the medial longitudinal arch of both feet. His family history was significant, in that his father had severely pronated but asymptomatic feet. The patient's foot had marked talonavicular bulging, forefoot abductus, a positive Helbing's sign and absent medial longitudinal arch. Excessive medial heel wear was noted in the shoes. Staheli arch index measurement* determined a value of 1.4 and the Rose valgus index** gave a value of 27. The boy also had recurvatum of both knees and elbows. While standing with knees fully extended, he could touch the floor with both palms, and his thumb and fifth fingers could be hyperextended past 90°, indicating ligamentous laxity.

The symptoms were considered to be due to overuse and an aphasic tibialis anterior muscle which failed to decelerate excessive pronation of the forefoot. Chronic soft tissue strain of the structures of the medial longitudinal arch was also diagnosed in association with tissue tenderness.

A Cobra insole was prescribed as the first line of treatment. The patient returned 4 weeks later. The insole was easily tolerated and the pain in the anterior tibia had resolved, although the child still complained that the feet ached after standing.

A neutral cast was then taken and a UCBL device was fabricated from polypropylene. When supplied to the patient, this device could not be tolerated because of irritation in the arch area of the foot. The positive neutral cast was then modified with plaster in the longitudinal arch to lower the orthotic plate. A Root orthosis was manufactured and this time the medial longitudinal arch pain responded to treatment as the orthosis was tolerated.

Review should continue every 6 months; arch and valgus index are measured at each follow-up. The objective of treatment is to prevent further subluxation of the talonavicular joint and alleviate all soft tissue strain. Neither child nor parents expect correction of the foot, only prevention of further symptoms.

*Staheli arch index—normal values in this age group 0.5–1.2.
**Rose valgus index—normal index of 0.20.

Rigid flat foot

Not all flat feet respond to orthoses. Failure to achieve an arch form when the hallux is extended (Jack's test), or when the patient is asked to stand on tiptoe, implies that some resistance is present. This resistance can often be associated with spasm, articular limitation or abnormal early development of the foot. Three conditions can be included within this category: tarsal coalitions with peroneal spastic flat foot, convex pes valgus and neurological conditions where the muscle tone is markedly affected, as in rare cases now of poliomyelitis. X-rays are indicated as mentioned previously to ensure that the diagnosis includes any of the serious conditions described next.

Tarsal coalitions

Pain in the region of the subtalar and midtarsal joints may in rare circumstances relate to tarsal coalition. This is a fibrous, cartilaginous or osseous union of two or more tarsal bones and is of congenital origin. The union or bar which bridges joints is not visible on plain X-rays until ossification is complete. Calcaneonavicular and talocalcaneal coalitions are the most common forms of coalition and their presence often leads to peroneal spastic flat foot, where the foot assumes a rigid pronated position. Other types of coalitions are rarely reported (Fig. 15.11). In approximately 50% of cases, the coalition is bilateral; conditions such as *Apert's syndrome* can produce extensive coalitions, making treatment not only difficult but unpredictable.

The patient usually presents in the second decade of life with a complaint of mild deep pain in the subtalar joint and stiffness of the foot. The onset of pain is determined by the age at which the cartilaginous coalition begins to ossify. Complaints of foot pain may be aggravated by activity and relieved by rest.

A middle facet talocalcaneal coalition is more likely to lead to severe pronation of the foot than any other coalition. Concomitant spasm of the peroneal muscles may occur intermittently or continuously. This may result from intra-articular effusion within the subtalar joint, causing a protective reflex spasm of the peroneals.

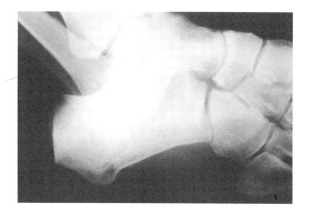

Figure 15.11 A talonavicular coalition. This is a very rare form of tarsal coalition, with few cases having been reported in the literature.

This is thought to occur because the posterior subtalar joint intra-articular pressure is less in eversion than in inversion. Alternatively, spasm may be a consequence of adaptive shortening of the peroneal tendons secondary to the pronated position of the foot, or the result of synovial irritation caused by the disturbed mechanics of the foot irritating the peroneal tendons. The spasm may be diagnosed by injection of local anaesthetic into the common peroneal nerve just below the neck of the fibular. This may relieve some but not all of the child's discomfort, the residual pain being resolved by an injection of local anaesthetic directly into the sinus tarsi.

Orthoses which reduce the pronated position of the foot may also relieve the pain. In cases of more severe pain, the use of a below-knee walking cast is indicated for 3–6 weeks, followed by the use of orthoses designed to hold the rearfoot in inversion. Approximately one-third of patients who have been treated in this manner have reported relief of symptoms (Mosier & Asher 1984). Two variations on orthotic management include producing a hard shell orthosis from a pronated cast, as inversion is not achievable; and using a zero post with a high heel cup modification to maintain the hindfoot in a position to deter further pronation.

If pain persists, surgical resection of the coalition with interposition of fat or extensor digitorum brevis muscle is the preferred operative treatment for the calcaneonavicular coalition. This is easier to manage surgically than the talocalcaneal coalition, which requires an arthrodesis because the joint cannot be salvaged. Severe unremitting pain may require a triple arthrodesis.

Convex pes valgus

This condition shows extensive mechanical derangement and is often known as 'rocker-bottom foot' because of the medial convex shape along the medial border creating the most severe form of flat foot. The only other condition associated with this foot shape is the equinus foot, where compensatory pronation causes severe flattening of the arch. Both foot shapes, once developed, can cause significant management problems. The incidence of this pathology varies between 0.76 and 2.2%; however, convex pes planus is less common than calcaneovalgus.

Complications associated with this condition may arise with concomitant problems such as spina bifida with myelomeningocele, neurofibromatosis, arthrogryposis and unilateral limb shortening. Multiple defects have been noted which may include congenital dislocation of the hips, atresia of the auditory canals and hypertelorism. The presence of such problems means that management becomes multidisciplinary. Problems associated with the foot include poor walking ability due to skeletal dysfunction and retarded skin viability over pressure areas.

Convex pes valgus is congenital—the newborn's foot appears everted and the forefoot may be abducted with some forefoot rotation. The heel will appear smaller and rounded proximally. The medial arch will have full contact with the ground because the talus will have adopted a vertical position. Because much of the pathology arises during development, the soft tissue structures are contracted laterally and stretched medially. Three approaches to treatment exist. Manipulation will assist to stretch the soft tissues, surgical reduction will prevent long-term cartilage damage and growth problems, and soft orthoses will protect the skin from adverse pressure within bespoke shoes.

Manipulation. Early stretching is essential and most effective at 3–8 days after birth (Becker-Anderson & Reimann 1974). In one case where treatment did not start until nearly 4 years, the case did less well. Radiographs are important to identify the extent of pathology and monitor the effects of manipulation. The talar bisection normally passes through the inferior body of the cuboid (usually present at birth), whereas the appearance of the cuboid is delayed in convex pes valgus. In the abnormal foot, the bisection passes well below the cuboid.

The objective of conservative treatment is to reduce the talonavicular dislocation, concentrating on the following areas:

- the equinus factor
- pronation of the hindfoot
- stretching the peroneal muscles
- adduction of the forefoot
- toe extensors and ankle dorsiflexors.

The technique involves dorsiflexing the calcaneus with the triceps surae (tendo Achilles) stretched for the count of 10. The calcaneofibular ligament is also stretched by pulling the calcaneus distally. The ankle dorsiflexors are stretched by plantarflexion of the forefoot with adduction.

Manipulations are performed for 15 minutes each, to the count of 10 before release in the newborn child. Tincture of benzoin is painted on the skin and the deformity placed in a cast for maintenance of correction. A thermoplastic splint can be used to continue tension on the contracted structures.

Surgery. As with club foot (CTEV), surgery succeeds if undertaken early and before 2.5 years. Beyond 6 years of age the deformity will become rigid, and cutaneous pressure problems will start to occur. Soft tissue release is preferred without articular interference; the forefoot is corrected first and the rearfoot last. Excision of the navicular has been used with some success, the talus being pinned through to the first metatarsal (Clark et al 1977). Casting is essential to maintain correction. Tight structures such as the tendo Achilles must be lengthened and the medial structures must be shortened by plication. The use of the above procedure, however, can lead to shortening of the medial side of the foot. Any aggressive disturbance of the blood supply to the head of the talus will create avascular necrosis.

Orthoses. Specialised footwear will be required to accommodate the deformity. It is essential that the shoe has no shank. Severe deformities will shorten the life of the shoe. A soft orthosis ranging from foamed polyethylene (Plastazote: density, 44–54 kg/cm^3) to polyurethane foam (Poron) will protect excessive pressure along the medial structures associated with the vertical talus and navicular, and should be ordered with bespoke footwear.

Juvenile rheumatoid arthritis

The problems and risks associated with this systemic autommimune disorder of collagen will be dealt with in Chapter 18. Unfortunately, not only is the subtalar joint affected by this disabling condition but so are toes at the metatarsophalangeal joints. While treatment of the disease requires multidisciplinary management, orthoses designed to prevent soft tissue deterioration are essential. Pronation is a common feature of this condition and intensive care and monitoring by the practitioner are essential.

Foot orthoses worn during the day and at night are required to protect the foot, which will be prone to excessive pronation with its attendant secondary cutaneous lesions. Where orthoses cannot be used, bivalved casts offer the same function and can be removed by the patient. These well-padded modalities protect joints and relieve spasm. No forceable correction should be used as soft tissues can rupture. The great toe can be splinted with soft replaceable and adjustable splints. Exercise is maintained together with any drug regimes and gentle manipulation. During active phases of the disease, when effusion is greater, weight-bearing should not be undertaken.

Surgical correction is rarely indicated in children, although partial synovectomies may be performed in the subtalar joint and ankle when conservative treatment has failed.

Rigid high arch (pes cavus)

Pes cavus usually does not present as a problem until adolescence. The main cause for concern is associated with the degenerative implications of neurological disease. Pes cavus is usually progressive and the foot becomes more rigid. The symptoms associated with pes cavus are a consequence of:

- the inverted rearfoot position which leads to instability and a tendency for lateral ankle sprains
- rigid plantarflexed first and fifth rays which lead to excessive ground reaction forces being directed at the first and fifth plantar metatarsal heads, resulting in hyperkeratosis
- clawing of the digits causing skin lesions on the dorsum of the proximal interphalangeal joints
- footwear fitting difficulties due to the dorsal hump of the midfoot caused by the high medial longitudinal arch.

Any neurological cause should be investigated; conditions such as Charcot-Marie-Toothe are hereditary. Treatment is largely palliative, directed at tissue viability and managing discomfort associated with digital and plantar hyperkeratosis. An attempt can be made to reduce the supinated position of the foot by providing an orthosis which will force the foot into a more pronated position and may even delay the progression of the pes cavus. These treatments are not effective if the foot is already rigid. Flexible high arch problems associated with plantarflexed first rays and everted forefeet are described further in Chapter 14.

Footwear advice is essential. Training shoes, which extend above the ankle, will limit the likelihood of lateral ankle sprain. A deep toe box with a thick cushioning midsole will alleviate digital and plantar lesions. Further relief of plantar lesions, as well as of the symptoms associated with poor shock absorption, may be obtained by providing a 6 mm neoprene insole, e.g. *Spenco*, within the shoe, although this intervention can fill up the toe box of the shoe and exacerbate digital lesions. This effect can be avoided by removing the section of the insole which lies distal to the plantar metatarsal pad.

In order to minimise discomfort, hyperkeratotic lesions should be regularly debrided, with occasional intensive periods of treatment to relieve any deeper tissue changes. Debridement, keratolytics and re-directive padding or appliances can all be used. The uncompromised patient should also regularly use emollients and a foot file or pumice stone to retain skin suppleness and reduce hyperkeratosis by abrading the surface lightly.

HALLUX VALGUS

Perhaps the commonest digital deformity to cause concern in the forefoot is that of hallux valgus. The condition is very significant in the child because, although it begins as an isolated abnormality of the first metatarsophalangeal joint, it will inevitably progress to involve the whole forefoot, causing deformity of the lesser digits, splaying of the forefoot, footwear fitting problems and degeneration within the first metatarsophalangeal joint.

Screening and monitoring

It is in recognising the progressive nature of hallux valgus that the practitioner can be most useful. Monitoring the progress of the condition is imperative and should be undertaken annually by measuring the first metatarsophalangeal joint angle with a digital goniometer while the child stands in their angle and base of gait (Fig. 15.12). More information can be obtained from weight-bearing radiographs which will show the first–second intermetatarsal angle, first metatarsal sesamoid position and the first metatarsophalangeal joint space.

These three components of hallux valgus can be evaluated with serial weight-bearing radiographs and will readily be seen to change if the condition deteriorates (Fig. 15.13). As a rule, X-rays should not be

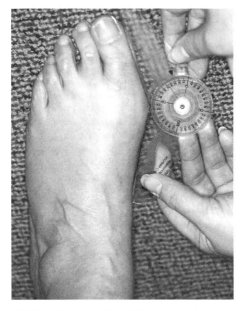

Figure 15.12 Measuring the first metatarsophalangeal angle with a digital goniometer.

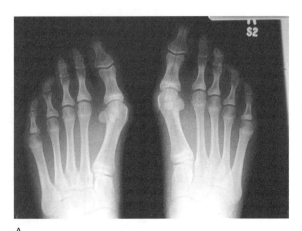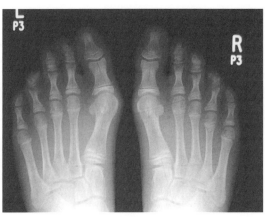

A   B

Figure 15.13   A, B: Deterioration in juvenile hallux valgus between open (B) and closure of the epiphyses (A). Note the changes in first–second intermetatarsal angle, first metatarsal sesamoid position and first metatarsal-phalangeal joint space.

used routinely in children and serial exposures may be 2–3 years apart. The importance of X-rays lies in the fact that the severity of the first–second inter-metatarsal angle and the lateral displacement of the sesamoids correlate directly with the severity of the hallux valgus angle (Hardy & Clapham 1951). The metatarsophalangeal joint space will reduce with the onset of degenerative joint disease, an important cause of pain in the condition and almost certainly a consequence of maltracking of the joint.

Orthotic management

The aetiology of hallux valgus is uncertain. Until the cause of the condition is known, it seems unlikely that treatment will be successful in all cases. The suggestion that hallux valgus could be linked to excessive pronation of the foot has been shown to be unlikely because there is no difference between the arch height of children with hallux valgus and normal children (Kilmartin & Wallace 1992). Apart from the common presence of a plantarflexed first metatarsal, there is also no consistent biomechanical abnormality between normal and hallux valgus feet (Kilmartin et al 1991). Moreover, in a 4 year study of the effect of a functional orthosis on 122 children with hallux valgus, it was found that the orthosis, which was de-signed to prevent excessive subtalar joint pronation, did nothing to prevent progression of the condition in the majority of the cases studied (Kilmartin et al 1994).

While orthoses may relieve the first metatarsopha-langeal joint pain associated with hallux valgus, parents and children should be counselled that pre-sent evidence suggests that such orthoses may not prevent the development of hallux valgus. Night splints have however been shown to be an effective treatment for hallux valgus (Groiso 1992).

In an uncontrolled trial of night splints in 25 Argentinian children, the night splints, which were worn for 3 years, corrected the hallux valgus angle by an average 3°.

Commercially made night splints are cheap and readily available and should be considered initially for children with hallux valgus. The child should be reviewed regularly to monitor both improvement and deterioration. Surgery may be considered where the deformity has advanced to Hardy & Clapham's (1951) critical angle of lateral deformity where the hallux abuts against the second toe. It is at this point that the condition really begins to progress rapidly. The first to second intermetatarsal angle widens as the proxi-mal phalanx of the hallux begins to act like a wedge to drive the first metatarsal into varus. As the deformity advances, the lateral pressure of the hallux may cause deformity of the lesser toes.

Surgery

The use of surgery to manage hallux valgus may be appropriate to improve footwear fit and prevent secondary problems. The selection of the appropriate procedure is critical to preserve epiphyses and blood supply in the growing foot. The decision to undertake surgery is best left to those conditions in which the deformity is marked, where the child is experiencing continual pain in the presence of footwear fitting problems, and where secondary changes arise, such as a second toe subluxing at its MTPJ. The appropriate surgical management of this condition is discussed in Chapters 7 and 14.

LESSER DIGITAL DEFORMITY

Digital abnormalities associated with the second to fifth toes are very common and can affect very young children. They cover a spectrum of deformity from mild burrowing of the fifth toe to adductovarus of the lateral three toes, or dorsal displacement of the second toe (Fig. 15.14).

Slight malalignment of the fourth and fifth digits may be considered innocuous. Treatment, however, should be instigated if the digital deformity meets the following criteria:

- *apical weight-bearing*—the deformity is severe enough to shift the toe purchase from the dense plantar pad to the poorly protected apex of the digit and nail edges.
- *adjacent toes*—where a deforming influence affects an otherwise normal adjacent toe. Transverse plane deformity of digits can sometimes lead to underriding of adjacent toes. In the case of the second toe, this can lead to loss of the buttress effect that the second toe normally exerts, predisposing toward lateral deviation of the hallux.

Digital deformity is difficult to treat in children under 5 years of age because the digits are small and difficult to hold in a corrected position. After 5 years of age, compliance will improve and treatment should be instigated if the above criteria are present. Toes may be splinted into a corrected position by taping (strapping), silicone devices (orthodigita) or using a latex band (rubber dam) (Fig. 15.15). Treatment should also utilise the other adjacent digits which can provide a splinting effect.

Deformity in the sagittal plane corrects earlier than other planes, which may resist correction. The objective of treatment must be to restore toe purchase and realign the sagittal position of the three phalanges. Once the proximal phalanx is restored to a neutral position (neither plantarflexed nor dorsiflexed), relative to the metatarsal head, the lumbrical muscles will often produce better dynamic equilibrium between the flexor and extensor muscles.

Splinting should be initiated for 1 month and the child should be encouraged to wear the device day and night. Progress should be reviewed and treatment continued if correction is identified. If after 3 months there is no change in the digital position then surgical treatment may be considered.

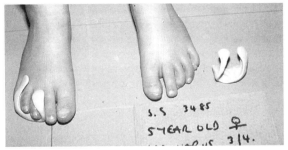

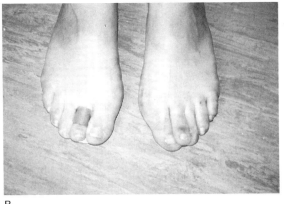

Figure 15.15 A: Silicone splints for lesser digit deformity. B: Rubber dam for correction of a dorsiflexed digit.

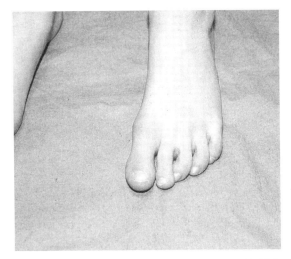

Figure 15.14 Lesser digit deformity in a 7-year-old child.

Polydactyly and syndactyly

These two conditions are less commonly observed. Polydactyly is best dealt with in the infant. Surgical excision of the accessory digit is required in most instances, although in poorly formed digits, devoid of bony or cartilaginous structures, the tourniquet amputation, where a tight thread is drawn around the base of the digit, works well.

Syndactyly is rarely a significant problem in the foot, unlike the hand where it will affect dexterity. The most common presentation is syndactyly of the second and third toes up to the level of the proximal interphalangeal joint—this is known as *zygodactyly*. The concern is usually cosmetic only and reassurance should be given. Desyndactylisation can only be achieved surgically and carries a high risk of inter-digital necrosis because of the proximity of the syndactyly to the neurovascular bundle of the digit.

Surgery

Surgical correction of digital deformity appears to be highly effective (Ross & Menelaus 1984, Hamer et al 1993). Flexor tenotomy or transfer is performed when the digits are flexible and easily corrected by manual manipulation. Arthrodesis of the distal or proximal interphalangeal joint is indicated when the deformity is rigid. An arthrodesis is reserved for when the toe bones are large enough. Painful apical weight-bearing is a reasonable justification for such intervention. Arthrodesis is considerably more complicated than a flexor release performed alone. The simple flexor release is very successful if undertaken before the joint becomes ankylosed, usually under 12 years of age. Flexor stab incisions can be performed through a plantar approach or, preferably, from the side, thus avoiding delicate vasculature. Orthodigital splinting with silicones can be used to maintain additional correction following surgery.

PAIN IN THE LOWER LIMB

FOOT PAIN

Foot pain is relatively rare among children. While the history of the complaint will often provide the diagnosis, radiological investigation is also vital to complete analysis because so many causes of juvenile foot pain are developmental abnormalities of bone and joint. Unremitting pain of a non specific nature must be considered seriously with early referral to the appropriate specialty.

Osteochondroses

Sever's disease

This condition is not a true osteochondrosis but an apophysitis. Heel pain in children is commonly a consequence of Sever's disease. This characteristically affects children between 8 and 15 years of age. Treatment involves reducing the traction that may be created by a tight tendo Achilles acting at the developing calcaneal epiphysis.

The child should be encouraged to wear training shoes; a shock-absorbing insole or heel pad made from polyurethane (*Poron*) may also be fitted inside the shoe. Wedging the heel into varus will reduce some traction from the tendo Achilles, while the calf muscles should be stretched to reduce the tension associated with tight posterior calf muscles. These measures may not completely relieve the pain from Sever's disease. The child should be reassured that the pain will resolve once the calcaneal epiphysis closes (see case history in Box 15.4).

Box 15.4   Case history: apophysitis

A 12-year-old boy presented with pain in his left heel after games. As a keen footballer, he had already consulted another practitioner who considered the problem to be a result of the studs on his football boots. Subsequently the patient had been playing football in normal shoes but found the problem was no better. Although the parents had at one time thought that the problem was nothing more than growing pains, they were becoming increasingly concerned about the chronic nature of the condition.

Examination revealed poor flexibility of the posterior calf muscles, with restricted ankle joint dorsiflexion. Upon palpating the calcaneus, the pain produced was similar to that brought on by activity.

The patient was advised to embark upon regular but gentle gastrocnemius stretching exercises. He was also advised to wear running shoes as much as possible. A *Poron* insole was placed in the shoes with a 6 mm sponge foam heel pad. Four weeks later, the child was reviewed. He reported that while the pain had improved considerably, the heel still ached after football. The patient was advised that complete resolution would occur in time.

Clinical comment. Unresolved pain in the heel will require further investigation to exclude bone cysts and avulsion fractures. Casting is reserved for intractable apophysitis for 6–8 weeks. Extended periods of immobility may benefit from bivalved casts or stock prefabricated casts (Air Cast).

The result of a severe apophysitis or rearfoot varus can leave children with a large retrocalcaneal lump at the back of the heel. This condition is known as Haglund's deformity and affects adults as well as children. As described in the previous chapter, this condition can be managed conservatively. The main problems associated with Haglund's deformity for children are the symptoms associated with chilblains, bursae and blisters. The condition arises more frequently in females and shoes often exacerbate the problem. Other forms of common heel pain can be related to verrucae; this area of management is dealt with later in this chapter.

Kohler's disease

Localised tenderness and swelling over the navicular bone in children aged between 3 and 5 years of age should lead the practitioner to suspect Kohler's disease. The onset of the pain in the midfoot can coincide with unusual physical activity or trauma to the area. If Kohler's disease is suspected, the foot should be radiographed. The characteristic radiographic features of increased density of the navicular bone with sclerosis and flattening help to confirm the diagnosis. This is largely a self-limiting condition.

A felt or foam pad inserted into the shoe will reduce some of the immediate tenderness. If the condition is not improved by such simple remedies, immobilisation of the foot in a below-knee plaster of Paris cast will reduce the acute pain. The cast should be left in place for between 2 to 6 weeks in the first instance. If pain is not resolved or recurs soon after removing the cast, another cast may be applied, or alternatively soft arch supports may provide sufficient immobilisation of the midtarsal joint to relieve discomfort and be continued in association with appropriate footwear.

While in some cases the navicular may settle in shape and density within 3–7 months, others may take 2–4 years (Ferguson & Gingrich 1957). What is significant is that the navicular always returns to its normal shape and density. Repeated radiographs may allow the practitioner to monitor pathological changes and deterioration. The relief of tenderness and swelling with immobilisation of the foot is the first priority of treatment.

Sever's and Kohler's disease are both the product of a developmental problem that resolves with maturity without long-lasting effects. The anticipated satisfactory outcome should be conveyed to anxious parents.

Freiberg's disease

Freiberg's disease is a degenerative aseptic necrosis of the secondary ossification centre of a lesser metatarsal head. It affects females more commonly than males around the age of 10–15 years, although it has been found in older patients. The condition frequently causes chronic pain and, in the long term, it causes osteoarthritic changes within the metatarsophalangeal joint (Fig. 15.16). In two-thirds of cases, the second metatarsal head is affected, while the third metatarsal head accounts for approximately another 25% of the incidence. Affectation of the fourth metatarsal head is rare, while involvement of the fifth is unlikely (Gauthier & Elbaz 1979).

Freiberg's disease presents as a history of aching or sharp pain localised to the metatarsal head which is aggravated by physical activity and characterised on examination by a palpable thickening of the metatarsal head. Radiographic examination shows a square, flattened metatarsal head and marked reduction in dorsiflexion, sometimes exhibiting a loose body.

Immobilising metatarsophalangeal joint motion can be assisted again by the use of a below-knee or below-ankle rigid fibreglass cast. The outcome is not easy to predict and may depend upon how much damage is allowed to continue before being appropriately diagnosed. Unlike apophysitis, small cartilage and osseous fragments may produce synovitis as they become compressed with movement of the metatar-

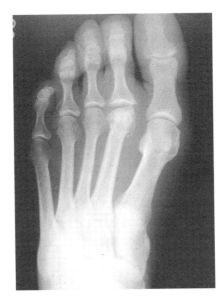

Figure 15.16 Freiberg's disease of the second metatarsal head. Note the classic flattened head compared to the other metatarsals.

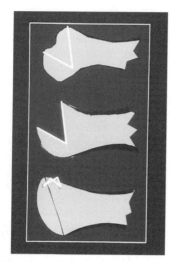

Figure 15.17 Removal of a wedge of bone from the metaphyseal area of the metatarsal will rotate the articular surface of the metatarsal head so that the healthy cartilage-covered plantar condyles articulate with the base of the proximal phalanx. The wedge of bone resected from the metatarsal neck is triangular in shape, with the apex of the triangle directed plantarly (Tollafield 1993).

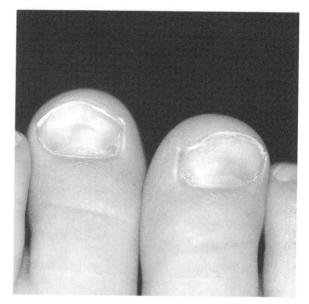

Figure 15.18 A spoon-shaped great toenail. While the nail is concave dorsally, it involutes steeply at the sides, predisposing to ingrowing nails.

sophalangeal joint. Smith et al (1991) found that some 50% of those examined improved with conservative treatment. The other half required an operation to decompress the joint.

Surgery. Smillie (1967) recommended the use of autogenous bone chips grafted into the damaged metatarsal head, recreating the articular dome. Often the surgeon sees Freiberg's disease too late for this to be effective, as radiographic changes are poorly identified on plain X-rays. Gauthier & Elbaz's (1979) procedure has proven successful where the disease has developed. A dorsiflexory osteotomy can restore joint function, remove diseased and deformed bone, and decompress the joint (Fig. 15.17). Early recovery offers one of the greatest benefits and internal hard fixation is not necessary provided that close attention to capsular repair is undertaken (Tollafield 1993).

Nail pathology

The general management of onychocryptosis (ingrowing nails) has already been covered in considerable depth in Chapter 6. The principles of management vary little between adult and child. However, ingrowing toenails can present in the young baby. In many cases, the problem is related to the shape of the hallux nail (Fig. 15.18). The spoon-shaped nail appears too wide for the toe, with obvious curvature of the nail sides. The sides irritate the sensitive soft borders and cause inflammation of the sulci, which then further engulfs the nail edge, forming an enlarged ungual labia or hypertrophied nail fold.

Partial nail avulsion with phenolisation of the nail matrix, performed under local anaesthetic, is not appropriate in the baby because of the technical difficulty of injecting a baby's toe. Moreover, the instruments which are usually used to perform such a procedure are far too big for the infant's toe. Treatment is directed at reducing the inflammation of the nail sulci and preventing the progressive cycle of inflammation leading to further trauma, ulceration and infection.

Operative treatment should be delayed as long as possible to allow for natural resolution of the problem, which usually occurs around 5 years of age when the nail shape spontaneously improves. Palliative measures include the use of topical antiseptics and prevention of the nail fold from nail edge irritation. The parents should also be advised to keep the hallux nails correctly trimmed by using an emery board to file the nail, rather than scissors. Cutting down the side of the nail should not be performed by the parents, as a spicule of nail may be left. Moreover, the use of scissors in the area will probably inflame the sulci further.

> **Box 15.5** Case history: ingrowing toenail
>
> A 7-year-old male attended clinic to have an ingrowing nail affecting the medial side of the right hallux treated. Recurrent pain along the groove was remarkable and an abnormal phalanx was demonstrated by X-ray. The proximal phalanx appeared to have developed a unilateral sided abberation during the growth process, previously unidentified at birth. The skin crease (Fig. 15.19A) suggested an abnormal problem. The crease became inflamed repeatedly, requiring frequent antibiotic management. The patient also had a dysfunctional kidney. Treatment required incision of the toe and removal of the isolated bone (Fig. 15.19B). Seven months following surgery, some tenderness was occasionally appreciated but the condition was otherwise comfortable with spacious shoes and no abnormal sequelae were suspected. Twelve months after surgery, the toe had settled. The nail plate showed no deformity and the sulcal crease was no longer evident (Fig. 15.19C).

If recurrent onychocryptosis and sepsis occurs in the baby, partial nail avulsion may be performed under short-acting general anaesthesia. It is considered poor practice to undertake any treatment by force. While very rare, children forced into having treatment may develop a vasovagal collapse, which may occur suddenly with dramatic consequences.

When an adolescent presents with onychocryptosis, there is little justification for anything other than partial avulsion with phenolisation, performed under local anaesthetic. Where hyperidrosis, injudicious self-care and involution present together, treatment may be time-consuming and intractable. The case history in Box 15.5 reports an unusual case of an ingrowing nail related to a growth defect.

Verrucae pedis

Verrucae pedis, or 'foot warts' (*verruca*: wart), are endemic amongst schoolchildren. During the 1970s and early 1980s, most NHS foot health departments treated children in large numbers. The former policy of managing all verrucae has now given way to a general policy in the UK of only treating those cases in which discomfort is the chief concern—pain is therefore the main justification for treatment. The use of verruca socks, now available from most pharmacists, attempts to reduce epidermal abrasion and hence entry of the viral infection. In the child, verrucae will eventually spontaneously resolve and it is suggested that once this has occurred reinfection is less likely (Bunney 1983).

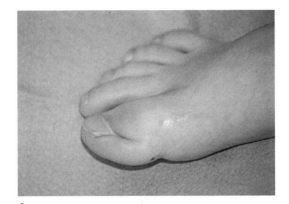

A

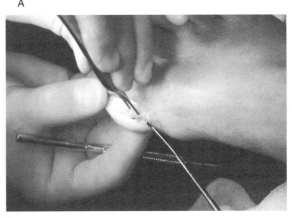

B

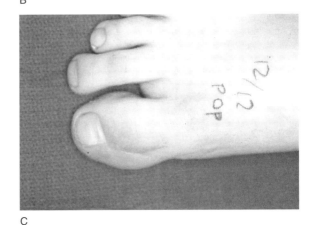

C

Figure 15.19 A: The toe shows a deep crease along the medial border. B: Intra-operative identification of the separate bone poorly defined. C: Twelve months after surgery, there is good recovery and narrowing of the toe.

Verrucae will often present as a single lesion on the sole of the foot (verruca) and are usually painful when located over a weight-bearing area. When present on non-weight-bearing areas, the lesion, often complicated with a thick keratin covering, is raised and appears nodular, and if large can become fissured. Dorsal lesions are often less resistant to treatment as epidermo-dermal changes are less involved. In this respect, hands are easier to treat than plantar foot lesions, which can penetrate some 6 mm into the underlying tissues (Fig. 15.21).

Mosaic verrucae are more superficial than the common wart (*Verruca vulgaris*); large weight-bearing areas of the foot can be involved. Less commonly, verrucae will affect the dorsum of digits and sometimes can occur in the sulci, eponychial fold or nail bed. When not compressed by weight-bearing forces, growth of verrucae can be quite florid.

Treatment

Treatment options range from home treatments to minor surgery. Treatment can be divided into groups as shown in Box 15.6.

Some treatments are relatively inexpensive, such as occluding the wart for several weeks. *Minor surgery* with curettage and excision (Figs 15.20 and 15.21)

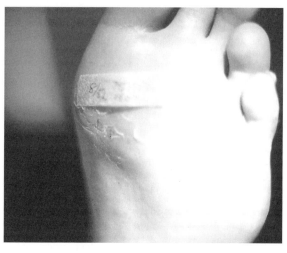

Figure 15.20 Wide excision of multiple verrucae is advised, but recurrence can lead to disappointing results, with further viral infection (Koebner phenomenon) along the line of the wound. This result does allow further successful treatment with chemicals to clear the residual infection.

Box 15.6 Methods of treatment for verrucae

- Caustics
- Desiccants
- Keratolytics
- Cryosurgery
- Cautery
- Curettage
- Laser

---

forms a low cost method of treatment but needs to be used judiciously as regrowth is possible along the excised margins. *Laser treatment* is experiencing a resurgence now that cheaper models are available. The diversity of laser models, however, means that some sources require local anaesthetics, while others do not. Anecdotal experience in the US suggests that laser is no more beneficial than other treatments and new UK research is awaited. Most departments will have *cryotherapy equipment* such as liquid nitrogen or a nitrous oxide gun system (Fig. 15.22). Nitrous

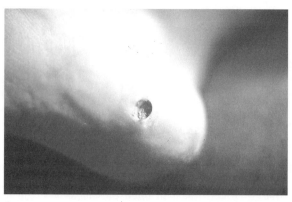

A

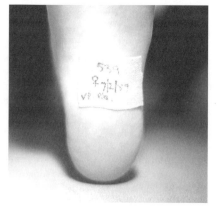

B

Figure 15.21 A: Excision of single well-defined verruca in a 6-year-old boy under ankle block local anaesthesia. B: Eighteen months later there is minimal scarring.

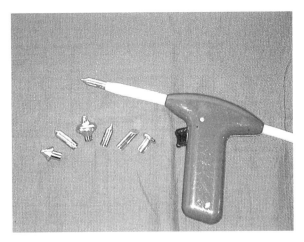

Figure 15.22 Common systems for freezing warts use liquid nitrogen or nitrous oxide. Variable nozzles shown here with the 'Spembly' nitrous oxide system.

oxide emission gases must be removed from the treatment room by special exhaust pipes; this precaution is particularly important in the case of pregnant women.

Cautery can be highly effective, but such methods require considerable skill in local and regional anaesthesia and knowledge of the cautery technique, together with the relevant safety aspects.

Isolated lesions. In cases of painful single verruca pedis, the patient should be informed that all treatment measures are tissue destructive in nature and no 'one-off' treatment can guarantee a cure. Treatment will usually damage the healthy tissue which surrounds the lesion before the infection will clear. Aggressive treatment with caustics must be applied carefully and clear instructions given to the parent or older child.

Monochloroacetic acid, often applied using an acid crystal, can cause localised inflammation and even cellulitis. The appearance may mimic infection, although cultures of such breakdowns are sterile (Tollafield 1979). Caustics are often mixed with keratolytics to create delamination of keratin. Sensitive skin will react within several hours and the dressing must be removed and attempts made to limit caustic action by the application of sodium bicarbonate (1 in 80 aqueous solution) or sodium chloride as a strong salt footbath.

Single lesions in children respond remarkably well to between two and six applications of caustic-keratolytics combined or applied separately on a weekly basis. Younger children may find the reactive treatment too aggressive and cryosurgery too uncomfortable at the time of application. The need to maintain a moist-free environment is essential with caustic

acids. This, of course, will require abstinence from swimming. The use of keratolytics works well in young children, however, resilient infections can be treated using regional anaesthesia and curettage or cautery.

Mosaic lesions. A much gentler approach is required because of the larger area affected. A strong astringent will dry the verrucae to the point where the infected tissue can simply be debrided. Although not a commercially available preparation, formalin 10% solution is particularly effective, especially when combined with alcohol or glutaraldehyde (Glutarol).

Multiple single warts. These can cover large areas of the weight-bearing plantar surface. Treatment of central sites, often known as 'mother centres', can have a remarkable effect upon the peripheral, less symptomatic, lesions. Heels and metatarsal head areas on the sole are particularly resilient; scarring is often a complication that may be inevitable but undesirable. Excision should be avoided for all but well-defined areas. Incomplete excisions have a high recurrence rate, producing a Koebner phenomenon such as occurs in psoriasis. Secondary scarring may cause further pain.

Verrucae in children resolve more rapidly than in adults. The practitioner will ultimately select the most effective treatment. For this reason, no one method can be recommended for all lesion types. Patient psychology is essential when determining which approach to select. The range of medications and methods available is extensive. Prior to restrictive use, even smallpox vaccines were used in the USA. At one point this was thought to provide immunological stimulation against the papova virus. Table 15.1 provides a summary rather than a definitive approach to treating children for this condition. The practitioner, no matter how experienced, does not always meet with success. Patients and their parents can become quite anxious about the recalcitrant nature of this lesion. A break from treatment may improve the anxiety that arises from long periods of treatment. Varied treatment methods can also help the patient; aggressive methods such as acids, cautery or cryosurgery can be punctuated with applications of keratolytics. Because these lesions can almost disappear spontaneously, some psychological influence may be suggested. Stress at school can affect the immunological system. Ceasing treatment can also reduce stress. The practitioner may suggest that the patient is deliberately given no treatment for 4–12 weeks, to allow the skin to recover as well as reduce the weekly drudgery that treatment can bring.

Large areas of infection may need to be managed in stages. *Staged management* may require the application

Table 15.1 Summary of methods in treating verrucae.

Method	Indications	Preparations/methods	Complications	Action
Desiccants				
Formaldehyde	Used on all type of warts. Good for young children. A plastic applicator should be used	Formaldehyde is also prepared in solutions and a water-miscible gel base	Caution on sensitive skin. Glutaraldehyde stains skin brown	Cease application. Patient to alert practitioner
Bromine complexes	Used for all types of warts	Benzalkonium chloride-bromine 25% applied similarly to keratolytics (see below)	Sensitivity	Cease application. Patient to alert practitioner
Keratolytics				
Salicylic acid with lactic acid	Small and larger areas of warts, and corns depending upon medication strength. Applied to single or multiple warts—protect surrounding skin. Useful on young children. Must be debrided occasionally	Available as pastes/ointments and in plasters. Common compound salicylic acid 10–60% with lactic acid 4–17%	Increase sensitivity from repeated use. Infections can arise if heavy loss of epithelial tissue arises. Cannot be neutralised effectively. Commonly misused by patients & GPs for corns	Cease application. Patient to alert practitioner
Podophyllum	Single warts, or multiple where well defined and on thicker (sole) epidermis. Applied in apertured pad to protect skin. Pastes should be occluded with polythene cover	Salicylic acid (25%) with 10% Podophyllum (Posalfilin). Preparations also available in alcoholic base (0.5%) and resin (15%) with tincture of benzoin. Weaker agents used for a wider area: Condyline/Warticon and Podophyllin paint BP	As salicylic acid. Skin will become white or black/brown and expand with moisture. Dark colouration will arise, regular debridement is recommended	Cease application. Patient to alert practitioner
Caustics and acids	Resistant warts with good thickness of tissue; avoid in young children, sensitive skins, low pain threshold, and thin soft and atrophic skin. Caustic agent will create tissue atrophy and epidermal layers will breakdown. Used on isolated areas rather than large areas at one time. Management in stages is useful with varying strengths. Preparations cannot be purchased as standard preparations from pharmacy. Care should be used and applications made by the practitioner *not patient*. Must be checked every 7–14 days as highly penetrative	Monochloroacetic acid, trichloroacetic acid. Can be mixed in conjunction with 40–60% salicylic paste as liquid/crystals with correct skin protection	Sensitivity to surrounding skin can give rise to marked breakdown with brown/white discharge. May present erroneously as cellulitis	Contact practitioner. Neutralise (see text) with bicarbonate of soda 1 in 80 solution or salt foot bath if at home. Administer mild analgesics as required and rest foot, release breakdown, dry dressing, review 2–7 days

Table 15.1 (contd)

Method	Indications	Preparations/methods	Complications	Action
Silver nitrate	Used to deal with superficial warts, and bleeding points. Has poor penetrative power as forms a self-resistant eschar. Less toxic than acids, but can cause problems in patients with sensitive skin. Useful for mosaic lesions or remnants of lesions, post cryosurgery treatment to reduce blistering. Best applied as a stick moistened with water or alcohol. Contact with skin causes instant oxidisation (white appearance initially), which turns black over next few hours. Must be debrided for further penetration	Styptic stick, solutions are difficult to come by as silver content makes them expensive	Must not be used on soft skin webs between toes, on sensitive skin, or on weak fragile skin. Uncontrolled application can cause solution to run	Neutralisation with sodium chloride solution or as a salt footbath
Thermal agents Cold/cryosurgery	Single warts, satellites, nodular types on digits. Ideal for soft skin. Causes blisters. Not affected by water—patients can still swim. May be too painful for very young children if long freeze upheld. LA may be useful in selected cases. Several applications made directly to lesion until white halo. Rapid freeze and thaw thought to be critical to effectiveness; several freezes recommended. Postapplication—silver nitrate stick or simple adhesive dressing. Can be used on most age groups but exclude in sensitive/anxious children. Repeated freezes every 2–6 weeks/1–6 treatments, depending upon type of lesion	Liquid nitrogen, nitrous oxide gas, carbon dioxide gas. All these agents are highly damaging if uncontrolled, will cause instant cellular destruction below −20°C. Handling and ventilation of gases is essential. Products may comes as jets, simple swabs for liquid N_2, or piped gases through fine tubes (Fig.15.22). Gaskets and washers need monitoring, equipment will come under Health & Safety Regulations	Large bullae which should be released and dressed. Treat infection/pain as indicated under cautery	
Cautery	May be used on wider areas of infection or single clusters. Local anaesthetic is indicated in all cases. May be used in suitable patients from 6 years upwards. Indications on single, mosaic areas. Multiple wide areas require staged management (see text). Postoperative medication (mild analgesics required). Attempt to limit damage to dermis. Scarring will occur but usually only as superficial fill in	Heat desication (hot wire) and electrical diathermy (current). Bipolar best for electrical safety, monopolar with earthing. Many models available	Ulceration due to deep penetration or too much electrical/heat destruction. Electrical shock due to poor earth (monopolar), caution in patients with metal, implants, pacemakers, delayed healing. Treat infection with antibiotics and antiseptics as appropriate. Use mild to moderate analgesics depending upon symptoms	

Table 15.1 (contd)

Method	Indications	Preparations/methods	Complications	Action
Laser	See text and Chapter 9. Useful for treating portions of large verrucae at a time. Penetration depth varies. Some do not require local anaesthetic.		Many safety features to regard. Different source than cautery	
Surgical	Procedures undertaken under local regional block or direct infiltration with or without 1 in 200 000 adrenaline (for haemostasis). Single lesions indicated usually from 6 years if child tolerates anaesthetic—avoid direct infiltration in this age group, offer ankle block for plantar surface. Multiple lesions may be curetted, large lesions best treated with methods above	Curettage—scooped out Excision—surgical dissection with sutures Stippling—multiple punctures with needles	Techniques not applicable for large areas or multiple infections. Swelling, pain and infection. Treat clinical signs and symptoms as above. Bleeding with curettage can be assisted with styptic (haemostatic) dressings packed into wound. Should heal quickly	

Note: The above treatments will depend upon practitioner skill, adequate training and knowledge when using the medications described above. Manufacturer's instructions should always be read first. Lesions should be debrided initially. Patients should have oral and written instructions where appropriate, emergency telephone numbers (pagers) and written discharge information to avoid inappropriate counter measures. Equipment should be approved, correctly serviced and all medications professionally prepared. Complications MUST be discussed in each case before treatment is undertaken and measures to neutralise agents should be covered in any post-treatment instructions given. All the agents cited are applicable to children and need to be used with caution, especially in any patient with a doubtful healing capacity.

of several methods in order to prevent aggressive skin breakdown (see Table 15.1).

The objective of treatment remains the stimulation of the body's own defence mechanism to deal with these viral infections.

Tumours

After verrucae, the commonest swelling to affect children, next to ingrowing toe nails with their paronychial granulation, is the subungual exostosis. This condition affects children from adolescence to young adulthood, frequently presenting with a cartilage cap. While termed an osteochondroma, these are not true osteochondromata as they lack a well-defined perichondrium and their cytology is different. Subungual exostoses with cartilage caps are reactive, usually non-malignant, lesions which show a gradual change from fibrous to proliferating cartilage, and which then undergo irregular enchondral ossification. The growth that ensues may take many months, but eventually the skin is stretched causing pain with deformity (Fig. 6.8B).

Surgery

Once an exostosis has been diagnosed, surgery is indicated, particularly if there is paronychial distension of the hallux or lesser toe.

LEG AND KNEE PAIN

While the diagnosis and treatment of the foot may appear isolated, the influence of the leg, acting superiorly to the foot and ankle, cannot be excluded from treatment. Common conditions affecting the leg and knee will be discussed, together with differential diagnostic considerations. Orthoses are commonly used to manage non-specific disorders of the leg successfully, but a judicious approach is always important and a second opinion is suggested if doubt arises with the primary diagnosis. The reader is therefore recommended to refer to texts dedicated to the lower limb for further details of treatment, as many conditions that affect the leg are outside the scope of this book.

Pain in a child's legs should always be taken seriously; growing pains are a problem for many children who have to deal with periods of discomfort. The origin of the pain should always be assessed. Pain arising from the CNS or autonomic nervous system, vascular changes, tumours or from trauma or infection, especially haematogenous osteomyelitis,

must be excluded during the examination. In many cases, the problem is one of poor muscle flexibility during periods of growth between 6 and 12 years of age.

Treatment

Growing pains. Tight hamstrings will often lead to nocturnal discomfort in the posterior knee. Stretching exercises shown to the parent, to be performed on the child, will help to alleviate the complaint. In some cases, nocturnal sedation and pain relief with paediatric strength elixir such as Calpol may help relax muscles. Massage and warmth from flannels or thermal packs which retain their heat will reduce spasm. Where pain continues unabated, a second opinion from a paediatrician is worthwhile. Investigative tests should commence with urine analysis. Other conditions that may need to be excluded include osteomyelitis, apophysitis and knee pain.

Haematogenous osteomyelitis. The bones most commonly affected by this condition include the tibia, femur and humerus. Onset of symptoms is rapid and the patient will report malaise. Previous minor injuries or even boils should be considered as a source of this pyogenic disorder, most commonly related to *S. aureus*. If this condition affects the superior tibia, unattended disease may spread to the knee, although it is more commonly spread from the inferior femur. The area is hot and very tender and such symptoms, combined with pyrexia, should be managed as an infection until proved otherwise.

Blood cultures may not show raised leucocytic activity initially. Erythrocyte sedimentation rates and C-reactive protein assays should be undertaken together with plain X-rays and bone scans. A C-reactive protein blood test is more sensitive in the early stages of inflammatory processes (Lodwick et al 1995). If this is negative, then a bone scan is indicated, as skeletal changes may take several weeks to show rarefaction and periosteal alteration consistent with the disease. Treatment per se will require bed rest and systemic antibiotics as a combination of flucloxacillin and fusidic acid until the organism can be isolated. Analgesics should be used to reduce pyrexia and control pain. Surgical drainage is indicated only where the results of antibiosis are unsatisfactory.

Osgood-Schlatter. This condition affects males between 10 and 15 years of age. While the literature has supported different aetiologies, the pathogenesis seems to suggest that the condition is similar to an apophysitis. Rest from sporting activities forms the first line of conservative care. In severe cases, a cast to immobilise the knee is recommended. Where the tendinous insertion of the patella tendon is acutely involved, 3–4 ml of hydrocortisone with local anaesthetic has been considered valuable (Tachdjian 1972). Surgical options are not recommended, although changes such as early fusion of the tibial epiphysis have been rarely reported, leading to the need for osteotomy following genu recurvatum. The enlarged tibial tubercle indicated old Osgood-Schlatter. Resection of bone might be used if the bone was particularly deformed. As with most apophysitis, the condition will resolve in time.

Anterior knee pain. This is very common among mid-adolescent girls (see case history in Box 15.7). Treatment will aim to:

Box 15.7 Case history: anterior knee pain

An overweight 14-year-old girl complained of aching behind her knee caps. The pain had been present for at least a year and appeared to be deteriorating. She had been excused from all field games because the knee kept 'giving way' and was made more painful by activity. Since developing the knee pain, she had also missed many days from school because she had found that climbing the school staircases aggravated the pain. Ibuprofen had been prescribed by her GP in order to keep her pain-free at school.

On examination, both knees were very sensitive to patella compression; flexing the knee and lateral pressure aggravated the symptoms. Palpation of the posterior medial facet of the patella indicated no fissuring suggested by the absence of crepitus. The patient was asked to stand and squat; she flexed the knees slowly but only achieved half squat position because the pain became unbearable.

On standing, marked squinting of both patellae were demonstrated. The thighs were thin with little muscle definition of the quadriceps. The Q angle was 30°. Walking revealed a tendency to walk with the knee slightly flexed. The hamstrings were tight when the 90:90 or SLR test was performed; knee was recorded at 40° flexion at maximum extension.

Treatment was planned to deal with the high Q angle; muscle imbalance, i.e quadriceps weakness and hamstring tightness; and obesity.

A neutral suspension cast was taken of both feet, and functional orthoses were prescribed. The patient was asked to perform hamstring stretching exercises by simply touching her toes. Straight leg raises were also recommended to improve the tone of the quadriceps muscles. An appointment was made for her to see a dietician. The orthoses were fitted in her shoes some 2 weeks later and good reduction in the Q angle was noted. At subsequent follow-up, the knee pain was greatly reduced by the use of the orthoses and exercises, but had not resolved completely. The patient was referred on for knee arthroscopy or release of the lateral patella fascia.

- improve patella position
- restore normal muscle equilibrium to the quadriceps and hamstring muscle.

A high Q (quadriceps) angle is thought to result from internal femoral position. A high Q angle can be reduced when an orthosis is placed beneath the foot (Fig 15.23; D'Amico & Rubin 1986). The orthosis is thought to supinate the subtalar joint producing external rotation of the leg. With reduction of the Q angle, the patella may be positioned more satisfactorily in the intertrochanteric fossa of the femur. This will alleviate the shearing of the patella against the femoral condyles associated with patella malalignment. Shearing of the patella against the femoral condyles is thought to be an important cause of pain (Fox 1975).

Poor alignment of the patella can also be more directly treated by strapping the patella into a correct position. The *McConnell technique* seeks to realign the patella in the transverse, sagittal and frontal planes. This technique involves the application of rigid strapping to the patella and around the side of the knee to correct any medial or lateral deviation of the patella.

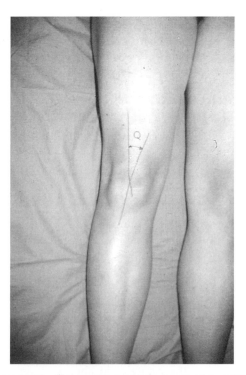

Figure 15.23 The quadriceps angle described by a line drawn from the anterior superior iliac spine to the centre of the patella, and a line drawn from the tibial tuberosity to the centre of the patella.

Tilting of the patella, which may increase compression on the medial and lateral surfaces, is also dealt with in this manner (Hilyard 1990).

The vastus medialis muscle provides an important stabiliser for the patella. If the muscle is weak, due to injury, inherited tendency or biomechanical dysfunction, the patella will be pulled laterally and superiorly by the dominant vastus lateralis. Shearing of the patella against the lateral condyle will result. The vastus medialis must be strengthened by exercises which will seek to increase muscle bulk. Straight leg raise assessment (SLR) is useful when the knee is acutely painful. SLRs can be performed by exercising the vastus medialis, without the need for any knee flexion, thus obviating shearing behind the patella. SLRs, however, will not exercise the vastus medialis muscle in isolation from the quadriceps muscle group. The vastus medialis muscle only comes into effect in the last 30° of extension. Extension exercise, with a heavy weight on the foot, extending the knee from 30° flexion to full extension, will exercise the vastus medialis and assist in improving patella tracking.

COMMON GAIT PROBLEMS

Of all conditions presented to practitioners, the pigeon toe gait raises greatest concern.

Gait variations associated with in-toeing and out-toeing, rather than those causing pain, tend to produce a problem of stability, ungainly stance, tripping and shoe wear contrary to normal expectations. The foot specialist is concerned with more than just mere gait problems, in that the foot is thought to compensate adversely during development, heralding problems later in life. While hard scientific evidence is perhaps less than convincing, empirical experience suggests that the midfoot should be protected against pronatory changes.

IN-TOEING

While many paediatric complaints originate within the foot, abnormalities associated with the leg are also common. In-toeing is a particularly common lower limb problem which does not become apparent until the child begins to walk at around 13–18 months (Figure 15.24). Thirty per cent of 4-year-old children walk with their feet pointing towards the body midline; however, the condition persists in only 4% of adults (Svenningsen et al 1990).

Spontaneous resolution of the complaint usually

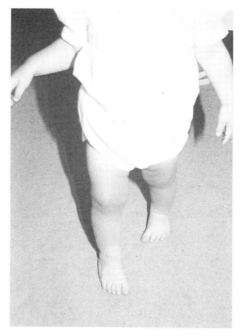

Figure 15.24 The in-toeing child. Note in this case that the feet are severely adducted while the knees face forwards; therefore, the cause of in-toeing is below the knee.

occurs between the ages of 4 and 11, a factor which must be borne in mind before treatment is planned. The condition is considered significant when the child constantly trips over their own feet. Often this will lead to numerous injuries and much distress for the parents and the child; in these cases treatment is required.

The type of treatment instigated will be largely determined by the cause of the in-toeing. One of the most common causes is hamstring shortening. Diagnosis is made with the leg straightened at the knee in extension (straight leg raise, SLR—this is also known as the 90:90 test; Fig. 15.25). In children up to 12 years of age, it should be possible to fully extend the knee when the hip is flexed to 90° as the child lies supine. In many asymptomatic children, however, this test may reveal some tightness as normal bone growth between the ages of 9 and 12 can outpace muscle lengthening. Where there is a history of problems and the knee will not extend beyond 70°, stretching exercises should be instigated to improve hamstring flexibility.

Treatment

Treatment can be directed at soft tissue, osseous

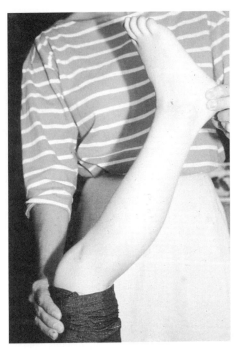

Figure 15.25 The straight leg raise (SLR) or 90:90 test to establish hamstring flexibility.

and articular relationships which cause the adducted position of the foot (see the treatment algorithm in Fig. 15.26).

Soft tissue relationships

Compliance from young children is poor when asked to undertake stretching regimens. It is more appropriate to ask the parents to perform the exercises on the child. The stretching exercise is quite similar to the diagnostic test. With the child lying flat on their back, the hip is flexed to 90°; the parent stabilises the thigh and, while grasping the back of the child's heel, extends the knee. The child counts to 30 and then the leg is allowed to relax. The exercise is then repeated at least another 10 times on both legs. Thirty days of intensive hamstring stretching are usually recommended. The child is then reviewed. If full extension of the knee upon repeating the SLR test is still not achieved, then another 30 days' stretching should be considered.

Re-education. Even when the hamstrings are stretched out, the child may continue to in-toe. In such cases the parents should be reassured that there is no structural reason why the child should not walk straight; they are simply assuming a habit. The habit

may be broken by reminding the child to walk straight or regularly playing games which require the child to walk with feet out-toed. A useful exercise that can be played out by the child involves placing footprint shapes on the ground and tracing their own feet onto the footprints while walking and running.

Gait plates. Abduction of the foot can be encouraged by limiting toe-off from the lateral side of the forefoot (Fig. 15.27). The gait plate alters the natural metatarsal break at the 4/5 metatarsophalangeal joint where flexion takes place. Propulsion from the lateral side of the foot is thwarted so that the child will rotate the leg to offer foot contact from the medial side. In order to achieve propulsion, the child must abduct the foot and roll off from the medial forefoot; the effect is to alter gait, producing straighter alignment. Gait plates cannot treat rotational problems, they can only realign the foot at contact whilst in use.

The gait plate is fabricated in much the same way as a Root or Shafer orthosis. The anterior edge of the orthosis, however, is extended distally to a point just short of the 4/5 toe sulci. The gait plate can be prescribed in 3–4 mm polypropylene or 3 mm acrylic. A deeper heel seat can be made from polypropylene and a high medial flange fabricated. Gait plates are not recommended for the apropulsive gait under 4 years of age as the device will not work as effectively as in older children. Muscles in the child should be continuously stretched during development in combination with gait plate prescription. Repeat stretching programmes are indicated, although a long-term programme is likely to result in non-compliance.

Osseous and articular relationships at the hip

In-toeing may also be a consequence of limited external rotation at the hip joint. Torsion within the proximal head and neck of the femur must be excluded, although diagnosis is difficult from clinical examination alone. Recent diagnostic aids now include ultrasound scanning. Serious rotational 'torsion' should be referred on to the orthopaedic specialist; however, in these cases the effects of rotation should be serious with the foot in-toeing in a marked fashion. Osteotomy of the femur is still the main treatment for these conditions. Corrective osteotomy is far from being a minor procedure and is known to carry important complications such as postoperative compartment syndrome as well as recurrence of the original condition.

Articular, soft tissue limitations and minor torsions may still benefit from a prescription gait plate. It has been suggested that the improvement in walking may

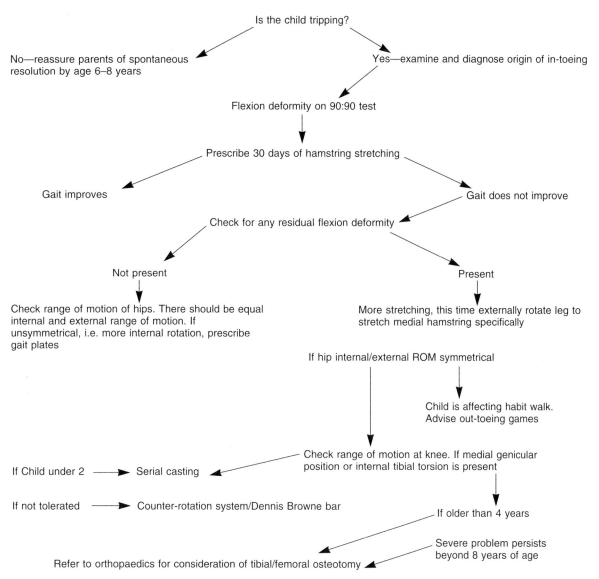

Figure 15.26   Algorithm to help determine the most appropriate treatment strategies for in-toeing gait. The practitioner is particularly interested in managing foot problems associated with recognisable developmental variations. Any suggestion of hip or knee disease warrants a different management. Orthoses are strictly contraindicated until an accurate diagnosis has been undertaken.

be a consequence of the child being forced to pronate off the orthosis; as the foot abducts with pronation, the tripping ceases. To date, there is no evidence to confirm that the gait plate will cause such an effect. In some cases a gait plate will produce no obvious benefit and alternative treatment must be considered. In the past, twister cables and Dennis Browne bar and boots have been used. These devices are worn at night and hold the legs in an externally (laterally) rotated position. Their value has been seriously questioned by Fabry et al (1973), who found that these devices actually retarded the rate at which children grew out of the condition.

Holding the legs in external rotation with a device worn on the feet primarily exerts a corrective force on the foot, and also exerts a force on the knee joint, which in under-5s is quite flexible and easily rotated. If the cause of the in-toeing is proximal to the knee

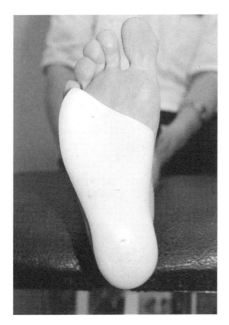

Figure 15.27 A gait plait for in-toeing children.

joint, the corrective force is obviously not being applied at the appropriate level.

Knee and tibial relationship

The effect of treatment on the knee joint may, however, be useful in the treatment of medial genicular position or internal tibial torsion, both of which are causes of in-toeing. Medial genicular position occurs when the entire tibia is internally rotated at the knee joint. Internal tibial torsion, however, is caused by a lack of normal external rotation of the distal end of the tibia relative to the proximal end of the tibia.

The prognosis without treatment for medial genicular position has not been determined. It seems, however, that those children with no external rotation available at the knee joint tend to show little sign of spontaneous resolution by 5 years of age. Those with external motion available must be considered as being capable of walking straight but choosing, out of comfort or habit, not to.

Both medial genicular position and internal tibial torsion can be very successfully treated by above-knee serial casting. This intervention aims not to cause a bony rotation of the tibia but a rotation at the tibial–femoral interface which is then maintained by soft tissue adaptations within the knee joint.

Serial casting. In applying a plaster of Paris cast, the area should first be protected from irritation with a

pre-cast wrap of green line Tubifast covered by orthopaedic wool. The Tubifast should extend 10 inches beyond the distal ends of the toes and up as far as the groin. Special attention should be paid to protect the malleoli, extensor retinaculum, posteroplantar calcaneum and the dorsum of the toes. Double-thickness orthopaedic wool may be applied to those high pressure areas or alternatively silastic sheeting can be used.

The cast is applied as three cylinders, the first from the foot to just below the knee joint and the second around the thigh. When these are set hard, they are joined together by a third cylinder which encircles the knee. As the third cylinder of plaster sets, the knee is extended and the tibia rotated externally.

Once the limb has been protected, the first section of the cast is applied. Two 7.5 cm rolls of plaster of Paris are applied from the foot to the tibial tuberosity. Rather than smoothing out the end of each roll, the ends are turned over, forming a convenient tag (Fig. 15.28). In this way, the end of each roll can later be found and the plaster unravelled by the parents. While the first section of the cast is drying, the foot is held at 90° to the leg to prevent any accommodative shortening of the triceps surae muscle group. The rearfoot is also held in neutral or very slightly

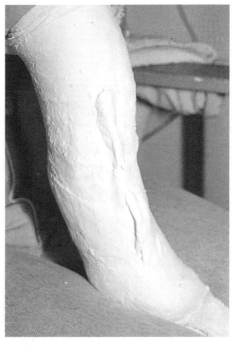

Figure 15.28 Above-knee plaster of Paris serial casting. The plaster tags allow parents to remove the cast.

supinated to prevent the foot adopting a pronated position. The second cylinder is then applied around the middle of the thigh. Once dry, the two sections of the cast are then connected by a third cylinder. Once this is applied, the tibia is externally rotated on the knee joint, the corrected position being maintained while the knee section of the cast dries.

Once the cast is complete, the ends of the Tubifast are pulled down over its proximal and distal edges. Sharp edges of the cast can be protected by the over-turned Tubifast; this can be assisted by placing an adult's sock over the cast to protect it further from damage with walking. The cast should be left in place for 1 week. The parents should be advised that if the child is overly distressed, they should not hesitate to remove it. The cast is removed by placing the child in a bath of warm water and soaking the plaster of Paris for at least 20 minutes. The tags at the end of each roll are then found and the rolls of plaster un-wound. Cutting the cast off with a cast cutter is not really appropriate for young children and should be avoided.

Three weeks of casting is usually sufficient to correct the in-toed gait, although another 3 weeks of casting is often employed to guard against recurrence. Use of the Dennis Browne bar and boots may also prevent recurrence, although many children will not tolerate having both feet secured by a single bar (Fig. 15.29). The counter-rotation system is better tole-rated because it allows independent movement of both legs and can also be used when the child is non-weight-bearing.

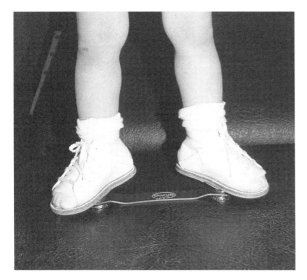

Figure 15.29 The Dennis Browne bar and boots.

Serial casting and counter-rotation devices can be employed to good effect in cases of inferopatellar in-toeing. Their value in the treatment of conditions originating above the knee is questionable, because it is difficult to achieve a corrective effect at this level. In suprapatellar in-toeing, gait plates and hamstring stretching forms the mainstay of intervention. The prognosis for most children with an abnormal angle of gait is good, with clear evidence that this devel-opmental problem is outgrown by the age of 6 to 8 years. However, if problems persist beyond 8 years of age, referral to an orthopaedic specialist to consider osteotomy of the tibia or femur is appropriate.

OUT-TOEING

Out-toeing or markedly abducted feet may also be a cause of parental concern because of cosmetic appearance and the apparent clumsiness. Causes of out-toeing include:

- external femoral position
- lateral genicular rotation
- external tibial torsion
- excessive subtalar joint pronation in the presence of a high subtalar joint axis.

All out-toeing will respond to orthotic treatment

Box 15.8 Case history: out-toeing

An 8-year-old boy attended clinic because his mother was very concerned about his 'Charlie Chaplin' style of walking and clumsiness. The mother claimed that the boy rarely participated in football because of an almost complete inability to run and kick a ball at the same time. The child walked with severely abducted feet. Both patellae, however, faced forwards, indicating that the origin of the abducted angle of gait was below the knee. On further examination it was found that the child had a lateral genicular position.

Gait plates were prescribed after taking plaster casts. Upon fitting the gait plates, the walking style improved immediately. The child assumed a reduction in the abducted angle of gait. The devices were worn constantly for 2 months. The anterior projection of the plate was then machined off to prevent the first metatarsophalangeal joint being adversely affected. The standard orthosis that remained continued to positively influence the child's gait.

One year later, the mother reported that the child was now participating in field sports; the only time she noted a return of the poor style of walking was when he walked along the side of a swimming pool. The child was reviewed every 6 months and orthotic treatment was continued until adolescence.

which seeks to supinate the foot and thus create adduction (see case history in Box 15.8). The forces which are to be resisted by the orthosis require very effective control of the foot—in particular, a deep heel seat of up to 40 mm and high medial flange are indicated. Shoes must be adequate to accommodate a high heel cup.

SUMMARY

Pain is not the only reason for consulting a practitioner. Abnormal foot shape may have the potential to progress and lead to pain in the future, and it is important that early developmental aberrations are recognised. Many of the locomotor problems affecting the child's leg and foot require long-term monitoring and some will require treatment. Few treatments lead to instant correction; most act as a medium to provide the right circumstances for normal development. It is with this in mind that treatment should only be provided where necessary.

In some cases, this chapter has reflected on problems that might not always fall to the practitioner specialising in feet. It would be inappropriate not to examine disease entities that could arise from a higher source other than the feet and cause confusion with a diagnosis. It would be expected, however, that any condition arising elsewhere would be referred to the appropriate specialist, as not all problems are amenable to orthotic management. Treatment that is provided should have clear goals and measurable objectives.

REFERENCES

Becker-Anderson H, Reimann I 1974 Congenital vertical talus. Reevaluation of early manipulation treatment. Acta Orthopaedica Scandinavica 45: 130

Berg E E 1986 A reappraisal of metatarsus adductus and skew foot. Journal of Bone & Joint Surgery 68-A: 1185–1196

Bunney M 1983 Viral warts. Churchill Livingstone, Edinburgh

Clark M W, D'Ambrosia R D, Ferguson A B 1977 Congenital vertical talus. Journal of Bone & Joint Surgery 59-A: 816

D'Amico J C, Rubin M 1986 The influence of foot orthoses on the quadraceps angle. Journal of the American Podiatric Association 76: 337–340

Fabry G, McEwan G D, Shands A R 1973 Torsion of the femur (A follow-up in normal and abnormal conditions) Journal of Bone & Joint Surgery 55-A: 1726–1738

Ferguson A B, Gingrich R M 1957 The normal and abnormal calcaneal apophysis and tarsal navicular. Clinical Orthopaedics 10: 87–95

Fox T A 1975 Dysplasia of the quadraceps mechanism. Surgical Clinics of North America 55: 199–225

Gauthier G, Elbaz R 1979 Freiberg's infraction; a subchondral bone fatigue fracture. A new surgical treatment. Clinical Orthopaedic and Related Research 142: 93–95

Groisso J A 1992 Juvenile hallux valgus. A conservative approach to treatment. Journal of Bone & Joint Surgery 74-A: 1367–1374

Hamer A J, Stanley D, Smith T W D 1993 Surgery for curly toe deformity; A double blind randomised prospective trial. Journal of Bone & Joint Surgery 75-B: 662–663

Hardy R H, Clapham J C R 1951 Observations on hallux valgus based on a controlled series. Journal of Bone & Joint Surgery 33-B: 376–391

Hilyard A 1990 Recent developments in the management of patellofemoral pain: The McConnell programme. Physiotherapy 76: 559–565

Kilmartin T E, Wallace W A 1992 The significance of pes planus in juvenile hallux valgus. Foot & Ankle 13: 53–56

Kilmartin T E, Wallace W A, Hill T W 1991 First metatarsal position in juvenile hallux abducto-valgus – a significant clinical measurement? Journal of British Podiatric Medicine 46: 43–45

Kilmartin T E, Barrington R L, Wallace W A 1994 A controlled prospective trial of a biomechanical orthosis in the treatment of juvenile hallux valgus. Journal of Bone & Joint Surgery 76-B(2): 210–215

Kite J H 1950 Congenital metatarsus varus. Journal of Bone & Joint Surgery 32-A: 500–506

Lodwick D, Tollafield D R, Cairns J 1995 Laboratory tests. In: Merriman L M, Tollafield D R (eds) Assessment of the lower limb. Churchill Livingstone, Edinburgh, ch 13, p 311

McPoil T, Cameron J, Adrian M 1987 Anatomical characteristics of the talus in relation to forefoot deformities. Journal of the American Podiatric Medical Association 77: 77–81

Mereday C, Dolan C, Lusskin R 1972 Evaluation of the University of California biomechanics laboratory shoe insert in "flexible" pes planus. Clinical Orthopaedic and Related Research 82: 46–57

Mosier K M, Asher M 1984 Tarsal coalitions and peroneal spastic flat foot. Journal of Bone & Joint Surgery 66-A: 976–984

Penneau K, Lutter L, Winter R 1982 Pes planus: radiographic changes with foot orthoses and shoes. Foot & Ankle 2: 229–303

Pentz A S, Weiner D S 1993 Management of metatarsus adductovarus. Foot & Ankle 14: 241–246

Ponsetti I V, Becker J R 1966 Congenital metatarsus adductus, the results of treatment. Journal of Bone & Joint Surgery 48-A: 702–711

Rose G K 1958 Correction of the pronated foot. Journal of Bone & Joint Surgery 40-B: 674–683

Rose G K 1962 Correction of the pronated foot. Journal of Bone & Joint Surgery 44-B: 642–647

Rose G K, Welton E A, Marshall T 1985 The diagnosis of flat foot in the child. Journal of Bone & Joint Surgery 67-B: 71–78

Ross E R S, Menelaus M B 1984 Open flexor tenotomy for

hammer toes and curly toes in childhood. Journal of Bone & Joint Surgery 66-B: 770–771

Rushforth G F 1978 The natural history of the hooked forefoot. Journal of Bone & Joint Surgery 60-B: 530–532

Smillie I S 1967 Treatment of Frieberg's Infraction. Proceedings of the Royal Society of Medicine 60: 29–31

Smith T W D, Stanley D, Rowley D I 1991 Treatment of Freiberg's disease. A new operative technique. Journal of Bone & Joint Surgery 73-B(1): 129–130

Staheli L T, Chew D E, Corbett M 1987 The longitudinal arch. Journal of Bone & Joint Surgery 69-A: 426–428

Svenningsen S, Tierjesen T, Auflem M 1990 Hip rotation and intoeing gait. Clinical Orthopaedic and Related Research 252: 177–182

Tachdjian M O 1972 Pediatric orthopaedics. Saunders, Philadelphia, vol 1, p 410–421

Tachdjian M O 1985 The child's foot. Saunders, Philadelphia, p 556–557

Thomson S A 1960 Hallux varus and metatarsus varus. Clinical Orthopaedics 16: 109–111

Tollafield D R 1979 Disinfection in chiropody, a two part study. Northamptonshire Area Health Authority

Tollafield D R 1993 Freiberg's infraction: surgical management by osteotomy; a forgotten technique? British Journal of Podiatric Medicine & Surgery 5(2): 2–5

Tollafield D R, Pratt D J 1990 The control of known triplanar forces on the foot by forefoot orthotic posting. British Journal of Podiatric Medicine & Surgery 2: 3–5

Wenger D R, Mauldin D, Speck G 1989 Corrective shoes and inserts as treatment for flexible flat foot in infants and children. Journal of Bone & Joint Surgery 71-A: 800–810

Wynne-Davies R 1964 Family studies and the cause of congenital clubfoot, talipes equino-varus, talipes calcaneo valgus and metatarsus varus. Journal of Bone & Joint Surgery 46-B: 445–456

FURTHER READING

Kite J H 1967 Congenital metatarsus varus. Journal of Bone & Joint Surgery 49-A: 338–397

Romanowski C A, Barrington N A 1991 The accessory ossicles of the foot. The Foot 2: 61–70

16

Sports injuries

T. D. Prior
D. R. Tollafield

INTRODUCTION

In recent years there has been a general increase in the number of people participating in sport for recreation, leading to a subsequent increase in sports injuries. Improved knowledge of injuries and greater public awareness have led to a large number of centres and clinics specialising in the treatment of these conditions. Many disciplines are involved with sports injuries, of which a significant proportion relate to the lower limb. This has resulted in greater collaboration and sharing of knowledge between health professionals.

This chapter will look at managing some of the common 'wear and tear' problems affecting sports performance. A single chapter cannot purport to contain all the mechanisms of sports pathology, and so this chapter emphasises common foot injuries. Inevitably, there will be some overlap between this and other chapters of the book, as some conditions are common to different client groups.

An orderly approach to management should be taken. The treatment plan is designed to suit the type of pathology, whether chronic or acute. Surgery and drugs have a minimal role in the plan—surgery causes unspecified periods of disablement, while drugs are even less popular, partly because of stringent blood testing. For the most part, the practitioner will attempt to use treatment methods that combine the principles of rest, stabilisation, manipulation, mechanical and physical therapies.

TREATMENT AND TRAINING REGIME
Defining fitness

The healthy, fit athlete provides the practitioner with a paradox—although the athelete may appear fit, abnormal mechanical factors may still affect sports performance.

Fitness forms an essential part of the assessment 'chain'. Without fitness, injuries and pathology are more likely to occur. When treating the sportsperson, attention must be paid to both biomechanical and physiological function. Fitness does not rely on being healthy alone. The athlete may be physiologically sound and yet have a mechanical problem. For example, a sportsperson might have a limb length discrepancy. The limb length discrepancy does not always require managing. While the practitioner will recognise that this structural abnormality exists, the sportsperson might nevertheless be able to perform adequately. The practitioner's skill lies in determining when to treat and when to leave alone.

Compensation can arise within the musculoskeletal system for some types of dysfunction; limb length discrepancy is one example. The long-standing limb length discrepancy may be inappropriate for treatment because of the possibility of introducing a new condition. Prevention of compensation in the first place might be appropriate where such compensation is functional. Simply put, functional adaption may arise in part of the body to create stability elsewhere. However, stabilising the pronated foot in the case of a forefoot varus is better than allowing a functional limb length discrepancy to arise. The leg shortens on the side of the pronated foot.

Individuals can function with small compensations; however, when an injury due to direct trauma or overuse arises, direct treatment is required to offset problems due to poor healing. Because sportspeople use their anatomy beyond the usual ranges of the average person, the tolerance adopted by the tissue of the body has to be greater. Examination of the whole musculoskeletal system is necessary to avoid omitting abnormal mechanical faults.

Physiological ageing reduces the body's resilience to fend off insult, especially in the absence of training. If a motor car is pushed beyond its usual requirements, having functioned well without problems for years, components start to wear. The knock-on effect of strain on other components can lead to further unreliable episodes. The sportsperson must not only be aware of the mechanism, but must also know how to maintain each component for reliable function. Good muscle strength and flexibility, adequate joint motion and proprioception will also be required to maintain a healthy fit body.

Aids to diagnosis

Taking a history is essential and forms a prerequisite to diagnosis—this has been dealt with elsewhere (Merriman & Tollafield 1995). Investigations should be undertaken to clarify a problem that has an unclear origin.

Gait analysis is particularly useful, assisting the practitioner not only in the process of determining a diagnosis but also in providing re-education. Video playback can provide the runner with visual evidence of any potentially faulty running styles that might lead to pathology. Video replay can be used to analyse patients with and without shoes, and with and without an orthosis, as well as to determine the efficiency of old and new footwear. Another useful feature of video recording of gait lies in the evaluation of orthotic control. *Control* is a term applied to minimising inappropriate frontal and transverse plane motion, usually identified in the hindfoot. The forefoot is influenced by hindfoot instability and many patients will find orthotic management beneficial.

The effect that the shoe has on mechanical function can be assessed by looking at the frontal plane angle between the heel counter and the leg during running. The posterior aspect of the lower third of the leg can be bisected with a marker pen. The shoe can be marked with the patient shod by placing a coloured strip to coincide with the calcaneus. The eversion or inversion angle of the shoe to leg can be measured from video replay on the screen at the point of maximum pronation.

Many other appropriate diagnostic aids, such as Doppler flow, X-rays and blood tests, can be used to assess medical problems in sportspeople in a similar way to other patient groups. This chapter assumes that the physiology of the patient is normal.

Restoration of function is based upon the practitioner's subjective or objective assessment of the problem and on preventing prolonged or further injury. Factors associated with dysfunction may have an intrinsic or extrinsic origin. Intrinsic problems may be confined to local tissue repair, inflexibility around joints, diminished muscle strength and proprioception affecting joints (ligaments). Extrinsic problems are associated with the manifestation of increased forces that disadvantage the efficiency of foot and lower limb function. The practitioner is concerned with the cause of abnormal forces associated with stress and strain. Footwear and orthoses play a large part in diminishing the adverse effects to a level where performance in a particular sport can be restored. Exercises to strengthen muscles that are weak must consider the patient's general state of flexibility. A sportsperson with unyielding connective tissue would have to maintain a higher awareness of stretch and warm-up technique than those who were more flexible.

The most common group of foot problems associated with dysfunction arise from abnormal pronation and supination. Pronation creates abnormal torque (twisting forces) through the knee, as well as straining the foot and ankle. Many higher problems in the leg, the hip and sacroiliac joint may arise from foot instability resulting from abnormal pronation. Supination reduces natural shock attenuation through the body, and adverse effects can arise in the knee and hip as in pronation.

Tissue repair

Local treatment to the foot will depend upon the type of inflammation present (Table 16.1). All sports injuries involve acute or chronic inflammation. As a result, the management of these conditions follows the same pattern, according to the structure involved and the extent of injury. It should be remembered that all tissues have a predetermined healing rate which cannot be altered and that treatment aims to promote this process. Figure 16.1 outlines the phases of inflammation (Evans 1980). As chronic conditions involve all the stages of inflammation simultaneously, a number of modalities should be employed together. Many of the physical modalities have been described in Chapter 9, although orthoses, medication and surgery may have a part to play in rehabilitation.

Flexibility and strength

Inflexibility of muscles and ligaments prevents normal joint motion and will decrease the available shock absorption through the foot. Such a dysfunction creates stress within the joint and associated structures. Similarly, muscle weakness prevents normal function, creates muscle imbalance and exposes the foot and ankle to injury. Whether inflexibility or weakness occurs, each will aggravate the other, establishing a vicious circle which delays return to pain-free activity. The injured athlete must therefore have any inflexibility or weakness addressed as part of rehabilitation in order to resolve the problem and prevent any recurrence.

There are several methods of assessing muscle strength. Active assessment involves resisted movement against the practitioner. Alternatively, there are various forms of *isokinetic* testing machines which provide a computerised quantitative assessment. However, these machines are expensive and will not be considered further, but it should be noted that they do offer a quantitative method of illustrating improvement following injury, and as such are a potential tool for determining treatment effectiveness.

Stretching of muscle tendons should commence during the rehabilitation period and continue when the athlete returns to activity. When exercising, warm-up and warm-down periods are essential to prevent further injury.

Proprioception is associated with autonomic awareness of position or movement change. Injury and trauma, particularly affecting joints, can reduce the level of proprioception. A good example of this occurs with lateral ankle sprain. Trauma to the stretch receptors within the joint structure may lead to further injury. By re-educating the musculature around the

Table 16.1 Aims and methods of treating inflammation

Phase	Treatment	Aim
Injury/inflammation	Rest	Prevent further damage. Bone injuries require immobilisation to promote alignment; 6–8 weeks required
	Ice	Constrict arteriolar capillaries, reducing local blood pressure and thus decreasing haemorrhage and inflammatory exudate. This will reduce fibrosis
	Compression	Increase tissue pressure and thus reduce swelling
	Elevation	Decrease local blood pressure, thus reducing haemorrhage. Increase lymphatic and venous drainage to limit oedema and pain
	Gentle movement	Gentle muscle contraction will increase venous and lymphatic drainage
	Drugs	Non-steroid anti-inflammatory tablets can interfere with the chemical mediators in the acute inflammatory phase
Repair	Heat	Increase local blood supply to encourage healing
	Ultrasound	Similar to heat action; improves fibroblastic repair
	Movement	Normal movement encourages natural tension in healing tissue to promote strength

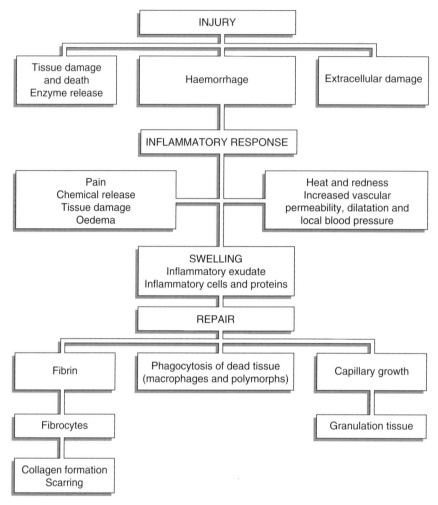

Figure 16.1   The phases of inflammation.

ankle joint, improved balance can be obtained, hence improving joint protection.

A simple test to determine proprioceptive function involves the patient standing on the affected foot. If the patient can do this comfortably for 30–60 seconds, the exercise should be repeated with eyes closed. The examination should include standing on tiptoes, and finally tiptoes with eyes closed. Poor proprioceptive control can be managed by a 'wobble board'. The wobble board is a flat surface with a central pivot such as a half circle about which the board will tip randomly. The patient stands on the board and tries to balance with both feet placed on either side of the pivot centre. The objective of the exercise is to move the board to the four compass points in a controlled manner. Balancing on one foot can be initiated when

this is successfully achieved. The wobble board is particularly valuable for re-educating ankle and knee weakness. In the case of the knee, a small trampoline can be used as an adjunct to the wobble board.

Flexibility exercises may include two main techniques: passive static stretching and proprioceptive neuromuscular facilitation.

Passive static stretching. This technique can be performed without special equipment. The muscle is placed under gradual tension until a pulling sensation is experienced. The muscle is then held for 15–30 seconds. When the stretch is being performed, sudden jerky movements or bouncing (ballistics) should be avoided. Figure 16.2 shows examples of common stretches employed for the lower limb.

Proprioceptive neuromuscular facilitation. Although

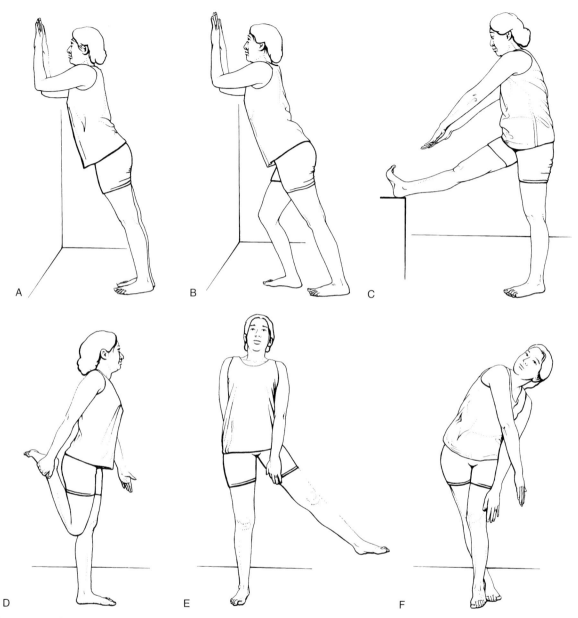

Figure 16.2 Common exercises used to increase muscle flexibility should be held for 20–30 seconds. These exercises should be performed before and after sporting activity (warm-up and warm-down). A: A gastrocnemius stretch. If the foot is allowed to pronate, the plantar fascia will also be stretched. If pronation is prevented, a more effective stretch is placed on the muscle. B: A soleus stretch. C: A hamstring stretch. Care should be taken to avoid bending the spine with forward movement from the waist. This exercise can be performed by lying on the floor, placing the leg up against the wall, thus protecting the spine. D: A quadriceps stretch. The pelvis should be pushed forwards while the leg is pulled backwards. E: An adductor stretch. F: An iliotibial band stretch.

this is not just a stretching technique, the flexibility of the muscle can be increased (Norris 1993). It incorporates active contraction of the muscle whilst in the stretch position against resistance for 5–8 seconds; this is followed by relaxation and further stretching of the muscle for 15–30 seconds. Proprioceptive neuromuscular facilitation using resistance and stretch can be achieved either passively, with an assistant, or actively.

Specific muscle groups

The two main muscle groups that have the most significant effect on lower limb function are the hamstrings and gastro-soleus (triceps surae) muscles. Straight leg raises (SLR), often known as the 90:90 test, provide an indication of hamstring tension as well as knee extension. The expected range of knee extension is 170° with the hip flexed, although 155°–160° is a more realistic target. The posterior calf muscles may be assessed similarly by ankle dorsiflexion. When examining the ankle for foot dorsiflexion, the subtalar joint (STJ) is placed in neutral with the foot at right angles to the leg and the knee extended and flexed appropriately. It is important not to obtain false dorsiflexion by including additional subtalar pronation. The values vary with the position of the knee: 10° of foot dorsiflexion beyond right angles, with the knee extended, including stretch on the posterior group with gastrocnemius influence, and 20° of foot dorsiflexion with the knee flexed excluding the gastrocnemius.

Inflexibility due to any reluctance of the hamstrings to stretch appropriately can influence the balance between knee flexion and foot dorsiflexion. Increased knee flexion during activity will not only cause greater ankle dorsiflexion but will also increase the pronatory force on the foot. Similarly, tightness of the medial or lateral hamstrings can influence the position of the leg, promoting an internal or external rotary bias, respectively. This bias can affect foot function by creating additional pronation at an inappropriate point during stance. In addition, inflexibility may stress the lower back by causing a posterior rotation of the pelvis.

Gastro-soleus inflexibility can be compensated abnormally by increased knee flexion or hyperextension (genu recurvatum), an early heel lift or increased foot pronation. An alternative method used to examine and consequently stretch this muscle group is to use an inclined slope.

In order for a muscle to function effectively, it must have sufficient power, strength and endurance for the activity required. Power and strength allow the muscle to support and overcome the forces required of it; endurance allows this to continue for the duration of the sporting activity. Muscles should be assessed with a graduated strengthening regime. With regard to knee injuries, particular attention should be paid to the quadriceps and hamstrings, whilst foot conditions involve all the extrinsic muscles of the lower limb.

Where the subtalar/ankle joint is otherwise normal, the excursions of inversion and eversion of the foot can often be inhibited by reduced muscle strength and endurance. If the muscles are weak, there is little hope that they can support the forces acting through them. Alternatively, the muscle may have sufficient strength but may be unable to continue the activity for a sustained period of exercise. Failure of either strength or endurance results in a loss of intrinsic support and stability. Soft tissues, joints and bone may be exposed to increased stress, resulting in inflammation, fractures, skin pressure and progressive deformity. There is little hope that an orthosis will provide effective assistance where muscles function abnormally.

Use of exercises

Sports enthusiasts will find that different activities use different muscles and therefore switching activities requires muscles to be re-educated, first, to enable safe continuation in that sport. The older enthusiast will find this harder than a teenager. The most popular method of strengthening muscles and increasing their tone is by the use of weight-training machines which are available at reputable clubs. Free (unattached) weights should be avoided as an injury may occur if the weight is too large. The muscles responsible for inversion, eversion, plantarflexion and dorsiflexion can be exercised by means of a length of elasticated rubber. There are commercially available varieties (Cliniband and Theraband) or, alternatively, a bicycle inner tube can be used. Figure 16.3 demonstrates the technique to be used for these exercises (band not shown).

Certain movements such as hopping and jumping require a muscle/tendon to be stretched and then contracted powerfully in a short period of time. This stretch–shortening cycle is known as plyometric exercise. In addition to the above strengthening exercises, plyometric exercises (Albert 1991) should be included where necessary. Achilles and patellar tendon exercises are particularly involved in this movement. Strengthening and re-education of muscles can begin initially with specialised weight machines; the weights are gradually increased. Following this, hopping exercises, in both forward and backward directions, straight lines and zig-zags, can be performed to improve proprioception. These exercises should not be commenced, however, until sufficient strength and endurance have been established.

Adverse neural tension. Although not a common phenomenon, adverse neural tension (ANT) is a recent development in physiotherapy (Butler & Gifford 1989) and should be considered within the context

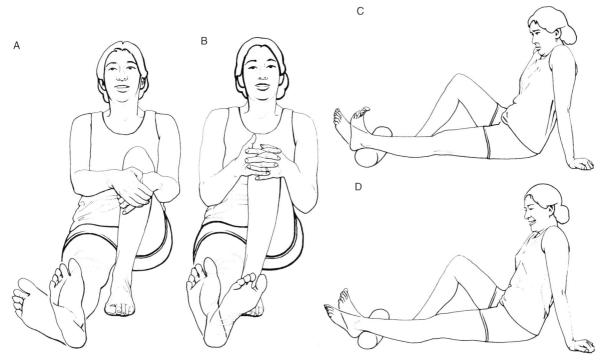

Figure 16.3 Cliniband strengthening exercises (band not shown). The band is attached to the foot which is then moved against the tension. A: Eversion/abduction. B: Inversion/adduction. C: Dorsiflexion. D: Plantar flexion of the foot. The leg should be straight and the ankle placed on a small cushion to allow movement.

Instructions. Care should be taken to move only the foot and not the leg. A 6 foot length should be tied into a loop and anchored around something solid. The patient then performs 20 repetitions on a light stretch, 15 on a medium stretch, and 10 on a strong stretch for endurance, strength and power, respectively. Each circuit should be repeated three times, with exercise performed three times per week. This will not be possible initially, but once it is achieved with the high strength band, a further increase in strength is unlikely.

of flexibility. Misdiagnosis may result in the failure of any strategies to assist the patient with ANT. ANT is a syndrome in which there is mechanical restriction of extraneural origin, or physiological damage to the nerve associated with an intraneural origin along the spinal or soft tissue route of the nerve. When this occurs, normal function is limited and pain can result. Neural tension can explain muscle inflexibility or leg and foot pains that have peculiar presenting symptoms. By stressing the neural pathway, as in Figure 16.4, adverse neural tension (ANT) can be assessed. However, when conducting this manoeuvre, great care should be taken to prevent damage to the spine. Patients can suffer from considerable distal discomfort, without any significant spinal symptoms, yet still have adverse neural tension. Suspicion of this condition should warrant an appropriate referral to a physiotherapist or osteopath for a more thorough examination.

Activity levels after injury

Educating the sportsperson to return to sport following an injury is essential to prevent early repetition of the same problem. A training regime will include monitoring sports activity, careful selection of running surfaces and balancing the direction of track running. In the latter case, surface camber can affect the symmetry of shoe wear. The number of hours of activity will have to be recorded to ensure that only a measured amount is permitted. A 30% increase in activity might be allowed every 2 weeks. Swimming, running in water with a buoyancy aide, or cycling can maintain fitness levels by preventing muscle atrophy while minimising compression load on joints. Alternation between the different activities often provides the best training programme. Any activity level should be based on the degree of pain present. An example is outlined in Figure 16.5, emphasising rest, walking

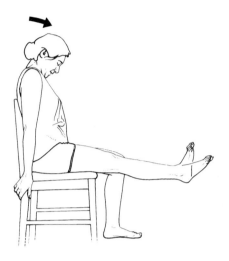

Figure 16.4 This demonstrates a *slump test*. The practitioner asks the patient to slouch at the waist and put their head on their chest. The practitioner then extends the knee and dorsiflexes the foot. If symptoms are reproduced, and relaxation of the foot or extension of the neck changes the symptoms, the test is positive. Internal or external rotation of the leg at full stretch may illicit symptoms, as may gentle downward pressure on the shoulders.

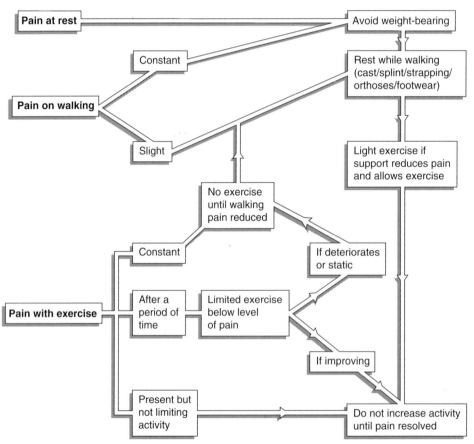

Figure 16.5 A structured approach to planning activity level based on the level of pain experienced. Treatment may be implemented or continued at all stages.

and exercise within the planned return to activity. An increase in activity level prior to the restoration of satisfactory intrinsic and extrinsic function is not advisable. Footwear selection forms an essential part of education. Although footwear in general has already been covered in Chapter 13, the wide variety of sports footwear requires further comment.

Footwear and sports

The evaluation and treatment of any foot condition should include examining the type of footwear worn by the patient. When assessing the athlete, the practitioner must consider the suitability of footwear worn for different activities. Practitioners have experienced treating injured athletes who have tried to run a marathon in a cheap pair of tennis shoes.

Evaluating footwear

Shoe construction should be checked in general, noting a few essential anatomical points in shoe design. Whilst it is difficult to generalise about which shoes to advise, many practitioners like to compile a list of shoes that they regularly suggest to patients. Selection is based upon assessing the components of the shoe and robustness of design seen from wear patterns.

The design of the shoe should be checked for any factors that may lead to an injury. The heel flare and heel tabs must be examined to rule out potential heel tendon irritation. The upper of the shoe can often be set incorrectly on the sole (Fig. 16.6). If a poor quality shoe is detected, the patient should return the shoe unworn to the shop. The amount of torsion (twist) within a shoe created by inversion and eversion of the sole is important. A shoe with marked inversion and eversion movement within its structure is unlikely to control a foot with excessive motion.

When checking shoes that have been worn for a period of time, the upper, insole, midsole and outer-sole should be examined for signs of wear. Evidence of deformity in the upper, midsole collapse, insole destruction, compression, cracking or excessive sole wear will indicate that the shoe has come to the end of its natural life. In extreme examples, patients can be found to wear a deformity into their trainers; one common effect is to produce a varus position (Fig. 16.7). Injury can occur when a new pair of shoes is used resulting in an altered adverse gait. If the sole or the upper of the shoe provides insufficient support, the shoe may show signs of medial deformation, suggesting abnormal pronation. An antipronator shoe that controls this force should be appropriate.

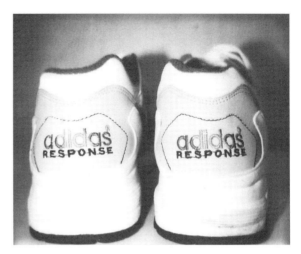

Figure 16.6 This demonstrates poor quality control during shoe construction. Note how the upper of the right shoe has been placed in a pronated (everted) position on the sole. This is demonstrated by the angle of the lettering which is in the same direction for both shoes.

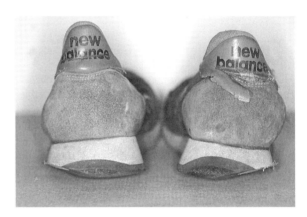

Figure 16.7 A pair of severely worn shoes taken from a runner. The heel is worn into a varus position. The runner developed an injury when new shoes were obtained.

Sizing and fitting

It is easy to forget to check the adequacy of fit of the shoe when treating an athlete. Adults frequently have not had their feet re-measured since they were children, and have subsequently bought the same size shoe for years thinking that size does not alter. It is not uncommon for an adult to think that it is perfectly normal for the hallux to 'jam' against the upper of the shoe—the indent in the toe box easy to spot.

The shoe should be long enough to allow adequate room between the longest digit and the end of the shoe. As a rule-of-thumb, there should be one finger's width between these two points. The toe box should represent the shape of the forefoot and provide sufficient room at the ends of the toes to prevent trauma.

The widest part of the foot is usually the metatarsophalangeal joint (MTPJ) line, which should correspond with the widest part of the shoe and will ensure that the toe break of the shoe coincides with the foot. This may be checked by asking the patient to go onto tiptoe and ensuring that the toe break and foot coincide. If this does not happen, metatarsalgia may develop.

Laces

A correctly fitted shoe should not have the lace eyelets touching centrally. This would indicate that the shoe is too broad for the foot. If this occurs, or is unavoidable, addition of soft padded material to the tongue of the shoe will provide a better shoe fit. A shoe that is too narrow will have a large gap between the lace eyelets. As a rule-of-thumb (or finger perhaps), there should be approximately one finger's width between the eyelets.

Footwear adaption

Modifying footwear alone can improve symptoms. Considerable discussion regarding modification has already been presented in Chapter 13.

Insoles

The insole of the shoe often plays an insignificant role in the control of foot function, although some include a valgus filler to improve wear comfort. Many insoles are removable, allowing either the addition of materials or replacement with an orthosis to improve foot control.

Running shoes

The wide assortment of styles, shapes and designs is bewildering. To add to the selection difficulty, many manufacturers discontinue lines on a regular basis; this means that a runner who has found a good pair of shoes has to start all over again. For those experienced in treating runners, it is not uncommon to find patients who have bought several pairs of shoes, at considerable expense, in an attempt to find one suitable pair. An awareness of the principles involved will assist the practitioner far more than committing each shoe design to memory. Some guided advice can be invaluable to the patient. One source of help is *Runners' world* magazine, which prints an assessment of the differing running shoes available on the market every April. This will at least provide the practitioner with an initial basis for selection. Table 16.2 describes the effect of each shoe component on function (Anthony 1987, Heil 1992).

Racing shoes and spikes

These shoes are light-weight so as to promote increased speed and minimal energy expenditure. The use of lighter materials will subsequently reduce the degree of control and shock absorption. Sharp spikes are used to produce maximum ground purchase in the forefoot region, as this part of the foot maintains greatest ground contact. Most spikes offer little control of the foot, but a small degree of in-built heel raise is useful for when heel contact does occur.

Hockey/football

One major problem with hockey and football boots relates to the flat sole construction with no heel raise. Although heel strike occurs less frequently in these sprinting sports, some manufacturers now produce shoes that incorporate a heel. Additionally, a rigid sole can be a problem, as these shoes may place an increased stress on the Achilles tendon as the foot fails to flex the sole of the shoe across the metatarsal break point (see case history in Box 16.1).

The length of studs worn by players may also influence injury patterns. A wet, soft surface requires longer studs to maintain adequate ground purchase. Insufficient grip increases the risk of injury as the player has less stability. On firmer ground, shorter studs should be worn. Studs can either predispose players to joint injuries, due to too much purchase as the player twists on a firmly planted foot, or reduce ground contact if the short stud results in slippage. Moulded soles and shoes are generally more appropriate for artificial surfaces, but unfortunately the shock-absorbing properties required from shoes on harder terrain are either absent or insufficient.

Box 16.1 Case history: rigid soles

A female hockey player, while responding to treatment for recurrent Achilles tendinitis, re-injured herself, despite careful training, whenever she played. Examination of her match shoe revealed a rigid sole, and treatment simply consisted of shoe advice, changing to a flexible design.

Table 16.2 Components of the running shoe and the effect on function

Shoe section	Function	Comments
Upper	Supports the foot within the shoe	A firm upper is required to control abnormal foot function. Leather is firm but heavy. Lycra is lighter but has no support. Mixed synthetics are best
Heel counter	Supports the calcaneus	Weak materials deform easily and provide little support. A firm heel counter is recommended
Heel tab	Support and pulling on shoe	High heel tabs can cause trauma and injury to the tendo Achilles. Remove tab
Midsole	Strength and shock absorption	Can be one or composite materials. Higher density will increase control and lower density decreases shock impulse
Varus wedge	Rearfoot control	Located at the medial rearfoot. Density varies to achieve best supportive position
Heel flare	Stability	Heels are commonly flared to increase surface contact and increase pronation speed. One adverse effect causes increase of lever arm and may require grinding down on lateral side
Outsole	Contact, strength and grip	To provide light composition, materials are carbon or blown rubber
Ripple tread Waffle tread		Linked to less injuries. Design may attract dirt and increase weight of shoe
Straight		Traditionally for pronated foot
Semi-curved		Traditionally for supinated foot or faster runners
Upper/sole attachment Slip lasted	Allows motion, shock absorption provided	Upper stitched to the sole. Reduces control and softer base tends to wear more than others
Combination lasted	Good rearfoot versus poor forefoot control	Rigid board stitched into rearfoot, forefoot slip lasted. Rigid base for orthoses at rearfoot, but soft forefoot is susceptible to wear
Board lasted	Good control, reduced flexibility	Rigid board throughout glued to the upper and stitched to the sole. While this is the best base for orthoses, weight is increased

Tennis and squash shoes

These require sturdier upper and sole components. The shoe must be able to withstand the multidirectional turning and pivoting involved in these activities. An ideal shoe is one that provides hindfoot stability and cushioning. Orthoses can improve adverse instability and may help to reduce high levels of friction placed on the forefoot.

Aerobic shoes

The popularity of aerobic exercise has resulted in a whole spate of previously unrecognised foot injuries. The classic aerobic shoe is more akin to an ankle boot which aims to reduce the risk of ankle sprains.

However, this also reduces ankle function, subsequently affecting foot and leg function. The development of aerobic shoes has not yet progressed to the same state of high technology as running shoes. Some manufacturers have made an attempt to provide shock absorption and hindfoot foot stability; those shoes that do not have these attributes can lead to a greater incidence of overuse injuries. The patient should be advised of the increased risk of ankle sprain and should change to a good running shoe for this activity.

Ski boots

The basic aim of ski boots is to provide rigid support around the ankle whilst allowing a degree of sagittal plane motion. Many ski boots are angled in this plane with a spring-loading mechanism to allow active dorsiflexion of the leg over the foot. If there is an underlying equinus abnormality, or the angle and tension of the boot is too high, compensation of the foot in the boot can occur. Such compensation for equinus arises at the STJ or MTJ, although the knee can also be forced into hyperextension. Subsequent foot pathology is brought about by twisting of the foot against a non-resilient material. Whilst exercises to stretch the tendo Achilles and orthoses may be considered, adjustment of the boot is indicated. Control of excessive pronation within the boot can increase the efficiency of the skier when turning the skis, but this may increase the stress on the knees.

In conclusion, practitioners who ignore the patient's shoes do so at their peril. Attention to many of the simple principles can have great benefits and significantly assist treatment. However, the practitioner should always remember that the majority of manufacturers have commercial concerns and as such tend to cater for fashion and gimmicks rather than function alone.

Orthoses

Although much has already been written on orthoses and prescribing in previous chapters, further comment on this subject is required because of the specific needs of the sportsperson.

Control is a term frequently used with orthoses and represents the ideal outcome as a gain in foot stability. Control can refer to reduction of unwanted hindfoot movement. Most additional, unwanted motion arises by compensation. If this motion is not limited by orthoses or strapping, symptoms will arise. Table 16.3

illustrates the types of control that can be used in the form of clinical, stock and prescription orthoses.

When deciding on the type of orthosis to prescribe, factors that should be taken into account include financial implications, the level and type of activity performed, patient expectations and shoe fit. Many patients, having benefited from a temporary orthosis following an injury, may not require expensive orthoses. The same result can be achieved by using a stock orthosis. One has only to consider the number of athletes with unsatisfactory biomechanical alignment who do not suffer injury to realise that orthoses are not essential for all athletic performance! If, however, the injury does not fully respond to simple devices, or if it recurs, then more sophisticated orthoses may be required on a long-term basis to prevent constant replacement.

Evaluating the effectiveness of orthoses

The best way to evaluate the effect of orthoses on foot function is to strap the orthosis to the bare foot and video the patient exercising. While this is advantageous, the process is time-consuming. Unfortunately, at present, no method exists to assess orthoses within the shoe without computerised technology. The shoe-to-leg measurement is a useful indicator to show that the orthoses have reduced the speed of pronation and thus have decreased the stress to the limb (Fig. 16.8).

When examining the inside of the shoe, the indentations made into the insock by the distal orthotic edge should be evenly worn. Excessive medial indentation at one point suggests that pronation has not been sufficiently controlled; likewise, with a single point of lateral indentation, too much supination exists.

Table 16.3 Types of orthotic control

Orthotic type	Method	Advantage/disadvantage
Clinical (temporary)	Felt adhered to the foot or shoe allows benefit to be assessed	Inexpensive, short term only, 2–5 days
Soft (stock)	Synthetic rubbers (polyurethane) adhered to an insole base (e.g. Frelon)	Effective at low cost. Not moulded to shoe, possibly bulky
Preformed (stock)	Preformed moulded orthosis, e.g. AOL, Alpha and Multi balanced orthoses (variable clip-on wedges); control can be varied	Improved appearance, may be bulky, lasts longer than above, moderate cost
Casted prescription	Thermoplastic materials moulded to cast taken of foot. Requirements to a written prescription	Long-lasting, relatively expensive and has to be sent away to a laboratory. A pair for each activity may be necessary

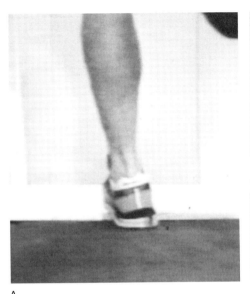
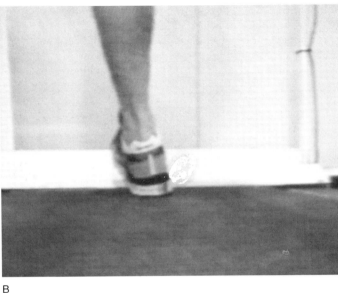

A   B

Figure 16.8   A: This demonstrates the compression of the lateral sole of the left shoe of a runner with an inverted calcaneus at heel strike. B: The addition of orthoses with a medial rearfoot post supports the deformity and therefore results in a more even distribution of sole compression.

Fitting problems. Because manufacturers use their own inserts, orthoses are not always easy to accommodate in sports footwear. Standard inserts should be removed and the patient should be told not to use the insert under or over the prescribed orthosis. Replacement orthoses may cause damage to the inner shoe because the materials used are harder than the manufacturer's soft polyethylene foamed inserts. The patient needs to give approval before embarking upon this alteration. Many orthoses, particularly those made from hard polypropylene and their modifications, can weigh as much as a modern light sports shoe. Newer lighter materials, such as carbon fibre, promise to overcome this problem. Practitioners need to be aware of the effects of this unwelcome weight gain, which will not be appreciated by the serious athlete.

The effects of orthoses on joints

Joint limitation. Experienced practitioners find that, despite following a clear programme of action using orthoses, not all patients will tolerate their prescription. In part, selection of a stock or temporary orthosis may alert the practitioner to predictable problems likely to be experienced later with prescription devices.

A patient with a small range of subtalar motion, for example, may notice the limiting effects of movement more than a patient with a larger range of motion. Material selection and sensible prescription modification are essential. One common complaint arises when the foot pronates against an orthosis causing rubbing and blistering of skin. The orthosis should be modified to provide greater flexibility from the material selected.

Some of the problems resulting from the use of orthoses arise at specific anatomical sites, such as the first ray, ankle and knee joints. Assessment prior to orthotic prescription must consider the suitability of each joint. A few points are worthy of discussion.

First ray. The position of the first ray should be carefully assessed. The first metatarsal has to be able to plantarflex in order that the metatarsophalangeal joint can dorsiflex during late stance. The position of the first metatarsal at this point in the gait cycle is different to the position observed when the foot is non-weight-bearing in neutral. As a result, an orthosis that simply balances the forefoot position compromises the position of the first ray. While this may not usually cause problems, it may aggravate injuries associated with the first ray such as in the case of flexor hallucis longus tendinitis. In addition, an orthosis places increased stresses onto the first metatarsophalangeal joint and further reduces the effectiveness of the peroneus longus tendon. The dynamic equilibrium between the invertors and evertors of the foot may be altered causing foot instability.

A common misconception involves the practitioner ordering a medial addition to the positive cast to increase first ray plantarflexion. This adaptation merely moves the orthosis away from the arch on the cast only to allow the foot to fall back on the plate when it is weight-bearing. The orthosis may need to have a first ray cut-out made to alter the point of contact beneath the second ray. Softer orthoses will limit the first ray less if used together with lower values of correction.

Ankle equinus. There are a number of problems that can arise following the dispensing of orthoses to patients with an ankle equinus. Orthoses designed from a neutrally balanced cast can create unwanted compensation—the heel will lift up out of the shoe, the foot will pronate off the orthotic plate, or the knee will hyperextend. The tendo Achilles will require stretching before a cast is taken, or it may need to be lengthened surgically.

Knee problems. Reduced compensation within the foot may well result in abnormal rotation at the knee. This problem occurred in a top class runner and is discussed in the case history in Box 16.2.

Effect at late stance. A large proportion of orthoses finish just behind the metatarsal heads. This design provides control particularly when the foot is in ground contact ('flat foot'). When the heel lifts as it does in sprinting, the control offered by an orthosis diminishes. In an attempt to improve control, orthoses can be extended onto the plantar aspect of the metatarsophalangeal joints or even to the digits.

Box 16.2 Case history: orthoses aggravate a knee injury

After a runner had been successfully treated with orthoses, a replacement pair appeared to aggravate a knee injury associated with attenuation of the anterior cruciate ligament. Pain was elicited in the knee when the patient was examined weight-bearing with the knee flexed. Pain increased when the patient was examined with the orthoses fitted.

Careful questioning revealed that a period of high intensity sprint training had preceded the problem. Posterior inflexibility was demonstrated.

The increased control provided by the new orthoses, combined with faulty training, had resulted in knee trauma. The symptoms associated with the new orthoses were repeated with a varus wedge placed under the whole foot. When the first ray was excluded, by placing a varus wedge under the rearfoot and the second to fifth metatarsals, the symptoms ceased immediately due to the increased motion allowed.

Specific treatment

Some discussion regarding other treatment interventions, such as surgery and drugs, has been included for completeness.

The management of sports problems with surgery

Where physical therapies fail to stabilise pathology, intervention using surgery may be appropriate. Urgent intervention using surgery should be considered in the case of fractures requiring open reduction to provide early mobility and restoration of function. Repair of ruptured tendons with an internal repair often provides a much faster rehabilitation and return of strength than rest and casting. Compartment syndrome should be dealt with early to avoid vascular complications. These procedures are used initially to prevent future problems. Surgery has a place in minor cases where the problem has a chronic nature. Surgery offers a rapid solution to some of these problems but the practitioner must bear in mind that surgery may produce an unacceptable delay in returning to sporting activities for most patients. Unless the athlete can be offered a quick resolution by surgery, this option is less favoured. The types of problem that can be resolved quickly are small painful lumps and bumps, such as mucoid cysts, fibromata, warts and corns. In the case of corns, underlying bone can be resected where a phalanx has a well established deformity. Arthroplasty/arthrodesis can offer some beneficial resolution to a fixed toe deformity. Surgical decisions should not be undertaken if they only address part of a problem. First ray surgery affecting the MTP joint may be inappropriate in a young patient if more extensive surgery is required later on to deal with the underlying cause. Problems that relate to toenails, such as onychocryptosis, expansive sub-

---

Box 16.3 Case history: surgery and therapy combined

An example of a combined conservative (mechanical) and surgical approach concerned a 16-year-old male with chronic knee problems. While orthoses provided by podiatry led to 75% improvement in recovery, with return to sporting activity, arthroscopy of the knee by an orthopaedic surgeon provided both diagnostic and surgical management which allowed full restoration of intrinsic function.

This case history illustrates the beneficial roles played by podiatry and orthopaedics as components of an example of multidisciplinary management.

ungual exostoses, recalcitrant intermetatarsal neuromata or a Freiberg's condition, should be managed more aggressively.

Combined therapy with surgery can often bear fruit, as illustrated in the case history in Box 16.3.

Surgical intervention is considered again briefly later on in this chapter, when specific conditions affecting the foot and lower leg are discussed.

Management of problems using drugs

The use of oral, injectable or cutaneously applied medication may have a place in treating the sportsperson. Usually, long-term use of drugs is undesirable and such management is best applied simultaneously with physical therapy and orthoses. The purpose of most medication for foot problems relates to managing pain and inflammation, although infection may occasionally arise in the foot, requiring antibiotics.

Injections of local anaesthesia and corticosteroid medications can provide direct reversal of pain and inflammation, respectively, to joints, soft tissue areas and paratenons. The use of local anaesthetic prior to some steroid injections reduces the discomfort of the injection. Many inflammatory problems can be reversed by using small doses (0.1–0.7 ml) to allow the body to continue the reparative process. Corticosteroids may have a short or long action—phosphates provide a shorter duration of action than acetates. When the frequent use of corticosteroids shows limited or no improvement, the practitioner would be better to use alternative therapies. If one to two injections fail to create a favourable response, it is unlikely that further injections will improve matters. In some cases, repeated injections may make the pain worse.

The use of corticosteroid injections to treat acute inflammation around tendons is controversial. A popular opinion suggests that a steroid injection around the tendon may cause degeneration, with an increased risk of subsequent rupture. Mahler (1992) concluded that steroid injection into the tendon of animals resulted in collagen necrosis, but little evidence has been gathered to support problems arising from injections into the paratenon. A retrospective study of 83 patients with tendo Achilles pain concluded that corticosteroid injections had a role to play in paratenon injuries (Read & Motto 1992). Cortisone injections have a role in the treatment of paratenon lesions, in that they reduce symptomatology, but do not necessarily provide an earlier return to match fitness (Read & Motto 1992). Currently, the practitioner must show caution with injudicious use of steroid injections around any powerful tendon.

Indications of injectable steroid use. These include synovitis, capsulitis, peritendinitis, bursae, neuroma, clonic joint spasm with a history of non-infective trauma (e.g. affecting the first MTPJ), painful arthritides where no other treatment is planned, and subtalar sinus tarsi pain syndrome.

Contraindications. In most cases, injectable steroids should not be injected into undiagnosed tumours or areas of infection, and should not be used repetitively into or around any tendon, intravascularly (except where indicated as specifically intended to reverse anaphylaxis) or over bony prominences. In the latter case, atrophy of the skin can arise and is difficult to reverse. Problems associated with such treatment may require surgery to excise reactive tissue. Unfortunately, in a small percentage of cases, unremitting 'flare-ups', and particularly small inclusions, necessitate surgical intervention.

Oral medication. Analgesic medication should be selected for its specific action, effectiveness and lack of side-effects. A good history should be taken before prescribing any drug, taking into consideration current medications and gastrointestinal problems first. The lowest available dose and frequency should be used initially.

NSAIDs form the main group of anti-inflammatory drugs and range from common acetyl salicylic acid (aspirin) and ibuprofen at one end of the anti-inflammatory spectrum, to diclofenac sodium and indomethacin as middle-band strength drugs. Other NSAIDs are described elsewhere, but strong NSAIDS should be reserved for systemic disease. The dual analgesic/anti-inflammatory action forms a valuable management tool, but side effects from long-term use should be avoided. Drugs are not alternatives to rest and good rehabilitation.

Paracetamol (acetaminophen) and codeine compound drugs are best used for pain following injury, from minor strains to stress fractures. The moderate to severe categories of pain drugs will usually include opioids (>15 mg codeine), which should be used appropriately and, again, only for limited periods.

Infection should be controlled with systemic antibiotics only where an organism has been identified first or where systemic changes are noted or localised spread is evident in the form of cellulitis. Principal treatment should always include rest, elevation and drainage of the wound first. Good wound protection and antiseptics such as chlorhexidine and cetrimide should be used more frequently to avoid blind use of broad-spectrum antibiotics. Before prescribing any drug, as much diagnostic evidence should be gathered as possible.

INJURIES AND PATHOLOGY RELATED TO SPORT

Most conditions affecting sportspersons relate to overuse problems rather than acute injuries, typified by open fractures, torn ligaments, tendons and infections. For the most part the acute problem finds its way to the accident and emergency department of a hospital rather than the consulting room.

The 'acute' forms of sports injury requires discussion in more detail elsewhere because such injuries tend to have complex attending problems, such as blood loss and nerve involvement, which require careful assessment before treatment. Some of the common overuse (chronic) problems are discussed below.

Shin splints

This is a commonly misused term which describes pain along the tibial shaft; hence, it is perhaps more correctly termed *medial tibial stress syndrome*. Shin splints have been described as myositis, tendinitis and periostitis due to abnormal stress placed on the associated muscles and their bony attachments (Subotnik 1976). Common aetiological factors include overuse, lack of shock absorption, a sudden increase in training levels, poor footwear, muscle imbalance, running on banked or hard surfaces and biomechanical abnormalities. Microtrauma in tendon and muscle fibres causes inflammation. Chronic cases may develop into a stress fracture or compartment syndrome (due to oedema within the compartment). Tibialis posterior is the most common structure associated with shin splints (Rzonca & Baylis 1988), with pain often occurring 12 cm proximal to the medial malleolus—any muscle may be involved (Table 16.4). Initially there will be pain and tenderness over the muscle belly or tendon. In mild cases, this may only be present during or after exercise. Pain coincides with exercise and the site of pain may be located over the tibia and not directly over muscle/tendon. Occasionally there may be some swelling of the area involved.

Treatment involves rest, ice, non-steroidal oral anti-

Table 16.4 Shin splints: cause, symptoms and management. DIPJ = distal interphalangeal joint, TA = tendo Achilles, FDL = flexor digitorum longus, PB = peroneus brevis, STJ = subtalar joint, T. post = tibialis posterior, T. ant = tibialis anterior, FHL = flexor hallucis longus, PT = peroneus tertius

Muscle	Cause	Function	Symptoms reproduced	Treatment
T. Ant	Tight TA	Increase dorsiflexory pull	Resisted dorsiflexion, uphill running	TA stretch, heel lift
	Inverted forefoot	Short tendon stretched or excessive firing to slow foot slap	Passive plantarflexion, downhill running	T.Ant stretch, forefoot control
PT	Tight TA	As above	Resisted dorsiflexion and eversion	As above
T. post	STJ pronation at heel strike and midstance	Tendon stretch and excessive firing to slow pronation	Resisted adduction and plantarflexion	TP stretch, STJ control
	Tight TA	Increases pronation		TA stretch
Soleus	As T. post	As T. post	Passive dorsiflexion	As T. post
FHL	STJ pronation, flexible plantar-flexed first ray	Pronation and internal tibial rotation at midstance and propulsion stress muscle and tendon	Resisted plantarflexion of hallux whilst dorsiflexed	Orthotic control allowing plantarflexion of first ray
FDL	STJ pronation, FDL inflexible	Resisted dorsiflexion of toes during running	Resisted plantarflexion of toes at DIPJ	FDL stretch, orthotic control
PL	Cavoid foot	Excessive firing to slow late supination. May increase first ray plantarflexion, causing a functional forefoot valgus	Resisted abduction and eversion	Orthotic control, either lateral or medial balance to allow for plantarflexed first ray control
PB	Supination or pronation	PB helps to stabilise the lateral border as it may fatigue	Resisted abduction and dorsiflexion	Orthotic control

inflammatories, ultrasound, exercise to increase flexibility, shock absorption, footwear advice, orthoses, strengthening exercises and training advice. Shin splints associated with pronation respond quickly to strapping (low-dye taping) and temporary orthoses.

Stress fractures

Closed hairline fractures can arise from overuse or repetitive stress, particularly, but not exclusively, in long bones such as the tibia, fibula or metatarsals. As part of the differential diagnosis, any underlying bone disorders should be ruled out.

Two possible pathological processes have been considered. Firstly, muscular weakness results in a lack of shock absorption, causing the redistribution of the forces within the bone, thus increasing the stress and causing subsequent fracture (Rzonca & Baylis 1988). Secondly, bone responds to stress by remodelling. There is initial bone resorption (from osteoclasts) followed by bone formation (from osteoblasts). The bone is therefore weaker when the rate of bone resorption is greater than the rate of bone formation. If the bone is subjected to stress at this stage, a fracture may then result (McBryde 1989). Research has suggested that increased plantarflexor strength can cause anterior bowing, predisposing the tibia to a stress fracture in the lower third (Gehlsen & Seger 1980).

Localised pain from a stress fracture becomes less intense and eases upon rest but an ache may remain. In the leg, symptoms commonly occur 6–8 cm above the medial malleolus or at the proximal tibia. If the fibular is involved, pain will radiate along the bone creating soft tissue swelling and pinpoint tenderness. No pain is found on joint movement or with muscle tests against resistance. Pain may be elicited by using a tuning fork or ultrasound to vibrate across the fracture, or by physically moving the bone on examination. An X-ray taken early will prove negative unless bone callus formation is apparent at 2 weeks following trauma. A Technetium[99] bone scan is rather more sensitive to cellular change and will provide results earlier than plain X-rays.

A 4-year study of soldiers in basic training (Pester & Smith 1992) revealed that common sites affected in the foot are the second and third metatarsals and the calcaneus. The navicular, cuboid, sesamoids and talus are less commonly involved. Of these, the sesamoids may be the hardest to diagnose as they can be present in more than one fragment (bipartite and tripartite). The cortex of the bone may be disrupted. Foot bones can create greater difficulties in diagnosis than long bones such as the tibia and fibula. This is particularly likely where stress fractures are hidden by overlapping metatarsals and bones of the midtarsus, or where a fracture arises within the subtalar joint. Since the foot has been subject to newer refined imaging techniques using computerised tomography (CT) and magnetic resonance imaging (MRI), clearer cross-sectional bone anatomy pictures have been possible. Inevitably, it appears that pathology now appearing in these overlapping joints has been previously missed by plain films. High costs and lack of available appointments in NHS hospitals mean that other problems take higher priority than foot imaging.

Treatment. In all cases of bone fractures, plain X-rays should be reviewed if the initial X-ray is negative and symptoms continue after 2–3 weeks. Rest for 8–12 weeks is necessary, although training may commence if symptoms resolve quickly. A below-knee cast or a cast designed as a backsplint may be used by orthopaedics for stress fracture of the leg, but in many cases below-knee casts are unnecessary for metatarsal and other stress fractures. Ice may be used initially for swelling, followed by NSAIDs with rest. Exercises should be used to avoid disuse atrophy during the recovery process. Orthoses and footwear advice should be implemented to increase shock absorption.

Education and alteration in training or running surfaces may be required. Attention to any underlying bone deficiency or disease should be addressed in case a pathological fracture should develop. If the problem is severe and casting does not reduce the pain within the foot, surgical fixation or excision of loose bones such as a fractured sesamoid may be required.

Compartment syndrome

This is usually characterised by pain in the leg and foot due to increased pressure in the muscle compartments of the calf. Research suggests that anterior and lateral compartment syndromes are relatively rare compared to the deep posterior compartment syndrome (Styf 1988). Activity causes the muscle to increase in size as water diffuses into the compartment due to lactic acid build-up. Muscular activity produces increased metabolites and muscle size. The increased pressure within the muscle compartment is resisted by the fascia surrounding the compartment. This fluid build-up compresses vital vascular and nerve structures, causing ischaemic symptoms. The chronic state is more common amongst runners, while an acute compartment syndrome poses a medical emergency with surgical intervention necessary to reduce the internal pressure.

A chronic shin splint may develop into a compartment syndrome. Symptoms of compartment syndrome include a tense, swollen muscle compartment, erythema, diffuse pain on foot movement about the ankle, claudication-type pain on exercise, distal paraesthesia with occasional foot drop and herniation of the fascia. Pulses are often present, as the condition is generally described as small vessel occlusion. Symptoms are made worse by exercise and relieved by rest but persist until the pressure drops.

In the foot, compartment syndrome, while rare, can create obstruction to the blood supply as in the case of a flexor hallucis longus which subsequently atrophied (Lehto et al 1988). The compartmental pressure subsequently reduced, together with the symptoms, without intervention.

Treatment. Diagnosis is undertaken by measuring compartment pressures. Chronic cases may be treated conservatively with a reduction in activity level and exercise. Muscular overuse may be improved by controlling any abnormal foot function. Conditions failing to respond to conservative care require surgical intervention; dividing the fascia to produce decompression of the soft tissues around the muscle.

Compression of the superficial peroneal nerve

The superficial peroneal nerve may be compressed between the fascia and muscular tissue where the nerve emerges from the deep fascia (Malay et al 1987), approximately 8–15 cm proximal to the ankle on the lateral aspect of the calf. Upon exercise, this causes pain and paraesthesia on the dorsum of the foot;

furthermore, a positive Tinel's sign may be elicited. Pain is created by pressure at the point of emergence with active dorsiflexion and eversion, or by passively plantarflexing and inverting the foot to pull on the nerve, thus exciting the effect of entrapment.

Treatment. Local treatment with ice, frictional rub, massage and ultrasound may reduce inflammation and limit scar adhesions. Injection therapy initially with steroid may further reduce such pathological changes. If symptoms dictate sufficient urgency or intensity, surgical release may be necessary.

Achilles tendon overuse

The Achilles tendon does not have a true synovial sheath but is surrounded by paratenon. The injury to the tendon is classified by the tissue involved (Lemm et al 1992), as summarised in Table 16.5.

Overuse, abnormal foot mechanics and shoes with a high heel tab or rigid soles are the most common causes of tendon pathology. It is common to find inflexibility in the calf muscle and abnormal foot function associated with the condition. Localised pain and stiffness may occur the day after injury and will be eased initially by gentle stretching exercises. Unsatisfactory management may lead to an increased intensity and duration of pain until it is present all the time. Pain may be present on passive dorsiflexion, active plantarflexion against resistance and standing on tiptoe. There may be swelling, tendon thickening, crepitus (crackling), nodular formation due to small ruptures, and an inability to perform exercise. Thompson's test is positive when, upon squeezing

Table 16.5 The classification and clinical diagnosis of Achilles tendon injuries

Tissue	Pathology	Diagnosis
Tendinitis	Inflammation at the insertion of the tendon on the calcaneus	Pain located on palpation at this site. Increased with ankle dorsiflexion
Peritendinitis	Inflammation of the paratenon similar to tenosynovitis	Generalised enlargement which does not move with the tendon. Painful on palpation with the tendon both taut and relaxed
Peritendinitis and tendinosis	As above, plus small areas of degeneration or partial tears	Mixture of peritendinitis and tendinosis
Tendinosis or partial rupture	Poor blood supply to tendon and inactive fibroblasts can cause asymptomatic tendinosis which may present as a partial or complete rupture	May present as a small nodule which moves with the tendon. Pain on palpation often reduces with tension of the tendon, possibly due to protection of damaged tissue by superficial taut fibres
Total rupture	Central necrosis and rupture may be due to one major or several intermittent events	Severe pain and swelling. Negative Thompson's test. Loss of Kagar's triangle on lateral X-ray

the calf muscle belly, the foot fails to plantarflex. The test is indicative for a muscle–tendon rupture.

Treatment. This involves rest and may include a below-knee cast or backsplint following an acute episode of injury. Casts will reduce tendon activity, although activity is essential once the acute phase has settled. After the cast has been removed, care must continue, with partial restriction of ankle movement with strapping, plastic ankle stirrups (e.g. Air Cast) and orthoses designed to lift the heel to reduce tension in the tendo Achilles. Ice can be used to reduce local inflammation with friction prior to casting. Ultrasound is only of benefit with peritendinitis, as the tendon has a poor blood supply. Strength, flexibility and plyometric exercises with appropriate orthoses are essential to restore normal function.

Footwear and training advice will help prevent recurrence. Corticosteroid injections have been used as mentioned earlier.

Surgery may be necessary in severe cases with paratenon stripping, excision of necrotic tissue or suture of ruptured fibres.

Retrocalcaneal bursitis

Inflammation of the bursa located between the Achilles tendon and the calcaneus has a similar aetiology to the aforementioned tendon injury—careful differentiation is required. Enlargement of the posterosuperior aspect of the calcaneus may predispose to discomfort located distally and slightly anterior to the tendon. Swelling of the bursa may be evident and lateral pressure may cause discomfort.

Treatment. Rest, ice, heel raises, orthoses, footwear and training advice. Ultrasound may be beneficial, offering early resolution. Corticosteroid injection can provide rapid relief but caution is advised where the skin is already thin. Further atrophy may cause sensitised skin, which may be intractable to pain-relieving methods as illustrated by the cautionary tale in Box 16.4.

Peroneal tendons

Subluxation or dislocation of the peroneal tendons may occur anteriorly and proximal to the fibula malleolus in association with a violent contraction of the peroneals. This may occur in many sports (Brage & Hansen 1992), when the effect of the restraining retinaculae has been overcome. The patient may present with an acute or chronic condition, complaining of pain, swelling and bruising along the sulcus behind the fibula malleolus. Diagnosis may be difficult as the symptoms often reduce spontaneously. Subluxation of a tendon is a chronic condition which may result in a snapping sensation with episodes of the ankle giving way. Stress to the tendons by active eversion and dorsiflexion against resistance will reproduce symptoms. Examination of the ankle should be thorough, as concomitant ligament and osseous injuries can occur.

Peroneal tendon problems may be aggravated if increased stress is placed on the peroneal tendons. This may occur in the foot which has an unstable plantarflexed first ray and functions in a pronated position. At toe-off, the first ray will give way to the increased ground reaction forces from pronation, resulting in increased stress to the peroneus longus tendon. Control of pronation, while leaving the first ray free, will limit this type of problem.

Treatment. This involves rest, ice, compression and elevation in the acute stage, with 3–6 weeks of non-weight-bearing activity in a cast. Strapping can be used but a cast is preferable. Surgical correction is extremely effective for this condition once stress X-rays confirm a positive lateral instability. MRI imaging can also assist in determining the precise area of pathology. Effective correction by surgery can be achieved by re-routing the tendons under the calcaneofibula ligament, re-grooving the peroneal groove on the fibula or repairing the peroneal retinaculum.

Ankle sprains

A traumatic injury to the ligaments supporting the ankle joint can cause extensive damage, depending on the severity of the injury (Roy & Irvin 1983). A partial or complete tear of a ligament may occur, affecting the bone at the point of attachment. Depending upon the speed of injury, an avulsion fracture may develop. The joint capsule and retinaculae are usually involved if bony injury is included.

Box 16.4 Case history

A 29-year-old female presented with a tender nodule over her left heel. Two injections of 0.2 ml Depo-Medrone left the area with an element of epidermal tenderness. Surgical investigation demonstrated a traumatic neuroma which required further surgery to remove atrophied skin. The condition showed a slow improvement despite multitherapy. A hydrogel-type pad along the lines of Silipos had to be used to allow daily comfort. Caution must be taken with surgery around the heel because the tissue around the calcaneus lacks good protection once damaged.

The fibula malleolus is commonly associated with inversion injuries, predisposing to lateral instability. The anterior talofibular (ATF), calcaneofibular (CF) and posterior talofibular ligaments will become involved, in this order, depending upon the severity of injury and position of the ankle joint. Previous rupture of the ATF ligament will predispose the CF ligament to trauma if further injury occurs. A supinated foot type may aggravate this injury.

The tibial malleolus is less commonly affected by an eversion injury than the fibular malleolus. Stress is better tolerated by the deltoid ligament than by the lateral ligaments. A pronated foot type may aggravate this injury.

Treatment. The acute stage presents with pain, swelling, bruising (ecchymosis) and loss of function. In the chronic stage, these symptoms persist, causing the patient to move the ankle less. In both cases there will be pain on direct pressure and on stressing the affected ligaments. An X-ray should be taken to rule out the possibility of a fracture, as well as quantifying the lateral stability using stress tests or a TELOS. The latter system uses a predetermined pressure to stress the ankle in the anteroposterior direction and in the frontal plane. A common peroneal block is used to limit the influence from discomfort and muscle spasm.

If a severe injury has occurred, plaster of Paris immobilisation for 4–6 weeks may be indicated where the bone does not require open reduction. Nonsteroidal oral anti-inflammatories will control pain and inflammation, whilst rest for 2–3 days is essential, with ice, compression and elevation in the acute phase. Felt material in the shape of a horseshoe should be placed around the malleolus to prevent skin shear and increase compression. Following felt protection to the malleolus, a bandage is firmly wrapped around the ankle to support the joint.

In the absence of a fracture, gentle mobilisations should be initiated after 48 hours, with wobble board exercises to improve proprioception, and then continued throughout rehabilitation. Local friction manipulation will reduce scarring, while ultrasound and laser will reduce inflammation. H-wave and interferential therapy can be used to reduce pain and swelling.

Exercise of damaged ligaments can be supported with strapping or ankle supports, although the functional benefit is controversial. Exercises to promote ankle and subtalar joint mobilisations are important. It is not uncommon for the subtalar joint range of motion to be reduced as a result of the swelling and inactivity. This results in abnormal and decreased function. Inversion and eversion strengthening exercises are important to restore muscular support, as well as actively exercising the subtalar joint. Once swelling has receded, orthoses are ideal for rehabilitation to influence frontal plane motion (inversion); modifications such as flaring the lateral post may assist treatment. When an unstable ligament ruptures, repair or surgical reconstruction of the structure is usually indicated.

Some athletes, especially soccer players, will experience discomfort when sudden loads are placed on the joint during the rehabilitation process. If movement reduces and pain becomes intense and starts to course throughout the ankle joint, strapping will help. Exercise should be modified when discomfort is severe; when the sensation reduces in severity and frequency, exercise can then be increased.

Synovitis of the ankle joint

This is inflammation and fibrosis of the synovial lining of the joint with or without degeneration of the articular cartilage. This condition, usually associated with a traumatic origin, may be aggravated by abnormal foot function or ankle equinus. The patient will report chronic ankle pain, usually on the lateral side, which is increased by exercise and presents with intermittent swelling.

Treatment. The same treatment used for an ankle sprain should be considered. Intra-articular steroid injection may be of use, with arthroscopic debridement necessary for chronic cases.

Footballers ankle

This involves the formation of an exostosis over the anterior border of the tibia and the neck of the talus. Excessive traction (plantarflexion) or excessive compression (forced dorsiflexion) results in the formation of an exostosis with possible ankle impingement. Pain, especially on exercise, and intermittent swelling are reported by the patient. An ankle equinus with or without excessive pronation can exacerbate the condition because of the relative bid for further dorsiflexion around the subtalar complex.

Treatment. Management should aim at reducing inflammation by physical therapeutic techniques such as ultrasound. Any underlying mechanical influence should be managed either by encouraging stretching exercises or by orthoses to limit further damage. Surgical excision of an exostosis may be required where symptoms cannot be relieved by conservative methods and where the extent of pathology is too far advanced. The anterior margin of the ankle joint will then be reduced by open surgery or closed (arthroscopy) technique.

Os trigonum syndrome

This condition involves pain at the posterior aspect of the ankle due to a disorder of either an enlarged posterior process of the talus (Steida's process) or an accessory ossicle (os trigonum). Excessive plantar-flexion is common in such activities as dancing.

The result of forced movement can lead to irritation around an os trigonum, prominent Steida's process, or a fracture of the process may develop. Pronation and supination have been implicated as aggravating factors in this condition (Blake et al 1992). Pronation results in adduction and plantarflexion of the talus, which will cause the posterior talocalcaneal ligament to tighten against the os trigonum or Steida's process. Eversion of the calcaneus may increase the compression between the tibia and calcaneus contact surfaces. In supination, the posterior talofibular ligament also tightens, allowing the lateral process of the talus to move inferiorly, again increasing the compression between the tibia and fibula.

The flexor hallucis longus tendon may rub against an os trigonum or prominent Steida's process as it passes between the bifurcation of the posterior tibio-talar and talocalcaneal ligaments. This is more likely in activities such as ballet that rely on the flexor muscles, and may result in a tendinitis. Pain at the posterior aspect of the ankle will be experienced at toe-off, or when the foot is plantarflexed. Eversion or inversion movements may cause discomfort.

Treatment. A definitive diagnosis depends on imaging techniques; a plain X-ray will reveal an os trigonum or a Steida's process. If a fracture is suspected, an MRI or CT scan may be necessary to establish the extent of partition.

When pain results from irritation and no fracture has been identified, rest, ice, massage and ultrasound will moderate inflammation. Orthoses will reduce pain by limiting excessive movement. Exercises to maintain flexor muscle strength and flexibility will help to restore function. A corticosteroid injection may be indicated to improve immediate inflammation. In the case of fracture, a below-knee cast is used for 4–6 weeks to allow the break to settle. Surgery is reserved for a united os trigonum where symptoms fail to settle.

Traumatic myositis ossificans

Trauma to muscle results in haematoma formation.

If subsequent fibroblastic growth exceeds myoblastic tissue growth, calcification of the newly laid down collagen results (Kaminsky et al 1992). It may involve other soft tissue structures, such as fascia, subcuta-neous fat, aponeurosis, tendons or periosteum. Pain, swelling and inflammation at the site, atrophy of tissue bulk, calcification and ossification of the associated muscle will occur.

Treatment should aim to minimise haematoma for-mation by standard physical therapy techniques: rest, ice, non-steroidal anti-inflammatories to prevent organisation of the haematoma. Accommodation within footwear may be a problem. Excision is only necessary if the mass affects joint motion or causes pressure within footwear.

Cuboid pain

Pain and discomfort at the calcaneocuboid, cuboid fourth and fifth metatarsal articulations commonly arises and is infrequently reported. The major cause has been attributed to subluxation of the cuboid (Helal 1986), whereby the cuboid is displaced either dorsally or laterally. This can occur by favouring the outside of the foot, as in running on a slope or during an inver-sion sprain. The osseous displacement would appear to be more of a rotation, with the medial plantar aspect of the cuboid moving more plantarly. The patient reports pain on weight-bearing around the cuboid joint line, extending along the outer border of the foot. Symptoms can be elicited by direct pressure and stress to the respective joints. Cuboid/metatarsal discomfort can radiate to the metatarsal heads, although pain is not present on palpation of the metatarsal heads. The pain can be intense and may limit walking.

Treatment. In severe cases, rest for 1–2 weeks in a below-knee cast will often resolve the pain. In less severe cases, reducing activity with strapping and orthoses to limit movement may be adequate. Physical therapy would include ice, ultrasound, infrared, inter-ferential and joint mobilisations and manipulations. Activity can often be resumed within 1–2 weeks with appropriate control and footwear advice. A corticos-teroid injection is sometimes indicated. Mobilisation can be performed by grasping the midfoot with the patient kneeling and the thumbs placed on the plantar aspect of the cuboid. A whip-like motion is produced to rapidly plantarflex and adduct the foot, while pressing the cuboid into position. A useful orthotic modification can be ordered where a small raise can be incorporated into the orthosis by cutting away plaster from beneath the cuboid. When the orthotic plate is pressed at the time of manufacture, the raise in the plastic coincides with the cuboid to exert an upward lift.

Lisfranc's joint injury

The five metatarsals articulating with the cuneiforms and cuboid constitute the Lisfranc's joint. Trauma to this area can result in dislocation with or without fracture (Arntz & Hansen 1987). Major trauma from a motorbike road traffic accident or entrapment of the foot within the stirrup in an equestrian fall may present with considerable displacement requiring open reduction. More subtle injuries may occur in sport from trampolining or simply from a misplaced step. These injuries occur in all patient groups, and such manifestations can become chronic unless dealt with appropriately.

Pain and swelling of the midfoot with an inability to bear weight is common with pain on palpation around the Lisfranc's joint. This is accentuated on inversion and eversion of the foot. The patient reports pain associated with a severe foot deformity from a collapsed or pronated foot due to ligamentous injury. An excessively pronated foot will further aggravate the condition and arthritic degeneration of the midfoot is common.

Treatment. A below-knee cast is required for 6 weeks to reduce swelling and settle acute symptoms. The chronic condition may be treated conservatively, with local therapy for pain and inflammation and with orthoses and footwear modifications for the foot position. Persistent pain can be treated by arthrodesis of the affected joints; any major displacement must be managed as a priority by open reduction.

Metatarsalgia

Intermetatarsal neuroma is a benign enlargement of the intermetatarsal nerve, commonly associated with the third–fourth space (Morton's neuroma), which has been described earlier in Chapter 14. Tight footwear and activities such as ballet can contribute to this condition.

Bursitis is an inflammation of the intermetatarsal bursa due to trauma (usually microtrauma) or infection. The symptoms are very similar to that of a neuroma, although there is less interdigital paraesthesia.

Treatment. Management for both conditions is much the same. The treatment and conditions are dealt with more fully in Chapter 14.

Capsulitis (forefoot). Inflammation of the joint capsule can affect any joint. The condition is associated with direct trauma, poor footwear, a sudden increase in training loads, prominent and overloaded joints or infection. In the latter instance, all the associated signs of sepsis will be present: Metatarsophalangeal capsulitis will present as pain on walking, and is reproducible on direct pressure and movement of the joint. Pain is often present on the plantar aspect but may also be present on the dorsum. Lateral compression of the joint may cause pain which mimics a neuroma or bursitis. Both these aetiologies and Freiberg's disease must be ruled out during the examination. There may be swelling and inflammation. The second and fourth MTP joints may be predisposed to trauma with increased loading secondary to abnormal foot function or inefficient first and fifth rays, respectively.

Treatment. A local anaesthetic injected into the capsule will provide confirmation, and corticosteroid agents injected into the joint (0.1–0.3 ml) will eradicate most symptoms. If two injections fail to improve symptoms, the practitioner should not persist with this line of management.

Antibiotics are necessary if infection is suspected, although this is rarely a cause of capsulitis. Aspiration of the joint will confirm infection as a cloudy aspirate as well as reduce any intracapsular pressure causing pain.

Rest, ankle strapping, ice and protective padding will reduce trauma and inflammation in the first instance. Ultrasound, orthoses and footwear advice may all be of benefit within the management plan. Subluxed MTP joints will have to be reduced surgically.

Management of this type of problem may resist treatment. An MRI may be useful to determine any rupture to the flexor plate which underlies the metatarsal head. Alternatively, a radio-opaque dye may indicate any loss of flexor continuity, as the dye will leak out and show up on plain X-ray. Surgical repair is indicated.

Sesamoiditis. This is an often misdiagnosed inflammatory condition of the sesamoid associated with overuse, worn footwear or a flexible plantarflexed first ray (Potter et al 1992). The latter is subjected to increased force during multidirectional games such as squash and tennis, as well as from vertical repetitive compression forces associated with jumping and squat thrusts. The condition is aggravated by posterior muscle tightness and excessive pronation.

The patient reports a sharp intense pain around one or both sesamoids. Symptoms arise on weight-bearing and with direct pressure on examination. Pain may be elicited by traction on the flexor hallucis brevis tendon. Symptoms may arise on the medial side of the tibial sesamoid if the ligament has been affected.

An X-ray may reveal a fracture, a plantar prominence or degeneration of the sesamoids (axial view). A syndesmosis or bony bar may exist between multipartite sesamoids. Forced distraction of the syndesmosis has been implicated in turf toe (see below).

Treatment. Management involves rest, ice, redistributive padding or functional orthoses. Care must be taken not to apply pressure against a tight medial band of the plantar fascia. In order to avoid aggravating symptoms, forefoot padding can be restricted to the lateral four metatarsals. Footwear advice is important and chronic cases may require a walking foot cast with an aperture to the painful area. Surgical removal of the sesamoid or any fragments is necessary if the condition remains unresponsive to treatment.

Turf toe. This is a traumatic soft tissue injury to the first MTP joint caused by forced hyperextension to the joint. The condition results in plantar capsular and ligamentous injury and occasionally disruption of components of the medial sesamoid. It is more common in sports played on synthetic surfaces and presents as a hot, swollen, painful, bruised joint. Any bony injury should be excluded from the diagnosis.

Treatment. Management consists of rest, ice and strapping to limit pain, movement and adverse effects of inflammation likely to predispose to long-term osteoarthritic changes. Protective padding and orthoses may be of benefit and shoes with a firm sole will reduce the dorsiflexory force at the joint. Surgical repair of the soft tissue is sometimes indicated.

Dermatological anomalies

Blisters form within the epidermis or epidermal-dermal junction. Fluid will form with or without haemorrhage due to a rise in friction over areas not used to such stresses. Footwear and hard surfaces are usually the cause in inexperienced athletes and those attempting to break in new shoes. Excessive motion due to pronation or decreased motion in a foot may predispose to blisters. Symptoms arise because sacs of clear fluid create tension against fine nerve endings, resulting in pain. A brown/black discoloration indicates haemorrhage. One common site for blister formation is beneath the first metatarsal head or great toe.

Treatment. The skin should be protected from the trauma of friction. Advice regarding correctly fitting footwear should be considered as part of education. Redistributive or cushioning protective padding, or hydrogel skin products, e.g. 'second skin' Spenco, can be used to reduce friction at common sites of blister formation. Two pairs of socks, with the pair next to the skin made of cotton, can be used, or an application of vaseline to the skin to limit surface damage. Moist skin arising from hyperhidrosis should be corrected by desiccants and powders.

When managing the blister, the roof may be punctured or removed. Removal is based on size, turgor and pain. If the blister has reduced in size and discomfort is minimal, no action other than protection should be undertaken. If the blister is painful, the fluid should be drained via two sterile puncture holes in the roof. If the athlete is likely to perform in the near future, or the blister is deep, removal of the roof of the blister is likely to be painful. In this instance, it should be left intact. However, trauma to the area may result in the roof being ripped away, necessitating good protection. A weak mixture of sterile saline and Betadine solution (in alcohol) dries the blister and allows an early return to activity. The application of the weak mixture is achieved by injecting the fluid through the holes that were made to drain the blister—protection is still required. If the blister is smaller, or the roof of the blister has already become loose, the roof should be removed.

Athlete's foot. This condition is associated with a superficial infection of the skin (Table 16.6) which occurs in dry or moist skin and is often associated with poor foot hygiene. When a breach in the skin occurs due to a fungal infection, a secondary bacterial infection may occur.

Athlete's foot can present in many forms, which include dry, flaky skin, vesicular and pustular formation, interdigital maceration with skin loss, and partial or complete involvement of one or more nail plates. The area may be localised or widespread and is often pruritic.

Pitted keratolysis is a condition commonly affecting young males. The skin has a moth-eaten appearance

Table 16.6 Athlete's foot. Aetiology, species, organisms and incidence

Incidence (%)	Species	Infecting organism
25–30	Dermatophytes	*Trichophyton, Microsporon* and *Epidermophyton*
50	Saprophytic yeasts	*Candida, Hendersonula* and *Aspergillus*
20–25	Gram-negative	*Pseudomonas, Proteus, Escherichia*
	Gram-positive	*Corynebacterium, Dermatophylis*

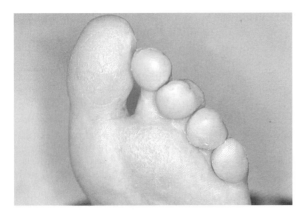

Figure 16.9 A case of pitted keratolysis.

and is saturated. Infection with a Gram-positive bacteria, *Dermatophilus congolensis*, has been identified (Conner & Gibson 1988). Pitted keratolysis is related to hyperhidrosis and is commonly found on the heels, toes and the ball of the foot and can cause discomfort (Fig. 16.9).

Treatment. The best form of treatment is prevention. This involves advice on foot hygiene, such as alternating shoes daily where possible, wearing clean cotton socks and washing feet daily, ensuring that the skin is dried thoroughly. An antifungal powder in the shoes may be useful and oral antibiotics for bacterial infections would be appropriate. Dry skin lesions are best treated with an antifungal cream or ointment. Moist skin lesions are best treated with surgical spirit or a desiccating antifungal product, such as potassium permanganate. A few crystals should be dissolved in a warm footbath sufficient to add a coloured tinge to the water. Too many crystals will cause skin discoloration. Salicylic acid (3–5%) in spirit is particularly effective for pitted keratolysis when applied on cotton wool twice daily. Powder application on the feet has no role to play for macerated skin as the interdigital spaces become clogged.

Skin tone should be maintained either by an emollient or surgical spirit as appropriate. However, symptoms will invariably recur, at which time treatment should recommence.

Mycotic nails may be treated with a topical lotion, although these may take several months to work. Similarly, oral antifungals are available, but are required for 3–12 months depending upon the type selected. These will have the advantage of treating any skin infection at the same time. Pharmacological preparations are described in Chapter 8.

Purpura. Haemorrhage within the epidermis and dermis, associated with trauma, commonly occurs around the medial and lateral aspects of the heel. Damage may be associated with a rough sole/upper interface within the shoe. It is particularly common in soccer players and may be aggravated by the heel position, brought about by increased forces acting on the medial side of the foot in association with pronation, or on the lateral side with supination. The small areas of black discoloration usually consist of many pinprick haemorrhages and are often mistaken as verrucae. There may be associated callus formation, which is the usual cause of pain if present.

Treatment involves debridement of the callosity, control of foot position, attention to the inside of the shoe and emollient application.

Subungual haematoma. This is caused by single or repetitive blows to the nail plate. Footwear is often incriminated when found to be too short. Patients with a hyperextended distal phalanx may be predisposed to this condition. Pain and throbbing around the nail area will be evident, with a black/red discoloration beneath the nail plate. Treatment is discussed in Chapter 6, but correctly fitting footwear is essential to prevent reoccurrence.

SUMMARY

The management of the sportsperson can be both challenging and rewarding. Involvement of other professionals encourages multidisciplinary collaboration, ideally leading to the best concept of care. This chapter has concentrated on the foot, but the whole body should be considered in a treatment programme. As always, an accurate diagnosis and thoughtful planning provide the basis for successful management. The patient's lifestyle, types of sport and attitude towards the problem will equally contribute to the likely success of any planned management.

In designing a treatment plan, the competent practitioner should be prepared to make unpopular decisions. It may be appropriate to advise athletes to reduce or cease some activities in order to prevent serious or long-term injury. However, a car cannot be driven for long distances at high speed indefinitely without some sign of stress. The same is true of the human body, which cannot be pushed beyond a point when adverse symptoms are likely to arise. The best mechanic in the world cannot prolong a car's life for ever, similarly, it is not possible for the practitioner to maintain a patient at a high performance level indefinitely.

REFERENCES

Albert M 1991 Eccentric muscle training in sports and orthopaedics. Churchill Livingstone, New York, p 45–73

Anthony R J 1987 The functional anatomy of the running training shoe. The Chiropodist 42(12): 451–459

Arntz C T, Hansen S T 1987 Dislocations and fracture dislocations of the tarsometatarsal joints. Orthopaedic Clinics of North America 18(14) 105–114

Blake R L, Lallas P J, Ferguson H 1992 The os trigonum syndrome. Journal of the American Podiatric Medical Association 82 (34): 154–161

Brage M E, Hansen S T 1992 Traumatic subluxation/dislocation of the peroneal tendons. Foot & Ankle 13 (7): 423–430

Butler D, Gifford L 1989 The concept of adverse mechanical tension in the nervous system Part 1: Testing for dural tension. Physiotherapy 75 (11): 622–636

Conner D H, Gibson D W 1988 Infectious and parasitic diseases. In: Rubin E, Farber J L (eds) Pathology. J. B. Lippincott, Philadelphia, p 394

Evans F 1980 The healing process at cellular level: A review. Physiotherapy 66(8): 256–259

Gehlsen G M, Seger A 1980 Selected measures of angular displacement, strength and flexibility in subjects with and without shin splints. Research Quarterly for Exercise and Sport 51(3): 478–485

Heil B 1992 Running shoe design and selection related to lower limb biomechanics. Physiotherapy 78(6): 406–412

Helal B 1986 Foot problems. In: Helal B, King J B, Grange W J (eds) Sports injuries and their treatment. Chapman and Hall, London, p 444

Kaminsky S L, Corcoran D, Chubb W F, Pulla R J 1992 Myositis ossificans: Pedal manifestations. The Journal of Foot Surgery 31(2): 173–181

Lehto M, Rantakokko V, Kormano M, Jarvinen M 1988 Flexor hallucis longus muscle atrophy due to a chronic compartment syndrome of the lower leg. British Journal of Sports Medicine 22 (1): 41

Lemm M, Blake R L, Colson J F, Ferguson H 1992 Achilles peritendinitis, a literature review with case report. Journal of the American Podiatric Medical Association 82(9): 482–489

McBryde A 1989 Stress fractures in runners. In: D'Ambrosia R D, Drez D (eds) Prevention and treatment of running injuries, 2nd edn. SLACK International Book Publishers, New Jersey, p 45–47

Mahler F 1992 Partial and complete rupture of the Achilles tendon and local corticosteroid injections. British Journal of Sports Medicine 26(1): 7–14

Malay D S, McGlamry E D, Nava C A 1987 Entrapment neuropathies of the lower extremities. In: McGlamry E D (ed) Comprehensive textbook of foot surgery, 1st edn. Williams & Wilkins, Baltimore, vol 2, ch 21

Merriman L M, Tollafield D R 1995 (eds) Assessment of the lower limb. Churchill Livingstone, Edinburgh

Norris C M (ed) 1993 Sports injuries diagnosis and management for physiotherapists. Butterworth Heinman, Oxford, p 95–96

Pester S, Smith P C 1992 Stress fractures in the lower extremities of soldiers in basic training. Orthopaedic Review 21(3): 297–303

Potter H G, Pavlov H, Abrahams T G 1992 The hallux sesamoids revisited. Skeletal Radiology 21(7): 437–444

Read M T F, Motto S G 1992 Tendo Achilles pain: steroids and outcome. British Journal of Sports Medicine 26(1): 15–21

Roy S, Irvin R (eds) 1983 Sports medicine prevention, evaluation, management and rehabilitation. Prentice-Hall, New Jersey, p 380–402

Rzonca E C, Baylis W J 1988 Common sports injuries to the foot and leg. Clinics in Podiatric Medicine and Surgery 5(3): 591–611

Styf J 1988 Diagnosis of exercise-induced pain in the anterior aspect of the lower leg. The American Journal of Sports Medicine 16(2): 165–169

Subotnik S I 1976 Shin splints of the lower extremity. Journal of the American Podiatry Association 66(1): 43–45

FURTHER READING

Aston J W, Carollo J 1989 Normal patterns of walking and running. In: Subotnik S I (ed.) Sports medicine of the lower extremity. Churchill Livingstone, New York, p 173–174

Cimino W R 1990 Tarsal tunnel syndrome: Review of literature. Foot and Ankle 11: 47–52

D'Ambrosia R D, Drez D (eds) Prevention and treatment of running injuries, 2nd edn. SLACK International Book Publishers, New Jersey

Dockery G L, Nilson R Z 1986 Intralesional injections. Clinics in Podiatric Medicine and Surgery 3(3): 473–485

Duddy R K, Duggan R J, Visser H T, Brooks J S, Klamet 1989 Diagnosis, treatment, and rehabilitation of injuries to the lower leg and foot. Clinics in Sports Medicine 8(4): 861–876

Gerrard D F 1993 Overuse injury and growing bones: the young athlete at risk. British Journal of Sports Medicine 27: 14–18

Hay S M, Smith T W D 1992 Freiberg's disease: an unusual presentation at the age of 50 years. The Foot 2(3): 176–178

Hlavac H F 1978 Good shoes for bad feet. Journal of the American Podiatry Association 68(4): 248–251

Levitsky K A, Alman B A, Jevesevar D S, Morehead J 1993 Digital nerves of the foot anatomic variations and implications regarding the pathogenesis of interdigital neuroma. Foot and Ankle 14(4): 208–214

Pavlov H, Torg J S 1987 The running athlete, roentgenograms and remedies. Year Book Medical Publishers, Chicago

Philps J W 1990 The functional foot orthosis. Churchill Livingstone, Edinburgh

Rodeo S A, Warren R F, O'Brien S J, Pavlov H, Barnes R, Hanks G A 1993 Diastasis of bipartite sesamoids of the first metatarsophalangeal joint. Foot and Ankle 14(8): 425–4

Roy S, Irvin R 1983 Sports medicine prevention, evaluation, management and rehabilitation. Prentice-Hall, New Jersey

Subotnik S I (ed) 1989 Sports medicine of the lower extremity. Churchill Livingstone, New York

Sunberg S B, Johnson K A 1991 Painful conditions of the heel. In: Jahss M H (ed.) Disorders of the foot and ankle, medical and surgical management, 2nd edn. W. B. Saunders Company, Philadelphia, ch 47

Torg J S, Vegso J, Torg E 1987 Rehabilitation of athletic injuries, an atlas of therapeutic exercise. Year Book Medical Publishers, Chicago

17

The elderly person

A. M. Carr

INTRODUCTION

The elderly are, by far, the largest sector of society seeking health care. Practitioners need to be aware of some of the key issues which affect this group. For the purposes of this chapter, these issues are identified as:

- defining 'old age'
- the increasing elderly population
- the ageing process
- attitudes towards the elderly
- should the elderly be treated differently from other age groups
- problems that occur more commonly in the elderly.

Defining 'old age'

Difficulties arise in defining old age—at what point does an individual become 'old'? Most texts refer to those of pensionable age as elderly. Age categories can be useful in determining the 'normal' physiological and psychological changes that occur with age, but within these parameters the individuality of the person is lost. The current trend to subdivide older people into young-old (aged 60–74) and old-old (aged 75+) is too obtuse a classification in terms of the numbers and variations of persons within each category.

Laslett (1989) identified four ages of man within qualifying nations. He defined a qualifying nation as one where:

- there is a 50:50 chance of males aged 25 years reaching their 65th birthday
- one-tenth of the population is over the age of 65
- the gross national product is at least $7500 dollars per person.

Descriptors for the four ages, described by Laslett

Box 17.1 Laslett's (1989) four ages of man

- First age—an era of dependence, socialisation, immaturity and education
- Second age—where there is increasing independence, with growing maturity, responsibilities, earning and saving
- Third age—a stage of life in which there is a sense of personal fulfilment
- Fourth age—a period of final dependence, decrepitude and death

---

(1989), can be found in Box 17.1. It is obvious from these descriptors that many of those aged 60 plus are in the third age, the personal fulfilment stage of their lives, and not the fourth age.

Laslett's concept of four ages challenges traditional views about older people, who are often seen as sick, decrepit and dependent upon social services. As Bernard (1991) points out, 80% of elderly people do not suffer from senile dementia, 75% are in reasonably good health, 95% live in the community and almost 60% will be between 60 and 75 years old at the end of the century.

The increasing elderly population

Since the turn of the century, census data has shown that the general population is ageing. In developed countries, there has been a dramatic rise in the number of people aged 60 and over, and this number is set to increase by a further 1.3% by the year 2000 (Table 17.1). The important factor, illustrated in Table 17.1, is the underlying trend upward in the number of people surviving to age 80 and over. As women tend to live longer than men there has been, and will continue to be, an inevitable increase in the number of older women who live on their own.

The increasing proportion of the population who are elderly is primarily due to the effects of a falling birth rate and an improvement in the number of children who survive the first few years of life. Although

Table 17.1 Predicted population increases in the UK

Age range	1980	2000 (% increase)
Total population	55.9 million	55.2 million (−1%)
Over 60 years	11.1 million	11.3 million (1.3%)
Over 70 years	5.4 million	6.0 million (11.1%)
Over 80 years	1.4 million	1.8 million (28.6%)

Source: adapted from provisional projections produced by the United Nations Population Division (1980).

population numbers, as a whole, are declining, in developed countries the number of people living to an older age is increasing rapidly. As a result, the elderly will continue, as a group, to be the major users of health care services in the future.

The ageing process

The ageing process is slow, poorly understood and variable in its effect upon each individual. Chronological age is of little value in the accurate assessment of a person's health status, although decremental changes in the functional capacity of the body's organs and systems are generally associated with ageing.

Ageing is viewed as a continuum between normal physiological changes associated with age and abnormal pathological changes. The latter is often termed 'secondary' ageing and may be due to disease processes, misuse, stress and general environmental wear and tear. The end result is a decline in vitality. There is a reduction in the biochemical efficiency of the cells, a diminished response to environmental stress and a lessened ability, both physiologically and psychologically, to compensate for disease effects.

A number of criteria have been used to distinguish normal ageing from other biological processes:

- *Universality*. This means that all members of a particular species should experience a bodily process at approximately the same age, e.g. the menopause.
- *Internality*. The aetiological factors involved in the primary ageing process must be intrinsic, i.e. not from an exogenous source. Diseases that are caused by external factors cannot be viewed as being part of the ageing process.
- *Progressiveness*. This relates to the irreversibility (with drugs or otherwise) of the ageing process. In other words, disease effects will continue to worsen despite the intervention of medicine.
- *Harmful*. Ageing can be viewed as an evolutionary advantage by ensuring survival of the fittest and death of the unfit. It also serves as a means of population control. Ultimately, the normal ageing process will result in death.

So, normal ageing involves changes which will affect all older people, has an intrinsic cause that cannot be arrested by medical intervention and is ultimately harmful to the individual.

Attitudes towards the elderly

Apart from the inevitability of death and its relative nearness in elderly people, other fears and anxieties have been associated with growing old (Laslett 1989). These include:

- a fear of dying
- physical and mental decay
- disease
- social and economic dependence
- a feeling of general worthlessness.

All these factors stigmatise society's negative image of older people. The phenomenon by which the 'labelled' readily accept the insults that are written on the labels is well documented by those who study stereotyping (Laslett 1989). There is a tendency that the role and status ascribed by society for elderly people are those that they assume.

A number of authors have suggested reasons for this negative stereotyping of the elderly. Itzin (1986) believes that ageist attitudes, resulting in the formation of stereotypes, are acquired during childhood. Old people are treated as incompetent beings who have little of value to offer society as a means of compensation for the perceived burden their existence creates. Old people hold very similar attitudes, with feelings towards themselves of anger, disgust, embarrassment and exasperation (Phillipson & Strang 1986).

The situation is not helped by those who refer to 'the demographic time bomb' (Victor 1987, Bernard 1991). The notion that the rising number of elderly people will cause a social disaster, because of the high level of health and social services they will require, hypes up the negative image of the elderly. Supporters of this view consider that provision of such services will eventually lead to economic mayhem. This is a very one-sided view which perceives the elderly as 'parasitic' consumers who contribute little to society. Such a view demonstrates how the level of support afforded to the elderly is dependent upon their perceived worth and upon prevailing political and economic philosophies.

Health professionals are cited by Laslett (1989) as grave offenders in the perpetuation of negative images of ageing. Elderly peoples' self-perceptions of value and capacity are often based on comments made by practitioners in the consulting room. Campaigns to 'better the lot' of elderly people tend to focus on their disabilities and helplessness from a particularly negative angle that emphasises their dependence.

Older people will have contributed to the NHS throughout their lives, and at a time when they require most care, they can find they have to compete with younger people for limited resources. The average NHS expenditure by age is set out in Table 17.2.

Table 17.2 NHS expenditure related to age

Age banding	Expenditure (£)
0–4	196.60
5–14	97.17
15–44	89.27
45–64	148.66
65–74	414.76
75–84	926.88
85+	1452.35

Source: Social Services Committee (1988).

In the purchaser–provider context of 1990s health care, practitioners are increasingly being faced with the question of whether or not therapeutic interventions are justified for the elderly. 'Ageism' within health care is becoming increasingly apparent as the population ages and the NHS continues to move in the direction of the market place. Ageist clinical assumptions, such as older people having a poorer quality of life, decreased social worth, cognitive and sensory impairment and a poorer prognosis, are being used to justify why scarce resources should not be used to treat them, even though there is no evidence to suggest that these assumptions are correct (Whittaker 1991). Whittaker (1992) believes that the older the patient, the more likely they are to remain on a waiting list.

A more worrying trend is that health care practitioners, who might otherwise consider themselves egalitarian, can be provoked into ageist discrimination by limited resources. Health care practitioners can be guilty of encouraging acquiescence, compliant patients being favoured because they allow the practitioner to dictate their needs and treatment. It should always be borne in mind that age does not render individuals incapable of making appropriate choices regarding their health.

Stereotypical images brought about by ageist attitudes should be addressed. Remember that not all elderly patients will be confused, have multiple pathologies, chronic disease or hearing difficulties. The majority will be generally fit and healthy and well able to provide a comprehensive medical history, understand advice and the implications of their foot problem(s).

Should the elderly be treated differently from other age groups?

Practitioners will inevitably treat far more older patients because of the insidious and chronic nature of many foot-related problems. For many years, older people have been treated as a homogenous group rather than a diverse, complex mixture of individuals who will have had numerous different life experiences. The diversity of such experiences has a profound effect on the participation, expectations and potential of each individual. Each person's lifestyle will have an impact on their health status and sense of well-being. One could argue that all patients, whether young, middle-aged or elderly, should be treated as individuals and that no one age group should be treated as a special case. Practitioners should therefore get to know all their patients as individuals and tailor their treatment plans accordingly.

Effective communication is essential to any treatment. From the moment a patient enters the clinical environment, information and assistance should be available. An outline of the waiting, treatment, referral and return period systems should be given, particularly if a patient is to be kept waiting or requires the assistance of others to attend the clinic. Patients should be encouraged to discuss their needs, both short- and long-term, and relate their fears, hopes, likes, dislikes and preferences. They should be involved in treatment planning to ensure their individual needs are met and wishes respected. A humanistic approach should be adopted, empowering patients to choose and determine treatment outcomes in consultation with their practitioner.

A holistic and multidisciplinary approach is always in the best interests of the patient to ensure progressive patient care. Liaison with other health care practitioners reduces the possibility of conflicting management plans and enhances patient care. In general, treatment should be directed towards improving the quality of life of the individual.

PROBLEMS THAT OCCUR MORE COMMONLY IN THE ELDERLY

Although all people should be treated as individuals, there are certain factors that need to be taken into consideration when treating the 'elderly'. These factors are listed in Box 17.2.

Medical

Complex medical histories

Many diseases affecting the elderly manifest in later life, although the disease process may have started in the middle or earlier years. In older people, there is a tendency towards degenerative disorders of the neurological, skeletal and vascular systems. As people

---

> **Box 17.2**   Factors to be taken into consideration when treating elderly people
>
> - Medical
>   —complex medical histories
>   —polypharmacy
>   —gait abnormalities
>   —falls
>   —osteoporosis
>   —dementia
> - Social
>   —poor housing
>   —poverty
> - Personal
>   —bereavement

age, the effects of disease show an atypical and non-specific presentation. All health care practitioners should be aware that relatively minor illnesses can have serious consequences in older people. This is usually due to multipathological presentations, where chronic disorders influence the prognosis and management of an acute episode.

In determining an effective management regime, the medical history should incorporate details of the following:

- conditions suffered at some point in the past and which are now inactive, e.g. rheumatic fever. These are important in terms of the potential a patient may have to tolerate other disease processes or the degree of resistance to disease.
- pathologies which are currently controlled by drugs and lifestyle changes, e.g. diabetes mellitus. Consideration should be given to the effects of such pathologies on the presenting problem. Practitioners should be aware of the side effects of these drugs and the pathologies they may mask. Appointment times should be able to accommodate special needs, e.g. regular food intake.
- progressive or slow developing conditions, e.g. atherosclerosis. These conditions require constant monitoring as they can result in changes to the treatment plan. Such changes are necessary to accommodate the different stages in the pathological process of these conditions.
- cyclical conditions which have periods of relapse and remission, e.g. rheumatoid arthritis. The patients' needs may differ at particular points in the disease process.
- presenting pathologies causing concern to the

patient or the practitioner. Practitioners should aim to manage the presenting complaints by a system of direct treatment, monitoring or referral.

Inevitably, there will be pathologies which fit into more than one of the above categories, but the essential point is to ensure treatment plans are flexible enough to accommodate change.

Polypharmacy

As people age there is an increased likelihood that they will use prescribed medications. Drugs may be necessary to control disease states and allow a more comfortable life. However, there are a number of problems related to drug therapy in older people which health care practitioners, responsible for health monitoring, need to be aware of. Older people have an altered sensitivity to many drugs; the reasons for this may be pharmokinetic or pharmodynamic.

Drugs are carried around the body in the blood, and bind with plasma proteins, particularly albumin. With advancing age, there is less albumin in the blood for drugs to bind with; this results in an increase in the drug's pharmacological effect (Trounce 1994). Liver function is less effective in older people and so drugs that are metabolised by this route have a tendency to accumulate, e.g. lignocaine, tricyclic antidepressants and caffeine. Renal dysfunction can also lead to drug accumulation, as drugs are not excreted effectively, e.g. digoxin, propanolol. New drugs may cause particular problems for elderly people, as this age group tends to be under-represented in drug trials.

A number of drugs may be taken by the older person suffering from multiple pathologies. Sharpe & Kay (1977) found that 7% of geriatric complaints were being treated with four or more drugs. Sometimes the drug mixture is incompatible or even contraindicated. In some instances the patient may not understand the necessity for each drug or may make errors in dosage. Complex dose schedules for chronic conditions usually cause the most problems, especially in those with poor vision and impaired dexterity. Incomplete instructions related to drug dosage and timing may lead to poor levels of compliance. A patient may also be taking drugs from previous prescriptions plus over-the-counter medicines for the same complaint. The practitioner should work towards a level of cooperation with patients regarding drug therapy. This should include an understanding of the prescribed medication in terms of its therapeutic objective, potential side-effects and administration.

During the initial patient assessment, a complete record of drug therapies, used on a regular or an occasional basis, should be noted. This should include prescribed and over-the-counter drugs used topically or systemically. This listing should be checked and updated at every subsequent appointment. Although not an exhaustive list, those drugs listed below are of particular importance to the practitioner:

- *Antihypertensives.* These drugs are used to treat high blood pressure (hypertension) and may cause postural hypotension resulting in an increased risk of falling.
- *Minor tranquillisers, sedatives, hypnotics.* Mild depression and anxiety are most commonly treated with these drugs. Their side-effects include postural instability due to their depressant effect on the central nervous system. Some hypnotics, which have a long half-life, can give hangover-like symptoms many hours after their therapeutic effect. This is especially so with long-term use, e.g. nitrazepam has a 20 hour half-life in young people and up to a 60 hour half-life in the older person (Swift 1983).
- *Non-steroidal anti-inflammatory drugs (NSAIDs).* Used in the treatment of inflammatory disorders, these drugs can produce symptoms of dizziness and fluid retention in older people (Goodwin & Regan 1982). Fluid retention can result in oedema with subsequent foot health problems; for example, shoes no longer fit correctly and cause pressure lesions on the foot. Dizziness can cause falling, with risks of fractures, loss of confidence, immobility and subsequent dependency.
- *Tricyclic antidepressants and other major tranquillisers.* Used for more severe depressive states and anxiety, these drugs can cause postural hypotension and have a depressant effect on the central nervous system.
- *Diuretics.* These drugs are often used in the treatment of hypertension as well as heart failure. Their side-effects include dizziness, fainting and black-outs. Due to the increased frequency of micturition associated with these drugs, patients may be anxious that they will not reach a toilet in time.
- *Corticosteroids (systemic).* Used mainly to reduce the symptoms of inflammation, these drugs can increase the degree of bone loss, resulting in osteoporosis and an increased risk of fracture (Downton 1993). Steroids can also lower the body's natural resistance to invading microorganisms.
- *Corticosteroids (topical).* These preparations are especially useful in the treatment of inflammatory dermatoses. However, they must not be applied to

fungal, viral or bacterial infections, as spreading may result. Care should be taken in the use of combined preparations where corticosteroids are mixed with antibacterial or antifungal agents in one preparation.

Gait abnormalities

Bipedal posture is less stable than quadripedal posture. The support base in the biped is small and requires a complex neuromuscular system to maintain balance. The important areas of sensory input which play a vital role in maintaining balance are:

* visual
* proprioceptive
* vestibular.

Information regarding the position of the body in space and in relation to the rest of the body is constantly being transmitted by proprioceptors in muscles, tendon, ligaments and joints. Visual clues and the vestibular apparatus enhance this information, so that rapid corrective responses can be made to maintain balance. Age affects balance by:

* increasing the threshold for excitability of proprioception
* decreasing spatial visual sensitivity
* reducing the effectiveness of vestibular function (Downton 1993).

In a study by Puykko et al (1990) it was concluded that 'muscle spindle proprioceptive sensitivity is poorer in very old subjects than in younger age groups, and disruption of proprioception has a greater effect in the very elderly than in younger subjects'. Responses to movement, in order to maintain balance, are therefore slower in older individuals.

Older people tend to take shorter steps, thus maintaining a longer period of stance phase; as a result the speed of gait is slower (Wolfson 1992). The angle and base of gait is obtuse, therefore providing a wider base for support. According to Downton (1993), old men show a slower walking speed, shorter stride length, greater degree of out-toeing, longer stance phase, shorter swing phase, slightly greater stride width, less hip rotation and knee flexion (during swing), and less ankle extension at the end of stance phase than young men.

As described by Broe (1992), senile gait disorder is a multifactorial syndrome without an identifiable pathological basis. It is thought to be a subclinical manifestation of age-associated disease processes. It affects about 4% of people aged 65–74 and about

---

Box 17.3 Characteristics of senile gait

* Flexed position
* Ataxia
* Slowness
* Reduced upward gaze
* Absent ankle reflex
* Reduced distal vibratory sense
* Action tremor
* Mild cognitive impairment

25% of those aged 75 plus. The characteristics of this disorder are listed in Box 17.3.

Idiopathic Parkinson's disease is closely associated with ageing. There is an increasing incidence with age, and about 2% of the population over 70 is affected. Parkinson's disease progresses slowly, with symptoms becoming more marked with duration. Patients are unable to control their balance effectively and display a resting tremor, bradykinesia and rigidity. Stride length is reduced and gait is slower, with limited arm and torso movement. Patients are unable to control balance effectively and make sharp, rapid corrections to movement (Wolfson 1992).

In non-idiopathic Parkinson's disease, prescribed drugs are the most common cause of gait abnormalities, e.g. prochlorperazine used for vertigo, metoclopramide used for nausea, and thioridazine used for anxiety, confusion and insomnia (Broe 1992). Improvement of symptoms can be seen with the use of dopamine-increasing drugs. Failure to respond to such drugs suggests either a misdiagnosis or that the patient is becoming tolerant to the drug (Trounce 1994).

Weakness, clumsiness and impaired voluntary motor control are signs that the descending corticospinal tracts are affected. Unilateral disruption of the tract is often caused by a cerebral vascular accident (stroke). The lower limb appears circumducted and the foot plantarflexed. Bilateral lesions may result from severe osteoarthritic changes in the spine which compress spinal nerves. This results in a scissor-type gait, hyperadduction and spasticity, where the feet appear everted and plantarflexed (Wolfson 1992).

Ataxia is more common in the elderly, with its characteristic wide-based, unsteady gait and lurching steps. One of the primary causes is infarcts either in the cerebellum or cerebral cortex. Bilateral frontal lobe lesions cause a halting gait, with sliding of the feet along the floor (magnetic gait; Wolfson 1992). Changes in movement are laborious and minor corrections to balance are ineffective, resulting in falls. Examination of the patient often reveals spasticity of the lower limb and the Babinski sign.

Falls

Falls are usually multifactorial in origin, resulting from a combination of intrinsic and extrinsic factors. Visual and vestibular impairments are common factors in the epidemiology, as are drug therapy, cognitive dementia and environmental factors.

The consequences of falls for the older person and society in general are wide-reaching. Serious injury and fractures are most commonly caused by falls (Melton & Riggs 1987). Post-fall syndrome, characterised by hesitancy, irregularity of progress and reluctance to move, exacerbates the risks of further falls. Immobility has severe economic consequences, with increased levels of dependence on health and social services. In studies carried out by Blake et al (1988) and Downton & Andres (1991), it was found that between 28 and 35% of those aged 65 and over, and between 32 and 42% of those aged 75 and over, had fallen. Morris et al (1987) found that subjects with dementia were up to three times more likely to fall than those without dementia. Sloman et al (1982) found that depressed people walked slower, with a shorter stride length, and are predisposed to falling because of associated psychomotor changes. Table 17.3 lists the likely causes of falls in the elderly population.

Table 17.3 Potential causes of falls in older people

Cause	Examples
Neurological	Epilepsy
	Parkinson's disease
	Cerebral vascular accident (stroke)
	Peripheral neuropathies
Vestibular	Ménière's disease
Visual impairment	Senile cataracts
Myopathies	Polymyalgia rheumatica
	Polymyositis
	Dermatomyositis
Bone and joint disorders	Cervical spondylosis
	Osteomalacia
	Hypercalcaemia
	Paget's disease
Endocrine	Hyperthyroidism
	Hypothyroidism
Dementia	Alzheimer's type
Environmental	Uneven walking surfaces
	Poor lighting
	Loose carpeting
	Ill-fitting footwear
Drug therapy	Hypotensives

Footwear is an important factor when considering prevention of falls. Shoes with non-slip soles should be recommended. Fastenings can pose a problem for older people. Slip-on shoes are easier to put on, but are liable to slip off the foot, whereas laces, straps and Velcro may be unmanageable. Special consideration needs to be given to the footwear needs of older people (see Ch. 10).

Walking aids such as sticks and frames are useful in broadening the support base and providing extra security for the patient. Camouflage can be used where patients do not wish to appear disabled. For example, umbrellas can be adapted so that they serve as walking sticks; shopping trolleys can be used as a replacement for walking frames. Visual impairments can be improved by the wearing of appropriate lenses and provision of adequate lighting. Environmental hazards such as loose carpeting and insecure step stools should be avoided.

Where possible, the aetiological factors resulting in falls should be controlled or eliminated. Careful assessment and monitoring of the patient, in consultation with a multidisciplinary care team (including social services and voluntary care workers), should provide the best possible outcome. With the increasing elderly population, it is essential that action is taken to reduce the incidence of falls.

Osteoporosis

This is a metabolic disease which predisposes bone to fracture with limited amounts of trauma (Brazel 1979). The skeleton is composed of two distinct types of bone: cortical (compact) and trabecular (cancellous). The former comprises the outer layer of the long bones and the cortex the remainder of the skeleton (approximately 75% of total bone mass). Trabecular bone is a honeycomb-like lattice of intersecting bone plates that form the central portion of the bone. Cancellous bone is, therefore, more subject to blood-borne metabolic influences (Ryan 1983).

During childhood and adolescence, new bone formation exceeds resorption, leading to net increases in bone mass. This peaks at about 30 years of age and then resorption rates begin to overtake formation rates, resulting in decreased bone density and calcium loss. The mechanism by which maximum bone mass is achieved in early life is related to genetics, activity levels and nutrition. At a cellular level, the rate of bone loss is influenced by gonadal hormones, calcium intake and bioavailability, vitamin D synthesis, parathyroid hormone, thyroid hormone, growth hormone and calcitonin (Riggs & Melton 1986).

A number of body systems are involved in the maintenance of bone mass. Pathology relating to any one of these systems could lead to the onset of osteoporosis. For example, osteoporosis may occur due to an age-related decline in the renal conversion of vitamin D to its active form (Rossman 1983). According to Gallagher et al (1979), the dietary intake of vitamin D_2 (ergocalciferol) and uptake of vitamin D_3 (from sunlight) is reduced in old age. This may be due to poor diet or immobility, both of which are associated with older people.

Women are at greater risk of suffering from osteoporosis than men. They have a lighter skeleton than men (lower peak bone mass) and suffer oestrogen deficiency at the menopause. Both are associated with an increased predisposition to osteoporosis. Females lose about 60% of their trabecular bone and 35% of their cortical bone during life, whereas males lose only 40% and 25%, respectively (Riggs & Melton 1992). The resultant instability can lead to hip fractures, where between 25 and 30% of victims in the UK are dead within 6 months.

Trabecular bone loss renders a person more susceptible to vertebral crush fractures and hip fractures, with resultant immobility and potential neurological implications. Wrist fractures are more common in younger osteoporotic sufferers than in older sufferers. This is because younger patients will try to break their fall by putting out their hands. With older people this reflex action is lost and hence they tend to fall suddenly and fracture their hips.

Immobility due to disability or a lack of exercise is an important factor in the development of osteoporosis. Exercise programmes for older people should be prescribed and encouraged. Any exercise regime needs to be maintained. Dolsky et al (1988) cited evidence to suggest that exercise-induced gains in bone mass are lost within months once the exercise regime is discontinued.

Dementia

Dementia refers to a disorder where there is an acquired impairment of intellectual and memory functions due to brain disease. As well as memory disturbances, patients with dementia demonstrate defects in abstract thinking, judgement, personality, language, praxis and spatial skills. By definition, these affects must be of a significant magnitude to interfere significantly with work or social activities (American Psychological Association 1980).

The causes of dementia are many, and onset is accordingly variable. Sudden onset is associated with head injury or a stroke, whereas a reversible dementia may be due to polypharmacy, depression or a subdural haematoma. Sometimes these are referred to as treatable dementias, in that there is an associated disorder which can be treated to relieve the symptoms of dementia. Cardiovascular disorders can affect cerebral blood flow, causing dementia, and should be treated promptly to avoid permanent brain damage. Disorders that interfere with the metabolic homeostasis of the brain can also manifest as dementia, e.g. diabetes mellitus, hypothyroidism and anaemia.

The incidence of dementing illnesses increases with advancing age, with Alzheimer's disease being the most common cause in the UK. It affects approximately 0.1% of people between 60 and 65 years, 1% of those aged over 65, and 2% of people over 80 years (Friedland 1992).

Alzheimer's disease is associated with early amnesia developing to consistent amnesia as the disease progresses. Spatial skills are limited, while language and social skills can remain intact, often giving the casual observer a false indication as to the extent of the disease. Physically it may resemble Parkinsonism, but more often there is no visible change. Patients may be depressed, apathetic and easily irritated. Behavioural changes are so variable that health professionals will need to assess each individual case using careful history taking and well-structured questioning.

Approximately 15% of Alzheimer's cases have a hereditary link, thought to be associated with chromosome 21 (Friedland 1992). Also, all Down's syndrome sufferers will develop pathological evidence of Alzheimer's disease if they survive beyond 35 years of age. Clinically, dementia is evident in about half of Down's syndrome sufferers aged over 35 years. Pathologically, there are neurofibrillar tangles, neuritic plaques, amyloid infiltration of vessel walls, granulovascular degeneration and Hirano bodies. Chemically, Alzheimer's disease is associated with deficiency in neurotransmitter substances.

Due to the overlapping features found in Parkinsonism and Alzheimer's, the presentation may be clinically confusing. Both can be associated with joint rigidity, faltering gait and an inability to comprehend even simple instructions. Health professionals need to use discretion in prescribing treatment regimes that involve self-care. Where assistance from relatives or other carers is available, it should be utilised with respect to the care needs of the patient and life patterns of the carer. In the case of severe Alzheimer's disease, the person may require 24-hour care. The social circumstances of an individual suffering from dementia are of paramount importance, the emphasis being on cooperation rather than compliance.

Social

Poor housing

Housing which lacks one basic amenity such as a hot water supply, an inside toilet or bath/shower is classed as 'unfit' (Office of Population Censuses and Surveys 1993). Almost half of such properties are occupied by those aged 65 and over. In the UK, about 60% of people over 55 years are owner-occupiers, being entirely responsible for the standard of basic amenities in their homes. Practitioners should be aware of the housing conditions of their elderly patients. For example, foot problems causing pain and discomfort can discourage weight-bearing, so preventing ease of access to an outside toilet. This may precipitate problems of incontinence. Lack of hot water can result in an inappropriate standard of personal hygiene, which can result in placing a patient at risk of secondary infections by opportunistic microorganisms.

Poverty

Old people are better off now than they were in 1948 when the current compensation scheme of benefits started. However, one in three of those living on or below the (socially agreed) standard poverty line are over pension age, despite this section of society making up only one in five of the general population. Proportionally, women make up the greatest percentage of poor pensioners. Elderly women are far less likely to have been in employment when they were younger.

Financial poverty relates to other areas of deprivation. Older people are less likely than younger people to own consumer durables. They are also less likely to eat fresh meat on a regular basis. Financial dependence on the state is closely associated with wider notions of dependence. Many elderly experience social isolation, which is exacerbated by lack of money. Fewer old people own cars, which restricts mobility and social interaction. Isolation can lead to feelings of worthlessness and so heighten depression. This may result in some elderly people failing to take proper care of themselves. The elderly need to be encouraged to maintain their personal well-being, to take pride in their appearance and ability to remain fit despite the financial burdens they may be facing.

Health practitioners should always take into con-sideration the social and financial restrictions of their patients. An awareness of the widespread nature of poverty, especially in advanced age, will facilitate sympathetic and successful treatment regimes.

Personal

Bereavement

The term bereavement is most often associated with the death of a relative or close friend, although the reaction to 'loss' of any 'love' object may be defined in similar terms. Throughout the course of life there are numerous instances where an individual has to adapt to change in order to continue the process of living; death is usually the most disruptive influence and can have a traumatic effect on the life of an older person.

Following death, there is a period of grief and mourning. The bereavement period passes through a number of experiential stages leading to final acceptance and a reorganisation of their lifestyle (Parkes 1970, Morris 1971, Worden 1982).

Grief can be divided into three areas: feelings, physical sensations and behaviour. Initially the bereaved person is in a state of emotional shock and is unable to accept the loss (denial). Later, there is anger, frustration and pain, which may be associated with feelings of incompetence at their inability to have prevented the death. The second stage brings depression and apathy and the final stage brings recovery and accommodation. Parkes (1975) further qualified the stages of grief by identifying 'determinants' of grief:

- mode of death
- nature of attachment
- who was the person
- historical antecedents
- personality variables
- social variables.

The mode of death relates to cause and location. Death from 'natural causes' tends to lead to fewer problems related to acceptance of death than if it was due to traumatic causes (Wright 1991). Bowling & Cartwright (1982) found that adjustment to loss and acceptance of death were better in older people, possibly due to the fact that elderly people talk about death more openly than other age groups in society. Glick et al (1974) found that anticipation of death was an important determinant of recovery.

The relationship that existed between the dead person and the bereaved is important in terms of acceptance of loss. If the bereaved person's life revolved around nursing a sick spouse prior to their death, as is often the case with older people, the loss of this role may be a significant factor in the bereavement process. In order to come to terms with loss, the bereaved person must weaken and eventually break the ties they have to their past and future that involved the dead person. Only when these ties are broken can new ones be made, enabling the bereaved person to become involved with life again.

Personality variables and past experiences affect the bereaved and influence their individual ability to cope with loss. It would be realistic to suggest that, as a person gets older, they should become more adept at coping with loss, having learned, over time, how to move on to the next stage of the grieving process successfully.

Social variables revolve around religion and culture. In modern Western society, death is a taboo subject. There is a somewhat squeamish reaction to displays of open grief. In many respects, death has been sanitised and health professionals are unsure of their role. Many, unless specifically trained to deal with bereavement, try to avoid the subject and the dead person's name. This is done with the intention of avoiding upset to the patient, but the impact of this social denial and repudiation of mourning is to heighten the chances of the bereaved person becoming emotionally disturbed due to an overlong period of grief (Kubler-Ross 1975).

Closely linked to cultural and religious issues are those of ethnicity. Ethnic identity affects values, beliefs and behaviours, rendering people sensitive to social, personal and life span developments. In a study carried out by Luborsky & Rubinstein (1987), the bereaved re-formed their identities around central ethnic values.

Depression and anxiety are commonly associated with mourning but can seriously affect daily living. There is an increase in mortality among the widowed in the first year after bereavement. This is attributable not only to anxiety and depression but also to physical complaints. Some of these may be stress-related. The level of stress caused by having to readjust to a new life pattern can magnify feelings of inadequacy, which in turn affect levels of dependence, subsequently having a detrimental affect on adjustment.

Elderly people who lose their spouse through death must come to terms with losing a loved one, which may explain the great difficulties encountered by elderly people in adjusting to their new single role. The rate of suicide is higher in the first year post-bereavement. The sense of frustration following death of a spouse can result in anger suicide. Fear suicide occurs when the intensity of the emotion a person feels about being alive becomes greater than the fear of death.

The manifestations of normal grief vary in intensity and time-span depending upon the circumstances of the individual. However, prolonged or delayed grief is referred to as 'abnormal grief'; this is where the person is unable to pass through the experiential stages of grief and is therefore unable to resolve it on an emotional or social level. Worden (1982) describes specific behaviours that can persist for abnormally long periods of time and which could indicate an abnormal grief response; sleep disturbances, overactivity, visiting places or carrying objects belonging to the deceased, avoiding reminders of the deceased, dreams of the deceased.

Health practitioners should be aware of the effects of death and be on guard for signs of abnormal stress. Referral for counselling is an option, but many just need time to adjust and access to allow them to vent their emotions without fear of ridicule.

SUMMARY

Practitioners should consider how they will cater for the increasing number of elderly people that may present with a variety of needs related to primary and secondary ageing processes. Ageist attitudes among health care practitioners should be addressed to ensure equality and non-prejudicial treatment. It should not be automatically assumed that old age is synonymous with ill health. Older people should be consulted and empowered to allow them to live as independently as possible. Consider the words of Thompson (1977) who wrote:

It is not unimportant to have read George Grissing and Kipling, to have heard Elgar or to know something of the old British Empire and the battles of the First World War. These are not ordinary people, wrestling with inflation or especially concerned with the great debate on education. They represent an age whose influence is still there, though attenuated. They are people whose stage of life I have not reached or may not reach… I can only try to understand old age by an effort of imagination, and it is therefore distinct and unique, yet infinitely diverse in manifestation.

REFERENCES

American Psychology Association 1980 In: Evans J G, Williams T F (eds) 1992 Oxford Textbook of Geriatric Medicine. Oxford University Press, Oxford, p 483

Bernard M 1991 Vision for the future. Nursing the Elderly Jan/Feb: 10–12

Blake A J, Morgan K, Bendall M, Dallosso H, Ebraham S, Arie T, Fentern P, Bassey E 1988 Falls by elderly people at home, prevalence and associated factors. Age Ageing 17: 365–372

Bowling A, Cartwright A 1982 Life after death. A study of the elderly widowed. Tavistock, London

Brazel U S 1979 Common metabolic disorders of the skeleton in ageing. In: Reichel W (ed) Clinical aspects of ageing. Williams & Wilkins, Baltimore

Broe G A 1992 Parkinson's disease and related disorders. In: Evans J G, Williams T F (eds) 1992 Oxford Textbook of Geriatric Medicine. Oxford University Press, Oxford, p 546–556

Dolsky C R, Stock K, Etiansi A 1988. Weight bearing exercise training and lumbar bone mineral content in post menopausal women. Annals of International Medicine 108: 824–828

Downton J H 1993 Falls in the elderly. Edward Arnold, London, p 49, 59

Downton J H, Andres K 1991 Prevalence, characteristics and factors associated with falls among the elderly living at home. Aging 3: 219–228

Friedland 1992 Dementia. In: Evans J G, Williams T F (eds) 1992 Oxford textbook of geriatric medicine. Oxford University Press, Oxford p 483–489

Gallagher J C, Riggs B L, Eisman J 1979 Intestinal calcium absorption and serum vitamin D metabolites in normal subjects and osteoporotic patients: effects of age and dietary calcium. Journal of Clinical Investigations 64: 723–734

Glick I O, Weiss R S, Parkes C M 1974 The first year of bereavement. John Wiley, New York

Goodwin J S, Regan M 1982 Cognitive dysfunction associated with naproxen and ibuprofen. The Elderly Arthritis and Rheumatism 25: 1013–1014

Itzin C 1986 Ageing awareness training: A model for group work. In: Phillipson C, Bernard M, Strang P (eds) Dependency and interdependency in old age: theoretical perspectives and policy alternatives. Croom Helm, London, p 114–139

Kubler-Ross E 1975 Death – the final stages of growth. Prentice Hall, New Jersey

Laslett P 1989 A fresh map of life: the emergence of the third age. Weidenfeld & Nicolson, London

Luborsky M, Rubinstein 1987 Ethnicity and lifetimes: self and identity among elderly widowers. In: Gelford D, Barnes C (eds) Ethnicity and ageing. Springer, New York

Melton L J, Riggs B L (1987) Epidemiology of age related fractures. In: Alvioli L V (ed) The osteoporotic syndrome. Grune & Stratton, New York

Morris S 1971 Grief and how to live with it. George Allen & Unwin Ltd, London

Morris J C, Rubin E H, Morris E J, Mandel S A 1987 Senile dementia of the Alzheimer's type: an important risk factor for serious falls. Journal of Gerontology 42: 412–417

Office of Population Censuses and Surveys 1993 The 1991 census, persons aged 60 and over. HMSO, London

Parkes C M 1970 The first year of bereavement. A longitudinal study of the reaction of London widows to the death of their husband. Psychiatry 33: 444–467

Parkes C M 1975 Bereavement: studies of grief in adult life, 2nd edn. Penguin, Harmondsworth

Phillipson C, Strang P 1986 Training and education for an ageing society: new perspectives for the health and social services. Health Education Council/Department of Adult Education, University of Keele

Puykko, Jantti P, Aalto H 1990 Postural control in elderly subjects. Age Ageing 19: 215–221

Riggs B L, Melton L J 1986 Involutional osteoporosis. New England Journal of Medicine 314: 1670–1686

Riggs B L, Melton L J 1992 Involutional osteoporosis. In: Evans L G, Williams T F (eds) Oxford textbook of geriatric medicine. Oxford University Press, Oxford, p 405–411

Rossman I 1983 Physician as geriatrician. In: Cape R, Coe R, Rossman I (eds) Fundamentals of geriatric medicine. Raven Press, New York

Ryan K 1983 Oestrogen replacement therapy. In: Cape R, Coe R, Rossman I (eds) Fundamentals of geriatric medicine. Raven Press, New York

Sharpe D, Kay M 1977 Worrying trends in prescribing. Modern Geriatrics July: 32–39

Sloman L, Berridge M, Homatidis S, Hunter D, Puck T 1982 Gait patterns of depressed patients and normal subjects. American Journal of Psychiatry 39: 94–97

Swift C G 1983 Hypnotic drugs. In: Issacs B (ed) Recent advances in geriatric medicine. Churchill Livingstone, Edinburgh, p 123–146

Thompson K 1977 Why I get a kick out of looking after older patients. Modern Geriatrics July: 24

Trounce J 1994 Drugs at the extremities of age. Clinical Pharmacology for Nurses. Churchill Livingstone, Edinburgh

Victor C 1987 Old age in modern society: a textbook of social gerontology. Chapman Hill, London

Whittaker P 1991 The dangers of ageism in clinical decision making. Geriatric Medicine 21: 51–55

Whittaker P 1992 Rationing, ageism and the new look NHS. Geriatric Medicine 22(1): 53–58

Wolfson L I 1992 Gait and mobility. In: Evans G J, Williams F T (eds) Oxford textbook of geriatric medicine. Oxford University Press, Oxford, p 585–594

Worden D W 1982 Grief counselling and grief therapy. Routledge, London

Wright B 1991 Sudden death. Churchill Livingstone, Edinburgh

18

The management of foot ulcers

J. Mooney

INTRODUCTION

The normal physiological state ensures that the optimal internal environment is maintained by homeostatic feedback mechanisms. When normal homeostatic responses are altered, physiological efficiency is lost and pathophysiological processes supervene. This happens with ulceration; tissues become increasingly delicate, and subject to deterioration and loss of function, resulting in loss of tissue viability. This situation is further compounded, as the factors which led to tissue breakdown in the first place are also likely to result in delayed or impaired healing.

Changes to the normal homeostatic mechanisms may be caused by a range of local and/or systemic pathologies (Box 18.1). Local factors, such as trauma,

---

Box 18.1   Local and systemic causes of ulceration

- *Local*
  Trauma—from footwear, nail pathology, minor knocks
  Deformity—lesser toe and first ray problems
  Chilling
  Vasospastic disease—Raynaud's disease
  Peripheral vascular disease
  Infection
  Neuropathy—motor, sensory, autonomic

- *Systemic*
  Diabetes mellitus
  Hansen's disease
  Peripheral neuropathy
  Neurological disease
  Rheumatoid disease
  Generalised ischaemia and arterial disease
  Chronic venous insufficiency
  Immunodeficiency and AIDS
  Ageing and debility
  Pharmacological regimes, e.g. steroid therapy
  Disseminated and terminal cancers
  Chemotherapy and radiation therapy

deformity, chilling and poor fitting footwear, predispose the patient to breakdown of superficial tissues, ulceration and infection, and exacerbate poor healing. Areas of previous ulceration, known as 'atrophie blanche', are particularly at risk of further breakdown if the predisposing local and systemic factors re-establish, are not addressed, or if there is a deterioration in the patient's general health.

This chapter explores the generic principles and treatment strategies associated with the management of ulceration, followed by an examination of the management of the specific types of ulcer which may affect the foot.

PROCESSES ASSOCIATED WITH TISSUE BREAKDOWN

One or more of the following features are likely to be associated with ulceration.

Ischaemia

Ischaemia is a reduction or deficiency of blood flow, due to contraction or constriction of an artery or arteriole in association with vascular disease; or restriction of superficial blood flow in areas of high external pressure, leading to hypoxia of affected tissues. Tissues function inefficiently under conditions of ischaemic hypoxia and tend to break down.

Neuropathy

Neuropathy results from degeneration of nerve function (Box 18.2). It may affect the peripheral nervous

---

Box 18.2 Causes of neuropathy in the lower limb

- Demyelination of peripheral nerve fibres
- Biochemical abnormalities of the neurone
  - sorbitol accumulation leading to oedema of nerve fibres in association with hyperglycaemia
  - reduction in free myo-inositol concentrations
  - reduction in nerve ATPase
  - intracellular accumulation of glycogen
- Thickening of the basement membrane of endoneurial blood vessels
- Metabolic abnormalities secondary to endoneurial hypoxia
- Trauma to nerve fibres
  - neurapraxia
  - axonotmesis
  - neurotmesis
- Ischaemia

---

system, as is seen in diabetes mellitus, Hansen's disease (leprosy) and multiple sclerosis, or it may affect the central nervous system, as in cerebrovascular accident (stroke) and spinal injury. The more severe the damage or degeneration of the nerve, the more severe the effects of neuropathy. In extreme cases, patients may present with loss of all (motor, sensory and autonomic) neural modalities (Table 18.1).

Mononeuropathy causes abnormality of function in the dermatome or myotome subserved by a single nerve, whereas polyneuropathy is a widespread, symmetrical abnormality of many nerves, involving all types of nerve fibre, usually in a 'glove and stocking' distribution. Neuropathies may arise from direct nerve damage, or as the result of failure of neural development in utero, e.g. spina bifida. More commonly, neuropathy presents in progressive demyelinating disease, such as multiple sclerosis, or as the long-term complication of diabetes mellitus (Tillo et al 1990). Neuropathic patients may present with plantar ulceration due to polyneuropathy, the combination of uneven weight-bearing in the foot (from motor neuropathy and arthropathy) on dystrophic and poorly perfused skin (from autonomic neuropathy) causing extensive but pain-free ulceration (due to sensory neuropathy) in areas of decreased tissue viability.

Muscle function and limb reflexes are reduced or lost in motor neuropathy. This can result in profound effects on gait, unbalanced movement and even joint contracture. Sensory neuropathy may involve loss of proprioception (awareness of joint position) and loss of pain. These factors, either singly or combined, may result in unconscious tissue damage. Autonomic neuropathy may result in loss of sweat production and imperfect arteriolar function. Loss of sweat production can cause skin dystrophies, cracks and fissures. Imperfect arteriolar function is one of the earlier indications of autonomic neuropathy. Patients may have apparently good pedal pulses, but poor superficial and skin perfusion, as arterial blood is diverted away from peripheral tissues through shunt mechanisms, creating a relative ischaemic hypoxia in superficial tissues. There is a concomitant increase in blood flow through deeper tissues and bone, which can lead to osteoporosis, with bone softening and fracture, particularly in joint areas. The combination of microfracture and loss of proprioception leads to the development of neurarthropathy (Charcot's arthropathy).

Infection

Infection occurs as the result of direct colonisation of dermal and deeper tissues by resident or transient

Table 18.1 Effects of neuropathy in the lower limb. Note—these problems may be seen in any combination in the neuropathic patient

Effect	Outcome
Loss of normal sensation	Paraesthesia
	Numbness of part or all areas of the foot
	'Glove and stocking anaesthesia', with the greatest sensation loss distally
	Pain-free, deep 'trophic' ulceration, especially of the plantar skin overlaying the metatarsophalangeal joints
	Pain-free fracture to bone, associated with neuroarthropathy (Charcot joint)
	Painful neuropathies and hyperalgesia
Loss of normal motor function	Isolated mononeuritis and loss of function of the subserved muscle
	Multiple mononeuritis with loss of function of all muscles within the affected neurotome
	Loss of intrinsic foot muscle function, causing development of the 'diabetic claw foot'
	Gait abnormalities and unequal loading of the plantar surface
	High plantar pressures
Loss of normal autonomic function	Loss of sweating and atrophy of sweat glands
	Loss of function of erector pili muscles—no 'goose pimples'
	Dry skin, prone to fissuring
	Loss of vasomotor tone, with shunting of arterial blood away from skin arterioles
	Loss of proprioception (loss of stereognosis)
	Increased blood flow through bone, leading to osteoporosis and neuroarthropathy (Charcot joints)
	Impotence

Table 18.2 Common microorganisms that may cause infection in the debilitated or susceptible patient

Classification	Infecting organism
Bacteria	
Aerobes	Staph. aureus
	Staph epidermidis
	Strep pyogenes
	Corynebacteria minutissimum
Anaerobes	E. coli
	Pseudomonas
	Clostridia
Viruses	Herpes simplex
	Herpes zoster
	Papova virus
	Molluscum contagiosum
Fungi	Trichophyton ssp
	Microsporum ssp
	Epidermophyton ssp
	Candida ssp
	Actinomycoses ssp

skin flora (Table 18.2). The infecting organism usually invades via a break in the skin, such as an interdigital fissure or ulcer, although it may arise indirectly in the foot or limb from blood-borne pathogens (see case study, Box 18.3). Infections in areas of reduced tissue viability can establish quickly and spread rapidly. Local spread involves contiguous extension of the infection along tissue planes. Distal spread occurs where emboli of infected material are carried through the narrowing arteriolar tree. Prostheses are potential sites for the spread of infection (see case study, Box 18.4).

Susceptibility to infection depends on host resistance and medical status, state of the skin, the nature and virulence of the infecting organism, and the blood supply of the affected tissues. The medical history may reveal diabetes mellitus, autoimmune disease, hepatitis, congestive heart failure, renal disease, sickle cell anaemia, cancer or hypertension. The skin surface is more likely to be colonised by opportunistic microorganisms in areas where normal secretions and sweating are reduced or absent. This situation is associated with autonomic neuropathy. Areas of poor tissue viability, due to ischaemia, will not show the normal response to invading microorganisms, and are therefore more prone to infection. Exudate and serum, found in ulceration, are ideal culture media for aerobic bacteria. The presence of ulceration also allows anaerobic bacteria access to deep structures, such as tissue planes, tendon, fascia and bone.

Polypharmacy

'At risk' patients, that is those patients who have systemic and local pathologies which result in their tissues being particularly prone to ulceration, may

Box 18.3 Case study: foot infection due to bacteraemia

A 56-year-old Caucasian was diagnosed as having rheumatoid arthritis at 34 years of age. Over the last 22 years, her symptoms have been controlled by prednisolone (10 mg daily). Six years ago she was diagnosed as an insulin-dependent diabetic.

Both feet showed severe hallux abductovalgus, subluxation and deformity of the lesser toes, and pronounced plantar rheumatoid bursae. Surgical shoes were made for her, but she prefers to wear a more fashionable style when she can.

Two years ago, she contracted influenza and severe bronchitis; this deteriorated to pneumonia. She was admitted to hospital for 6 days to bring the chest infection under control. A month after coming out of hospital, she developed an infected bursitis in the tissues overlying the left first metatarsophalangeal joint (MTPJ). There was no history of ulceration at this site and no apparent break in the overlying skin. The infection was controlled by systemic antibiosis with flucloxacillin for 21 days. The skin overlying the left first MTPJ ulcerated after the course of antibiotics had been completed. At the same time the diabetes became increasingly difficult to regulate, requiring larger doses of insulin night and morning.

In this instance, infection from the upper respiratory infection spread via the circulation to another site. The presence of two systemic diseases (rheumatoid arthritis and diabetes mellitus) plus dependence on steroids and insulin placed this particular patient at considerable risk of infection and ulceration. Patients with diabetes often find glycaemic control difficult in the presence of infection.

The ulcer was dressed daily, initially with hydrogel dressings, changed every 2 days for 10 days, and later with semi-permeable film, changed every 4–5 days. The area healed after 3 months.

Box 18.4 Case study: sporadic soft tissue infection and bone infection

A 41-year-old Caucasian was in excellent general health but subject to unexplained episodes of severe soft tissue infection. Ten years ago, during his time as a regular serviceman, he injured his right knee. He sustained an open fracture at the distal end of the femur and extensive soft tissue injuries that caused severe disruption to the knee joint. He spent several months in hospital, undergoing a prolonged series of orthopaedic operations to rebuild the joint, and finally was given a total knee joint replacement. He left the army on medical retirement 2 years after the injury.

In the subsequent 8 years, he has suffered several bouts of severe lower limb infections, particularly affecting the lateral side of the right foot, which twice required hospital admission for intravenous antibiotic therapy. There were no signs of fissuring or breaks in the epithelium, and repeated tests for foot fungal infections were negative.

The episodes of infection became more frequent, with five episodes during the last year alone, two of which were life-threatening. These involved not just the right foot but also the right thigh and buttocks. He is now awaiting admission to hospital to have the prosthesis removed. There was no indication on radiograph or bone scan of osteomyelitis, but it was considered that a deep-seated infection at the site of the prosthesis was the only possible cause of the constant infections.

Box 18.5 Case study: iatrogenic onychocryptosis

A 58-year-old Caucasian has suffered from severe, chronic bronchitis for 45 years, for which she has been prescribed prednisolone for the past 30 years. As a result of the bronchitis, she has severe clubbing of the digits, involuted toenails and is chronically short of breath. She has iatrogenic, type 1 diabetes mellitus and severe hypertension.

The combination of digital clubbing, nail involution, peripheral oedema secondary to hypertension and long-term steroid therapy predisposed to her developing an infected ingrowing toenail on the tibial border of the left first toe.

After consultation with her GP, steroid and insulin doses were temporarily elevated, and she was given antibiotic therapy for 10 days peri-operatively. A Frost's procedure (surgical avulsion of the tibial side of the nail, together with excision of the local nail matrix) was carried out under local anaesthetic. Healing was slow. The wound was dressed twice daily—initially with an alginate, and then, as healing progressed, with a non-adherent dressing. Healing was complete by 8 weeks postoperatively, although the patient required an additional course of antibiotics at week 4 to control local soft tissue infection.

---

have to take a cocktail of medications. This is known as 'polypharmacy'. Polypharmacy can result in a number of iatrogenic problems (see case study, Box 18.5). Table 18.3 lists some common pharmacological regimes that are frequently prescribed for this group of patients.

Malignancy

Tissue breakdown and ulceration may arise as a result of neoplasia. Areas of long-standing ulceration, especially venous ulcers, can undergo malignant changes. Conversely neoplastic skin lesions can present as areas of ulceration. Characteristically, these lesions develop raised, rolled and ragged edges, and may initially present as scabbed nodules. Malignant melanoma are less common than basal cell carcinoma,

Table 18.3 Common pharmacological regimes associated with 'at risk' patients

Drug	Indication	Action	Common name	Complication
Soluble insulin	IDDM	Decrease hyperglycaemia	'Human' insulin	Hypoglycaemia
Oral hypoglycaemics	NIDDM	Increase uptake of glucose into cell	Biguanides	Gastric upset Lactic acidosis
		Augments insulin secretion from pancreas	Sulphonylureas	Hypoglycaemia in the elderly
Non-steroidal anti-inflammatories	Pain Inflammation due to arthritis	Inhibit prostaglandins	Aspirin Ibuprofen Paracetamol	Increase bleeding tendency Gastric upset Overdose leads to liver failure
Antirheumatoids	Rheumatoid arthritis SLE Polymyositis	Anti-inflammatory Analgesic Reduction of IgM antibody	Gold salts Penicillamine	Toxic (10%) Side-effects (40%), proteinuria, dermatitis
Immunosuppressants	Severe RA Severe SLE Autoimmune diseases Transplant surgery	Inhibits leucocyte action	Steroids Glucocorticoids Cytotoxic agents, Azathioprine	Depress bone marrow and renal activity; suppress responses to infection and injury
Vasodilators	Coronary and cerebral artery disease	Rapid onset, short-acting Marked coronary vasodilation Reduced cardiac oxygen consumption	Glyceryl ti-nitrate (GTN) Nifedipine Ca^{2+} channel blockers	Increases bleeding tendency Postural hypotension
	Hypertension	Lower arterial pressure		
Cardiac glycosides	Mild heart failure	Increase force and heart rate	Digoxin	Tachycardia
Beta-blockers	Hypertension	Block beta adrenoreceptors of heart	Propanolol Atenolol	Drowsiness Peripheral vasoconstriction Reduced peripheral perfusion, cold extremities
Diuretics	Oedema due to heart failure; reduction of high blood pressure	Inhibit sodium resorption at kidney tubule	Thiazides Loop diuretics	May aggravate diabetes and gout
Uricosuric agents	Gout	Prevent the accumulation of uric acid in joints and tophi	Allopurinol	Increases action of anticoagulants
Antibiotics	Bacterial infections	Prevention of replication of bacteria	Penicillin	Many patients show hypersensitivity
			Aminoglycacides, 4-Quinolenes Cephalosporins Macrolides	Effective against Gram −ve For septicaemia For penicillin-sensitive patients
			Tetracyclines Metronidazole	High bacterial resistance For anaerobic infections
Anticoagulants	Prevent or reduce venous thrombosis Aspirin	Prevention of fibrin formation within a clot Prophylaxis to CVA and MI	Warfarin Aspirin	Normal clotting mechanisms reduced Gastric bleeding, subconjunctive bleeding
Iron	Iron deficiency anaemia	Ensure normal haemoglobin formation	Ferrous sulphate	
HRT	Menopause	Menopausal vasomotor symptoms, 'hot flushes' Prevention of osteoporosis	Hormone replacement therapy	Increased peripheral blood flow

but show a relatively higher incidence on the legs. Both skin and nail areas may be affected. The lesion does not always arise from a 'mole', and not all malignant melanoma are pigmented. Changes such as ulceration or bleeding, in pigmented or non-pigmented skin lesions, may indicate neoplastic changes.

Areas of long-standing ulceration can undergo malignant changes. Squamous cell carcinoma can occur at sites of chronic trauma and may be seen in association with protracted ulceration such as venous ulcers. These lesions can metastasise, in contrast to basal cell carcinoma (rodent ulcer) which do not.

TREATMENT PRINCIPLES

The treatment of ulceration is primarily concerned with the promotion of the healing process and the eradication or control of the causal factors. Ulcers heal by secondary as opposed to primary intention (Fig. 18.1). It is essential that every effort is made to achieve optimum conditions in order that healing can take place. Many factors may be responsible for preventing or slowing the healing process; these are illustrated in Figure 18.2.

Treatment of ulceration involves:

- establishing optimum local conditions to allow healing by secondary intention to proceed in a smooth and uninterrupted manner
- reduction or control of the local and systemic factors which have caused or predisposed to the development or prolongation of reduced tissue viability
- education of the patient or carer to the many ancillary factors that predispose the patient to ongoing ulceration and the ways of avoiding or controlling these
- continuous monitoring, regular review and treatment of areas of previous or potential ulceration
- close liaison with other members of the hospital and primary health care teams.

Assessment of the ulcer

Prior to the implementation of the treatment plan, it is essential that a thorough assessment of the ulcer and the patient's general and local foot and limb health has been undertaken. It is essential that this information is updated at each subsequent treatment.

All details regarding the ulcer should be recorded: base, edges and walls, type of exudate and the state of surrounding tissues (Table 18.4). The practitioner should inspect, assess and note the size, number and site of actual and potential areas of tissue breakdown,

using reference points. One method is to record ulcer features in relation to a clock face, with a defined point as 12 noon. It is useful to record the exact dimension of the lesion(s) by tracing the outline on to a sheet of semi-permeable film which can be retained in the patient's record as an ongoing indicator of the progress of the lesion. In a similar manner, the cross-sectional shape of the ulcer, as well as the angulation of the ulcer walls in relation to the base, should be estimated and noted. All these aspects provide an indication of whether the ulcer is improving or deteriorating.

There are a range of systems which can be used to grade the extent of ulceration—an example of one of these can be found in Table 18.5. The presence and extent of infection, the degree of presenting neuropathy, and vascular status should also be noted (Wagner 1981). It must be noted that all ulcers, regardless of the stage of healing, may be subject to secondary infection. A supervening infection can be diagnosed by both local and systemic signs (Table 18.6).

Table 18.7 identifies the features one can expect to find in extending, chronic, infected and healing ulcers. Inwardly sloping walls indicate a healing ulcer, whereas undercut margins are a feature of an extending lesion. Vertical sides are seen with static or ischaemic ulcers. It is important to note the appearance of the base of the ulcer; whether it perforates to deeper tissues, is necrotic, sloughy, granulating or undergoing epithelialisation. The amount and type of discharge are indicative of the stage of healing. Extending and infected lesions show copious amounts of thick, smelly or purulent discharge which may relate to aerobic or anaerobic infections affecting soft tissues or bone. Static ulcers tend to produce moderate amounts of clearer, more serous discharge, and infilling ulcers tend to have only scanty clear discharge. The condition of the surrounding tissues (such as inflammation, cellulitis, raised temperature, oedema) will indicate the progress or deterioration of the lesion. Meticulous documentation of the ulcer progress is essential.

TREATMENT STRATEGIES

The following treatment strategies may be used in the management of ulceration:

- cleansing
- dressings
- mechanical therapy
- surgery
- advice.

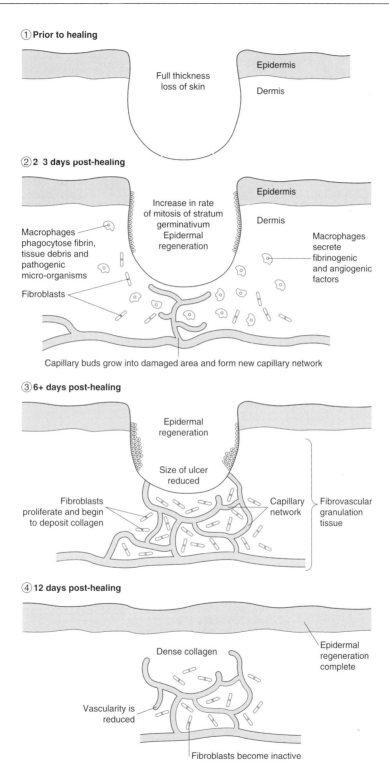

① Prior to healing

Epidermis

Full thickness loss of skin

Dermis

② 2 3 days post-healing

Epidermis

Increase in rate of mitosis of stratum germinativum Epidermal regeneration

Dermis

Macrophages phagocytose fibrin, tissue debris and pathogenic micro-organisms

Fibroblasts

Macrophages secrete fibrinogenic and angiogenic factors

Capillary buds grow into damaged area and form new capillary network

③ 6+ days post-healing

Epidermal regeneration

Size of ulcer reduced

Fibroblasts proliferate and begin to deposit collagen

Capillary network

Fibrovascular granulation tissue

④ 12 days post-healing

Dense collagen

Epidermal regeneration complete

Vascularity is reduced

Fibroblasts become inactive

Figure 18.1 Healing by second intention.

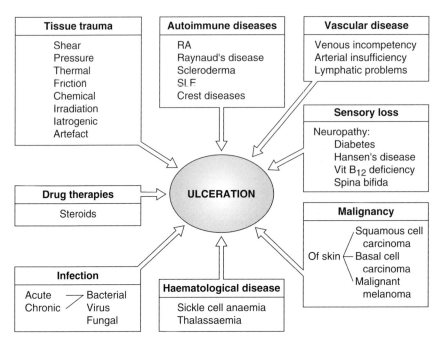

Figure 18.2 Factors that prevent or slow healing.

Table 18.4 Assessment of the ulcer

Feature	Appearance	Indication
Ulcer floor	Pink/white	Epithelialisation
	Pink/red	Granulation tissue formation, infilling and early healing
	Slough	Yellow jelly-like/fibrous matter on the floor of the ulcer indicating a static or regressing ulcer
	Necrotic	Black/dark burgundy discoloration of the involved tissues indicates infection, severe ischaemia or gangrene
	Infected	General signs of infection—pus, odour and copious thick exudate
	Perforating	Deep structures visible; tissue planes exposed
Ulcer walls	Undercut margins	Regression
	Vertical walls	Static ulcer, e.g. an ischaemic ulcer
	Saucer-shaped	Infilling and healing
	Rolled edges	Possible malignancy—biopsy
Exudate	Copious	Infection—take a swab
	Thick	Infection—take a swab
	Smelly	Infection—take a swab
	Light	Progress toward healing
Surroundings	Peripheral flare	Infection or inflammation
	Increased skin temperature	Infection or inflammation
	'Woody' oedema	Long-standing problem
	Haemosiderosis	Venous incompetency

Cleansing

Cleansing is essential to aid the removal of loose, necrotic or sloughy material, to reduce the likelihood of infection, and to aid the development of healthy granulation tissue. A sterile solution at 37°C of 0.9% sodium chloride (physiological saline) is the best cleansing solution. All cleansing solutions should be warmed to body temperature before being applied, in order to prevent the cooling of deep tissues, and to

Table 18.5 The Wagner system of ulcer classification (NB—This system classifies ulcers by depth. Other systems classify ulcers by site or by ulcer type)

Grade	Description
0	No open lesions with intact skin, but potential sites of ulceration such as hammer toes, bunions, prominent metatarsal heads or Charcot's joints are present; hyperkeratotic areas are classed as pre-ulcerative areas
1	Superficial ulcers penetrating through full skin thickness, but not to below the subcuticular adipose layer
2	Deep ulcers penetrating through superficial adipose tissue to tendon, capsule or bone, but without deep infection
3	Deep penetrating ulcers complicated by deep abscess formation or osteomyelitis. This classification also includes plantar compartment abscesses, tendon sheath infections and necrotising fascitis. Urgent surgical debridement together with intravenous antibiosis as a hospital in-patient is vital in order to prevent gangrene and infective thrombotic vasculitis developing
4	Areas of gangrene associated with ulceration. The gangrene commonly affects the toes, but the forefoot or heel may be affected. Surgical excision of the dead and infected tissues, such as a ray excision, together with intravenous antibiosis should allow the remainder of the foot to be salvaged
5	Areas of gangrene are so extensive that major amputation is necessary

Table 18.6 Signs and symptoms associated with tissue infection

Sign	Feature
Heat and redness	Local tissues are hot, with an increase in skin erythema There is a notable abrupt change in skin temperature, from normal to hot There may be a red skin flare extending proximal from the lesion, along the line of lymphatic drainage (lymphangitis)
Oedema	Local tissues are oedematous and the area swollen and tender There may be swelling of proximal lymph nodes (lymphadenitis)
Pain	The patient complains of pain (unless neuropathic) and acute tenderness; the patient may complain that the area throbs in time with the pulse. Pain is usually worse if the foot or limb is dependent
Exudate/pus	Pus accumulates in a pocket below the skin, or there is a purulent, malodorous exudate The nature of the wound exudate changes, from clear and sweet to cloudy, coloured or foul The amount of exudate from the wound increases
Malaise	The patient may feel feverish, complain of interrupted sleep and night sweats, and will have a raised temperature (pyrexia) The patient will feel unwell, ache, and feel as if she has the 'flu coming (general malaise)
Haematological effects	The erythrocyte sedimentation rate (ESR) and C-reactive protein levels are raised Leucocyte and lymphocyte counts are raised, indicating infection In septicaemia, bacteria can be identified from a blood sample

maintain optimal conditions for fibroblast activity and healing. The cleansing solution should not be applied with cotton wool, as the fibres of cotton detach and lodge within the ulcer. Rather, it should be delivered from a sterile syringe (without the needle) so that it can be directed into the depths of all cavities within the ulcer. In this manner, the ulcer can be flushed out under some degree of pressure, dependent upon the size of the syringe, without causing damage to the capillary network in the newly forming granulation tissue.

Granulation tissue is very delicate and very sensi-

tive to the toxic action of the chemical constituents of most disinfectants. The use of cetrimide-based cleansing agents is not recommended, even if the ulcer is very dirty, as their action is both cytotoxic and cytostatic, and will reduce or impede healing (Thomas & Hay 1985). The addition of antibiotics to the solution is not usually advised because of the development of resistant strains of bacteria.

Dressings

Dressings should be applied under aseptic condi-

Table 18.7 Assessment of the status of the ulcer

Feature	Extending	Chronic	Healing	Infected
Base	Slough/eschar	Slough and granulation tissue	Healthy granulation and epithelial islands	Deep, penetrating
Edges	Eroded/undermined	Rounded/raised	Covered by epidermis	Eroded, undermined
Walls	Steep/undermined	Steep/sloping inwards	Shallow	Steep, undermined
Discharge	Plenty/purulent/pongy	Scant/serous/non-smelly	None—may bleed with trauma	Copious, purulent
Surroundings	Clear inflammatory margin	Congested	Healthy	Acutely inflamed
Treatment	Clear slough/eschar	Clear slough as necessary	Care and protection	Antibiosis
Comment	Getting worse	No progress, may adhere to deep structures	Getting better, may leave a weak scar area (atrophie blanche)	May spread rapidly
Description	Active	Static	Decreasing	Spreading

tions. During the time it takes to change a dressing, the temperature at the ulcer site reduces due to the exposure of the deeper tissues to ambient temperature. It can take up to 3 hours for normal temperature (i.e. 37°C) to re-establish at the ulcer base. It is, therefore, important that ulcers are not exposed or left uncovered for longer than necessary.

Modern dressings are designed to encourage and enhance healing, and to minimise the local conditions that predispose to breakdown (Morrison 1994). However, the most ideal dressing, creating optimum local conditions, cannot counter the general and systemic factors that may have exacerbated low tissue viability. Treatment must always include identification and reduction of *all* the factors that have contributed to the formation and maintenance of the ulcer. Without such an holistic approach, the most perfect ulcer dressing cannot achieve its aim.

A wide variety of proprietary dressing materials is available to the practitioner. An 'ideal' dressing would assume all the functions of intact skin in terms of protection and control of infection: prevention of water loss; maintenance of pH; thermo- and osmo-regulation. To be used on the foot, the dressing will also need to conform well to curved surfaces, be comfortable when in position, pain-free at the dressing change, and easy to apply by the single-handed practitioner (Box 18.6).

An 'ideal dressing' suitable for the management of all types of ulcers, through all stages of the healing process, has not yet been invented (Thomas 1990). It is said that healing cannot be speeded up—its detractors can only be reduced. The research that sup-

Box 18.6 Characteristics of the 'ideal' wound dressing

- Non-adherent so that dressing changes cause minimal tissue trauma and pain
- Comfortable in place, with good conforming qualities and easy retention
- Protective against trauma
- Impermeable to bacteria
- Non-toxic and non-allergenic
- Maintains a high humidity at the wound surface but prevents maceration
- Allows gaseous exchange to ensure optimal oxygen levels within the wound
- Draws exudate away from the wound surface, but does not allow drying of the wound surface
- Maintains thermal insulation
- Retains all functions with infrequent changes, to reduce disturbance of newly formed tissues and to maintain optimal temperatures
- Reasonably priced, widely available, and has a long shelf life

ports the production of the wide range of dressings reports success with specific regimes for specific ulcer types, often under laboratory conditions. But the same degree of success cannot always be expected in the field.

Dressings react and integrate with the ulcer surface and influence the microenvironment of the ulcer. Each type of dressing has distinctive attributes and advantages, and it is important that these are taken into consideration when choosing the most appropriate dressing for a particular ulcer (Table 18.8).

The choice of dressing will change as healing

Table 18.8 Types of modern ulcer dressings

Dressing type	Composition	Action	Use	Examples
Hydrocolloids	Hydrophilic granules Hydrophobic matrix	Absorb exudate Liquefies Swells into ulcer	Rapid removal of slough and eschar Promotes granulation Moist environment Reduces pain Occlusive, but gas-permeable For light/medium exudate Initial increase in wound size *Not* with anaerobic infection Change weekly	Granuflex Tegasorb Biofilm Comfeel
Hydrogels	Water in agar or starch-based gel	Rehydrate eschar Reduce pain Cooling action Absorb exudate	Moist environment As a carrier for growth factors Gas-permeable Transparent—view ulcer For light/medium exudate *Not* with anaerobic infection Change every 3 days Wash off with saline	Geliperm Spenco 2nd skin Vigilon
Alginates	Firm gels (guluronates) Soft gels (manuronates) Some collagen Ca^{2+}	Aid all stages of healing Highly absorbent Conforms to ulcer Haemostatic	Moist environment Pain-free dressing changes (Moisten with saline) Fibres are biodegradable Change every 2 days	Fibracol Kaltocarb Kaltoclude Kaltostat Sorbsan
Foams	Polyurethane sheet foam	Hydrophilic inner Hydrophobic outer Conforms well	Absorbent Low adherence Bacteria-proof outer layer	Lyofoam Allevyn
Charcoals	Charcoal fibres within dressing pad	Adsorptive	Take up bacteria Adsorb purulent exudate Deodorising Do not keep wound moist	Actisorb Plus Carbonet Kaltocarb Lyofoam C

progresses and the environmental needs of the alter (Table 18.9). Deep sloughy ulcers requ dressing that will aid lysis of slough, and mair high tissue temperature and low oxygen tensio dressing should absorb high levels of exudate v allowing 'strike-through' (exudate soaking t the full thickness of the dressing) and should secondary infection. Granulating ulcers re non-adherent dressing that will absorb m amounts of exudate. It should also be gas-pe (i.e. permeable to water vapour) and mc insulating. Epithelialising wounds require that are gas-permeable, non-insulating, non and protective.

Once the ulcer base is no longer sloughy, has ceased, and the cavity has been inf healthy granulation tissue, unimpeded sation should occur. It is essential that th used at this stage of healing will retain th moist environment at the ulcer surface, yet

the newly forming tissues. Optimal epithelialisation conditions, at 37°C, in igh oxygen nd enhance nt dressings m dressings fficient tran- event macer- hey have the examination o remove the

erable risk of tegrity of the hed. Thus the rbating factors overdressings, ain over a semi- tional protection

Table 18.9 Choice of dressing in relation to the status of the ulcer

Appearance of ulcer	Dressing function
Ulcer filled with a hard, black, necrotic eschar. There is little exudate	Occlusion of area (encourage moisture retention to soften the eschar)
Ulcer filled/covered with yellow matter. There may be copious amounts of smelly exudate	Moisture retention Absorption of fluid/exudate Antimicrobial action (if infection present) Deodorising action (if ulcer smells) Insulation (maintain 37°C) Low oxygen tension in deep ulcers (low PO_2)
Ulcer clean and granulating, but significant tissue loss has occurred. Exudate should be reducing/minimal and should not smell. Healing is proceeding, but it is still at an early stage	Fluid absorption Inhibition of secondary infection Aid thermal insulation Minimise odour Low oxygen tension in deep ulcers (low PO_2)
Ulcer clean and superficial. Lost tissue has been replaced by granulation tissue, and epithelium is growing across the ulcer	Gas permeable —high oxygen levels at ulcer surface —gaseous water vapour retained at ulcer surface Low adherence —delicate new tissues are not traumatised when the dressing is changed Cooler surface temperature to encourage epithelialisation

Sterile gauze is probably the cheapest ulcer dressing and is readily available. It relies on the innate absorptive action of cellulose netting to draw away exudate from the ulcer surface. Several thicknesses of cotton gauze offer a minimum of protection from trauma, but gauze is only suitable for non-complicated ulcers. It is not indicated for the treatment of stubborn ulceration, as microscopic particles from the dressing tend to be shed into the ulcer and can promote a foreign body reaction, delaying healing. Where gauze is laid directly over an actively granulating ulcer, capillaries grow between the threads of the dressing, causing it to become adherent. When attempts are made to remove the gauze, damage and loss of newly generated tissues occur. The deeper the ulcer, the nearer its temperature should be maintained at core body temperature (37°C) to encourage fibroblast and leucocyte function. Gauze is a poor insulator and thus does not maintain this optimal temperature.

Fibroblasts are most active in conditions of low oxygen tension, and epithelial cells are most active in conditions of high oxygen tension. Sterile gauze does not maintain conditions of low oxygen tension when used to cover deeper ulcers. Healing ulcers should be kept moist but not macerated. Gauze is gas-permeable and thus does not retain water vapour at the ulcer surface. As a result, drying of the ulcer surface occurs. The converse situation can occur when gauze readily clogs with exudate, resulting in maceration of the ulcer.

Dressing regimes for specific complications

A range of complications are associated with ulceration and require specialised management (Table 18.10).

Necrosis and eschar formation (Fig. 18.3). Necrosis of the skin and deeper tissues ('dry' gangrene) may arise as the result of arterial disease; it tends to affect the tips of the digits, bony prominences and the heels. Areas of necrosis may become infected ('wet' gangrene) following colonisation by virulent pathogens, such as *Clostridia* and *E. coli* species, in tissue areas where the vascular supply is compromised, and particularly in debilitated patients. It is seen in association with the deep infections associated with foot ulceration in diabetic patients. The plantar surface of digits and metatarsophalangeal joint (MTPJ) areas are commonly affected, and distal vessels become blocked by emboli of infected material arising from a more proximal site of infection.

Healing will not proceed normally until all necrotic, escharotic and contaminating debris is removed from the area, as this provides an ideal culture media for colonising pathogens, and positively detracts from the healing processes by acting as foreign matter. There are a range of occlusive dressings and preparations that can help to clear necrotic material, eschar or slough, but removal is better achieved by quite radical excision back to tissue with a good blood supply. The mechanical removal of unwanted tissue

Table 18.10 The treatment of complications associated with ulceration

Problem	Action	Method
Necrosis and eschar	Debridement Soften	Dissection with scalpel; aseptic technique Occlusive dressings (hydrogels, hydrocolloids) for 48 hours (NB—*not* with infection), followed by debridement Enzymic dressings will soften hard tissue within 24 hours Acidic creams
Slough	Lyse	Occlusive dressings (hydrogels, hydrocolloids) or alginate dressings for 48 hours (NB—*not* with infection), follow by debridement Acidic creams Dextranomer/Cadexomer beads Sugar paste (see below)—change up to 5× daily Honey—change 2× daily
Exudate	Absorb	Occlusive dressings (hydrogels, hydrocolloids) Hydrocolloid paste or granules Alginate dressings Dextranomer/Cadexomer beads
Infection	Systemic antibiosis	Aerobic infections—fucidin, flucloxacillin or erythromycin Deep staphylococcal infections—clindamycin or co-amoxyclav (Augmentin, a mix of amoxycillin and clavulanic acid) Anaerobic infections—metronidazole
	Topical antimicrobial Debridement	Medicated tulles, metronidazole 0.8% gel (anaerobes) or impregnated beads Of all infected and necrotic material
Granulation and epithelisation	Uptake of exudate	Semi-permeable film, if there is only scant exudate. Foam dressings are used if there is moderate exudate. Hydrocolloids, hydrogels or alginates can be used if there is still considerable exudate but infection is *not* expected
	Prevention of infection Environment Protection	Sterile dressing Optimal for presentation From trauma

Sugar paste is very effective (Middleton & Seal 1985). It lowers the wound area to pH < 5, but requires dressing changes up to 5× daily

	Thin paste	Thick paste
Caster sugar	1200 g	1200 g
Icing sugar	1800 g	1800 g
Polyethylene glycol	1416 ml	686 ml
Hydrogen peroxide 30%	23.1 ml	19 ml

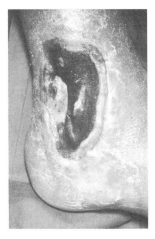

Figure 18.3 Necrotic eschar in association with venous ulceration.

is referred to as 'debridement'. It is best achieved by meticulous surgical dissection under aseptic conditions. In extreme cases, amputation of digits, excision of rays or removal of part or all of the foot may be necessary. The criterion for the decision of the level of amputation is based on the point in the foot or limb at which normal healing can be expected. Where large areas of tissue have been compromised or lower limb ischaemia is severe, proximal amputation is performed, for example, at the midpoint of the lower limb or thigh.

Areas of necrotic tissue should divide away from healthy underlying tissues by a process of autolysis. The area of slough and necrotic tissue will show an increasingly clear line of demarcation between the healthy and devitalised tissues, so long as the wound area can be kept free of infection and no further deterioration of the blood supply to the immediate area occurs. The process of autolysis will allow the necrotic material to come away leaving a healthy granulating ulcer base, which will heal in time. However, where tissue viability continues to deteriorate, the surface of the ulcer may dry out, forming a tough, adherent, hard and leathery eschar. This is very difficult to separate from the underlying tissues and autolysis tends not to occur. The hard edges of the eschar traumatise the delicate underlying and surrounding tissues, leading to extension of the necrotic process.

Rehydration of escharotic tissues was traditionally achieved using chlorine-based wet dressings, such as Eusol (Edinburgh University solution of lime), but since this both encourages skin maceration and predisposes to further tissue breakdown, its use has waned. The long-term use of hypochlorite or chlorine-based dressings is not advised, as they are tissue toxic. They destroy or inhibit fibroblasts, generally suppress healing, and are rapidly inactivated by blood, pus and serum. Their use should be reserved as a short-term adjunct to the treatment of dirty and heavily infected ulcers.

Occlusive dressings such hydrocolloids or hydrogels can rehydrate dried out tissue by retaining moisture that would otherwise be lost through evaporation, while preventing local maceration or incubation of infection. This process allows the escharotic tissue to soften and separate from the underlying healthy tissue. As the eschar comes away or is dissected off, the floor of the ulcer is seen as healthy granulation tissue. Both hydrocolloids and hydrogels need to be covered by a semi-permeable film dressing in order to maintain a high wound humidity. Some hydrocolloids and hydrogels include this feature. However, the use of occlusive dressings should be confined *only to those ulcers that are known to be non-infected*. It is difficult to be sure that deep foot ulcers are non-infected, as swab cultures can tend to identify the superficial and innocuous microorganisms and miss the deep-seated anaerobes. The use of occlusive dressings in these cases *is not indicated*, as it can lead to the creation of the ideal microclimate for culture of anaerobes and the rapid onset of life-threatening foot and limb infection.

Slough. Slough is a yellowish, necrotic, moist material that may fill the base of an ulcer (Fig. 18.4). It is made up of fibrin, pus, bacteria, leucocytes and DNA, and contains many inflammatory mediators. Since it is an ideal culture medium, its presence predisposes to infection. Slough may be very tough, fibrous and adherent, or jelly-like and more easily removed. It

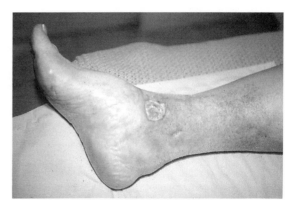

Figure 18.4 Slough. (Reproduced with permission from the London Foot Hospital slide collection.)

will interrupt and delay the healing process, and therefore should be removed before its surface dries out to form an eschar.

Polysaccharide (starch) beads can be used on small lesions to remove slough and absorb exudate. They are placed within the ulcer cavity once or twice a day, either dry or as a paste mixed with ethylene glycol. All traces of the previous application must be removed completely at each dressing change; this is best achieved by flushing out the ulcer with warmed (37°C) physiological (0.9%) sterile saline directed into the cavity from a syringe. An alternative formulation of polysaccharide bead dressing liberates 1% iodine for use in cases where infection is present. This type should not be used in conjunction with hydrogel dressings, due to a product–drug interaction, and is contraindicated in patients with thyroid problems, because of the systemic effects of liberated iodine.

Hydrocolloids (Rousseau & Niecestro 1991), hydrogels and alginate-based products (Hinchley & Murray 1989) can all be used to remove accumulated fibrin from the ulcer base. They all have the added bonus of being able to absorb large volumes of exudate, and aid debridement of slough.

Products that create a low pH within the ulcer will assist in slough separation. Acidic creams and lotions (pH 2.4) based on malic, salicylic and benzoic acids have antibacterial properties, as well as facilitating the cleavage between dead and living tissue. They may, however, cause irritation of the skin surrounding the ulcer. Honey has a low pH (2.5) and is useful in the care of some infected ulcers, as its hygroscopic action dehydrates bacteria. Honey is prone to contamination with clostridial spores and should not be used in diabetics (Zumla & Lulet 1989). All these types of dressing require frequent changes, a minimum of twice a day, and should only be used until the slough has come away, as conditions of low pH will depress the later stages of healing. Surgical debridement can be used to remove slough.

Exudate. Exudate, or discharge, acts as an ideal culture medium for infecting pathogens and causes maceration. Amounts of discharge vary with ulcer type and the presence of infection. Deep, neuropathic (trophic) ulcers, in particular, tend to produce copious amounts of exudate. The characteristics and volume of the exudate should be noted as part of the overall assessment of the ulcer.

Some dressings are designed to absorb large quantities of discharge, preventing strike-through of the overlying bandage. Heavily exudating ulcers require highly absorbent dressings such as hydrocolloids, hydrogels, cadexomer or dextranomer beads. Those with a significant degree of tissue loss respond well to light packing with alginate rope or ribbon. Foams, too, are highly absorbent and indicated for use with discharging ulcers, as well as for use during the latter stages of healing (Appendix 1).

It is not advisable to use a highly absorptive dressing on a drying ulcer as it will cause desiccation of the surface.

Plain unmedicated tulle, gauze and semi-permeable films are mainly used as dressings for superficial, healing ulcers.

Infection. Where secondary infection supervenes, as is likely in a long-standing ulcer, the use of systemic (oral or intravenous) antibiosis is indicated. Initially a wide-spectrum antibiotic is prescribed, which may be altered to a more specific regime after laboratory tests identify the nature and sensitivity of the infecting organism(s). Deep-seated and bone infections will require a combined therapy to counter both aerobic and anaerobic bacteria. Severe, acute infection can be treated with a combination of systemic antibiosis, with additional topical antibiosis for the first 48 hours, so that a high concentration of antibiotic is achieved in the affected tissues within a short time of the start of therapy. In cases of extensive arteriolar sclerosis and local ischaemia, topical antibiotic dressings may be used, especially if anaerobic infection is suspected (Thomas & Hay 1991).

The use of topical antibiotics and antiseptics is not universally welcomed, as bacterial resistance, local skin reaction and generalised hypersensitivity can result. Povidone-iodine has the broadest spectrum of activity of any topical antiseptic commonly available, although its effectiveness is reduced by contact with pus and exudate. It is only active so long as the characteristic orange colour persists, for the exudate will inactivate the liberated iodine. Alcohol-based iodine solutions should be avoided as these interrupt the healing process. Any iodine-liberating products should be used with care on subjects with thyroid problems, and may react with some hydrogels. Dressings or creams containing slow-release silver ions are reported to be useful in the control of local infection (Morgan 1992).

Infected, discharging ulcers have a characteristic and very unpleasant smell, which can cause the patient much embarrassment. Dressing pads which incorporate powdered charcoal can help control odour. Their use is aesthetic more than medicinal and while these dressings are useful to control the signs of a foul ulcer, the ulcer management regime must address the cause of the offensive discharge rather than mask it.

Other problems associated with healing. Collagenolysis/tissue breakdown may occur at the same time as epithelial regeneration, so that the ulcer becomes 'roofed', exudate is trapped within the wound and the ulcer increases in size (Fig. 18.5). This is frequently seen in neuropathic plantar ulcers in diabetic patients. The overlying callosity and unsupported peripheral epithelium should be debrided with a scalpel. Sometimes patients are unwilling to accept the need for such radical debridement as they think it will make the ulcer worse. The practitioner must explain the need to remove the overhanging edges in order to improve the likelihood of healing.

Some patients show an overexuberant response to injury leading to the formation of hypertrophic scars and keloid tissue. The use of pressure bandages has been shown to be of some benefit in controlling

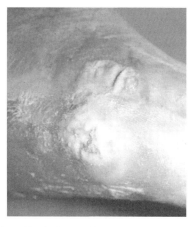

Figure 18.5 Roofed ulcer. (Reproduced with permission from the London Foot Hospital slide collection.) (See also Fig. 8.11.)

the generation of keloid, especially in burn cases. Excess fibrosis, as the result of ongoing fibroblastic activity over the course of months in long-standing ulcers, leads to scarring and inflexibility in the immediate area. The tissue may contract so that the area of previous ulceration, although fully epithelialised, is tied down to underlying structures. As it is essentially a scar, its blood supply is minimal, and thus it easily undergoes re-breakdown unless it is continuously protected.

Mechanical therapy

Removal of all pressure and shear from the site of the ulcer, via bed or chair rest, can aid healing. However, it is beneficial for the patient to continue to ambulate during the healing period to avoid the development of disuse osteoporosis and other complications that can ensue from long periods of inactivity. The most effective way to achieve this and maintain the normal bony architecture of the foot is to wear a well-padded, total-contact, below-knee cast or a padded rocker-soled 'slipper' or 'bootee' made from plaster of Paris or bonded resin. These are made to the patient's foot/limb and are removable or incorporate a window over the ulcer area to allow frequent changes of dressing (Fig. 18.6). Under such a regime, high vertical loading and shear stress at the ulcer site are prevented/reduced. This, in conjunction with the rapid reduction of local oedema, allows the majority of ulcers to heal usually within 4–6 weeks, regardless of their 'pre-cast' duration (Walker et al 1987, Laing et al 1991). However, the problem will quickly re-establish once ambulation recommences or the cast is no longer worn, unless appropriate footwear and orthotic control are provided. These devices are *not* indicated in cases of ischaemic or neuroischaemic ulceration.

Whereas, in the younger patient, it may be possible to achieve a degree of improvement in the position and alignment of the lower limb by the use of functional orthoses (see Ch. 12), in the older patient and those affected by arthritis, this is less likely. For these patients, it is important to accommodate the presenting problem, and redistribute pressure and shear away from the ulcer site (Ullman & Brncick 1991). A range of in-shoe or adherent devices suitable for this purpose are described in Chapters 11 and 12.

A triple-layered full-contact insole, made to a cast of the patient's foot, gives the optimum reduction in plantar pressures and minimalisation of shear stress (Janisse 1993). The selected materials should reduce surface shear stress, cushion vulnerable areas and

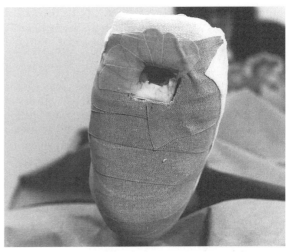

A

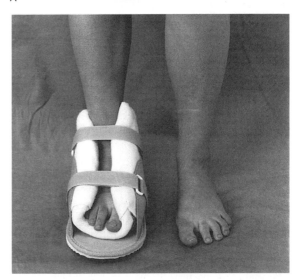

B

Figure 18.6 A: Scotch cast boot with cut-out to remove pressure and shear from the site of a neuropathic ulcer. B: Patient standing in Scotch cast boot with sandal. (Photographs reproduced with permission from Robert Wilson.)

deflect high plantar pressures away from areas of decreased tissue viability. The top layer is usually made from soft, mouldable polyethylene foam; the middle layer from urethane polymer for long-lasting shock absorption; and the bottom layer from cork or dense polyethylene foam for control (Laing et al 1991). This type of insole usually cannot be accommodated within a normal shoe, but can be used in conjunction with extra-depth ready-made shoes, bespoke

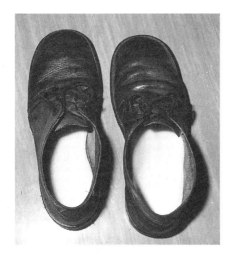

Figure 18.7   Surgical shoes with bespoke insoles. These shoes were made to a cast of the patient's foot to accommodate a triple-layer special diabetic insole. (Reproduced with permission from the London Foot Hospital slide collection.)

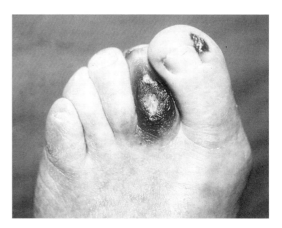

Figure 18.8   Mummified toe. (Reproduced with permission from the London Foot Hospital slide collection.)

or surgical shoes (Fig. 18.7). Many rheumatoid and diabetic patients can be quite well managed by wearing the triple-layer orthotic in roomy training shoes.

The role of surgery in the management of ulceration

As well as the excision of redundant dead or avascular soft tissue in the ulcer area, surgical excision or re-construction of misaligned or prominent bones can be carried out to encourage healing of ulceration, but only in a foot with a good blood supply.

Persistent ulceration of the plantar aspect of the forefoot may relate to the prominence of an under-lying metatarsal head, causing excess overload of plantar skin. The metatarsal is identified on radio-graph by applying a radio-opaque marker over the ulcer area. A simple sliding osteotomy performed at the neck of the relevant metatarsal via a dorsal incision can allow the metatarsal head to elevate so that it is no longer prominent (Addante 1970). Care has to be taken with this procedure as adjacent plantar metatarsal areas either side commonly become subject to overload and subsequent ulceration. Alternatively, an ulcer may form in relation to an underlying Charcot's joint with abnormal overload in the medial longitudinal arch. Removal of part of the underlying abnormal bone may lead to resolution (Brodsky & Rouse 1993).

If a toe has become mummified through ischaemic gangrene, but incipient infection makes it necessary to undertake surgery, the line of excision should be made at a level where the vascular investigation indicates that the blood supply is sufficient to allow healing (Fig. 18.8).

In cases of intractable painful ulceration and pain associated with rheumatoid disease, surgical excision of the distended bursa, metatarsal osteotomies, re-moval of the metatarsal heads (Fowler's procedure) or corrective surgery for hallux abductovalgus is indicated. Severe ankle and subtalar joint pain and distortion may require a triple arthrodesis (Fig. 7.6).

Any amputations of the foot leading to the loss of individual digits, and ray excisions in diabetic subjects are unfortunately, in 50% of cases, an omen for involvement of the contralateral foot (Kucan & Robson 1986). Amputation involving the hallux will cause considerable alteration in the biomechanics of the foot, and therefore, should be avoided if at all possible. Ulceration of the plantar pulp of the hallux, due to compensation for hallux rigidus, may heal following a distal hemiphalangectomy at the head of the proximal phalanx of the hallux. This procedure creates a greater range of movement at the inter-phalangeal joint, and, thus compensates for the hallux rigidus. A Keller's procedure is advocated to allow healing of a neuropathic ulcer on the plantar aspect of the first MTPJ. Adequate resection of infected tissue is required in the case of ulcers complicated by metatarsal osteomyelitis, gangrene and extensive tissue destruction (Ger 1985). In either case, the sur-gical wound is left unsutured, but packed, to allow infilling with granulation tissue from the wound base. Very occasionally, where there is a good blood supply, virtually no remaining infection and absolutely all necrotic material has been excised, the wound may be closed by primary closure.

Patient and carer foot health education

Health care is not a one way process. By using the term 'patient', a passive role is imposed upon the subject. No matter how good the level of care offered in the outpatient clinical setting, it is unlikely to achieve more than 1 hour per week contact with the patient (and frequently a lot less than that). As the patient, or the carer, is in charge of his own health care for the remainder of the week, patient education plays a vital role in any treatment regime.

Patients with diabetic foot disease have been shown to have insufficient knowledge about the serious effects of diabetes and its complications (Delbridge et al 1983). Some seem guilty of wilful self-neglect or psychological denial (Walsh et al 1987). For these reasons, patient education cannot be overemphasised (see Ch. 5). Reports credit specific foot care teaching programmes with up to 85% reduction in below-knee amputations in diabetic patients (Assal et al 1985).

The patient and the carer must be, and ought to be, taught the elements of basic foot care. Appendix 2 gives a form of words that can be used as an advice sheet to patients in terms of domestic foot health care. The information sheet should contain 'do's' as well as 'don'ts', and if resources allow, coloured illustrations of what healthy tissue and unhealthy tissue look like should be included.

However, merely 'telling' the patient what he ought to do is not enough—if such a strategy worked, the Government's Chief Medical Officer would have stopped adding health warnings to cigarette packets years ago. Continuing education and evaluation of the effects of previous input are requirements of any health promotion campaign, to introduce new knowledge and reinforce previous teaching. They must form part of any ongoing care plan.

THE MANAGEMENT OF SPECIFIC TYPES OF ULCERS

Neuropathic foot ulcers

The most common cause of neuropathic ulceration is diabetes mellitus. Diabetic patients with neuropathy are prone to develop abnormally thick plaques of plantar hyperkeratosis which may mask underlying trophic ulceration. Some will develop Charcot joints, especially of the tarsal and tarsometatarsal area, and,

less commonly, of the ankle (Laing & Klenerman 1991). Soft tissue swelling, erythema and heat over the affected joint area indicate diabetic arthropathy, which if left untreated will lead to gross foot deformity and ulceration due to abnormal weight-bearing. Urgent action is necessary to splint and rest the affected foot whilst healing takes place during the subsequent weeks/months.

The typical neuropathic ulcer presents as a wide area of thick hyperkeratosis, usually on the plantar surface of the metatarsal heads or in areas of excess pressure, such as the interphalangeal joint of the hallux in cases of hallux rigidus or overlying the plantar aspect of the weight-bearing tarsal joints in Charcot's arthropathy. Once debrided, the extent of the ulcer is exposed and surrounding maceration revealed.

These ulcers are deep, and typified by a full-thickness loss of epithelium, with a deep base that is either necrotic, fibrous, sloughy or showing hyper-granulation tissue. Because of the underlying neuropathy, the ulcer is pain-free, and the patient may be unaware of its presence, especially if there is a degree of retinopathy. The base of the neuropathic ulcer is characterised by deeper areas that may penetrate to underlying bone or fascial planes, harbouring anaerobic infection. Slough is usually yellowish, adherent and fibrous. The discharge is copious and cloudy, unless secondarily infected when it will be frankly purulent. These ulcers are quite large, e.g. 2.5 cm in diameter, deep, and of a somewhat irregular outline. The walls of the ulcer are frequently undermined and thickened (Fig. 18.9). The surrounding skin and tissues may appear relatively normal. Foot pulses are readily palpable, and even bounding, but Doppler ultrasonography may demonstrate abnormally high systolic ankle pressures, so that the ankle/brachial index computes to >1.5, indicating a degree of arterial calcification.

The extent of the ulcer should be investigated by probing the deeper recesses with a sterile probe to determine the depth of penetration, the condition of tissues at the deep sites (bone, capsule, tendon or fascia), the extent of undermining at the ulcer walls, and the presence of any hidden tracts, sinuses or abscess cavities from which pus may be expressed.

All overlying and peripheral hyperkeratosis must be removed. Necrotic and devitalised tissue must be cut back with a scalpel to healthy, bleeding borders. The use of chemical agents to debride slough and dead tissue is questionable, since most involve soaking, are tissue toxic, cause further maceration of the tissues and depress healing.

Any abscess cavities or pus pockets should be

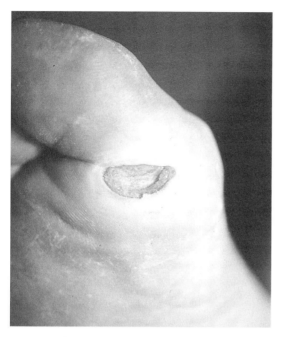

Figure 18.9 Neuropathic ulcer. (Reproduced with permission from the London Foot Hospital slide collection.)

opened, and a sample of the purulent exudate taken for microbiological analysis. The cavity should be flushed out with warmed (37°C) sterile saline from a syringe. Broad-spectrum antibiosis should be prescribed which will overcome both anaerobic microorganisms, e.g. metronidazole or ciprofloxacin, and aerobic microorganisms, e.g. flucloxacillin and amoxicillin. If necessary, the antibiotic regime can be altered once the sensitivity of the infecting organisms has been established. However, it should be remembered that the organisms obtained from the superficial discharge of an ulcer may not be the organisms that are causing the deep infection process. Likely pathogens will include *Staphylococcus aureus*, *Staph. epidermidis*, enterococci, Gram-negative enteric bacilli and *Bacteroides fragilis*. Areas of infected gangrene carry those microorganisms as well as populations of *Pseudomonas*, *Proteus*, *Serratia*, coagulase-positive and -negative staphylococci, methicillin-resistant *Staph. aureus* (MRSA) and anaerobic Gram-positive cocci. Where soft tissue infections occur, a 7–14 day course of antibiotics should suffice. However, with deep soft tissue anaerobic infections or infections involving bone, the antibiotic regime will need to continue for much longer—weeks or even months. Some authorities consider that the treatment plan for all neuropathic ulcers in diabetic patients, regardless of the type of tissue involved, should include long-term systemic antibiosis, as the presence of any infection will exert a deleterious effect on the healing process (Edmonds et al 1986).

The treatment of osteomyelitis always involves the combined approach of physical excision of necrotic or infected bone, sequestra and soft tissues, with the administration of antibiotics. Bone tissue culture is necessary to isolate the causative organism, as the exudate or the sinus tract does not usually yield the infecting organism that is the cause of the deep, anaerobic bone infection (Mackowiak et al 1978). The chosen antibiotic regime must be effective against aerobic and anaerobic Gram-negative and Gram-positive bacteria and *Pseudomonas*. It is usually delivered systemically, but successful infection control has been reported where, following excision of all infected bone, the postsurgical wound has been packed with antibiotic-impregnated polymethacrylate beads for 1 or 2 weeks, until healthy granulation tissue is established (Schein & Black 1987). The drug therapy only needs to be continued until the soft tissue infection has been controlled, as the radical excisional surgery should have removed all traces of infective bone tissue. Where systemic antibiosis is used alone, it is usually maintained for a minimum of 4–6 weeks, and often longer. A third approach is to establish a high blood level of antibiotic, via an intravenous line for 48 hours, and maintain this level thereafter with oral therapy.

Patients with grade 3 ulcers or over (Table 18.5) will require admission to hospital for intravenous antibiosis and surgical debridement, with excision of necrotic, infected soft tissues and/or bone, or amputation of areas of gangrene back to the level of healthy tissue with a good blood supply. The degree of vascularisation of tissues surrounding the gangrenous areas will determine the outcome of surgery, with the toe/brachial systolic pressures giving a useful indicator of likely healing. Apelqvist et al (1989) reported that gangrene occurred in 20% of subjects with a toe systolic pressure of < 45 mmHg. No foot lesions healed when the toe pressure was less than 40 mmHg, but 85% of foot ulcers healed when the toe pressure exceeded 45 mmHg. In contrast, the ankle/brachial index (ABI) did not yield the same useful break point because it can be very difficult to determine where medial arterial calcification prevents compression of the posterior tibial artery by the sphygmomanometer cuff.

Care of neuropathic ulceration can vary from the simple application of inert absorbent material, such as sterile gauze, to providing the optimum healing environment for the specific stage of healing (Tables 18.8 and 18.9). There is no one simple answer, although sheet polyurethane foams, e.g. Lyofoam or Allevyn, in conjunction with a programme of frequent dressing changes and plantar pressure reduction seem to fulfil many of the criteria. The more proactive hydrocolloidal dressings are *not* suitable for plantar ulceration where there is the likelihood of infection. Whichever dressing is selected, it is not a 'magic bullet', and the other factors that affect healing rates must be addressed.

A high percentage of neuropathic ulcers occur on the plantar surface of the foot. It is essential that every effort is made to reduce pressure and shear at the site of these plantar ulcers. This can be achieved by non-weight-bearing ambulation or by redistributive insoles combined with bespoke or semi-bespoke footwear (Figs 18.6 and 18.7; Chs 11, 12 and 13).

In diabetic patients, attention must always be paid to the management of blood glucose levels. The normal range of values of fasting blood glucose is 3.6–5.6 mmol/l. The aim of the treatment of diabetes mellitus is to maintain blood sugar levels within this range. Type I diabetics (insulin-dependent diabetes mellitus, IDDM) achieve this by regular injections of 'human' insulin. Type 2 diabetes (non-insulin-dependent diabetes mellitus, NIDDM) is relatively common in the elderly, middle-aged Jewish, and Asian populations. In type 2 diabetes, particular attention should be paid to the dietary intake of carbohydrates and fats. In many cases, the administration of oral medications, which either increase the activity of the pancreatic beta-cells (sulphonylureas) or increase the action of insulin at peripheral tissues (biguanides), is necessary.

The long-term complications of diabetes mellitus (regardless of the controlling regime) tend to occur some 20 years after the initial diagnosis. However, type 2 subjects may have a 'borderline' pathology for some years before the diagnosis is made, and thus the secondary complications may appear to arise earlier in this group. The long-term complications which designate the patient 'at risk' include neuropathy, arthropathy (Charcot joint), arterial and peripheral vascular disease, lowered resistance to infections, hypertension, nephropathy and retinopathy. Patients become increasingly prone to developing persistent foot ulceration and infections. The classic skin lesion associated with diabetes mellitus is necrobiosis lipoidica diabeticorum, which may cause ulceration of the anterior aspect of the leg, or of the dorsa of the foot and toes. Good glycaemic control unfortunately will not prevent these long-term secondary complications but poor glycaemic control will undoubtedly exacerbate them.

The multidisciplinary approach to diabetes foot care is essential. Liaison between professions—members of the primary health care team: GP, district nurse, health visitor, diabetologist and podiatrist—is essential for patients with systemic and multiple pathologies. But the team approach to patient management is incomplete if the local (i.e. within the foot and lower limb) and general factors leading to the initial formation of the ulcer are not addressed. These include impeccable glycaemic and pharmacological control, avoidance of infection, good vascularisation of the area, conservative podiatry, and footwear and orthotic management.

A key area to preventive management of the diabetic foot is the specialist foot clinic, where conservative, podiatric, orthotic and footwear therapies are provided. Pharmacological intervention and health education are available, and the clinic should have an 'open access' ethos (Jones et al 1987). Such a proactive approach is endorsed by the World Health Organization and the International Diabetes Federation, who, in the *St Vincent Declaration* of 1990, published the intention to reduce by 50% the rate of limb amputation for diabetic gangrene by the better use of known effective measures (World Health Organization 1990), as it is proven that foot care saves more limbs than reconstructive vascular surgery (Lippman 1979).

Practitioners can be guilty of making only a cursory examination of the diabetic foot (Payne et al 1989). The foot screening programme, in which every new case is inspected and fully assessed at the first visit, and ongoing cases are inspected, progress is reviewed and the care plan is evaluated at least annually, forms a vital part of ongoing preventive care of any 'at risk' patient. It is stressed that these are minimal requirements. The screening programme should include a visual examination (with record of deformities and skin lesions), vascular and neurological tests and assessments (and levels recorded), together with dynamic foot pressure measurements. This will allow the patient to be allocated to an appropriate 'risk status', which will be reflected in the formulation of the ongoing preventive care programme.

Ischaemic ulcers

Ischaemic ulceration tends to occur over bony prominences, at the tips of the digits (Fig. 18.10), at the periphery of the heel in conjunction with fissuring, and on the lateral aspect of the styloid process

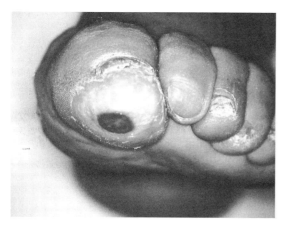

Figure 18.10 Ischaemic ulcer. (Reproduced with permission from the London Foot Hospital slide collection.)

and lateral malleolus in patients with peripheral or generalised arterial disease and in diabetic patients with microangiopathy. These ulcers are seldom complicated by overlying callus formation, although the exudate may form an occlusive crust. The base does not granulate readily, and may be covered by a very tough 'wash leather' slough. They are deep in relation to their diameter, with vertical walls, giving the ulcer a 'punched-out' appearance. Exudation is persistent, serous and relatively scanty, unless secondary infection supervenes. The exudate may dry to a hard, crystalline crust, giving the patient the impression that the wound has healed. In the foot, ischaemic ulcers are usually small (<5 mm diameter) and circular. The area is exquisitely painful, unless the patient has a sensory neuropathy, and patients may complain of ischaemic pain at the site long before the skin breaks down. The superficial tissues surrounding the ulcer are atrophic and cold. The patient usually has a degree of dependent oedema in the lower leg and complains of rest pain. In cases with major arterial pathology, pedal, and often limb, pulses are weak or absent, or monophasic on Doppler ultrasonography. However, in patients with microangiopathy, pedal pulses may be easily palpable, as the ischaemia of the superficial tissues relates to shunt mechanisms diverting blood away from the skin capillary plexus.

The management of ischaemic ulceration is difficult. Because of the paucity of oxygenated blood reaching the ulcerated tissues, healing is depressed and protracted. The care plan must include a full assessment of the vascular supply of the lower limb, with referral to the vascular surgeon for reduction of the proximal stenosis in narrowed arteries by balloon angioplasty, atheromectomy or arterial grafting. Healing may

occur spontaneously in time if a collateral arterial supply to the limb establishes. Local treatment is concerned with the prevention of secondary infection by the use of sterile dressings, together with the maintenance of optimal tissue viability by the reduction of any immediately exciting causes (such as excess foot pressures) with orthoses and bespoke surgical shoes (see Chs 11, 12 and 13). Hydrocolloid dressings can be of help, especially for malleolar ulcers that are complicated by eschar. Other useful interventions include raising the head end of the bed to improve foot perfusion during the night, and analgesics to control pain. Stopping smoking is mandatory.

Venous ulcers

Venous ulcers are the most common form of skin ulceration (Fig. 18.11). They occur as part of the quintet of signs of venous incompetence: varicosed deep and superficial veins and venules, dependent oedema, hemosiderosis and varicose eczema. These ulcers commonly affect the anteromedial surface of the lower third of the leg, as a result of the breakdown of eczematous skin and superficial tissues or due to local trauma. They first present as a small reddened area of skin that forms into a tiny blister, breaks open and then extends slowly to form a large shallow area of ulceration. They are rarely seen on the dorsum and never on the sole of the foot. They are persistent and slow to heal, and as with any ulcer, subject to secondary infection. The ulcer base is frequently seen to be made up of a mixture of sloughy and granu-

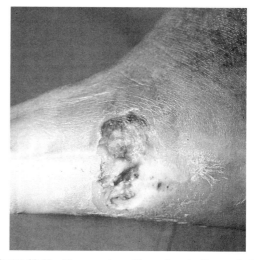

Figure 18.11 Venous ulcer. (Reproduced with permission from the London Foot Hospital slide collection.)

lating areas. Exudation is copious because of the wide area of exposed tissue. The surrounding tissues are oedematous and the immediate edge of the edge of the ulcer is raised and rounded.

The keystone to their treatment is the reduction of oedema and the restoration of venous return. Limb elevation assists in the reduction of oedema, and it is helpful to raise the foot end of the bed on blocks to aid venous return during the night. Compressive hosiery, which should be put on before the patient gets out of bed, prevents the accumulation of fluid within the tissues during the day. Venous function can be restored by surgical stripping or sclerosing of the varicosed superficial veins. The control of incompetent communicating veins is more difficult, and is addressed by the application of pressure bandages (Falanga & Eaglstein 1995). However, as the oedema may have been present for weeks, or even years, its reduction is difficult, especially if there is also any concomitant systemic pathology, such as hypertension or cardiac failure. The immediate ulcer is treated according to its stage of presentation (Table 18.9). Surgical procedures, such as split thickness skin grafting, may be used to close the ulcer area so long as the area is free of infection and the local blood supply is sufficient to allow healing to take place. The treatment of this type of ulceration costs the NHS many millions of pounds each year and forms the bulk of the workload of many district nurses. It is not surprising, therefore, that a considerable amount of ulcer-related research is focused on finding a dressing that will bring about more rapid healing, and require less hands-on, week-by-week care.

In cases of severe and extensive venous ulceration with undermining at the periphery, surgery is usually necessary to cut away the unsupported tissues, so that healing may take place from the deepest parts. Alginate rope may then be laid into the hollow created by the surgical debridement to take up excessive amounts of exudate, but all remnants of the dressing must be removed at every dressing change. Where there is no deep track or sinus linking the ulcer base to deep or underlying structures, and it is certain that there is no trace of infection, the ulcer cavity can be dressed with an amorphous hydrogel or hydrocolloid in granule or paste form. It is important that all traces of these dressings are removed at each dressing change by irrigation with warmed saline delivered from a syringe. The primary dressing may be left in place for 2–7 days, depending on the amount of wound exudation, but the overlying absorbent dressing should be changed daily to reduce the chance of strike-through.

Pressure ulceration

Pressure sores are the classic example of compromised tissue viability. The soft tissues of the foot are prone to breakdown in the debilitated patient by a similar pathological process to that which causes pressure or bed sores. In these cases, the foot tissues are likely to ulcerate, by virtue of hypoxia, chilling, poor perfusion or oedema, in association with trauma, shoe pressure, corn and callosity, and unkempt or thickened nails, in the elderly, immobile, or bed-bound patient. The heel and subungual areas are especially vulnerable.

The treatment of this type of ulceration is related to the control of the immediate cause of the problem, the assessment of underlying exacerbating or contributing factors, and, of course, local dressing therapy. Specifically, attention to the podiatric care of the affected foot is vital, with careful debridement of hyperkeratosis and reduction of thickened and distorted nails. Shoes should be of sufficient depth and width to prevent pressure over bony prominences, and all forms of plastic or nylon shoes or hosiery should be avoided, as their inherent elasticity will allow them to stretch to accommodate the deformity yet exert a continuous pressure over the area. The use of Plastazote and cushioning insoles in surgical sandals may be necessary to reduce pressure over prominent metatarsal heads in ambulant patients. The use of sheepskin bootees is indicated to prevent ulceration in bed-bound subjects, but those with pressure ulcers on the heels are best nursed on a water bed or ripple mattress.

Once healed, the area of tissue breakdown should continue to be protected to prevent re-breakdown, by the use of deflective padding materials, specially made insoles and bespoke shoes that will accommodate the foot and digital deformity. The scars left by heel pressure sores will need ongoing debridement of overlying callosity to prevent re-ulceration.

Ulceration in patients with rheumatoid arthritis

Vasculitic ulcers are a feature of autoimmune diseases, such as rheumatoid arthritis. The disease process is characterised by circulating immune complexes, which form microemboli within the smaller arterioles, with resultant formation of tiny patches of gangrene. Where these occur in the nail bed, they form splinter haemorrhages. In skin, they manifest as pinpoint areas of necrosis, which may coalesce to form a vasculitic ulcer. Steroids are often prescribed to patients who suffer from autoimmune disease to suppress the accompanying inflammation. The long-term use of these medications causes atrophy of the skin and a proneness to ulceration. The rheumatic process causes severe inflammatory hypertrophy of the synovial membrane within affected joints, and tendonitis, leading to gross joint deformity such as gross hallux abductovalgus (bunion) formation, excess pronation at the subtalar joint, flat foot (pes planus), abnormal weight-bearing and the formation of large painful bursae over the plantar aspects of the metatarsopha-langeal joints. Thus the rheumatoid foot is liable to undergo ulceration as a result of the underlying disease process, the medication that is administered to control the pathology, and the effects of abnormal weight-bearing and bursa formation that result from joint distortion.

The management of rheumatoid ulceration cannot eradicate the underlying vasculitic process nor the effects of long-term administration of corticosteroids. Thus the practitioner must concentrate on reducing the excess pressures that occur in association with foot distortion, thereby promoting tissue viability. This is achieved conservatively by regular podiatric treatment, together with the provision of cushioning insoles made to a cast of the foot, or extra-depth or bespoke surgical shoes (see Chs 11, 12 and 13).

Ulceration of mixed aetiology

Some patients present with ulceration that is of mixed aetiology—e.g. combinations of neuropathy and ischaemia (neuroischaemic; see case study, Box 18.7), neuropathy and infection, and ischaemia and infection. The treatment of these lesions is difficult. Initially, it is directed towards the pre-eminent symptom, such as control of infection, with later interventions being directed towards the underlying pathology, such as surgical revascularisation of the limb. It is not usually possible to reinnervate neuropathic tissue. The management plan is further complicated in the care of ulcers that have a combined arterial and venous aetiology (see case studies in Boxes 18.7 and 18.8).

SUMMARY

The management of foot ulcers cannot be directed solely towards the local repair of ulcerated tissues, but must take an holistic approach. Local factors such as vascular insufficiency, oedema, abnormal weight-bearing, local foot deformity and superficial infections must be identified, analysed and corrected where possible. Topical medicaments which can suppress the healing process should be avoided. The treatment

---

Box 18.7 Case study: neuro-ischaemic ulceration

A 74-year-old Caucasian has been an insulin-dependent diabetic for 31 years and has moderate essential hypertension which is controlled by diuretics.

She presented with bilateral hallux valgus, hammered second toes and Tailor's bunions on both feet. Areas of ulceration over medial aspects of both the first MTPJ and the right fifth MTPJ had been present for 4 weeks prior to referral. Both feet and lower limbs showed glove and stocking anaesthesia, with the patient being unable to detect touch or vibration below the knees. Vascular assessment confirmed that pulses in both feet were severely compromised, and the tibialis posterior pulse was virtually inaudible on Doppler ultrasonography. The ankle brachial index (ABI) of the right ankle was 0.3, and that of the left was 0.4, and popliteal pulses were very difficult to palpate.

Angiography revealed stenoses of both femoral arteries, just above the bifurcation at the knee. These were treated by balloon angioplasty, which was most successful. Foot pulses became audible and palpable, although those on the right foot were still worse than those on the left foot (ABI 0.65 and 0.8, respectively).

The areas of ulceration were treated weekly, with meticulous debridement of any overlying callosity and slough, and covered with non-adherent dressings. Triple-layer, full-contact orthoses were made to a cast of the patient's feet, and these were worn in surgical shoes. The areas of ulceration healed well. The ulcer over the right fifth MTPJ closed 2 weeks after the angioplasty, and both first MTPJ ulcers were healed within a further 4 weeks. Six months later, the patient developed an acute Charcot arthropathy of the right tarsal area, leading to collapse of the medial longitudinal arch. She remained ambulant during the healing phase in a rocker-soled walking cast, and did not develop further ulceration.

---

plan must include regular assessment of the patient's overall medical condition, including a review of body systems, drug therapies and social circumstances. A multidisciplinary approach is vital in order to improve the patient's general and foot health. The practitioner must involve the patient and, where pertinent, carers and other support services in the overall care plan. Without their compliance and cooperation, treatment is unlikely to succeed.

For the more routine cases encountered in podiatric practice, it may be possible to offer an intensive course of treatment, coupled with orthotic or surgical therapy and foot health education, to achieve a cure and allow the patient to be discharged from the active treatment register. However, it is *never* appro-

---

Box 18.8 Case study: ulceration of mixed aetiology

An 80-year-old Caucasian was diagnosed as having rheumatoid arthritis (RA) at the age of 76. Prior to this, she had been a very healthy and busy person. She tripped whilst boarding a bus 6 years previously and injured the lateral aspect of the lower right leg. A skin graft was used to aid healing. Both legs showed a degree of impaired venous drainage, with varicosities of both the long and short saphenous veins.

On diagnosis of the RA, she was prescribed ibuprofen to control pain and inflammation. This treatment had only minimal effect, and she was placed on a regime of weekly gold injections 1 year later. There was a dramatic improvement in the rheumatoid condition, but she developed dermatitis-like symptoms 8 months later affecting the skin on the right upper arm and particularly the lateral border of the lower left leg. The skin eruptions were treated with hydrocortisone cream. The gold therapy was stopped 2 months later, because she developed anaemia and proteinuria.

The rheumatoid condition worsened dramatically. Ibuprofen and co-dydramol were used in an attempt to control the pain and inflammation. The outer border of the left leg developed an ulcer, at the site area of the earlier dermatitis.

Over the next 2 years, the ulcer steadily deteriorated, until it was 8 × 5 cm in size, and 1.5 cm deep, with steeply sloping sides and an adherent sloughy base. Vascular assessment demonstrated that there were both venous and arterial pathologies. Soft tissue infections were a regular complication, requiring two short stay admissions to hospital.

The ulcer was dressed daily, and various types of dressings were tried. The patient refused to join a trial using topical growth factors. Her main complaint was of agonising pain from the, by now, excessively oedematous, discoloured limb, which was partially controlled by oral diamorphine. At this point in time, the leg ulcer is no better. It is treated daily by a maintenance therapy of absorbent and charcoal-based dressings and careful bandaging. Regular infections are treated symptomatically with topical antibiotic beads and systemic antibiosis.

---

priate to discharge an 'at risk' patient. Even when all ulcers are healed, and the patient's foot is appropriately protected by orthoses, housed in bespoke shoes, the foot is *still at risk*, as tissue viability is suspect and underlying debilitating factors persist.

The provision of foot health services should allow patients 'at risk' to have regular, ongoing and frequent 'routine foot care' and 'open access' to a foot clinic, so that any incipient lapses of foot health or early pathologies can be identified and treatment initiated at the earliest opportunity. It has been demonstrated that good, regular podiatry treatments cut the rate of lower limb amputation (Edmonds et al 1986), so the cost of running such an open service is well justified when compared to the fiscal implications of major surgery—in-hospital stays, rehabilitation costs, ongoing disability and the load imposed on social services and carers. A proactive approach to the maintenance and optimisation of foot health is the keystone of treatment of foot ulceration.

REFERENCES

Addante J B 1970 Metatarsal osteotomy as an office procedure to eradicate intractable plantar keratosis. Journal of the American Podiatric Association 60: 397

Apelqvist J, Castenfors J, Larsson J, Stenstrom A, Agardh C D 1989 Wound classification is more important than site of ulceration in the outcome of diabetic foot ulcers. Diabetic Medicine 6: 526–530

Assal J P, Mulhauser I, Pernet A et al 1985 Patient education as a basis for diabetes care in clinical practice and research. Diabetologoa 28: 602

Brodsky J W, Rouse A M 1993 Exostectomy for symptomatic bony prominences in diabetic charcot feet. In: Jacobs R L, Fuchs M D (eds) Clinical orthopaedics and related research. Lippincott Co, Philadelphia, p 269, 21–26

Delbridge L, Appleberg M, Reeve T S 1983 Factors associated with the development of foot lesions in the diabetic. Surgery 93: 78

Edmonds M E 1986 The diabetic foot: pathophysiology and treatment. Clinical Endocrine Metabolism 15(4): 889–916

Edmonds M E, Blundell M P et al 1986 Improved survival of the diabetic foot: the role of a specialist clinic. Quarterly Journal of Medicine 60: 232, 763–771

Falanga V, Eaglstein W H 1995 Exogenous agents in leg and foot ulcers. Martin Dunitz Ltd, London, p 143–155

Ger R 1985 Prevention of major amputations in the diabetic patient. Archives of Surgery 120: 1317

Hinchley H, Murray J R 1989 Calcium alginate dressings in community nursing. Practice Nurse 2: 264–268

Janisse D J 1993 A scientific approach to insole design for the diabetic foot. The Foot 3: 105–108

Jones E W, Peacock I et al 1987 A clinico-pathological study of diabetic foot ulcers. Diabetic Medicine 4: 475–479

Klamer T W, Towne J B, Bandyk D F, Bonner M J 1987 The influence of sepsis and ischaemia on the natural history of the diabetic foot. American Surgery 53: 490

Kucan J O, Robson M C 1986 Diabetic foot infections: the fate of the contralateral foot. Plastic Reconstructive Surgery 17: 439

Laing P, Klenerman L 1991 The foot in diabetes. In: Klenerman L (ed) The foot and its disorders. Blackwell Scientific Publications, Oxford, p 149–151

Laing P, Cogley D I, Klenerman L 1991 Neuropathic foot

ulceration treated by total contact casts. Journal of Bone and Joint Surgery 1: 133–136

Lippman H I 1979 Must loss of a limb be a consequence of diabetes mellitus? Diabetes Care 2: 432

Mackowiak P A, Jones S R, Smith J W 1978 Diagnostic value of sinus-tract cultures in chronic osteomyelitis. Journal of the American Podiatric Association 239: 2772

Middleton K R, Seal D 1985 Sugar is an aid to wound healing. Pharmacology Journal 235: 757–758

Morgan D A 1992 Formulary of wound management products. Media Mercia Productions, Chichester

Morrison M J 1994 Which wound care product? Professional nurse. Austen Cornish Publishers, London

Payne T H, Ganella B A, Micheal S L et al 1989 Preventive care in diabetes mellitus. Diabetic Care 12: 74

Rousseau P, Niecestro RM 1991 Comparison of the physicochemical properties of various hydrocolloid dressings. Wounds 3(1): 43–48

Schein C S, Black J R 1987 Implanted gentamycin beads in the treatment of osteomyelitis. Journal of the American Podiatric Medicine Association 77: 563

Thomas S 1990 Wound management and dressings. The Pharmaceutical Press, London

Thomas S, Hay N P 1985 Wound cleansing. Pharmacology Journal 235: 206

Thomas S, Hay NP 1991 The antimicrobial properties of two metronidazole medicated dressings used to treat malodorous wounds. Pharmacology Journal March 2nd: 263–266

Tillo T H, Giurini J M et al 1990 review of metatarsal osteotomies for the treatment of neuropathic ulceration. Journal of the American Podiatric Association 80(4): 211–217

Ullman B C, Brncick M 1991 Orthotic and pedorthic management of the diabetic foot. In: Sammarco G J (ed) The foot in diabetes. Lea & Feibiger, Philadelphia, p 207–224

Wagner F E, Jr 1981 The dyvascular foot – a system for diagnosis. Foot and Ankle 2: 64–122

Walker S C, Helm P A, Pullian G 1987 Total contact casting and chronic diabetic neuropathic foot ulcerations: healing rates by wound location. Archives Physical Medicine Rehabilitation 68: 217

Walsh C H, Fitzgerald M G, Soler N G, Malins J M 1987 Association of foot lesions with retinopathy in patients with newly diagnosed diabetes. Lancet 1: 878

World Health Organization (Europe) and International Diabetes Federation (Europe) 1990 Diabetes care and research in Europe: the St Vincent Declaration. Diabetic medicine 7: 360

Zumla A, Lulet A 1989 Honey – a remedy rediscovered. Journal of the Royal Society of Medicine 82: 384–385

Appendices

Appendix 1

Management of exudation in ulcers

No exudate	Light exudate	Moderate exudate	Heavy exudate

←——————————————— Hydrogel (e.g. Intrasite) ———————————————→

←—————— Hydrogel (e.g. Wet Geliperm) ——→ ←—— Hydrogel (e.g. Dry Geliperm, Vigilon) ——————→

←—— Low adherent dressings ————————————→ ←———————— Alginates ———————————→
(e.g. Tegapore, Melolin, Melolite, Metalline,   (e.g. Fibracol, Kaltocarb, Kaltostat, Kaltoclude,
Cutiplast, Ete, NA, Interface V-C, Perfron,   Sorbsan, Tegagel)
Telfa, Release, Silicone N-A, Tricotex)

←————— Foams —————→ ←———— Foams ————→
(e.g. Tielle, Lyofoam)   (e.g. Allevyn)

←—— Tulle-gras dressings ——→
(e.g. Jelonet, Paranet, Paratulle,
Periflex, Unitulle, Sofra-tulle,
Bactigras, Fucidin Intertulle)

←——— Hydrocolloids ———→ ←——— Hydrocolloids ———→
(e.g. Comfeel, Granuflex extra thin)   (e.g. Biofilm, Granuflex E)

←—— Semi-permeable films ——→
(e.g. Omniderm, Opraflex, Opsite,
Ensure-it, Ioban II, Tegaderm,
Cutifilm, Dermafilm, Transite,
Bioclusive, Transigen)

←——— Beads and powders ———→
(e.g. Debrisan, Iodosorb)

←——— Sugar paste ———→

Appendix 2

Foot care advice for people with diabetes

Diabetes can affect the circulation to your feet and make them go numb. This means that you must take particular care of them. In order to avoid infection and prevent foot ulcers from forming check your feet daily.

1. Wash your feet carefully every day. Use warm water and mild soap. Do not soak your feet. Dry gently and thoroughly. Dab surgical spirit between the toes. Rub moisturising cream onto the rest of the foot, especially the heel areas.

2. Wear clean socks/stockings every day. Make sure that there are no holes in them, and wear them inside out if the seams are prominent. Socks/stockings should be made of cotton mixture, and should fit your feet—try to avoid stretch-fit socks, and never use those made from man-made fibres.

3. Ask the fitter to measure your feet whenever you buy new shoes. Try to shop for them in the afternoon, as feet tend to swell during the day. Choose a pair made with soft leather uppers, and check that the lining is smooth. Make sure that the shoe is wide enough, deep enough and long enough, and avoid high heels. If you have insoles, check there is room for them in the shoe before you make a purchase. Try to get a pair with some form of fastening, such as laces or 'T' bar, and avoid slip-on or court shoe styles.

4. Consult a state registered chiropodist regularly (the practitioner will have the letters 'SRCh' after their name). They will examine and treat your feet, and advise you on how best to look after them. Use clippers to carefully cut your toenails after a bath, keeping the end of the nail level with the top of the toe. Do not cut down the sides. Don't cut away hard skin, and never use corn plasters.

5. Check your feet every day for any signs of skin problems, such as blisters, cuts, abrasions or infection. Any blistered, broken or inflamed skin should be washed with warm water, dried gently, and covered with an antiseptic cream such as Savlon and clean gauze. Consult your state registered chiropodist if it does not heal within a few days.

6. Do your best to control your blood sugar levels. Poorly controlled diabetics are much more likely to develop serious foot problems. STOP smoking.

Appendix 3

Using crutches

Crutches offer a useful method of immobilising the foot and ankle, while allowing the patient the benefit of movement. However, crutches should not be used indefinitely without good reason. Disuse of the limb may cause atrophy of muscle and demineralisation of bone. The following information may be useful when guiding patients in the use of elbow crutches, probably the most common type of crutch issued today. Such instructions should always be issued with a visual demonstration before the crutches are dispensed to the patient.

Crutches are available in a number of designs. Remember, not all patients will be able to use them, and alternative methods such as wheelchairs may have to be used instead. The instructions given below have been assumed for patients who will be using such aids for short periods only. Patients with disability and chronic conditions should seek the advice of a state registered physiotherapist.

Patients using the aluminium elbow style crutch would be expected to be able to manoeuvre without difficulty, compared with other designs. This type of crutch is therefore to be used as an aid, using the good side for additional stability. Patients with poor balance coordination and weak muscles affecting the contralateral side often progress poorly with the aluminium elbow crutch. Negotiating stairs and inclines should be discouraged until the foot has undergone

some recovery. The hollow aluminium crutches are popular because they are economical, light, strong and adjustable. Tall, heavy patients can bend the aluminium stem and each crutch must be checked for such damage before being dispensed. Other styles of crutches do exist—these are discussed briefly.

'Gutter crutches' provide more support for those patients with wrist and shoulder problems. The gutter forms the arm support and does not require the same amount of wrist strength as other crutches.

Where patients obviously would be unstable using crutches, 'Zimmer frames' are very beneficial. These provide four stable supportive legs, reducing the likelihood of falling over.

'Axillary crutches' may be beneficial for younger stable patients where the body can be lifted up. These crutches need greater energy than elbow crutches and can cause discomfort to the shoulder or axillary region.

Elbow crutches—information for patients

Crutches are adjustable for your arm length and leg height. While the crutches provided are made of hollow aluminium, they can be abused and will bend if used incorrectly. Follow these instructions to help you move about safely:

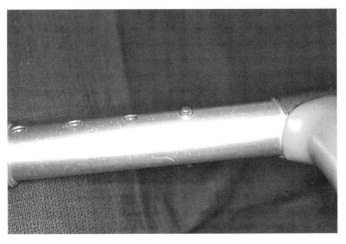

Fig. 19.1

1. Always adjust the arm length to coincide with a comfortable wrist position. The length of the upper section should be adjusted between the elbow and wrist. using the press-in stud/buttons (Fig. 19.1) to shorten or lengthen the stem.

2. The lower section is similarly adjusted so that the hand support comfortably drops beside the thigh. The wrist should be extended and rested on the handle without strain (Fig. 19.2).

3. The hand support is best used facing forwards. The point just below the elbow sits in a shaped rest, designed to support the lower arm.

4. Never attempt to take long steps or try to move quickly. If you have no existing heel pain, the use of heel contact will assist stability while keeping pressure off the forefoot.

5. Crutches may not suit you if you have weak arms or painful shoulders. An alternative system may have to be arranged. It is often better to use a walking stick than a single crutch.

6. If you cannot get on with your crutches, contact your practitioner.

7. Do not allow anyone to play with your crutches.

8. Stop using your crutches if you notice that they are damaged or bent.

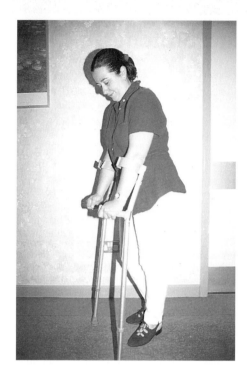

Fig. 19.2

Index

Page numbers in bold type refer to illustrations and tables.